CORPORATE
TIES THAT BIND

CORPORATE
TIES THAT BIND

*An Examination of Corporate Manipulation
and Vested Interest in Public Health*

Edited by **Martin J. Walker**
Foreword by **David O. Carpenter, M.D.**

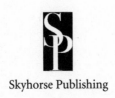

Skyhorse Publishing

Skyhorse Publishing books may be purchased in bulk at special discounts for sales promotion, corporate gifts, fund-raising, or educational purposes. Special editions can also be created to specifications. For details, contact the Special Sales Department, Skyhorse Publishing, 307 West 36th Street, 11th Floor, New York, NY 10018 or info@skyhorsepublishing.com.

Skyhorse® and Skyhorse Publishing® are registered trademarks of Skyhorse Publishing, Inc.®, a Delaware corporation.

Visit our website at www.skyhorsepublishing.com.

10 9 8 7 6 5 4 3 2 1

Library of Congress Cataloging-in-Publication Data is available on file.

Cover design by Rain Saukas

Print ISBN: 978-1-5107-1188-4
Ebook ISBN: 978-1-5107-1189-1

Printed in the United States of America

DEDICATION

DR. IRVING J. SELIKOFF

Dr. Irving J. Selikoff (1915–1992), a New York physician based at Mount Sinai Hospital, was the leading American medical expert on asbestos-related diseases between the 1960s and early 1990s. Selikoff was consistently demonized as a media zealot who exaggerated the risks of asbestos on the back of bogus medical qualifications and flawed science. Since his death, the criticism has become even more vituperative and claims have persisted that he was malicious or a medical fraud. However, most of the attacks on Selikoff were inspired by the asbestos industry or its sympathizers, and for much of his career he was the victim of a sustained and orchestrated campaign to discredit him.

From "Shooting the Messenger: the Vilification of Irving J. Selikoff,"
J. McCulloch and G. Tweedale[1]

DR. ALICE STEWART

Alice Stewart, (1906–2002) achieved worldwide fame, and changed medical practice, through her tenacious investigations and demonstration of the connection between foetal x-rays and child cancers. She went on to attract the enmity of the nuclear and health physics establishments—and the hostility of the British and American governments—by insisting that her studies showed that the adverse effects of exposure to low-level radiation were far more serious than had been officially accepted. . . . Stewart's entire life and career were devoted to social medicine, to the improvement of the lives of others, and to the bitter battles that have to be fought to ensure that findings contrary to policy or received wisdom . . . are investigated in a balanced and adequate way and, where necessary, acted upon.

From the Obituary of Alice Stewart by Anthony Tucker[2]

CONTENTS

PREFACE

David O. Carpenter

One of the greatest problems in scientific discovery is the perversion that can result due to conflicts of interest. While there are other possible bases for conflicts of interest, most are financial. Individual scientists may have financial conflicts of interest that influence the design of the studies they perform so that they obtain a result similar to that which they, or their funders, want. When funding for scientists comes from an organization or corporation with desires to present a clean bill of health to the public, there is strong motivation to give the funder what they want, if only to continue receipt of funding.

The most egregious epidemiological Judas in modern times is probably Sir Richard Doll, who for years took significant amounts of money from Monsanto, Dow Chemical, and the Chemical Manufacturers Association in return for making strong public statements denying that chemicals and radiation cause cancer. Because of his distinguished position, his views—though they fail to take into account the impact of hundreds of carcinogenic chemicals in our food, water, and air, and how these exposures increase rates of cancer in the general population—still have significant influence on public policy.

Corporations themselves have both more power and more money than most individual scientists to influence how scientific and epidemiological results are perceived by the scientific and general public, and especially by the regulatory and political bodies that determine whether restrictions are placed on products and their use. The financial return from development and sale of chemicals and some high-tech products can be enormous, and the temptation to ignore, hide, or deny problems by any means possible is great. This book offers an introduction as to how corporations can, and have, distorted knowledge and actions on health impacts of products in which they had financial interests.

There are a variety of ways that industry can pervert or manipulate knowledge of the toxicity of products in which they have financial interest. Many corporations have their own research units and actively participate in scientific meetings and the publishing of research results. But the outcomes of this research are often, indeed usually, controlled by the corporate management such that adverse effects of their product are not released, even if found by their own research.

Often adverse effects from internal testing are hidden under the ruse that the results are "proprietary." There are numerous examples of disease outcomes where industry-funded research failed to detect hazards but government-funded research showed significant adverse health effects. If research is carried out by teams beyond the corporation, they can still to some extent control the outcome by controlling the provision of raw data.

In the laboratory, it is always possible to obtain negative results if that is the desire. One can manipulate the assay sensitivity so as not to detect an effect. One can study a limited number of animals or people so that any results obtained are not statistically significant. One can fail to follow the animals or the people for a sufficient period of time so as to detect health effects, especially if the effect is something with a long latency, such as cancer. Or one can look for only acute effects, such as LD50, when the real concern is either a subtle change in cognitive function and behavior or a long-term alteration in reproductive function.

There are several common tactics used by industry to pervert or manipulate the results of scientific research and the way in which products are perceived after they come onto the market. Often independent researchers whose studies demonstrate adverse effects of an industrial product in which the corporation has a financial interest are described publicly as being "advocates," "fringe," or even "poor" scientists. This tactic is facilitated by the fact that any responsible scientist will always indicate both the strengths and weaknesses associated with their results in their publications.

Industry often inappropriately takes such "weaknesses" to publicly discredit the investigator while minimizing the importance of the results. When this is not enough, corporations can resort to harassment of independent scientists and others. This may take the form of accusations of misconduct or impropriety, or (at least in the United States) by demanding access to all unpublished data and documents through a Freedom of Information Law (FOIL). On occasion it means direct legal action against scientists, authors, journalists, or campaigners alleging defamation or loss of income as a result of statements concerning the dangers from the industrial product.

Corporations are often represented on national and international committees that make policy on environmental issues and use their voices on these committees to promote their own interests. The rationale for including individuals with such clear conflicts of interest on such committees is obscure. Often it is said that these individuals are clearly experts who have great experience with the products or their manufacturer. Such choices are also based on the concept of "balance." The result of such "balance" is usually that public health is compromised by the economic interests of the corporations. This is also common when it comes to comments from the press on environmental health issues. Reporters for newspapers or television often feel obligated to take a "balanced" view on health reports and go to industry for comments that mitigate or minimize the significance of the results showing risk. Corporate interests are used to attack and discredit independent writers and investigators.

Even more powerful interventions can be made by corporations in public health policy at the political levels. The situation in the United States is probably more egregious than elsewhere, but the problem occurs in every country and internationally to varying degrees. Except in circumstances where there is public financing of political campaigns, corporations contribute significantly to individuals running for public office who will support their views and corporate interests. These funds effectively buy influence that has impact on budgets for research, regulatory policies, and legislation. In the United Kingdom, money is poured into campaigning committees aligned to Parliament that influence the regulation and acceptance of questionably toxic products.

The net result of corporate influence on public health policy is that public health is inevitably compromised only to protect corporate profits. Through intentional lies, distortion of facts, corruption of individual scientists whose views are for hire to the highest bidder, and influence on the political system to protect profits, industry is responsible for significant morbidity and mortality of the world's citizens.

The history of smoking and cigarette manufacturers is a striking example. There was clear evidence that smoking caused lung cancer as early as the 1930s, but because of the political power of the tobacco industry, aided and abetted by health professionals, many of whom were either addicted to tobacco, held stock in tobacco companies, or were paid as consultants, there was no systemic effort to inform the public of the hazards of smoking or to restrict access to tobacco products until some forty years later. The costs in terms of lives lost and to the global economy are enormous. The World Health Organization states that tobacco kills nearly six million people each year worldwide and costs billions of dollars in excess health-care costs and lost productivity.

Even when developed countries did begin to regulate sale of tobacco products, the producing companies focused on developing countries, using the same advertising techniques that promoted smoking as something cool and without hazard. The magnitude of adverse health impacts of other chemicals and environmental exposures is less well documented than that of cigarettes and perhaps asbestos, but is increasingly significant.

Most collusive ties to industry in the area of research and the promotion of toxic products begin as secret ties, and by the time they have run their covert course, they have caused considerable damage. Turning around a single case and making even one individual responsible, regardless of the damage caused, is exceptionally difficult. Corporations and individually connected scientists have become adept at glossing over a system that can cause immense damage.

Once a product or an industrial process is questioned, the chances are that its defense will get more deeply embedded in the scientific fabric and that the truth about the damage it causes can become less easily challenged over time.

I have chosen to illustrate these phenomena with the story of PCBs, a subject not covered in any of the successive chapters. In point of fact, there are now so many such examples that the editor of this book must have had a difficult time choosing among them.

The Monsanto Company manufactured polychlorinated biphenyls (PCBs), sold as "Aroclors," in Anniston, Alabama and Sauget, Illinois from 1935 until 1977. While Monsanto had evidence for the toxicity of PCBs as early as 1937, little information on the degree of toxicity was provided to employees, government regulators, or the public even after manufacture and use of PCBs was terminated by federal action in the United States in 1976. As late as 2000, a company spokesperson stated, "The overwhelming weight of scientific evidence suggests there are no chronic human health effects associated with exposure to PCBs." However an internal memo dated September 4, 1953, stated "As I am sure you know, Aroclors cannot be considered nontoxic."

In 1969 an "ad hoc" committee was appointed to "(1) Protect continued sales and profits of Aroclors, (2) Permit continued development of new uses and sales, and (3) Protect the image of the Organic Division and the Corporation as members of the business community recognizing their responsibilities to prevent and/or control contamination of the global ecosystem." A 1975 memo regarding the reporting of results of a two-year study where rats were fed Aroclors made the following recommendation: "In two instances, the previous conclusion of 'slightly tumorigenic' was changed to 'does not appear to be carcinogenic.' The latter phrase is preferable. May we request that the Aroclor 1254 report be amended to say 'does not appear to be carcinogenic.'" While Monsanto had knowledge of the toxicity of PCBs, it was kept hidden. Later a jury found

Monsanto guilty of "suppression of the truth, negligence, trespass, nuisance, wantonness, and outrage," and they were held liable for damages.

One of Monsanto's major clients was the General Electric Corporation (GE), which used PCBs at a large number of sites around the United States primarily as an insulating fluid in capacitors and transformers. This led to releases into the environment at many plants. In 1976, GE is reported to have purchased about thirteen million pounds of PCBs from Monsanto and used about 5.6 million of those at two plants in Fort Edward and Hudson Falls, New York, communities on the Hudson River. Some five hundred thousand pounds of PCBs were escaping into the river each year, and all two hundred miles down to Manhattan were contaminated. Under threat from the federal government to require cleanup of the river, General Electric mounted an active research program, both internal and in universities, to document that anaerobic bacteria were capable of removing chlorines from the PCB molecule.

They argued that removal and cleanup was unnecessary because natural processes would solve the contamination. The GE publication, *River Watch*, stated in 1991 "GE scientists have announced laboratory findings that could lead to a simpler, cleaner way to get PCBs out of the Hudson River sediments. The findings show that all of the chlorine atoms on a PCB molecule can be removed by anaerobic bacteria." However, there was clear evidence that dechlorination did not result in destruction of the PCB molecule, only in a change in the congener distribution. These actions delayed the removal of PCBs from the river for more than thirty years. The upper part of the river is currently being dredged of PCBs; financed by GE, this is the largest and most expensive dredging project in US history.

GE funded a study of over seven thousand capacitor workers at the two plants along the Hudson River. However, to be included in the study required employment for only ninety days, and all secretarial staff and others not even working with PCBs were included in the study.

Not surprising under these circumstances, no elevation in cancer risk was found, even though PCBs are known human carcinogens. Later, a GE spokesperson said, "Public perception about the health risks of PCBs and the scientific facts are in conflict. Most scientists agree that PCBs are not the hazard to human health that was feared in the 1970s. PCBs produce tumors in some laboratory animals, but there is no proof—based on human exposure of more than forty years—that PCBs cause cancer or any other serious health problems in people." However, a recent study of 24,865 capacitor plant workers in three states, including those described above, performed by the National Institute of Occupational Safety and Health, found significant elevations in rates of all cancer—intestinal,

xiv CORPORATE TIES THAT BIND

brain, prostate, and stomach cancers, and malignant melanoma and multiple myeloma. In 2013 the International Agency for Research on Cancer (IARC) declared all PCBs to be known human carcinogens based on evidence including the GE-supported study.

In addition to being known human carcinogens, PCBs are known to increase risk of type 2 diabetes, hypertension, cardiovascular disease, hypothyroidism, and chloracne, and they cause cognitive deficits and neurobehavioral changes. If one depended upon Monsanto and GE, none of this information would be known. The length and persistence of arguments in favor of toxic products is demonstrated in the following book.

In 1735, Benjamin Franklin, one of the founders of the United States and authors of the US Constitution, stated, "An ounce of prevention is worth a pound of cure," (or in metric terms, "a gram of prevention is worth a kilogram of cure"). This old phrase captures the concept of the precautionary principle. The majority of chapters in this book show repeatedly that failure in preventing exposures to chemical toxins and various forms of radiation have resulted in human disease that could have been prevented.

The central issue is what level of evidence is necessary before steps are taken by individuals, scientists, and governments to prevent exposure of the public. A closely related question is at what point when there is incomplete information on a danger should the public be informed about the possibility of harm? It is often assumed by regulators as well as scientists that the public cannot deal with uncertainty and wants clear black-and-white statements (i.e., that something is either "safe" or "unsafe.") This condescension is most certainly not justified, as every person deals with uncertainty and risk at various levels all the time.

However, it is much more difficult to explain to the public the level of evidence in support of an issue, as well as the weaknesses in that evidence, than it is to make dogmatic statements about safety or lack thereof. Unfortunately, when there is uncertainty, too often the dogmatic statements made by persons in authority turn out in the long run to be wrong and have negative consequences at multiple levels. The effort to prevent fear of something for which evidence of danger is incomplete is fine when ultimately it turns out not to be dangerous, but is most certainly not fine when the incomplete evidence turns out to be correct or even an underestimation of the actual risk.

There are very different levels of proof used in the world today. In mathematics, it is possible to prove a theorem to an absolute degree of certainty. That is not possible in most other disciplines. Within the medical and scientific community, we use odds or risk ratios with confidence intervals (CI) as indicators of proof. Most epidemiological studies will present results with 95 percent confidence intervals, and occasionally with 99 percent confidence intervals. This approach acknowledges that there are associations that occur by chance and do not reflect causation. Thus, a 95 percent CI indicates that there is no more than a 5 percent possibility that the associations occurred by chance, whereas a 99 percent CI leaves only a 1 percent possibility of a chance association. However, regardless of the strength of association it is impossible to absolutely prove causation.

The variable one studies may, in fact, be tightly associated with something else that is not being directly studied, and it is the second variable that is causative of the association. Therefore, within the scientific community we rely on the "weight of evidence" from multiple sources and testing multiple variables in an effort, never totally achieved, to reach causation. In addition, we commonly attempt to apply the Hill Criteria (strength, consistency, specificity, temporality, biologic gradient, plausibility, coherence, experimental evidence, and analogy) when trying to distinguish causal from non-causal associations. This is in spite of the fact that Hill himself did not propose these as "criteria" but rather as considerations when drawing conclusions as to causation.

A very different standard of proof is that used in legal circles, which is "more likely than not." This is 50.1 percent level of proof, obviously much less stringent than 95 or 99 percent. Had this level of proof been applied to cigarette smoking and lung cancer and the results reported to the public, literally millions of lives would have been saved.

Scientists at Carnegie Mellon University developed the concept of "prudent avoidance" in the 1980s around concerns related to health effects of magnetic fields associated with power lines and household electricity. They outlined three distinctly different possible approaches for dealing with uncertainty. The first was to do nothing. This could be denial that there was anything of concern, or perhaps providing information in a passive manner. The second was to impose rigid regulation, even though there remains uncertainty as to the magnitude of the risk. This approach may not be in the best interest of society because of costs, inconvenience, and other adverse impacts. The third, intermediate course of action, and the one they recommended, was "prudent avoidance," which meant doing what could be done at both personal and societal levels to reduce exposures without undue costs and inconvenience. This approach involves providing information to the public and the regulators that accurately discloses what is known and what is unknown, allowing individuals to make their own decisions on whether or not to take steps to reduce their exposure.

The concept of "prudent avoidance" is good at a personal level, but it is much weaker than the basic tenants of the precautionary principle at a public or regulatory level. It should be the responsibility of governments to protect the public from exposure to hazardous exposures, and that decision should not be left to either the general, and often uninformed, public or those with vested interests.

The European Union's REACH regulations are an excellent example of application of the precautionary principle, in that they attempt to be certain that all toxicity of new chemicals is known before the chemical is allowed to be produced. And the possible toxicities are not only important to human and animal health, but also to the ecosystem.

Inevitably, corporations have a wide range of arguments about why a precautionary principle should not be invoked: if you scrutinize everything for safety, we will—they say—end up back in the Dark Ages; we will stifle freedom of production and the armchair observers will take control. Application of the precautionary principle does not mean stopping progress with development of new chemicals, new technologies, or new applications. It means only that we do not introduce a new exposure without having first determined exhaustively whether or not it poses harm to the human race or the ecosystem. The harm to human health caused by past mistakes—smoking, PCBs, asbestos, endocrine-disruptive chemicals—should motivate society to learn the tragedies of these errors and practice precaution.

A strong economy and growing economic and technological development are important to all societies, but such growth does not have to be at the expense of public health.

INTRODUCTION

Stories of data manipulation on the emissions from cars, which affected Volkswagen and other car producers, have recently been reported in the mainstream media. It could be said that the manipulation of "scientific" evidence by corporations has now come of age—a real and recognized factor in the litany of corporate malfeasance.

It is not surprising, however, that this issue has risen to the surface when automobiles—the testers' most loved product—are the subject; previously all kinds of faults and dangers in all kinds of products have been passed over by the mainstream media.

The chapters that follow in this book demonstrate clearly that data and science "bending" have a long history, which, because such incidents have apparently still been in the area of "doubt," have rarely been given space in the public media. This book scrutinizes this history, especially since the 1970s, in many different areas of corporate propaganda and the attempts to cover up public health risks.

It finds on the whole that, like most aspects of our world, corporate profit and corporate inquiry has taken the place of real scientific research. In almost every case the publicity given to the exposure of these research illusions has at best been brief and at worst non-existent. This book does its best to right that lack of balance.

The first chapters introduce readers to the way in which large companies, corporations, and individuals selectively produce, promote, and process products whose toxicity has been brought into question.

"A Dark Culture—the History and Literature of Health Damaging Production, its Exposure, and its Corporate Defense," the first chapter in the book, draws on the literature of toxic products and their production to look broadly and historically at the need companies and organizations, such as professional associations, have to promote good news while censuring the health damaging effects of products and their manufacturing processes.

In "The Basis of Bad Science," chapter 2, the authors provide a blueprint that describes the ways in which science and the information that flows from it, can be misused and manipulated in order either to ignore toxicity or reflect products and processes in a good light.

In chapter 3, "A Battleground— From Phenoxyacetic Acids, Chlorophenols and Dioxins to Mobile Phones—Cancer Risks, Greenwashing and Vested Interests," Lennart Hardell describes a personal career marred by attacks from industry and corporate epidemiologists. Hardell carried out the original research with the late Olav Axelson, which led to the banning in Sweden of a carcinogenic herbicide used by rail and forestry workers. Hardell describes how he has paid dearly for this contribution to the health of the public both in Sweden and other countries.

We are continuously subjected to the promotion of pharmaceutical medicines and often regaled with the news that science is defeating cancer in its global battle. In chapter 4, "Losing the War on Cancer," a senior cancer epidemiologist expresses his frustration at the gap that exists, especially in the developing world, between the claims of the cancer industry and the reality of improved health.

Giving damaging products and processes a clean bill of health is often termed "Greenwashing." This process is described in chapter 5, "Greenwashing: The Swedish Experience." Internationally renowned researchers utilize the authority of university-based research facilities and the media to promote research that reflects favorably on questionable processes and products.

In chapter 6, "Industrial Influences on Cancer Epidemiology," a researcher and author looks at the process of epidemiology and the ways that it might, by accident or by design, give a benign face to drugs, processes, and even adverse events.

In chapter 7, "Serving Industry, Promoting Skepticism, Discrediting Epidemiology," a Canadian civil rights and ethics worker looks in detail at one research worker whose work has been questioned on grounds of possible biases in the field of asbestos research.

The middle chapters of *Corporate Ties that Bind* introduce readers to a number of case histories and studies partly of individuals and partly of corporations or governments—the work that appears sympathetic to industry—and partly of institutions and industrial processes that promote products whose toxicity has been questioned.

Chapter 8, "Secret Ties in Asbestos—Downplaying and Effacing the Risks of a Toxic Mineral," is written by Geoffrey Tweedale, who throughout his career has written and researched extensively the effects of asbestos production and the way that its dangers and damage were veiled by the industry.

In "Kidding a Kidder," Martin Walker looks again at the work of the late Sir Richard Doll. Chapter 9 describes Doll's role in one of the biggest cases of toxic poisoning in Europe, which killed thousands of people in the Madrid region of Spain. Doll became the most important expert witness in this case against the distributors of cheap cooking oil, at the behest of the World Health Organization. However, not a word about the case was mentioned in his official biography.

"Escaping Electrosensitivity," chapter 10, is a personal account of undiagnosed illness that the medical profession and the corporations have attempted to delete from the research process of particular products and manufacturing processes. Christian Blom, a Finnish worker, paints a deeply observed picture of how he became electrosensitive and how he managed to live with this condition. He looks at length at the arguments used by industry to disabuse the medical profession and the public that there is such a phenomena.

Chapter 11 is concerned with undiagnosed and "invisible" illnesses. "Ignoring Chronic Illness Caused by New Chemicals and Technology" comes from a Scandinavian trade union journalist who covered from the beginning the damage done to workers by early computer screens. As with Christian Blom's chapter, Gunni Nordström looks at the affected workers and the attempts by companies to cover up the damage. The chapter is a complex account of the consequences of workers being beaten in the short-term by companies producing health-damaging high-tech equipment.

In her beautifully readable book, *The Woman Who Knew Too Much*, Gayle Greene describes the standoff that occurred at Oxford University between the committed, brilliant, and intuitive epidemiologist, Alice Stewart, and the industry-funded pragmatist, Sir Richard Doll. For chapter 12 in this volume, "A Tale of Two Scientists: Doctor Alice Stewart and Sir Richard Doll," Greene delves more deeply into Doll's attachment to industry and his seemingly continual desire to ensure that Stewart was not recognized as a leading voice in her profession.

Pharmaceutical corporations, because of their apparent altruism, take it for granted that they are entitled to shape government policy, especially in the field of vaccination. Increasingly, the pharmaceutical corporations in the United Kingdom and the United States have moved to take control of the supposedly independent vaccine regulatory agencies. In both the United Kingdom and the United States, regulators have made mistakes in licensing vaccines that have had serious adverse effects. In chapter 13, "The Corporate Hijacking of the UK Vaccine Program," Martin Walker looks at just one involvement of corporately sympathetic academics in vaccine regulation.

The major battles in Sweden over environmental toxins have taken place in relation to dioxin, a dangerous chemical that can infiltrate the environment in a number of ways. In chapter 14, Martin Walker and the late Bo Walhjalt look at the way this struggle developed, particularly with the intervention of US corporate agents and agencies.

Chapter 15, "Burying the Evidence—The Role of Britain's Health and Safety Executive in Prolonging the Occupational Cancer Epidemic," takes a hard look at Britain's Health and Safety Executive, its history, and recent attempts to reform and even remove it. It describes the inevitable outcome of the regulatory oversight of toxic industries as organizational bias. In particular, the lead author, Rory O'Neill, has exceptional experience and information of workers' illnesses and the failure of this organization, being the long-term editor of the trade union magazine, *Hazards*.

Chapter 16, "Spin in the Antipodes," takes us to Australia and relates how there is a serious emerging public health risk from the ubiquitous use of the cell phone and the increasing evidence for harm, including brain tumors, male infertility, behavioral disturbances, and electrosensitivity.

The nuclear industry is massive and monolithic; its interests stretch across many areas of the state and its security. During a period in the 1970s and 1980s all the resources of corporate defense were used to protect it from criticism. In an attempt to control academic information and attract expert witnesses to the civil claims that were rising against them, the nuclear industry set up the "independent" Westlakes Research Institute. In chapter 17, "Westlakes Research Institute," one of the long-term survivors of Sellafield and a founder of Cumbrians Opposed to a Radioactive Environment (CORE), Janine Allis-Smith, examines the "independent" Westlakes Research Institute, describing how this "academic" institution built a number of biases into their work.

The career of Devra Davis has been blighted by her honesty and its reception among academics. However she has continued with her populist and bestselling books while also researching the electromagnetic fields produced by mobile phones. In chapter 18, "Wilhelm Hueper and Robert Kehoe, Epidemiological War Crimes," which looks at the contrasting careers of Wilhelm Hueper and Robert Kehoe, she broaches the subject of how the views and acts of corporately guided epidemiologists can be corrected and sanctioned.

The final part of *Corporate Ties that Bind* looks at ways in which the conflicts of interest inherent in many of the previous cases might be avoided. It focuses on early warning systems and what happens when they are not in place.

In chapter 19, Pierre Mallia looks at the idea of the precautionary principle, which itself has become the butt of corporate criticism, and those who believe that entrepreneurs and producers should be able to do anything they wish in the name of progress, who argue that those who believe in precaution are stifling the freedom to produce and keeping us in the Dark Ages.

While science spends billions on harvesting and containing Earth's plant life, animal species can often fall prey to corporations. In chapter 20, "The Precautionary Principle in the Protection of Wildlife—the Tasmanian Devils and the Beluga Whales," Jody Warren looks at the failure to properly utilize the precautionary principle in the case of these two species.

Chapter 21, "Dust, Labor and Capital— Silicosis among South Africa's Gold Miners," looks at the legacy of the British and other countries mining asbestos in Africa. While it has been difficult for citizens in Britain and America to fight claims for damages against environmental or work toxicity, the legal struggle of those employed by corporations in their home countries is almost impossible. They have to fight not just the bent science but bent law and the legacy of imperialism.

In cases where whole communities are contaminated, the corporations that are responsible often fight to the death over that responsibility. With respect to research and evidence, corporations often seize the day. Amid a whole series of confounding tricks, they use their power to conduct epidemiological studies and buy up expert witnesses. One possible alternative to professional conflict of interest research in these cases is community epidemiology. In chapter 22, this subject is described by Professor Andrew Watterson.

Chapter 23, "Downplaying Radiation Risk," has been placed at the end of the book because it details one of the most pressing environmental problems in the contemporary developed world. It is an excellent example of how corporate production runs riot regardless of public health.

The short chapter 24, "You Have Cancer: It's Your Fault," which ends the book, is something of a rallying cry in favor of the cancer sufferer. While a whole army of disinterested academics find and promote bogus answers to the quickly expanding cancer statistics, Professor Sherman is absolutely sure that whatever the pressures, those who suffer from cancer should think long and hard before blaming themselves for their condition and understand the lengths to which corporations go in order to dodge responsibility, putting profit before health.

Chapter 1

A DARK CULTURE— THE HISTORY AND LITERATURE OF HEALTH- DAMAGING PRODUCTION, ITS EXPOSURE, AND ITS CORPORATE DEFENSE

Martin J. Walker

Day and night the telescreens bruised your ears with statistics
Proving that people today had more food, more clothes,
Better houses, better recreations—that they lived longer, happier,
more intelligent, better educated than the people of fifty years ago.
Not a word of it could ever be proved or disproved.[1]

George Orwell

Alex Carey's posthumous book, *Taking the Risk out of Democracy*, subtitled *Corporate Propaganda versus Freedom and Liberty*, was published in 1995.[2] Carey was a class-conscious Australian who for the last forty years of his life lectured mainly in industrial psychology and the psychology of propaganda. He realized, more than most, how industrialization had passed the door marked "Democracy" and was heading for rooms bare of choice.

Carey's book, a collection of published and unpublished chapters, gives a framework through which to view the problems of industry penetration of civil society and political democracy. The book throws open the political and cultural reasons for the drift of capitalism and representative democracy toward totalitarian corporatism. Carey's most famous quote is popularized by Noam Chomsky in the forward of Chomsky's book, *World Orders Old and New*:

> The twentieth century has been characterized by three developments of great political importance: the growth of democracy, the growth of corporate power, and the growth of corporate propaganda as a means of protecting corporate power against democracy.[3]

The following book principally focuses on the problem of distorted science or scientific information by those working directly for corporate interests. However, distorting epidemiology or other information and, as McGarity and Wagner term it, *Bending Science*[4] in order to ensure profit regardless of damage to workers, citizens, and the environment is not an isolated pursuit that takes place only within a refined academic environment.

The questions surveyed by science and open to reporting misinformation are not only questions of health and physical damage; they are also political questions. For example, while the matter of human microchipping undoubtedly has a health aspect[5] that research by corporate insiders might attempt to skate over, the political question of control of the social person is undoubtedly at the forefront of any debate and is perhaps more difficult for the corporations to argue, leading to more aggressive strategies to quiet any discourse.

Whether or not microchipping causes health damage, it is something that has to be contested or at least debated by a "free people" in a democracy. However, many health studies suggest it is not safe. Only a universal political campaign will take it off the corporate agenda; this same argument applies to other campaigns, such as that against genetically modified organisms (GMOs).

All techniques of propaganda exist within a social, economic, political, and cultural matrix, and it is important that those opposed to a corporate future realize this; otherwise, conflicts will be confined to the narrowest of criteria. Unfortunately it might be said that because of the nature of contemporary politics and the high technology means of production, the greatest of attention is paid by critics and reformers to the general situation of "censorship" and "disinformation" in occupational and public health "science" while such matters as the havoc wrought by the pharmaceutical cartels on, for instance, independent, natural forms of personal medicine have all but been written out of contemporary scientific history.

While the "scientists" who are victims of attacks use the language of science to defend themselves, the corporations frequently negate or completely abandon science in their attacks. Although, for example, there is no lack of science with which to address alternative therapies such as acupuncture and homeopathy, the pharmaceutical corporations, defending mass deaths from medicines, win without effort or proof by labeling practices as fraudulent, quackery, or simply of no therapeutic use.

The battles of clinical and research "scientists" with corporate industry and government have begun to hog the stage in the war with corporatism. Is it important to understand the scale and the "ballpark" of corporate industry's campaign to stop competition and the critical appraisal of products? Is it important to understand the distortion of information sociologically, historically, beyond science? I argue in this chapter that unless we understand the nature, the magnitude, and the strategies of corporations, we will be unsuccessful in challenging their illegality, immorality, and unethical behavior. After all, the strategies of the corporations are not only aimed at scientists, but at cutting-edge writers, campaigners, activists, and whistle-blowers, and, for example, medical practitioners who would not consider themselves first and foremost as "scientists."

The interesting juxtaposition of two reports emphasizes this concern about plausibility and recognition of the different streams of struggle involving corporations. "Heads They Win, Tails, We Lose: How Corporations Corrupt Science at the Public's Expense,"[6] was published by the Scientific Integrity Program of the Union of Concerned Scientists in 2012. It is an excellent report that depicts in detail the whole bag of tricks used by corporations to censor views and research results critical of corporate science, toxic production, and their effects upon health. While the report's message is radical, its apparent reliance upon the regulatory, political, and scientific establishment to solve or ameliorate the problems faced by science and scientists leaves one feeling that the scientific community has partially failed to understand the nature of corporatism.

The second report, "Spooky Business: Corporate Espionage Against Nonprofit Organizations,"[7] although sounding like a completely different report, in fact, addresses a very similar subject. It was published in 2013 by a single author, Gary Ruskin, with a PO Box number address in Washington, DC. Ruskin's very thorough research deals with the gathering of intelligence to inform attacks or containment on critics of corporations. One could say that this report deals with the groundwork that corporations carry out in order to campaign against individuals or groups.

The tactics outlined in the report are obviously used by and against people working well beyond the area of clinical or research science. I immediately recognized some of the tactics that had been used against me by pharmaceutical companies. "Spooky Business" tells the story of an intelligence community moving from the sanctuary of the dingy halls of the state to the more polished halls of the corporations. They are doing the same work for the private sector and their new targets are very similar, but now they are almost entirely those who critique corporations. "Spooky Business" updates one aspect of David Helvarg's brilliant book, *The War Against the Greens*,[8] and reports a new wholly more sophisticated war that is being developed by corporatism against democratic protest.

The report traces the growth of domestic private intelligence, which has grown up against any kind of opposition to corporations. It points to the fact that this domestic war economy is staffed by ex-police, federal agents, and the most skilled crisis PR management companies, all of whom have been head-hunted and poached by corporations and now have high-technology apparatus that are more sophisticated than those used by the US state.

Clearly independent scientists, clinical and academic, are to some extent burying their heads in the sand if they think that opposition to corporatism can succeed with a war fought only in the theater of scientific research.

Long before industrialization covered the developed world, there had been critics of the emergent industrial means of production. Bernardino Ramazzini (1633–1717) wrote the first cogent treatise on occupational health, which examined the potential sources of illness in more than forty-two occupations, both manual and sedentary. Titled *De Morbis Artificum Diatriba* (Diseases of Workers), it was published in 1700.[9] Ramazzini seemed to have faced little opposition to his accurate ideas about the damage done to workers by their working environment, and accepted as a teacher by two of Italy's best universities, he was highly respected academically.

One of Ramazzini's most quoted statements, however—"'Tis a sordid profit that is accompanied by the destruction of health"—and even his choice of subject to study hints at his concern about the workers and the moral stance of those who organized production. On other issues in Ramazzini's medical life, such as a cautious approach to the prescription of medicines, Ramazzini, a trained physician, did face opposition from the monopoly makers, sellers and providers of drugs, the apothecaries. When Ramazzini campaigned for the limited use of cinchona bark (from which the alkaloid quinine was derived) in the treatment of malaria, he was fought by the apothecaries who had been using the remedy in a typically "orthodox" manner for all kinds of fevers and making good profits from it. He also faced opposition from the ruling elite in medicine who were still following the idea of classic Greek physician, Galen, that all diseases were based on a balance of the humors.[10]

The turf wars in medicine between the apothecaries—the faint beginnings of the pharmaceutical industry—and independent healers were entrenched by the Inquisition of the late seventeenth century, which chose to see herbalism, for example, as diabolical. One of the first victims of these wars, although not apparently affected by the Inquisition, was Samuel Hahnemann, a trained physician born in Germany in 1755, who developed the theory and practice of homeopathy. At the time of his birth, treatments and diagnoses were chaotic from what we might today call a "rational perspective." There was no organized diagnostic procedure or treatment in the mid-eighteenth century; court physicians and other professionals believed in a ragbag of treatments from bloodletting and magic to a wide range of herbal and chemical elixirs that had rarely been tested.

Despite that today Hahnemann is ridiculed and derided, especially in the United Kingdom, he established himself prominently at the end of the eighteenth century as a scientific physician and medical researcher. He developed the already considered concept of "like curing like" and used a systematic and rigorous proving of a wide variety of natural substances on a large number of individuals.

Having chosen a substance that seemed likely to act as a cure, he would send out samples to students and colleagues with instructions for taking various quantities and to send back meticulous reports of all physical or psychological effects, a kind of scientific trial that was completely unknown for medicines at that time.

Hahnemann's most fundamental idea that has stayed relevant until the present day was that if you examined in detail the effects of a particular substance on the human mind and body, that substance could be used to "cure" those same effects when they were presented by a patient as an illness. What, however, was novel about Hahnemann's ideas for treatment, and what has attracted considerable attention since the late eighteenth century, for obvious reasons, was the idea that only the smallest dilution of the remedy was necessary to effect a cure.

Hahnemann came under heavy attack from the apothecaries who saw this rationally tried medicine as a serious threat to their irrational tricks. Also, of course, even at that time, money was a driving force of the apothecaries. Although training in homeopathy could take some time, the remedies themselves were cheap to produce and prescribe, or even free through a homeopathic hospital. Toward the end of his life Hahnemann came under severe attack.

His attitude to those who attacked him was clear. In a letter to a colleague, he wrote, "What is true cannot be minted into a falsehood, even by the most distinguished professor."[11] Seven years after this letter, he wrote the paragraph below, which stands as good advice today when facing shills on social media. Speaking of a colleague who was defending homeopathy, he wrote the following:

> I regret, however, that he should spend so much time and headwork on these sophistries. Believe me, all these attacks only weary the assailants of truth, and, in the long run, are no obstacle to its progress. We do well to let all these, specious, but nugatory articles alone, to sink of themselves into the abyss of oblivion, and their natural nothingness . . . All these controversial writings are nothing but signals of distress—alarm guns fired from a sinking ship.[12]

The scale, irrationality, and insensibility of these attacks on Hahnemann are evident in an 1825 quote from Christoph Wilhelm Hufeland, the most influential medical writer of that time, in an article about homeopathy:

> I consider it wrong and unworthy of science to treat the new doctrine with ridicule and contempt. It is in my nature to lend a helping hand to the persecuted. Persecution and tyranny in scientific matters are especially repugnant to me.[13]

The apothecaries, however, were determined to forge their monopoly and when they had done this, determined to enforce it. In his 1861 book, *The History and Heroes of the Art of Medicine*, J. Rutherfurd Russell traces the early attacks by the apothecaries on Hahnemann:

> The proverb says that "any stick is good enough to beat a dog," and the first stick the German apothecaries took up was a legal one. There was an enactment which prevented physicians from compounding their own medicines; this was brought to bear against Hahnemann and although he pleaded that he never actually mixed even two medicines, and that the law was never intended for such a practice as his, yet the stick came down on his back and he had to leave Leipzig in consequence.[14]

During the nineteenth century, both "orthodox" doctors and those who had gone over to homeopathy were pitted against recurring cholera epidemics that occurred across Europe. In the London cholera epidemic of 1854, of the 331 cases of cholera and simple diarrhea treated at the London Homeopathic Hospital, there was a 16.4 percent mortality rate. The neighboring Middlesex Hospital received 231 cases of cholera and 47 cases of choleric diarrhea. Of the cholera patients treated, 123 died, a fatality rate of 59.2 percent.[15]

In 1855, the treatment committee of the Board of Health compiled its major report for Parliament on cholera and its treatment. The treatment committee agreed among themselves to exclude the London Homeopathic Hospital statistics as they would "compromise the values and utilities of their average of cure, as deduced from the operation of known treatments, but they would give an unjustifiable sanction to an empirical practice alike opposed to the maintenance of truth, and to the progress of science."[16]

In a House of Commons debate on cholera in 1855, based on the report, Robert Grosvenor 1st Baron Ebury asks whether the Board of Health forms received from homeopaths were refused on receipt. Benjamin Hall replied that those forms returned by homeopaths had been systematically identified and excluded from the report.[17]

Perhaps one of the most transparent, even juvenile, attacks on homeopathy was practiced against Jacques Benveniste. Benveniste, a well-regarded researcher at INSERM, was the author of four papers previously published in *Nature* and some two hundred scientific articles, two of which were cited as "citation classics" by the Philadelphia Institute for Scientific Information.

In 1988, Benveniste submitted a paper titled "Human basophil degranulation triggered by very dilute antiserum against IgE" to *Nature*, which suggested that water conveyed the information of even greatly diluted substances and affected IgE. Benveniste waited a year for their agreement to publish.

The paper was published, but was accompanied by a disclaiming editorial by John Maddox, a leading pro-corporate skeptic. Soon after publication, the Committee for the Scientific Investigation of Claims of the Paranormal (CSICOP) began harassing Benveniste.[18] Despite the fact that other scientists in other laboratories replicated his results, CSICOP pressured Benveniste into giving them permission to send a team to "investigate" his experiments.

When James Randi—the showman magician with no science experience funded specifically to campaign against alternative medicine—turned up with John Maddox and the American, Walter Stuart, they behaved like three of the Marx brothers and proceeded to write up the results of their "research" for *Nature*.

On publication they claimed that Benveniste's work was a hoax. Benveniste, who had previously held Maddox in great respect, was to say later, "It was as if I had given the Pope my wallet to mind while I worked and he had stolen it."[19]

In concert with a massive propaganda campaign in the media, in every European country, Benveniste and his work were ridiculed. Within weeks he had lost his grants and his position at INSERM, while his very name became a byword for quackery.

With the pharmaceutical corporations having such control over journals and even news programs, Benveniste was unable to clear his name. Despite a continuing replication of his results, he was never able to regain a foothold in research before he died, ironically, during an operation in a French hospital.

It seemed that few "scientists" observing what happened to Benveniste were willing to take sides, insisting instead on seeing the case as one in which bona fide researchers outside the mainstream of medical research had misunderstood the science. In fact, Benveniste's results in particular were of enormous consequence to the pharmaceutical companies: were it possible to prove that very low doses of medicines could convey their information through liquids over distances, the fundamental premise of pharmaceutical medicine would be questioned and the premise of cheap universal "natural" health care could be partially established.

The examples of Hahnemann specializing in an idea of alternative medicines and Ramazzini who cottoned on to the damaging physical effects of industrial work processes, two forward-looking doctors in the seventeenth and eighteenth centuries set the stage for focusing on two strands of monopoly interests that have survived to the present day.

It was not until the middle of the nineteenth century that a movement against public and private environmental toxins began to coalesce. As the effects of environmental illness came to be noticed in a number of industries, reformers of various kinds began to question worker and consumer health safety.

Although in some occupations and industries, like the one that organized young chimney sweeps small enough to climb up chimneys, the movements for their protection were quickly effective; others had to wait until the end of the nineteenth century and the beginning of the twentieth for critical writings and campaigns. Even less easily proven, environmental health damage has stayed above the law and beyond reform until the present day.

Henrik Ibsen was one of the first writer critics to look at the question of what happens to someone, in this case a community-based doctor, who reports a public health threat caused by industry.[20] Ibsen finished *An Enemy of the People* in 1882, very close to the most energetic period of writing about vested interests and corporate denial of the toxic effects of industry in the United States.

The central character in *An Enemy of the People*, Dr. Thomas Stockmann, is the medical officer of health in a coastal town in southern Norway. His brother, Peter Stockmann, is the town's mayor, chief constable, and chairman of the municipal baths' committee, with his fingers in many local commercial concerns, including the local tannery which, it turns out, is polluting the new municipal baths.

When Dr. Stockmann links gastrointestinal illnesses suffered by his patients to the new "health-giving" spa baths, his brother reacts with a whole series of censorial dirty tricks that drive the town's population to hysteria, which is turned on the doctor. Throughout the play, Ibsen makes much of the fact that all party political systems expect individuals to subsume their own interests to those of the majority: a question particularly relevant to the contemporary battle over, for example, mass vaccination.

When Robert H. Sherard died in 1943, he left a legacy of thirty-three books, including fourteen novels, as well as many newspaper articles. Despite being born into an aristocratic milieu, Sherard, cut off from his inheritance by his father, plunged into the bohemian artistic fringe, writing biographies of famous authors, notably Oscar Wilde and Émile Zola.

At the turn of the nineteenth century, workers in the north of England found an unlikely champion in Sherard. From 1895 to 1901, in his mid-thirties, Sherard involved himself in a series of investigations that were published in Pearson's and The London Magazine: "The White Slaves of England," "The Cry of the Poor," "The Closed Door," and "The Child Slaves of Britain."[21] Whatever Sherard's driving feelings and purpose in these investigations, whether he wrote out of a sense of sympathy or socialist ideology or even in an attempt to live through the pain of the termination of a friendship with Oscar Wilde, the workers have rarely found a better advocate.

The White Slaves of England, first published in 1897, describes itself as a true picture of certain social conditions in England in the year 1897.[22] The book looks at, among others, the alkali workers, the nail makers, the slipper makers and tailors, the wool combers, the white lead workers, and the chair makers.

Sherard developed his own methodology to investigate working conditions: "The exploration of the factories was an easy task. One had often but to walk confidently in at the front door with firm steps and a brazen forehead. When this was impracticable there was the wall at the back. And there were other ways and means, which need not be detailed, lest helpful friends be molested."[23]

In the late nineteenth century, the alkali workers of Widnes and St. Helens represented the kind of health damage rarely seen even in the developing world today but recorded in the photographs of Sebastião Salgado[24] and chronicled in books like Disposable People: New Slavery in the Global Economy by Kevin Bales.[25] The damage done by chemicals to both the workers and environment was total. Sherard wrote the following:

The spring never comes hither. It never comes because neither at Widnes or St Helens, is there any place in which it can manifest itself. The foul gases which, belched forth night and day from the many factories, rot the clothes, the teeth, and in the end, the bodies of the workers, have killed every tree and every blade of grass for miles around.[26]

From the beginning of his investigations into the conditions of workers, and from the beginning he sided with them, Sherard seemed to have a built-in radar that kept him from playing any part at all on behalf of the employers, seemingly sure that to become involved with the employers was to directly undermine the workers' case.

Speaking of his involvement with the workers who shared small hospitalities with him, he says the following two sentences in relation to the employers—two sentences that might have become the slogans for any independent investigator into corporate power:

> I avoided contact with the masters as far as possible, and am in no way indebted to any of them for assistance in my enterprise. The factories I visit were visited by me as a trespasser, and at a trespasser's risk.[27]

Pearson, the magazine publisher, stood solidly behind Sherard when he was attacked by the bourgeoisie of northern England. Sherard's chapter on the slipper makers and tailors of Leeds came under incendiary attack by trade associations and retailers of Leeds. The *Leeds Times* doesn't waste any space in getting right to the point:

> Under the somewhat sensational general heading of the "White Slaves of England" in *Pearson's Magazine* for September, Mr. R. H. Sherard contributes to the current issue of *Pearson's Magazine* a rather highly coloured article.[28]

Despite on occasions "being on the run," "breaking into workplaces," and generally espousing a rebellious faith in the poor and the working class, when Sherard came up for air and his work was published, he had to fight off the industrial gentry who took every opportunity to slander and abuse him. Speaking of the main textile trade paper, he said the following:

> . . . have led it to commit . . . a series of very gross libels upon me. I am charged by the editor of the *Textile Mercury* with falsehood, slander, and "traduction." I presume traducement was meant.[29]

In the September 5, 1989, issue of the *Textile Mercury*, there appeared two leading articles, the first headed "Libels on the Nation." This article links Sherard's writing to the US muckrakers and then goes for his throat:

We were not, however, prepared to believe in the possibility of English journals joining in the lying and libelous attacks which have been made against *our industrial life generally* [my italics] by some American newspapers until we saw the current issue of *Pearson's Monthly*.[30]

The little known Sherard was one of the greatest investigative writers of the nineteenth century, a man completely wedded to a social cause who was not afraid of taking the brickbats of the new industrial middle class.

In 1888, there occurred a revolutionary strike in London that led to the first organization of a trade union for women. The matchgirls strike at Bryant & May in London's East End resulted from a number of conflicts between the company and their exploited workers. The working women, who made matches from white or yellow phosphorus, were as young as fifteen.

The strike began following the suspension of one worker on July 2 and developed within days. The women's demands covered a number of issues including the fourteen-hour working day, low pay, instant dismissals, the imposition of fines, refusal to allow breaks, and, perhaps the most serious of all: working with the deadly toxic, cancer-causing yellow phosphorus. The cancer was known colloquially as "phossy" jaw, and more formally "phosphorus necrosis of the jaw." The British Government was fully aware of the dangers of yellow phosphorus, which had been banned in Sweden and the United States, but argued that banning it would amount to a restraint of free trade.

Like many other political and labor disputes of this period, the strike, though won by the women employees, was progressed by outsiders of considerable political resolve. The first to join the workers was Annie Besant, a tireless campaigner for women who had already lost custody of her daughter to her clergyman husband, who had told the court that as Besant was not a Christian she was unfit to bring up her daughter. Besant was later to face trial at the Old Bailey after publishing a book about contraception.[31, 32]

On hearing about the strike, Besant published an article in June 1888 in *The Link*, a paper she had set up with W. T. Stead, a journalist. Her article titled "White Slavery in London," was, in the best tradition of investigative reporting, based on interviews with a number of women working at the factory.[33] The fact that Bryant and May had presided over the death and disfigurement of many young female workers did not stop them threatening a High Court action against Besant and her article. In the face of these heavy-handed tactics, Besant and others arranged for fifty-six matchgirls to march to the offices of *The Link* on Fleet Street and then on to the House of Commons.[34] The strike ended after a negotiated settlement on July 16 with most of the workers' demands being met.

It was, however, 1901 before the company announced that they had discontinued the use of yellow phosphorus, and it was not until the use of white phosphorus was prohibited by the international Berne Convention in 1906 and its provisions were implemented that industrial use ceased.

The most radical action of the campaigning group for the matchgirls, was the setting up of a matchmaking factory just round the corner from Bryant & May in 1891. This factory used the much safer, though more expensive, red phosphorus, and the company was soon producing six million boxes a year. Workers were paid twice the amount as those employed at Bryant & May and worked in better conditions. Salvation Army adherents campaigned with local retailers to get them to sell only red phosphorus matches.[35]

Twenty years after Ibsen's *An Enemy of the People*, and in the same decades Sherard and Besant were writing, a group of US journalists and writers emerged. Dubbed by Teddy Roosevelt as "the muckrakers," they were a non-hegemonic group of American writers who campaigned against corruption in City Hall, the boardrooms of the Trusts, and the personal lives of the great founding capitalists of the United States. Among their greatest exposés were Ida Tarbell's *The History of Standard Oil Company*[36] and Upton Sinclair's fictionalized horrors of the Chicago meat packing plants, *The Jungle*.[37] The muckrakers were, on the whole, more likely to be campaigners than today's academics.

Upton Sinclair was an active socialist when in 1909 he finished the manuscript for *The Jungle*.[38] Sinclair eventually got his manuscript accepted by Doubleday, where the editor was "a kind and extremely naive man" who: ". . . submitted the proofs to the managing editor of the *Chicago Tribune*, who sent back a thirty-two page report on the book, prepared by 'a disinterested and competent reporter.'"[39] When Sinclair exposed the report as meat packers' propaganda, Doubleday sent a young lawyer to investigate. He met a publicity agent for the packers who admitted that he knew of *The Jungle*: "I read the proofs of it and prepared a thirty-two page report." Upton Sinclair paid a high price for his critical campaign when, among other attacks, his communal home was burned down.[40]

The late Rachel Carson, a qualified marine biologist who had worked for the US Department of Fisheries, wrote the first "modern" book that gave a general picture of the damage that chemicals were doing to the environment and human and animal health. Her book, *Silent Spring*,[41] became the founding work of the environmental movement and the subject of a relentless campaign against environmentalists by the chemical companies.[42] To defend the DDT industry, the chemical companies developed a whole new lexicon of tricks.

The US producers of DDT, Velsicol, tried to stop publication of *Silent Spring*. In a letter to the book's publishers, they entreated

> In addition to the sincere opinions by natural food faddists, Audubon groups and others, members of the chemical industry in this country and in Western Europe must deal with sinister influences.[43]

The communists, they said, intended "to reduce the use of chemicals in this country . . . so that the supply of food will be reduced to East-Curtain parity."[44]

In defense of DDT, the American Medical Association sided with the US Nutrition Foundation, then supported by fifty-four companies in the food, chemical, and allied industries.[45] A "Fact Kit" sent out by the Foundation stressed the "independence" of those who attacked Carson, ". . . special interest groups are promoting her book as if it were . . . written by a scientist."[46] Of course, Carson was a scientist just not a corporate scientist.

Paul Brodeur has been one of the greatest writers and investigators in the area of public health. His life's work is a series of books about the health-damaging effects of different industries. His first book about the asbestos industry, written originally for the *New Yorker*, was published by Viking Press in 1973 as *Expendable Americans: The incredible story of how tens of thousands of American men and women die each year of preventable industrial disease*.[47]

Brodeur is a true original, one of the first writers to popularize the story of vested interests and manipulated science that damaged the health of thousands of workers and citizens. A quote from the *Newsletter of The Association of Trial Lawyers of America* places the book within the post-1968 era of the politics of industry and health: "This splendid exposé uncloaks the total callousness, stupidity, and deceit of the medical-industrial complex consisting of company doctors, industry consultants, and key occupational-health officials at various levels of the state and federal governments."

Brodeur went on to write books dealing with the cover-up of major health concerns in post-industrial society. Among these works are: *Currents of Death: Power lines, computer terminals, and the attempt to cover up their threat to your health*,[48] and *The Zapping of America: Microwaves, their deadly risk, and the cover-up*.[49] This latter book was published in 1977, again, well before its time.

The late 1960s and the 1970s was a period imbued with the spirit of investigation, a time when many sociologists—and indeed, scientists—saw and identified the damaging collusion that existed between the growing industrial complex and the health of the people. In 1977, the late Barbara Seaman and her doctor husband, Gideon, published their great investigation into hormone replacement therapy (HRT) and the use of hormones in birth control pills, *Women and the Crisis in Sex Hormones*.[50] The book was promoted as "the most important medical story of the 1970s." Unfortunately, the story of sex hormones, the doctors who pushed them, the companies that manufactured them, and the women they killed, remained one of the most "important medical stories of the next thirty years." When I wrote my book on HRT, *HRT Licensed to Kill and Maim*[51] in 2007, the best I could do was update Barbara Seaman's earlier work. Seaman's book, a solid five-hundred-page volume, charts in detail the collusion between industry and the medical profession and the adverse reactions that both groups continue to deny. Studies still repeatedly report on significant risk of cancer from HRT while manufacturers determinedly continue to produce it and doctors continue to prescribe it.[52]

We should always be grateful for the eccentrics and those who take on gigantic projects and pull them off. There are a few books that crop up "out of time," imbued with the spirit of the 1960s but published later. Sometimes, these authors might want to deny their progeny. I think of Geoffrey Cannon's magnificent book, *The Politics of Food*, published in the late eighties, in this way.[53] The book, that has no subtitle, is promoted on the front cover as describing, "the secret world of Whitehall and the food giants which threaten your health."

Like all good books of this genre, *The Politics of Food* was for a long period an excellent reference for any links between industry and the food we eat. When I found this book it was as if I had suddenly discovered another world, like that of Tolkien or the Borrowers.[54] The book is truly subversive, making nonsense of the fairy stories that a postwar generation had been told about food production and science's concern about health through food. More than anything else, however, Cannon's book gives names and specific details of vested interests and hitherto secret ties.

A more modest US book, of 260 pages, published in 1981 and announcing itself as *Industry Influence in Federal Regulatory Agencies*,[55] was written by Paul J. Quirk of Princeton University. Quirk, like Braithwaite in his stunning 1984 book *Corporate Crime in the Pharmaceutical Industry*[56] interviewed, in this case, regulatory officials, asking how they felt industry tried to influence policy. However, unlike Braithwaite, Quirk seems to flunk his conclusions.

In the 1970s, there was in sociology and the more specialized science of epidemiology—as there was in politics generally—a turn to the Right. This was very generally, a turn against the more human and small-scale observation of personal and group behavior in favor of a high-tech overview of large

populations. Such studies had serious disadvantages, tending to cut out or
delete the smaller clinical effects on human health, while describing in bland
terms the mass response.

This new epidemiologically based research shared goals between universities and business interests in what was first termed the "university-industrial
complex" by Martin Kenney in the title of his 1986 book, *Biotechnology: The
University-Industrial Complex.*[57] Kenney, an assistant professor of agricultural
economics at Ohio State University, raised concerns over the development of
close business ties between many universities and large biotechnology corporations and how this "university-industrial complex" would affect educational
institutions, agriculture, and society in general.

Sheldon Krimsky, in *Science in the Private Interest*, examined the ethical
quandary whereby university research has often become deeply entangled with
entrepreneurship and commercial interests—to become what Krimsky called an
"inevitable tide of corporate and academic partnerships and the commercialism
of knowledge."[58] Krimsky concluded: "As universities turn their scientific laboratories into commercial enterprise zones, and select faculties to realize these
goals, fewer opportunities will exist in academia for public interest science—an
inestimable loss to society."[59]

One main target for attack at the heart of the corporate science lobby has always
been what they consider alternative cancer treatments. It is abundantly clear
why this should be: cell-based cancer research is a booming multimillion-dollar
industry and, as in other environmentally caused illnesses, the occupational or
environmental roots of most cancers are being denied to the last. A small number of writers have pieced together the ways in which the cancer establishment
maintains a censorious grip over non-orthodox treatments and stymies preventative work.

Ralph W. Moss and Professor Samuel Epstein came at the problem of censorship from two different perspectives. While Epstein has tried valiantly to
bring the manufacturers of environmental carcinogens to book, Moss has drawn
attention to the considerable variety of treatments available and the "alternative"
treatments that have been censored. Ralph Moss has spent more than twenty
years investigating and writing about cancer issues and, like Epstein, has been an
activist in the sense that he has set up groups and organizations to pursue their
answers to the cancer problem.

In both cases, Moss and Epstein's first significant books, Moss's *The Cancer
Industry*[60] and Epstein's *The Politics of Cancer*,[61] presented information that
produced shock waves and tutored a generation. Professor Epstein has carried

the torch lit by individuals like Rachel Carson and the sociologist Edwin H. Sutherland, who wrote *White Collar Crime*,[62] in writing unambiguously about the corruption of science by corporations and large charities. Epstein has been exceptional among his generation of public health academics in his constant willingness to be involved in campaigning organizations, to name names and write about the reality of corporate liability. He has made frequent forays into Britain, inducing local authors to produce books echoing the analysis in *The Politics of Cancer*, such as *Cancer in Britain: The Politics of Prevention*.[63]

Although Moss's most renowned book, *The Cancer Industry*, was published in the 1990s, a more recent book, published in 2014, brings him full circle, from the initial incident after which he left Sloan Kettering, into the contemporary discourse about cover-ups and corporate shenanigans. *Doctored Results* tells the story of the suppression of the results of laetrile studies.[64] A promotional blurb on Amazon describes the book: "The first full-scale exposé of one of the major scientific scandals of the twentieth century by a man who was there at the time and who helped reveal the cover-up." Perhaps one of the clear distinctions between the work of Moss and Epstein is that Moss has always been interested in promoting alternative treatments, while Epstein has doggedly investigated the corruption of science in relation to prevention and the corruption of science in relation to allopathic treatments.

In 2005, Epstein published *Cancer-Gate: How to Win the Losing Cancer War*, a book packed with information that activists and critics of the cancer establishment need to fight back against the manipulation of epidemiology and industrial science.[65] More recently, Epstein has been working with congress trying to frame a bill that defines manipulation of research data as corporate crime, deserving of a criminal sentence.

The writer who best reflects the contemporary focus on consumer choice in the area of cancer is Barry Lynes. Lynes, who has written consistently about alternative cancer treatments since the 1970s, has plowed a lonely furrow; his books are far from academic texts, written with activists and sufferers in mind. Lynes became interested in suppressed cancer cures after studying Royal Rife. His first book, *The Cancer Cure that Worked*, has become a bestseller and looks at the life and times of Rife.[66] In 1990, aware of the lack of individual choice in the area of cancer care, Lynes wrote *Helping the Cancer Victim: Patient Rights, Medical Freedom & the Need for New Laws*.[67] This short book is a handbook for those affected by cancer and those seeing the need for campaigning for legal changes.

The late Christopher Bird, well known for his book *The Secret Life of Plants*,[68] also got involved in questioning the cancer establishment when he was the first person to recover one of Rife's microscopes. In 1996, Bird wrote the superb *The Persecution and Trial of Gaston Naessens*.[69] The book is excellent on-the-spot reportage enhanced by his description of arriving in town for the trial with his typewriter and returning to his hotel room every evening after the hearing to bash out his notes, which formed the basis of the book. Naessens was an experienced laboratory scientist and doctor who built a microscope similar to Rife's. Over a long period of scientific investigation, he discovered the life cycle of a microorganism present in the blood of people who contracted cancer. He developed a treatment that damaged the organism, and began to prescribe it, hence his prosecution by the Canadian medical authorities.

The reason Bird's book reflects on "secret ties" is because those who went as far as giving evidence against Naessens clearly did so for a reason: they were part of the massive international web that links industry to the regulatory agencies. Bird comments on these people and their evidence at length.

In academia and even within the more popular books and papers about "secret ties" and "vested interests," it is usual to report solely on the "positive" bending of science carried out by corporations to give a healthy gloss to their products. There is, of course, a whole other world of propaganda and PR crisis management that focuses on the negative attacks on those who appear to the corporations to hamper commercial competition.

One of the most science-saturated, technologically tumescent areas of modern production is pharmaceuticals. Given that in this area, science demotes the human being to the mechanistic level of the robot and that medicine's origins in science are lost in the mists and smoke of the industrial revolution rather than growing from an empathy with human life, it is not surprising that one of the greatest battlefields and the one in which disinformation is paramount is that of pharmaceutical medicine.

Two cancer therapeutic approaches that have come under constant attack over the last decades are those of Dr. Hulda Clark and Dr. Max Gerson. Gerson was a German doctor who fled to North America in the 1930s. Having worked on diabetes, mainly from a nutritional perspective, he turned his nutritional ideas to cancer. Like Rife and a number of other highly qualified practitioners, Gerson consistently wrote up his cases, as well as presenting reports and trials of his work to skeptical doctors and scientists. Unfortunately, these attempts at bridge building got nowhere, simply because his treatments did not involve chemical drugs that could be bought and patented by the pharmaceutical companies.

Gerson set up an institute to perpetuate his work and the publication of his writings. In 1958, he published *A Cancer Therapy: Results of Fifty Cases*.[70] Since his death, a number of people have written books based on their own cures using his treatment, most particularly Beata Bishop in *A Time to Heal: Triumph over Cancer, the Therapy of the Future.*[71]

Gerson's work has reemerged in the last thirty years in Britain. Aspects of the treatment were at the heart of the philosophy adopted by the Bristol Cancer Help Centre, which was mercilessly attacked by the cancer research "charities," their administrators, and scientists, and aligned "quackbusters" in 1991.[72] Then, in 2002, Michael Gearin-Tosh, a lecturer at Oxford University, wrote his exceptional book, *Living Proof: A Medical Mutiny.*[73] This book emerges in a very modest but self-assured manner as one of the best pieces of literature on a self-cancer cure, which stressed with great power the necessity and the problems of being free to make one's own treatment choices. Gearin-Tosh waited almost seven years after curing himself of cancer to validate his cure and publish his story. He died in July 2005, a full eleven years after he had been diagnosed with a fatal cancer.

In the United States, the National Council Against Health Fraud (NCAHF) and other quackbusters aligned to pharmaceutical and food corporations have, until recently, been much more energetic, making continuous attempts to shut down the clinics of the late Dr. Hulda Clark. Clark suffered a series of depredations, beginning with her arrest in 1999. This was followed by attempts to shut down her clinics and actions brought against people using her treatments or technology. Clark wrote a number of bestselling books in which she outlines her case for cancer being cured with detoxification and the application of electromagnetic fields. Quackbusters had an almost complete lack of success and were even humiliated in the US courts.[74]

One of my favorite books about cancer research and politics is by Evelleen Richards, an Australian writer and researcher. The book tells the story of what happened to Linus Pauling and Ewan Cameron when they suggested that vitamin C could be used, in part, as an alternative treatment for cancer. The book, *Vitamin C and Cancer: Medicine or Politics* is exceptionally good because it covers considerable ground, putting the controversy in a social, political, and cultural context.[75]

As an adjunct to Richards's book, it is informative to look at Sandra Goodman's writing about nutrition and cancer. This first arose in her book *Vitamin C: The Master Nutrient*[76] and was later developed in her extensive research review that she wrote originally for the Bristol Cancer Help Centre, "Nutrition and Cancer: State-of-the-Art."[77] Goodman, a genetic research graduate, was herself attacked viciously by British quackbusters after submitting a proposal to the Medical Research Council for research into the effect of germanium on AIDS-related illnesses.

Five cases that bear attention over and above that which was awarded them by authors who have worked on their cases are the German doctor Josef Issels; the Italian professor Luigi Di Bella; the French scientist Mirko Beljanski; Dr. Ryke Geerd Hamer, who spent almost three years in a French prison for advocating his theories about cancer; and Dr. Tullio Simoncini. All five of these qualified doctors became the target for disruptive attacks by the medical monopoly, their own governments, and those of other European countries. Behind these attacks one can sense not only the medical establishment but the pharmaceutical companies and other forms of corporate medicine.

I describe the work of Issels and the gross assaults upon him by the British medical establishment in my book *Dirty Medicine: Science, Big Business and the Assault on Natural Health Care*. But if you want to read a rounded and complete story of his life, you should turn to *Issels: The Biography of a Doctor* by Gordon Thomas.[78] Thomas is one of the great eclectic heroes of the struggle to get alternative cancer treatments to the public; he fought tooth and nail inside the BBC to get his film about Issels, *Go Climb a Mountain*, to the screen.[79] Issels had a great story to tell, having been tried and imprisoned in Germany and then attacked again by a gang of British cancer authoritarians in the pay of the British government. Also in relation to Issels, Peter Newton-Fenbow tells the story of Issels's Bavarian clinic from the patients' point of view in *A Time to Heal*.[80]

Vincenzo Brancatisano is a lawyer who, while defending the patients of Luigi Di Bella, the Italian cancer clinician, found another vocation: that of writer. In order to publish his monumental 735-page book about Di Bella, *Un po' di verità sulla terapia Di Bella*, Brancatisano linked up with the owner of a travel business.[81] With Brancatisano, as with Di Bella's career, we find the breakup of traditional political bases and a political consolidation around the right of patients to medical freedom of choice. For those ignorant people like myself who speak only English, Brancatisano has published one short book in English, *Di Bella: The Man, the Cure, A Hope for All*.[82] Brancatisano also showed his commitment to Di Bella's patients by publishing the provocatively titled "Sentenze di Vita" (Sentenced to Life).[83] In the Travel Factory, which published his work, Brancatisano and the late Professor Di Bella found a conscientious patron.

Unusual for that of a dissident cancer researcher attacked by the state and the corporations, the work of the Frenchman Mirko Beljanski, who died in 1998, is very well recorded, particularly in books by his wife, Monique Beljanski, and the work of his daughter, who runs an organization dedicated to his work. The Beljanski family also has their own publishing company that has produced a number of books telling the story of his life and research. These books range from short compilations of articles and essays, such as *Cancer: L'Approche Beljanski*[84] to the more comprehensive account of attacks upon him, such as *Mirko Beljanski, out La Chronique d'une "Fatwa" Scientifique* (Mirko Beljanski: story of a scientific fatwa).[85]

According to Dr. Hamer, the German physician, cancers are caused by a physical or psychological shock suffered by the patient. Dr. Hamer stands out among the "cancer doctors" in that, although he has published significant work on his theories about the origins and the treatment of cancer, his imprisonment in 2001 for almost three years for practicing medicine without a license—after his license had been taken away from him by the French State—has gone almost entirely unrecorded. In 2007, James McCumiskey published his book on Hamer, *The Ultimate Conspiracy*; this explains Hamer's theories but doesn't put his prison story into the context of his battles with the French authorities.[86]

Another doctor who stands out in a different way is the Italian Dr. Tullio Simoncini. He stands out for two reasons; first because he is absolutely straightforward about his treatment, and second because he is equally straightforward about the opposition he has faced from the orthodox cancer establishment. Simoncini has, for the last thirty years, treated cancers with bicarbonate of soda, with great success. He now finds himself in the same position as every other doctor or scientist who has insisted on following a path that diverges from corporate medical orthodoxy.

In an interview with Emma Hollister, when asked by Hollister "What has been the response of the medical authorities to your work?" Simoncini doesn't hesitate: "Suppression, plots, defamatory TV programs."[87] When a scientist has an effective and revolutionary idea, the medical institution attempts to suppress his work because he threatens the interests of the medical establishment and the pharmaceutical corporations. No matter how effective the therapy in question is, their aim will be to destroy the idea.

The case of Stanislaw Burzynski has become a cause célèbre in the United States, principally because the treatment that he has developed over forty years is based entirely on orthodox scientific research. Having left Poland in his postgraduate years, Burzynski developed a treatment that interferes with the ability of cancer cells to develop and divide. Following his administration of the treatment at his own research clinic in the early 1980s, the FDA began a war of harassment against him and his practice that has gone on for thirty years. Although the conflict has never been resolved, Burzynski has continued to treat patients with good results.[88]

The history of cancer research and treatment, especially in relation to the Nazi regime in Germany, has become the subject of focus of two books that

draw attention to the lack of resolve in this area of contemporary cell researchers sponsored by the biggest cancer research charities in Europe and America.
Devra Davis's latest book, *The Secret History of the War on Cancer*[89] and an earlier
one by Professor Robert Proctor, *Cancer Wars*,[90] both ask the question: "Why, if
there really is a war on cancer is it being lost over and again?" and, perhaps more
perceptively, "Why were the Nazis on the way to winning the war against cancer
by stifling its environmental triggers, while the US seems only to pretend to be at
war?" The Nazi regime took an interest even in the least known lay cancer curers across Europe and the tentative answer to the question could be that the war
against cancer in postwar Europe and the United States has perhaps been too
concerned with the profits of the leading corporations.

While the cancer industry establishment and the regulatory agencies fall
quickly upon qualified doctors who research alternative cancer treatments, they
tend to keep within the law when they harass them, while those who manufacture or practice with herbal cancer treatments can expect no mercy and are
treated like terrorists.

Kenny Ausubel, a US activist working for a better world, wrote perhaps the
best in-depth book about an herbal cancer cure, *When Healing becomes a Crime:
The Amazing Story of the Hoxsey Cancer Clinics and the Return of Alternative
Therapies*.[91] The book, published by Healing Arts Press of Rochester, Vermont,
is a thoroughly researched account of the life of Harry Hoxsey, who grew from
a small-time medicine salesman in the 1920s to the proprietor of a number of
popular clinics in the 1950s. Hoxsey fought a continuous battle with the medical
authorities and the larger organizations apparently protecting our health.

The story of Greg Caton and his herbal cancer treatments is stunningly similar in some details to the illegal acts performed by the US government in their
"War on terror." Caton and his wife are herbalists; they had a business in the
United States that ran afoul of an FDA campaign. Mark Lipsman wrote the first
complete account of Caton's earliest arrest in 2003.[92]

Caton was a victim of "Operation Cure.All," an initiative begun in 2001 by
the US Food and Drug Administration and the Federal Trade Commission. A
press release on the FTC's website says, "FTC, FDA, and other law enforcement
agencies move to stop Internet scams for supplements and other products that
purport to cure cancer, HIV/AIDS, and countless other life-threatening diseases."
Unfortunately, the FDA has used this as an excuse to shut down businesses and
arrest people whose products, though not recognized by conventional medicine,
actually work—and are inexpensive and have few, if any, side effects.[93]

The police "detained" Caton without charge for eight months in jail before
a sympathetic judge gave him bail. At the sentencing hearing, the judge rejected

the prosecution's contention that Caton had intended to cause harm with his products and sentenced him to the minimum possible under the sentencing guidelines: thirty-three months imprisonment. In all, Greg Caton estimates the FDA took (from him) $250,000 worth of materials and $400,000 worth of buildings. This doesn't include what he lost in the distress sale of PreservX and the one building he sold, his legal fees—which amounted to $50,000 for the criminal charges alone—or the ongoing revenue from PreservX and Alpha Omega.[94]

After his release, Caton decided to go to Ecuador with his wife and family; there he came to an agreement with the government to legally produce his herbal treatments. When the FDA realized that he was working in Ecuador and judged him to have broken his post-sentence probation conditions, intrepid FDA agents set out to arrest him.

In November of 2008, FDA agent John Armand tried to kidnap Caton in Ecuador and have him flown back to the United States, but he failed. However, Caton was arrested in Ecuador at a staged license checkpoint in February 2009, and false charges were brought against him: that he was in Ecuador illegally and selling herbal products illegally. At the first hearing before a judge, the judge accepted Caton's innocence of the charges and they were dropped.[95]

However, before he could gain his release from prison, the judge's order was countermanded by a police chief, and while the Catons were awaiting an appeal decision against the police chief's actions, Caton was kidnapped by US officials aiming to get him on an American Airlines flight to Miami. Caton's wife, Cathryn, called their attorney who called the judge.

This judge drove to the chief of police to release him of his authority. The judge then drove to the airport to stop immigration from deporting Greg. The US embassy and immigration officials heard of the judge coming and put Greg on the plane. They told the Ecuadorian federal judge that the United States had the legal right to deport Greg because he was on American property and could not be removed. The judge then talked to the airport tower to have the American Airlines flight stopped. American Airlines and the pilot would not listen. The judge called a general in the Ecuadorian military to have the plane intercepted and diverted to Quito, Ecuador. They could not react fast enough and the plane made it out of Ecuadorian airspace.[96]

I have no doubt that some readers will be asking what these stories of alternative practitioners and the growing list of cancer curers have to do with the core of this book. The facts are fairly clear, however, that when it comes to the pharmaceutical corporations, many of them are so powerful and highly capitalized, so integrated into the medical regulatory system and governments, so influential in the research charities and the education of doctors, so influential within the state, that the least of their crimes is skewing research results to protect dangerous products.

Moving away onto more even ground to look at academic work on the subject of manipulating information, in 2008 Harvard University Press published a seminal book on the subject of how corporations and scientists manipulate scientific and research results to protect commercial products, *Bending Science: How Special Interests Corrupt Public Health Research*, by Thomas D. McGarity and Wendy E. Wagner, two law professors.[97] The book gets my vote for best title; the authors' use of the word "bent" covers a multitude of sins and is used frequently in the text.

McGarity and Wagner pry open the presently tightly sealed boxes of science and opinion in regulation and on advisory committees, while at the same time addressing the problems in common language. Unlike some of the new-wave, activist writers, they do not shy away from focusing on pharmaceutical cartels. A paragraph from their conclusions makes the clear point that the matter of bending science, especially as this affects health, has to be tackled by the "citizen" who picks up the message through professional journals and popular media.

Both the scientific journals and the popular news media have a responsibility to probe the provenance of policy-relevant science and to expose to the public view the extent to which advocates' efforts have contaminated the process of generating policy-relevant science.[98]

It might be possible to have more faith in this optimistic conclusion were it not that both journals and the popular news media tend to be dominated by corporate interests.

The next contemporary book after *Bending Science* that deals with industry, science, and the regulatory agencies, David Michaels's *Doubt is their Product: How Industry's Assault on Science Threatens Your Health*, published in 2009, sums up in its title the way that the recent era has come to define the subjects of science, technology, and health.[99] It has to be said that academics have often been the last to come forward in such areas, possibly because much of their own work can be funded by the very people that they eventually come to criticize, and the whole university structure within which they work can owe industry big time.

The gap that exists between academics and activists is always worrying, but in the area of "secret ties" it can be very disturbing. Michaels, however, is that rare academic who has spent a part of his life at the center of the governmental machine and so should perhaps be considered a "whistle-blower" as much as a reflective academic.

Michaels's book follows a number of notable books that have put bad science and its distorted research at the very center of the growing toll taken by environmentally caused ill health. More recent books that posit the beginning of the crisis in environmental health occasioned by science place its origins in the early 1990s, coincident with the rise of the New Right and the governments of Reagan and Thatcher, both of whom gave the keys of government to the corporations and industrial science.

By the 1990s, it was clear that in relation to the industry manipulation of data, the gloves were off; a series of books explaining how industry, industrial science, and industry-embedded academics were endangering the health of the population began to appear. Inevitably, it was always partially the case that those who wrote about the results of corporatization sometimes didn't see the wood for the trees and failed to discuss corporations in the context of the development of capitalism.

In February 1993, Philip Morris (PM) and its public relations firm, APCO Associates, worked to launch a "sound science" coalition in the United States, with approximately $320 thousand budgeted for the first twenty-four weeks of the year.[100] Three months later, the Advancement for Sound Science Coalition (TASSC) had been formed.[101] TASSC described itself as "a not-for-profit coalition advocating the use of sound science in public policy decision making"[102] even though APCO created it to help Philip Morris fight smoking restrictions.[103, 104] One of the most important parts of this campaign was the Campaign for Good Epidemiology that tried, with some degree of success, to reroute epidemiology, essentially biasing it toward industry and making it much less sympathetic to citizens, workers, and communities.

The European "sound science" plans included a version of "good epidemiological practices" that would make it impossible to conclude that secondhand smoke—and other environmental toxins—caused diseases. Public health professionals need to be aware that an effort such as the "sound science" movement was not an indigenous effort from within the profession to improve the quality of scientific discourse but reflected sophisticated public relations campaigns controlled by industry executives and lawyers, whose aim was to manipulate the standards of scientific proof to serve the corporate interests of their clients.[105]

It can be observed that, while the last decade of the twentieth century introduced a steady debate about what became termed, in contemporary initialized language, COI or Conflict of Interest, over the following two decades up to the present, the doors of perception opened and many commentators began to see the massive gothic structures of industry manipulation in which conflict of interest was only one corridor.

With respect to the chemical industry, Fagin and Lavelle addressed all the important arguments, as can be seen by the title of their 1996 book, *Toxic Deception: How the Chemical Industry Manipulates Science, Bends the Law, and Endangers your Health*,[106] the style of which set the scene for the ongoing spate of books from Rampton and Stauber, starting with *Toxic Sludge is Good For You*.[107] Rampton and Stauber's books present a clearer more radical and straightforward analysis of vested and conflicting interests than previous more academic work. It was deeply and thoroughly researched, but it could be said that their books are the "graphic novels" of the literature on these topics.

Betrayal of Science and Reason: How Anti-Environmental Rhetoric Threatens Our Future, by Paul and Anne Ehrlich, was published in 1996.[108] The Ehrlichs are top-grade research scientists at Stanford and, as the title of their book suggests, they look closely at the language used by lobby groups and scientists tied to industry who have, for instance, denied global warming. One of the refreshing aspects of this book is that it states in the text all the dubious statements of deniers, and carefully picks them apart.

Only a year after *Betrayal*, in 1997, came Linda Marsa's book *Prescription for Profits: How the Pharmaceutical Industry Bankrolled the Unholy Marriage Between Science and Business*.[109] Marsa's book goes right to the heart of the matter, discussing how in the Reagan era everything was done to marry government research scientists to industry. The legacy of these policies, Marsa says, "is that the serpent has entered the garden: the quest for profits has poisoned science. The scientific culture is now so steeped in business that research is governed by the whims of the market place, not by good science."

A look at the bibliography at the end of Marsa's book reveals, I think, a worrying trend: almost all the references are to journal articles or newspaper reports. While the popularizing of scientific subjects in newspapers that began in the 1990s—and the trend away from serious, focused, lengthy books, has a definite upside—articles in newspapers and magazines, and papers in learned journals have a downside. With respect to newspaper articles, journalists are not the best analysts: they tend to write without references, slide over major content, and turn their minds to a completely different subject by the hour. But perhaps the more worrying thing about the growth of newspaper articles and more populist writing in some journals is that as soon as they are published they can disappear, leaving the reader searching only days later for a source. Also, we might assume that it has become more difficult for independent thinkers to get books about scientific controversies onto the market and some have resorted to publishing their own newsletters and magazines.

Despite these pros and cons, it was undoubtedly the trend toward the popularization of science in the 1990s, occasioned by timeless stories like that of Gallo's virtual claims on the AIDS virus, the rows that followed over-genetically modified crops, and the vaccine controversies that led industry-related liberal peers in Britain and other industry-compromised politicians to promote rules for newspaper articles about health, which favored industry rather than science or journalism.

On the other hand, were it not for those idiosyncratic journalists with sympathetic editors, we would never have had the great masterpieces of investigative writing on health like John Crewdson's *Science Fictions: A Scientific Mystery, A Massive Cover-Up, and the Dark Legacy of Robert Gallo*.[110] The book tells in immense and verifiable detail how HIV came to be "the probable cause of AIDS" and Robert Gallo's role in this theatrical promotion. Crewdson was very fortunate in being with a paper, the *Chicago Tribune,* that actually published the whole of his fifty-thousand-word prepublication manuscript.

In England, Lynne McTaggart, an Australian investigative journalist who originally wrote a groundbreaking book about foster care, has since 1989 been publishing the newsletter "What Doctors Don't Tell You."[111] Following this, she and her husband have been responsible for magazines and journals that look astringently at alternative therapies. In 1996, McTaggart published the book *What Doctors Don't Tell You: The Truth About the Dangers of Modern Medicine*.[112] The book contains a fifty-page chapter on vaccination that, as well as discussing adverse reactions, charts the cooperation between the British government and major pharmaceutical companies in vaccine development.

Those writing about secret ties have quite a different and perhaps more difficult job than those simply writing about freedom of medical choices and alternative therapies. Writing about secret ties involves deep research into companies as well as gathering evidence about the toxic companies' products, then showing how such information has been disguised.

Geoffrey Tweedale has written two books about the asbestos industry. The first, *Magic Mineral to Killer Dust: Turner and Newall and the Asbestos Hazard*, is a social, political, and health history of the industry and the arguments that raged around the safety of asbestos manufacture and its products.[113] The second book, *Defending the Indefensible: The Global Asbestos Industry and its Fight for Survival*, with Jock McCulloch, almost entirely investigates propaganda and front organizations set up to defend the industry against probing criticism of its record on health.[114] As an aside, both of these books are beautifully laid out and presented by Oxford University Press; this of course is important because the professionalism and status of the publisher lends extra authority to the possibly marginalized subject of both books.

George Carlo's book is one from an insider, written with Martin Schram, about the manipulation and deceit that have taken place around the science of cell phones, *Cell Phones: Invisible Hazards in the Wireless Age*.[115] As one of the first researchers who ran the cell phone industry's research program for six years and someone who came under immense pressure from the industry to report only profitable information, Carlo was ideally placed to write about the distortion and manipulation of research.

Charles Medawar and his long-standing British organization, Social Audit, have a special place in the hearts of British organizations and individuals interested in the philosophy and sociology of pharmaceutical marketing. In 1992, Social Audit published *Power and Dependence: Social Audit on the Safety of Medicines*.[116] The book is an all-out attack on the testing, licensing, and marketing of tranquilizers and sleeping tablets that were heavily marketed in Britain and the United States. Medawar writes in detail about the individuals and organizations responsible for pushing these drugs. The book contains reproductions of advertisements and promotional material. One hilarious advertisement has what is presumably a doctor's fingertips feeling the pulse of a female wrist, while the tasteful typographic slogan states, "Whatever the diagnosis—LIBRIUM."

Inevitably, some secret ties do not remain secret but are exposed by hardworking researchers and investigators. Battles over the leukemia clusters in Woburn, Massachusetts, went on for over thirty years, producing a number of court cases, books, and a major feature film, *A Civil Action*, starring John Travolta.[117, 118] The case, however, should be most notably remembered for the energy and the initiative that the community—the parents and friends of those children struck down by leukemia—have shown.

In the preface to Phil Brown and Edwin J. Mikkelsen's book *No Safe Place: Toxic Waste, Leukemia, and Community Action*,[119] Jonathan Harr, the author of the epic fictionalized account of Woburn, *A Civil Action*,[120] makes the point that after meeting Phil Brown four years into his own research into Woburn, he quickly realized that they were working on quite different projects and there was little need to be concerned about competition. To my mind, this is an important conclusion. Change is rarely moved solely by a single piece of academic work, studies, or even such things as Royal Commissions, but by a wide range of formal and informal, cultural and scientific exposures of important issues.

A Civil Action[121, 122] together with the film based upon it, remains one of the outstanding accounts of a community bent on defending itself, helped by a lawyer who, while earning his spurs in the field of toxic tort, bankrupts his practice and becomes completely converted to environmental activism.

Following close on leukemia clusters in Woburn, Massachusetts, and the story of the relationship between the lawyer and the community, is the film *Erin Brockovich*.[123, 124] It tells the true story of a legal assistant who, in 1993, lined up some 650 prospective plaintiffs from the tiny desert town of Hinkley, California, to sue Pacific Gas & Electric. PG&E's nearby plant was leaching chromium 6, a rust inhibitor, into Hinkley's water supply, and the suit blamed the chemical for dozens of symptoms ranging from nosebleeds to breast cancer, Hodgkin's disease, miscarriages, and spinal deterioration. In 1996, PG&E settled the case for $333 million.

In June 2009, Brockovich began investigating a case of contaminated water in Midland, Texas. "Significant amounts" of hexavalent chromium were found in the water of more than forty homes in the area, some of which have now been fitted with state-monitored filters on their water supply. Brockovich said "The only difference between here and Hinkley, is that I saw higher levels here than I saw in Hinkley."[125, 126]

Just as Braithwaite's book on the pharmaceutical companies is groundbreaking in that area, and my book *Dirty Medicine: Science, Big Business and the Assault on Natural Health Care*[127] has been considered groundbreaking in describing the activities of health lobby groups in the early 1990s, David Helvarg's 1994 book *The War Against the Greens*[128] is one of the most important books describing the growth of destabilizing covert groups in the United States. Helvarg's book is a beautifully readable account of post–Cold War covert warfare carried out by industry against the citizenry and democracy.

Out of the GM battles of the 1990s came Andy Rowell's book *Green Backlash: Global Subversion of the Environmental Movement*.[129] This timely book shared common ground with Sharon Beder's slightly later *Global Spin*.[130] Writing on LobbyWatch—a web site with yet another boring name—working to expose lobby groups, Rowell points out the bias of the UK Science Media Centre (SMC) on the subject of global warming and GM crops. Such groups set up by the lobby industry constantly publish what appears to be scientific information but which is actually industry propaganda.

Of the 120-odd press releases the SMC has issued—and which are on its web site—only about four have been on climate. This compares to over forty on issues to do with genetics and roughly another dozen each on animals in research and GM crops. The views of scientists critical of GM are all but absent, whereas pro-GM scientists are routinely quoted. The SMC also includes quotes from the chairman of the Agricultural Biotechnology Council (ABC)—a corporate lobby group for the biotech industry. Its chairman is clearly neither an eminent nor an independent scientist.[131, 132]

ON THE EDGE OF ACADEMIA

In 2002 Andy Rowell contributed to one of the books published in the US by Common Courage Press, *Battling Big Business*, which dealt with "Countering greenwash, infiltration and other forms of corporate bullying."[133] The book has a large number of contributors and plants its flag clearly in the complex ground of activists and the strategies they can adopt against all forms of corporate manipulation. A statement on the back of the book sums up just how broad the field of discovery and research is: "Battling Big Business reveals how corporate giants attempt to control their 'enemies'—and how groups and individuals can fight back." I get the impression, from brief remarks by the editor, Eveline Lubbers, that she had similar problems to those which I have had in both defining the area and trying to incorporate a growing number of contributors.

My lifetime interest in pulp fiction and contemporary crime fiction has more than paid off in relation to this book. Apart from *A Civil Action*, two books by John Grisham, himself trained as a lawyer and still a part of various trial lawyers' groups, narrate in considerable detail how vested interests act against claimants in toxic tort cases. In *The Appeal*, Grisham describes an appeal in a toxic tort case handled by a humane and altruistic husband and wife law practice.[134] The appeal is opposed by the chemical company involved and their network of public relations people, which reaches to the very heart of government.

The Runaway Jury, a fictional account of claimants against a tobacco company, lets the reader into the intricate world of private agencies that rig juries and press counsel into going beyond professional interests in acting for their industrial clients in complex suits.[135] Although Grisham does what many writers of fiction and drama have to do—that is, pack their stories with combined elements from a variety of cases—his approach to reality is rarely cavalier; he usually pursues the simplest and apparently least dramatic narrative track, which makes his stories correspond to reality.

One dramatist and writer of fiction in Britain who has tackled toxic tort cases in dramatic form is Gordon Newman, whose BBC *Judge John Deed* series drew on real-life legal situations.[136] Newman's work, prominent on British television since the seventies, has almost always dealt with legal situations, exposing the corrupt and manipulative side of vested corporate, political, and state interests.

One UK paper, the *Guardian*, got so far into crusading against the way in which GM crops were foisted on the population that one of its editors, Alan

Rusbridger, together with Ronan Bennett, the highly regarded Irish novelist and television and film writer, wrote a caustic television drama, *Fields of Gold*.[137] Lobbyists supporting GM crops tried to get this film stopped and after it had appeared they tried to damage it with bad reviews and letters to the BBC.

The lobbies and the GM companies learned a great deal from the campaign mounted against them between 1996 and 2005. When the dust settled, a complete regrouping was needed by the GM lobbies. The price that the newspaper paid seems to have been high; however, within months of their best writers giving a master-class in investigative journalism, Ben Goldacre, a non-writer, non-journalist, non-investigative, highly suspect "scientist," son of one of the "scientists" who had passed the damaging Urabe mumps strain MMR vaccination, was given a prestigious place on the paper, writing superficially about science. From this job, he was able to launch his "quackbusting" attacks on alternative medicine.[138]

Two researchers who have made a considerable impact in the United States, exposing secret ties and covert campaigns already mentioned in this chapter, are Sheldon Rampton and John Stauber. In *Trust Us We're Experts! How Industry Manipulates Science and Gambles with your Future*,[139] which followed *Toxic Sludge is Good for You*,[140] about promotion and PR companies, Rampton and Stauber pick through the whole field of distorted and manipulated science to expose many of those paid to assure us of industry safety while secretly juggling the science of toxicity. Rampton and Stauber are muckrakers in the mold, and it is almost impossible to find anyone in Europe or the United States who equals their diligent and detailed research. Their books are perhaps the most expert combination of journalism, research, and the critique of "science."

While a good deal of academic literature about the ties of vested interests remains relatively safe, even after years of research, a small number of investigative writers reach deep into the matrix of social and political culture. It needs the broadest view of how money, power, and military force link together to present this information in popular form to the public. One of the greatest exponents of this kind of intricate exposé is Greg Palast.

The titles of Palast's books signal their offbeat radicalism and might have come directly out of the Catch-22 period. The book that most influenced me and my contemporaries was *The Best Democracy Money Can Buy*.[141] The book has a section that details the selling off, after the Labour victory in 1997, of the most important publicly owned industries to private interests. In the investigation, Palast drew links between the new Lib-Labour functionaries, PR companies, and the new salesmen of Downing Street. Although some of Palast's targets were downed, he himself, though a British citizen, was deported. Palast's books are about "cover-ups" and distortions and how they are enacted. In their intimacy they disclose a constant stream of connected criminal and vested interests, which traverse across the urban landscape in the contemporary world.

When it comes to an environmental view of cancer and the extrapolations that industry uses to disguise its understanding of the role of its processes and products, the great majority of information now in circulation is reproduced in academic papers in journals. There are, however, a few exceptions apart from those, such as the work of Samuel Epstein quoted above. In 1979, Macmillan published a two-hundred-page book entitled *Cancer and the Environment*.[142] The book is very modest but novel in its form, using two columns with bold-type headings, like a continuous newspaper report. Its content, however, is quite spectacular. After a shaky start, when the editor, Lester A. Sobel, ensures that the industry view is more than adequately represented, the majority of the book is a compendium of all the information aired prior to 1980 about the environmental causes of cancer.

Even the long quotes from denialists of environmentally caused cancer are in themselves informative. This section of the book quotes Richard J. Mahoney, Executive Vice President of Monsanto, as saying in an unspecified speech in St. Louis, "We hear and read that a majority of human cancers—possibly as high as seventy percent to ninety percent—are due to environmental causes." Mahoney goes on to cite the classic industry argument, put forward by Richard Doll and probably quoted from Doll's unreferenced paper, "A . . . medical research paper noted that the overwhelming environmental causes of cancer are cigarette smoking and dietary considerations. . . . Control these two elements—cigarettes and diet—and you've controlled the cause of perhaps ninety-five percent of environmentally caused cancers."[143]

Nothing in Mr. Sobel's past—he served for four years in the US army during the Second World War in Patton's Third Army—as it is recorded on the back flap of the book, gives the reader any idea of why he adopted the form for the book that he did. The eclectic order of items reminds one of the kind of book Walter Benjamin, the great European intellectual, was preparing when he died in 1939. Items appear awkwardly under the general headings, but Sobel has done his level best to cover with real focus the swings both backward and forward of each new accusation of industry's role in the cause of cancer, apparently without bias.

On page 154, under the chapter heading "Radiation and Cancer," text below a subheading "Hanford, Portsmouth Studies" begins, "Alice Stewart, an epidemiologist at the University of Birmingham, England, said Feb 17 that her study of workers at the Hanford Atomic Reservation revealed that they died of cancer at a rate of 5 percent greater than the general population."[144] For those who know that Alice Stewart, a great British epidemiologist, was censored from academic recognition by, among others, her senior colleague Sir Richard Doll while they were both working at Oxford University, a text that repeats Alice Stewart's name and the conclusions of her work, time and again, is a refreshing change.

Gayle Greene, wrote the seminal biography of Alice Stewart, *The Woman Who Knew Too Much*.[145] In chapter twelve of this book, she goes more deeply into the comparison between the industry-embedded Doll and Stewart's epidemiology for the people.

Two books published during the first decade of the twenty-first century pull no punches in examining the question of industrial carcinogens and the environmental causes of cancer. *When Smoke Ran Like Water: Tales of Environmental Deception and the Battle Against Pollution*[146] and *The Secret History of the War on Cancer*[147] have got their author, Devra Davis, one of the most daring of the commentators on the causes of environmental cancer, into deep politically polluted water. Davis's books are very readable, interweaving the personal and familial with the objective and scientific in a traditionally feminine style. On the whole, the most rewarding subjective, or familial, personally contextualized accounts of cancer come from women, such as Sharon Batt in her *Patients No More: The Politics of Breast Cancer*[148] and Sandra Steingraber in *Living Downstream: An Ecologist Looks at Cancer and the Environment*.[149] Only rarely are men brave enough to introduce themselves into their narrative, as does Gearin-Tosh, who had a particularly feminine approach to his beautiful record of his own illness in *Living Proof*.[150]

This is not to say, of course, that some women's more academic accounts of cancer are not just as readable and perhaps more engaging than "scientific" writing by men. Liane Clorfene-Casten's *Breast Cancer: Poisons, Profits and Prevention*, one of the best journalistic accounts of the environmental causes of breast cancer, lays the blame directly on industry.[151] It is written, like *Silent Spring*, in a relaxed, engaging, but scientifically informative style, while campaigning, like Devra Davis, to shut down industrial polluters.

The information about a bogus campaign, funded by ExxonMobil, to influence the public and decision makers' opinions on global warming, first came to light in George Monbiot's autumn 2006 book *The Denial Industry*, later published as *Heat*.[152] Monbiot also published his research in the *Guardian*, which must have presented *Guardian* readers with some odd contradictions, for some of the people that Monbiot targeted as the criminal dross of the crisis PR industry were the very people lauded by his *Guardian* colleague and quackbuster, Ben Goldacre. The *Guardian* introduced Monbiot's articles on the ExxonMobil funding in the following way:

For years, a network of fake citizens' groups and bogus scientific bodies has been claiming that science of global warming is inconclusive. They set back action on climate change by a decade. But who funded them? Exxon's involvement is well known, but not the strange role of Big Tobacco.[153]

As if to a script written about modern America, from *Catch 22*, one of the heaviest and most critical reports of government and industry involvement in damaging the health of the people and then covering it up was the *Final Report of the Advisory Committee on Human Radiation Experiments*, published in 1996 by Oxford University Press.[154] This 620-page, large format book investigates the work that was undertaken by various agencies, but mainly covertly, in the United States and Europe between 1944 and 1974.

Inevitably, even the headings and subheadings are chilling, for example, "The Context for Nontherapeutic Research with Children: Children as Mere Means." This particular section of the report looks at research carried out by Massachusetts Institute of Technology (MIT) in the 1940s and 1950s in which breakfast food laced with radioactive iron and calcium was fed to "mentally retarded" children—referred to as "students" in the studies and the report—in a Massachusetts school. The research was funded by the odd triumvirate of US organizations: the Quaker Oats Company, the Atomic Energy Commission, and the National Institutes of Health.

The *Final Report* is an intriguing and extraordinary document; while one has to commend President Clinton on his initiation of the inquiry and the decision to publish the whole report through a high quality university press, it would take people with greater skills in language than mine to assess it. On my first and second reading of sections of the text, I could only marvel at the almost anodyne style of presentation that steers around any moral judgments like a world-class skier on a downhill slalom. To read the *Final Report* you might think that it was talking about the marketing of chocolate bonbons, or even, perhaps, something less health-damaging!

BEING DRAGGED INTO HAND-TO-HAND COMBAT

It is possible to criticize academic work on conflict of interest, vested interest, and the whole network of secret ties, firstly on the grounds that academics tend to draw only on previously published peer-reviewed information, which seriously restricts both their narrative and their conclusions, and secondly that articles and papers in journals about such subjects tend to keep important information within academia, where it is often not discussed with the same political edge it can be given outside.

Nevertheless, academic work on vested interests and conflict of interests is important, especially because many of those who write on these subjects are now involved in the academic equivalent of activism, perhaps writing beyond academia, perhaps investigating industry on behalf of campaigns, or even appearing for injured parties as expert witnesses. These then, are academics at the coalface, willing to get involved in the rough and tumble of legal actions against multinational corporations, or even campaign with activists.

One of the reasons why it is important to get out of the academic straightjacket when it comes to understanding and campaigning on the issue of the manipulation of epidemiological information, is that this kind of criminal behavior doesn't just affect academics. Nowhere has this been more the case than in the information spewed out by the pharmaceutical companies and the UK Department of Health over the MMR vaccination. In the United Kingdom, a war has descended on critics of vaccine policy and those whose children have been damaged.[155]

During the fifteen-year all-out assault on Dr. Wakefield, not one word was said in any even vaguely authoritative publication about either his scientific investigations or the science of MMR. He was character assassinated purely because he was preparing to appear as an expert witness for parents of vaccine-damaged children in a case brought by fifteen hundred claimants; a case that after a decade of work was pulled from the lists following the withdrawal of legal aid by a government department.

In Australia, the handmaidens of pharmaceutical cartels, the Skeptics, have kept up a program of torrential abuse, complaints to authorities, and physical threats against the leading support group for parents seeking advice on vaccination, the Australian Vaccination Network (AVN). The last chairperson of the group, Meryl Dorey, has suffered, and is suffering, quite public threats, lies, and abuse.[156]

Such attacks and campaigns cannot be answered solely within academia; however, many such groups and individuals drawn into battles with corporations and their acolytes do manage to attract the attention of academics who are interested in these areas of conflict. In Australia, Meryl Dorey and the AVN have found an objective academic willing to explore their circumstances in Professor Brian Martin.[157] Inevitably, Martin's academic observation on the character assassination of Meryl Dorey and the AVN attracted the swarms of pharmaceutical corporation microbes to Martin's University, where the chancellor received emails and letters complaining that Martin and some of his postgraduate students were supporting the anti-vaccination cause. Admirably, the university answered these criticisms by saying that they believed in academic freedom.

My book *Dirty Medicine: Science, Big Business and the Assault on Natural Health Care*, published in 1993, traced a number of cases where agents of the pharmaceutical corporations spent long periods, with the help of the corporate media, character assassinating those who proposed various alternative treatments or simply wrote objective accounts of the dangers of pharmaceutical preparations.[158] In my follow-up to the first *Dirty Medicine*, twenty years later, I published *Dirty Medicine: The Handbook*, in which I detailed the growth and spread of the pharmaceutical vigilante groups who spend their lives attacking critical campaigns and their supporters.[159]

The trade unions in both Europe and the United States inevitably have a very definite role in fighting hidden damage to workers. *Hazards Magazine* is a trade union–funded "journal," which takes the fight over health and danger to workers out into the broader society.[160] Inevitably, it steps over the line into civil society beyond the unions to publicize secret ties that endanger workers. Under the editorship of Rory O'Neill, it has become respected worldwide as an outlet for investigative journalism about health and safety in the workplace.

Professor David Egilman emerged, not for the first time, onto the public stage in 2003. Egilman is a doctor and a university professor whose lifetime fight has been on behalf of workers in dangerous industries who are adversely affected by environmental toxins. One gets the impression of Egilman as a "no-holds-barred" bare-knuckle fighter who, whether the opposition be a judge or a peer-reviewed journal, just does what he has to do. He is an academic who has frequently dragged his battles with corporately funded interests out into civil society.

In 2003, Egilman submitted an article for publication in the *Journal of Occupational and Environmental Medicine* (JOEM) that stated that Dow Chemical was covering up evidence that asbestos in a Texas chemical plant was causing mesothelioma, a lung cancer.[161] The conclusions of a Dow-funded study suggested that, despite eleven cases of mesothelioma among twenty-eight thousand employees, these were probably not related to the work environment.

The journal refused to publish Egilman's article, not because it found it of low quality, but because the subject was "not likely to be a high priority for the majority of JOEM readers." Egilman simply bought two pages of advertising space in the JOEM and ran the entire rejected manuscript anyway.

The journal's editor allowed Dow to publish a response but refused Egilman a rebuttal. This incident led to Egilman publishing, in April 2005, in the *International Journal of Occupational and Environmental Health* (IJOEH), an account of the suppression of his article and, later that year, a whole issue on the subject of conflict of interest. This October 2005 issue was groundbreaking.[162]

Its overall title was *Over a Barrel: Corporate Corruption of Science and its Effects on Workers and the Environment,* and it contained leading articles on conflict of interest by Egilman himself and a wide range of other academics; titles included "Abuse of Epidemiology: Automobile Manufacturers Manufacture a Defense to Asbestos Liability;" "Lifting the Veil of Secrecy from Industry;" "Funding of Nonprofit Health Organizations and Mining and Mendacity, or How to Keep a Toxic Product in the Marketplace."

The papers in this edition of the IJOEH show that for a long time there seems to have been an underground academia. Many academics have been writing in the wings about conflicting interests outside the tobacco industry but have been unable to present their work as part of an academic whole, or a movement.

Marco Mamone Capria, an academic mathematician from the Italian Perugia University, set up the web site and conference organization Science and Democracy in 2005.[163] It holds its triennial conferences in Naples and has published the proceedings so far in three books.[164] This is one way of bringing academia out into the public forum and anyone interested in conflicts in science and civil society should get involved in this group or one like it.

At the same time that affected individuals and some reporters were writing about the distortion of information around workers conditions, toxic processes, and products, a growing number of authors were beginning to write about corporations and their growth. Many of these writers pointed out that lies, deceit, and disinformation were necessary steps in the growth of corporate power.[165–172]

Few of these commentators, though—linking the death of democracy with this corporatism—address the issue of vested interests or conflict of interests in research, production, or health. While this is not surprising because it appears to be low in the food chain of the analysis of corporate growth, it is undoubtedly an issue that has to be brought to the fore; the issue of conflict of interests and vested interests and their resultant health-care issues is a major aspect of that failing democracy that accompanies corporatism.

I am ending this chapter with three books that do not focus on health but give a clear outline of the battles contemporary students, academics, and activists will inevitably find themselves fighting in the coming years. All three books cast light on what happens to people drawn almost accidentally into battles with vested interests. It would, perhaps, be difficult to find two books stranger than *Silencing Scientists and Scholars in Other Fields: Power, Paradigm Controls, Peer Review and Scholarly Communication,* by Gordon Moran,[173] and *Challenges* by the late Serge Lang.[174] The third book, *Battling Big Business; Countering Greenwash, Infiltration and Other Forms of Corporate Bullying*,[175] is perhaps a world away from the first two, a book that one imagines has been written before but discovers is completely original, written from the experience of political activists and investigators.

Silencing has a dull gray cover and fits into a series of some fifty books edited by Peter Hernon with such stimulating titles as: *Technology and Library Information Services* and *Microcomputer Software for Performing Statistical Analysis: A Handbook for Supporting Library Decision Making.*

Apart from *Silencing*, one other book stands out in the Ablex list: the editor of the series, Peter Hernon, added *Research Misconduct: Issues, Implications* and *Challenges* by the late Serge Lang. Reading *Silencing*, one gets the slightly uncomfortable feeling that Hernon and Moran have conspired to slip in a controversial text that might be read way beyond the intended librarian readership of the series.

To most mathematicians, the second book, *Challenges*, by the late Serge Lang, would probably appear even odder than *Silencing*. Written by one of the greatest mathematicians of the modern period, the book records in mesmerizing detail a number of "academic" political conflicts entered into by Lang in the course of his later academic life. Lang brings to these political conflicts the same spare analytical language that seems to come with the mathematician's mind. *Challenges*, which is over eight hundred pages and covers a number of battles, is published by one of the world's largest publishers.

Both *Silencing* and *Challenges* present us with a way of looking at, and dealing with, conflicts in academia and beyond, and the framework for both books grows from the personal experience of the authors. In 1977, Moran, an American, while a scholar at an Italian university, wrote a short article that questioned the provenance of a famous Italian painting. In the introduction to his book, Moran says about the conflict that developed over the origins of the picture:

> I did not expect that all other scholars would immediately agree that this famous painting was painted by someone other than Simone Martini, but at the very least I expected that any debate that ensued would proceed with a civility of discourse . . . Instead the Guido Riccio controversy . . . has been characterized by, among other things, insults, censorship, and falsifications, all directed towards silencing the new, unwanted hypotheses.[176]

In this intellectually exciting book, Moran looks at suppression of scientific work across the board, detailing how it is achieved. He comments on vested interests, skepticism, and whistle-blowing while drawing frequently on Serge Lang's work.

In *Challenges*, Lang lays out a way of going onto the attack; he lays down a strategy that he uses most usefully in attacking fabrication and political and funding bias in academic work. Rather than calling them controversies, he acts out "campaigns" in the military sense; he refers to them, as if a dusty bureaucrat, as "files." The point of this, I think, is to describe the very personal events of opening, recording, and perhaps closing a particular conflict. A file is also a small part of a larger program and this, too, might have been in Lang's mind.

Lang calls these battles "political" battles, yet he does not really approach them as a politician, not anyway as a party politician or even as a grassroots political activist, although there might be some similarity with the politics of a highly trained communist cadre struggling to organize and promote ideas in a hostile environment. He questions every word used by his opponents as well as their worldview, and most of all he looks at means of transmission. In his opening paragraphs he clearly states his purpose:

> For three decades I have been interested in the area where the academic world meets the world of journalism and the world of politics. On several occasions I have had the opportunity to study how political opinions are passed off as science or scholarship.
>
> I am bothered by the misinformation which is created and disseminated uncritically through the education system and through the media, and by the obstructions which prevent correct information from being disseminated.
>
> I am especially concerned when people who construct a reality askew from the outside world have the influence or power to impose their reality in the classroom, in the media, and in the formulation of policy, domestic or foreign. I find the situation especially serious when political opinions are passed off as science, and thereby acquire even more force.
>
> I am bothered by the way misinformation is accepted uncritically, and by the way that some people are unwilling to recognize it or reject it.[177]

In alluding to the title of the book, *Challenges*, the publishers say, ". . . Lang challenges some individuals and establishments, at the same time that he challenges us to reconsider the ways they exercise their official or professional responsibilities, and challenges us to form our own judgement."[178]

Lang's book does not look at corporations or the wider structures of social systems, perhaps because intimate knowledge and recorded discourse at a grassroots level clearly stood as "proof" to him. *Challenges* is an exceptional manual to be consulted during hand-to-hand fighting in academia. It also questions all the moral and professional judgments that underlie academic work, while analyzing what kind of interests determine the output of the social scientist.

Challenges is a call to academic arms, and while there are now many books written from an academic perspective that recount the ways in which corporations are stealing our liberty, few of those suggest anything other than an academic riposte. Little has so far been written for activists that shows how they might fight back—on the whole such discussions go on in campaign meetings and not in books.

However, *Battling Big Business*, which came out in 2002, is the book for activists and others that partners *Challenges*. *Battling* is a superb book that avoids the Hollywood dependence on mirages of foreign policy propaganda and comes right down to earth with chapters about the numerous ways in which it is possible to fight corporations exerting their power in your own backyard.

It is because of the spread of corporate ties, from the simple linear association between corporations and academics to connections deep in the community, that we have to see this phenomenon of influence and propaganda in its extended form. It is in light of these disinformation campaigns that we should understand how the growth of corporatism is eroding democracy.

It becomes, as well, increasingly important that those in the broader society, attacked in this way, learn the rules of engagement needed to defend themselves. It also becomes increasingly important that scientists who bear the brunt of academic attacks get down among the people and help organize campaigns with them, beyond the university, the research lab, and the learned journal.

It is not only the corporate media that have deserted their post. In the face of these battles for markets, we find, inevitably, that investigative and "trial" tribunals of various kinds, lower courts, advertising standards authorities, and prominently the criminal law and the police, mostly side with corporatism and refuse to take seriously complaints against corporately linked individuals and groups.

It is becoming clear that corporate intrusion into civil society is one of the major ethical problems of the twenty-first century; this issue is the door through which George Orwell's *1984* has and will enter silently and without fanfare. It includes all the relevant ingredients but, most specifically, includes the distortion of reporting on various social phenomena and the turning of light into dark on matters of the environment, technological advance, and health, safety, and personal peace of mind.

For those who have a political background, today when we think of authoritarianism or even fascism, we have to consider the rule of society by corporations, the retraction of social choice, and the implementation of product totalitarianism. We have to think more about corporate sciences controlling the means of production, culture, education, and the political system. The real future of the authoritarian society will not be through the fascism of the 1930s but through the control of society by postindustrial corporations that deny individual choice in a multiplicity of areas.

Vested interests and conflict of interest in industrial science production will be at the center of the new politics, discussion of these issues at the center of the new non-democracy. Although scientists should be at the fore in resolving these questions and regulating their own disciplines, cleansing it of financial influences and conflicts of interest they should also remember that the lay community clearly has rights—if not to be a part of discussions about detailed scientific matters, at least to discuss and determine the social uses of science and the general moral direction of research. Science as a new means of production is far too important to be left completely to scientists.

Looking to the future, it seems to me that there is little hope, as long as corporatism gains ground in the developed countries, of developing a fairness and objectivity in the research and promotion that examines industry-caused chronic illnesses. While liberal society looks to the Precautionary Principle,[179] the disintegrated nature of commercial competition in a capitalist system means that almost inevitably the freedom to produce is followed by the freedom to market. After this point it becomes impossible to turn the clock back.

Chapter 2

THE BASIS OF BAD SCIENCE[1]

David Egilman, Susanna Rankin Bohme, Lelia M. Menéndez, John Zorabedian

Corporations are human beings with empathy washed away.

David Egilman

While most of us have been taught to view scientific research as an unbiased source of knowledge that defies political or economic interests, in fact science plays a central role in corporate efforts to maximize profits. This has especially been the case in the fields of occupational and environmental health. Efforts to protect people and the environment are often expensive, and to the extent that corporations can avoid paying these costs, they stand to boost their profits. Due to its ostensible lack of a political or economic agenda, science engenders the public's trust, which corporations, in turn, can manipulate to make themselves seem trustworthy and objective. As a result, corporations often present themselves as impartial authorities, claiming to base their opinions on science. Science is pivotal to this dynamic, because it provides the most respected answer to the question of what constitutes a health or environmental danger. In order to circumvent liability and earn public favor, corporations can utilize "bad science" under the guise of objective and reliable science to convince the public and the courts in toxic tort lawsuits that their scientific "research" and findings are sound and do not endanger public health. Corporations thus use science to reduce expenditures on preventive measures or to avoid paying compensation to parties injured as a result of product manufacturing or use, thereby increasing their earnings and decreasing their liability.

CAPITALIST EXTERNALITIES

This chapter sets out to better understand "bad science" as a method used by corporations to shift onto victims the harmful costs of production. Proponents and critics of corporations alike have noted that a corporation's central and overriding mandate is to maximize shareholder profit.[2, 3] As economist Robert Monks puts it, a corporation "tends to be more profitable to the extent that it can make other people pay the bills for its impact on society." These costs are called externalities, and they often consist of practices that may either cause injuries to workers or consumers and/or degrade the environment. For example, when a company emits air and water pollution, it escapes paying its own "cleanup" bills. It instead externalizes the cost of that pollution—and its attendant health and environmental damages—onto individuals and governments who may suffer health risks, be forced to pay for cleanup, or pay for damages in indirect ways (such as fishermen who must buy fish because a manufacturing process exterminated the fish in their local stream). Corporations generally have the best information about their own products and are usually aware of the safety risks involved with their use. Many corporations are conscious of the risks involved in the production of dangerous commodities, yet they continue to devise ways to maximize the profitability of their products and minimize their liability.[4]

When they externalize health and safety costs to maximize profits, companies have two fundamental objectives: The first is to secure the least restrictive regulatory environment possible, and the second is to avoid legal liability for consumer and worker deaths or injuries caused by exposures to their products.

SCIENCE AND EXTERNALITIES

Science plays a key role in determining which health and environmental costs corporations must pay and which are externalized onto the broader society. Scientists are arbiters—sometimes inadvertent—in the fields of regulatory process, tort suits, and marketing. In each of these arenas, science is used to determine whether a corporation will pay for, or successfully externalize, health and safety costs by determining if there is sufficient evidence to show that a product caused a disease in an individual consumer, a pollutant presents a potential health hazard to a community, or if an exposure caused a worker's disease.

The key scientific question, then, that determines whether or not an externality really exists is, "Did the substance 'cause' the disease?" Based on the answer, science shapes the outcome: Will the cancer victim pay for the injury and bear the medical expense? Will the community pay for cleaning up the drinking water? Will companies be held responsible for producing, selling, and dumping carcinogens?

Science carries great legitimacy in the public decision-making process, because the widespread belief exists that the scientific method and the knowledge it produces are objective and reflect real truths about causes and effects. Most results of scientific inquiry, however, are not black and white, but gray. Certain scientific methods and results do not always universally apply to situations or populations. For example, the results of animal studies may not be applicable to humans. In the case of arsenic, exposure does not cause lung cancer in animals, but human epidemiologic studies have found cancer excesses in arsenic-exposed individuals. Although we know certain substances are harmful, no one can explain exactly how arsenic, tobacco smoke, or other carcinogenic substances cause cancer. Current scientific knowledge cannot fully account for the specific causal relationships between exposure to a carcinogen and the onset of disease. These problems are due, in part, to the absence of consensus on a set of criteria for determining cause-effect relationships.[5–8]

The public generally views science as objective and thus authoritative. In reality, however, science allows much room for uncertainty and debate. Corporations hoping to avoid responsibility for the harm caused by their hazardous production methods, manufacturing of dangerous commodities, or pollution, strategically use science to validate and justify their actions. Corporations manipulate the public perception of science as objective, truthful, and universal to convince regulatory bodies, the scientific community, the courts, the press, and the general public that, like science, they too are objective, truthful, and adhere to "universal" scientific methodologies and standards. Thus, in order to secure the least restrictive regulatory environment possible and avoid legal liability for worker and consumer deaths or injuries, corporations have created their own prejudiced body of "scientific" literature that is based on convenient—and not necessarily accurate—scientific information.

Over the past two centuries, many corporations and industries have developed a deliberate set of scientific, legal, and public relations tactics to influence science and avoid paying the costs of the disease and pollution they have caused. Viewed together, these strategies have enough commonality to be understood as part of the modus operandi of a large proportion of corporations in the United States.

Unlike well-conducted science, corporate-sponsored "bad science" does not seek to protect the public from harm by understanding and minimizing health and environmental risks. Corporations actively contribute to the production and dissemination of "bad science" with the aim of protecting their own interests. In order to achieve the objectives above, corporations use three strategies to capitalize on scientific uncertainty: (1) They create favorable scientific results, (2) They create and influence scientific organizations, and (3) They create public relations (PR) mechanisms to organize corporate-sponsored front groups, industry organizations, and think tanks to influence public perceptions of "scientific consensus" on the toxicity of their products or processes. These strategies achieve the externalization of costs by producing results that favor corporate interests or manufacture doubt about the health impacts of a substance.[9]

The dissemination of previously secret internal documents from tobacco, asbestos, beryllium, plastic, and chemical companies provides evidence that many of the industries' actions are both deliberate and ill-intentioned. The success of these strategies over many years is apparent in their continued impact on setting standards for exposures to toxic substances, limiting the ability to sue corporations for harm, and the defeat, delay, and weakening of regulatory oversight.

Such manipulative strategies are accomplished through self-serving partnerships between corporations, PR firms, and law firms that affect health, legal, and policy outcomes. This triumvirate lobbies for self-promoting policies and works together to avoid regulation and accountability. The strategies they employ for these purposes can culminate in worker and consumer fatalities and the long-term delay in arriving at an accurate assessment of damage.

CREATING FAVORABLE SCIENTIFIC RESULTS
Funding Science

Globally, industries spend trillions of dollars on research each year. They spend a great deal of this money in the United States, where, for example, in 1997 $157 billion was spent on industry-sponsored research of all kinds.[10] It is unclear how much of this total was spent on health and safety research, but we do know that industry far outspends the federal government on research in those categories. In 2014, The National Institute of Environmental Health Sciences, the federally funded agency charged with researching environmental health risks, had an extramural research budget of only $312 million. As the *Chronicle of Higher Education* reported, "an industry-sponsored study done ten years ago of risks in just one field ... cost about 'half' of the extramural research budget of NIOSH."[11]

Corporate funding can bias scientists to interpret results in favor of those who fund their research projects.[12] He who pays the piper may not have to directly pick the tune; academic researchers, under pressure to obtain funding, will often play the tune they know sponsors want to hear. Kjaergard and Als-Nielsen have demonstrated that the conclusions of researchers who received funding from a for-profit group were "significantly more positive toward the experimental intervention" than the conclusions of researchers without competing interests.[13] These results may reflect an unconscious bias in favor of sponsors even when no undue pressure is brought to bear on researchers.[14] Alternatively, companies can hire "experts" with known views and predictable perspectives and conclusions that endorse company policy. In some cases scientific consulting companies promise to generate research results that will favor corporate interests.[15] When these consulting companies publish their "research," they give it an imprimatur of scientific legitimacy and authority. To accomplish their ends, corporations and their consultants have, at times, falsified findings.[16–18]

Corporations rely on scientists and their research in a number of forums: influencing regulators by presenting corporate-sponsored articles that minimize the dangers of a product or process, arguing against liability in the courtroom, impacting subsequent scientific research, and swaying popular opinion through marketing campaigns. Corporations also depend on scientists to testify in both regulatory hearings and tort litigation.

Science for Hire: Science to Specification and Producing Doubt

One of the most common tactics used by corporations and law and PR firms involves contracting scientists to generate "controversy" over what would otherwise be clear-cut cause-effect relationships. David Michaels, the former Assistant Secretary of Energy for Environment, Safety and Health and current Assistant Secretary of Labor for the Occupational Safety and Health Administration (OSHA), convincingly presents this in his book, *Doubt is their Product*.[19] Michaels points out that research conducted by corporate-centered research firms such as ChemRisk frequently challenges regulations not by providing solid evidence that a product or process is safe, but rather by maintaining "that evidence is ambiguous, so regulatory action is unwarranted."[20]

Corporations employ science to specification (i.e., scientific work that is carried out with the express purpose of reaching a "conclusion" that supports a corporate or industry regulatory or litigation objective). This research may be conducted through in-house corporate labs, nonprofit research institutes, or for-profit "science-for-hire" firms. For example, in the words of the Chemical Industry Institute of Technology (CIIT)[21] a private, not-for-profit research organization created and funded by the chemical industry, this research is valuable because it "generates data which supports industry positions on risk analysis to modulate federal regulatory demands."[22]

The approach of ChemRisk illustrates how PR firms, lawyers, and research firms can manipulate science to construct doubt. Most of their research has been conducted for corporate clients who are faced with liability suits. For example, Exponent, a company that owned ChemRisk, described its business as related largely to impending litigation:

> Exponent serves clients in automotive, aviation, chemical, construction, energy, government, health, insurance, manufacturing, technology, and other sectors of the economy. Many of our engagements are initiated by lawyers or insurance

companies, whose clients anticipate, or are engaged in, litigation over an alleged failure of their products, equipment, or services.[23]

Similarly, ChemRisk advertises that its "scientists and engineers have served as technical advisers to lawyers in all aspects of environmental, occupational, toxic tort, and product liability litigation . . . including . . . technical strategy development, providing scientific advice, expert testimony, selection and preparation of expert witnesses, assistance in cross-examining opponent's expert witnesses."

ChemRisk claims that

> A distinguishing characteristic of our legal tort work is our emphasis on conducting original, field research which fills data gaps. This work is usually an essential component in resolving disputes involving chemical or radiological agents. We have provided support to litigants in some of the most publicized and complex major toxic tort law suits including silicone breast implants, developmental toxicants, beryllium, hexavalent chromium, benzene, asbestos, brake dust, dioxin, various pesticides, and many others.[24]

Following the publication of a paper by independent scientist, Thomas Mancuso, revealing that chrome was a carcinogen,[25] the Chrome Coalition, a group of chrome manufacturers, hired Dr. Dennis Paustenbach, the president and founder of ChemRisk, to begin "developing an anti-Mancuso manuscript."[26] In a 1996 meeting with the Chrome Coalition and their lawyers, Paustenbach described his approach to several "challenges." To delay benzene and 1.3 butadiene regulation, he claimed that he developed a critique based on the argument that missing information on the cancer dose-response relationship constituted a "data gap" that had to be filled before regulations could be finalized.[27] He recommended that "the [Chrome] Coalition may wish to approach the regulators with a program designed to fill a 'data gap,' thus entering into a data gap agreement, to forestall the rulemaking."[28] In the case of Paustenbach's research, "filling data gaps" means producing science with guaranteed results. Instead of beginning with a question and seeking the most accurate possible answer, this research starts with the desired "conclusions."

Paustenbach employed a similar approach in 1990, when he developed a proposal for the American Petroleum Institute (API) regarding benzene:

> McLaren/ChemRisk is pleased to provide this proposal to develop an alternative cancer potency estimate for benzene. It is our understanding that API would like us to develop a succinct, yet scientifically compelling, integrated position statement to

be used in comments to the state of North Carolina and as a possible springboard for future analyses that could be presented to US EPA and the State of California.[29]

The proposal goes on to explain some of ChemRisk's methodology, and indicates that comments from API member companies and other API consultants would be incorporated into final published papers:

> EPA and OSHA considered benzene to cause all types of leukemia in their development of cancer potency estimates for benzene . . . The objective of this task is to develop a succinct, compelling position that presents evidence that AML is the only type of leukemia induced by benzene exposure (task 4.1). A meeting with Dr. Richard Irons will be needed in order to discuss the molecular basis for benzene-induced AML (task 4.2).
>
> Deliverable to the API benzene task force: Draft manuscript, suitable for publication in *Fundamental and Applied Toxicology*. Comments from the Task Force and Dr. Irons will be incorporated into a final document.[30]

This work was published in the scientific literature without disclosing that the research was conducted with a foregone conclusion and was subject to editing by a task force of industry representatives.[31,32] The API continued to support scientific research that is favorable to industries, and in 2005 funded two other consultants—Drs. Irons and Wong—to develop research that "was expected to provide scientific support for the lack of a leukemia risk to the general population, evidence that current occupational exposure limits do not create a significant risk to workers, and proof that non-Hodgkin's lymphoma could not be caused by benzene exposure." In this case, the API held ultimate editorial control. They had the right to prevent the research from going forward if they did not like the interim results.[33]

Industry's Selection Process for Convenient Evidence and Causation Arguments

When confronted by evidence of the danger of their product or process, some corporations or industries have relied on a strategy of creating scientific doubt by raising general questions about the types of evidence on which one can rely to demonstrate causation. For example, company experts may opine that a study showing cancer in animals cannot be used to regulate human exposures because, they claim, animal studies can never be used as evidence of human causation. However, the same experts will rely on animal studies if it serves their interests.

There is no standard scientific method for determining cause-effect relationships between an exposure and a disease, and the type of evidence that can be used to establish a causation nexus has greatly changed over the course of the twentieth and twenty-first centuries. This evolving pattern is illustrated in Figures 1 to 3. Prior to the development of formal epidemiological studies, physicians relied primarily upon pathologic evidence and case reports to determine causation.[34]

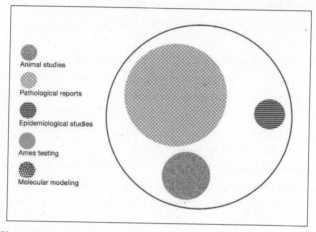

Figure 1—Circa 1930s (US): Representation of the relative importance of different types of information (adapted from Egilman 1992).[35] The diameter of each colored circle represents the relative importance of each type of information in this decade. The relative sizes and time frames are approximate.

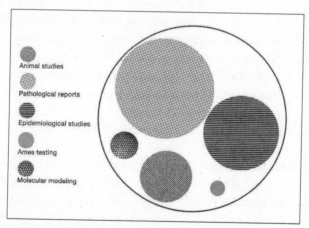

Figure 2—Circa 1970s (US): Representation of the relative importance of different types of information (adapted from Egilman 1992).[36] The diameter of each colored circle represents the relative importance of each type of information in this decade. The relative sizes and time frames are approximate.

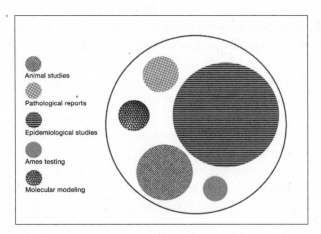

Figure 3—Circa 2006 (US): Representation of the relative importance of different types of information (adapted from Egilman 1992).[37] The diameter of each colored circle represents the relative importance of each type of information at this time. The relative sizes and time frames are approximate.

Corporations have used arguments about the validity of entire types of studies to dismiss whole categories of evidence that point to the harm resulting from their products. For example, tobacco companies questioned the consensus understanding that epidemiology could establish the cause-effect relationship between smoking and cancer. They argued that epidemiologic studies could not establish or "prove" causation because such studies could not prove that "cancer genes" were linked to "smoking genes." They then argued that smoking had not been found to cause cancer in animal studies. Finally, they argued that unless scientists could explain the exact mechanism through which smoking causes cancer, it could not be said that smoking was a cause of cancer. The companies also argued that since scientists admitted that they did not know exactly how cancer was caused, they could not say that smoking was a cause.[38]

Faced with epidemiologic evidence showing a link between cancer and smoking, the tobacco industry responded with the argument that greater weight should be placed on animal data and/or mechanistic understanding.[39] In his 1962 paper for R. J. Reynolds Tobacco Company (RJR), Alan Rodgman acknowledged that the "amount of evidence accumulated to indict cigarette smoke as a health hazard is overwhelming. The evidence challenging such an indictment is scant."[40] In his argument, Rodgman unwittingly revealed the systematic way in which the tobacco industry discounted evidence related to the "lung cancer/

cigarette-smoke proposition."[41] Each of Rodgman's four statements below served a particular function in discrediting various methodologies:

1. Statistical studies cannot prove cause-and-effect relationship between two factors; which criticized the epidemiology.
2. Mice are not men; which criticized the biological evidence
3. Metaplasia and hyperplasia do not become cancerous," which criticized the pathological evidence.
4. No experimental evidence exists to show that any cigarette smoke constituent is carcinogenic to human lung tissue at the level present in cigarette smoke, which criticized the chemical evidence.[42]

The chemical and tobacco industries have also stressed the appropriateness of a particular type of evidence, according to which type seemed most favorable to their respective case. The tobacco industry attacked epidemiology because results showed that tobacco caused cancer, while the chemical industry endorsed epidemiologic research because it is usually not available, it is expensive, and it often cannot be performed for technical reasons. The chemical companies, in contrast to the tobacco industry, have stressed the "unique" importance of epidemiological studies in establishing cause-effect relationships.[43, 44] The chemical industry's professed reliance on human epidemiological data stems from the fact that such data are difficult to obtain and, given that many toxin-related diseases have latency periods of twenty to forty years, are time- and resource-consuming; by the time the studies are completed, patient rights have expired, and chemical companies have new—or substitute—chemicals to promote.

In general, these companies claim that animal models, molecular understanding, and pathologic data cannot establish cause-effect relationships. According to the CIIT, industry-funded research has been successful in influencing regulators on the acceptability of animal evidence:

> In 1992 [the] EPA admitted for the first time that some chemicals causing cancer in laboratory animals are not relevant to human health risks. CIIT strongly influenced the EPA's change of attitude.[45]

Occasionally, when chemicals or other toxins, such as benzene or arsenic, are found to cause cancer in humans but not in animals, the chemical industry scientists reverse their arguments and, similar to tobacco companies, argue that causation in humans cannot be established until scientists produce positive animal studies and understand the exact mechanism of carcinogenesis.[46] In the end, each industry has asserted that the essential evidence required to justify regulatory action is the evidence that is not available. They are only satisfied by substantiation that is one step beyond the existing evidence, or is forever unattainable.

As early as 1965, in response to tobacco company duplicity, Hill argued that physicians had to consider all evidence for determining causation.[47] Since then, Hill's considerations have been well accepted and widely used by epidemiologists. Hill, however, recognized that, "All scientific work is incomplete—whether it be observational or experimental. All scientific work is liable to be upset or modified by advancing knowledge. That does not confer upon us a freedom to ignore the knowledge we already have, or to postpone the action that it appears to demand at a given time."[48]

Following Hill's example, unbiased scientists consider evidence from all types of studies in order to determine cause-effect relationships. Scientists often (consciously or unconsciously) utilize Bayesian analyses to integrate different types and quality of data. In a Bayesian analysis, a scientist shifts her perspective on the likelihood that a cause-effect relationship exists with the appearance of each new piece of evidence, whether it is a molecular, animal, or human study. A well-conducted study in a relevant animal model for a particular cancer showing that a substance causes cancer will enhance the scientist's position that the substance is a human carcinogen. For example, if prior to the study the scientist thought that there was a 30 percent likelihood that the substance caused cancer in humans, after the study she might change her view and believe there is a 60 or 70 percent chance that the substance is a human carcinogen. Different scientists have different views regarding the importance of animal or human epidemiologic data; however, an impartial observer will explain why she favors one form of evidence over another on a case by case basis. For example, a scientist may generally favor human data over animal studies, but might disregard a poorly conducted epidemiological study in favor of the findings from a well-conducted animal experiment.

While unbiased scientists consider all the data in a single integrated analysis, industry scientists often favor the type of data that supports their employer's position. For example, occupational and environmental studies that are directly or indirectly sponsored by multinational corporations disproportionately lead to results that fail to find that the exposure causes disease.[49–52] Epidemiologic studies may be designed by corporations to produce results that are favorable to them. These studies' findings tend to contradict the majority of independent scientific studies. For instance, the International Agency for Research on Cancer (IARC) considers exposures that occur in oil refineries to be "probably carcinogenic to humans."[53] This position is supported by a number of independent animal studies and human epidemiologic data.[54] While not all studies demonstrate "sufficient" risk for a particular carcinogen to cause a particular type of cancer, most studies noted by the IARC suggest possible, if not probable, risk.[55] Not surprisingly, industry-sponsored studies have not found any cancer increases or evidence of risk in oil refineries.[56]

Gennaro and Tomatis, whose work is important enough to be quoted at length in this chapter, enumerate a number of "critical points or errors to be avoided" that "may lead to falsely negative results" in epidemiologic studies.[57] They provide a list of "elements that do not meet the criteria for good epidemiologic practice oriented to the improvement of public health":

1. Privilege the use of descriptive instead of analytical statistics, and the adoption of cross-sectional instead of longitudinal epidemiological studies
2. Fail to study the single homogeneous subgroups of workers (in terms of exposure)
3. Consider only the exposure to one single substance, ignoring the possibility of exposure to multiple substances and their interactions
4. Keep the unexposed and exposed workers mixed (creating a dilution effect)
5. Compare the exposed workers, who are usually selected according to their overall positive health condition, with the general population (instead of unexposed workers), creating a healthy-worker effect and comparison bias
6. Take into consideration only one single disease (or disease family, [e.g., cancers]) rather than all diseases
7. Maintain disaggregation of homogeneous pathologies, thus making statistical significance more difficult to achieve
8. Fail to study reversible symptoms or serious sentinel abnormalities
9. Study neoplastic effects (usually having medium-long latency periods), at follow-up periods too short to allow for their development
10. Compare effects on the same target organ between groups of individuals exposed to different agents (e.g. asbestos workers vs. tobacco smokers) having the same target (e.g., lung)
11. Interpret the absence (or inadequacy) of both environmental (and biological) monitoring and epidemiologic studies as evidence of absence of exposure and negative health effects
12. Keep the measurements of exposures separated from the measurements of health effects
13. Privilege statistical significance rather than biological significance and consider the results of large and multicentric studies more important than other factors (biology, exposure, etc.)

14. Use the conventional two-sided statistical test instead of the one-sided statistical test, which appears to provide the greatest reassurance against missing an exposure-related effect
15. Use univariate analysis instead of a multivariate analysis that permits the simultaneous study of all the relevant variables (e.g. age at hire, sex, area, job, calendar period, length of employment, latency, etc.)[58]

Gennaro and Tomatis further describe the misclassification of exposed and unexposed workers by corporate-sponsored studies that obscure the relationship between risk of exposure and disease.[59] As they demonstrate, corporate-sponsored epidemiologic studies misclassify exposed workers with disease as unexposed controls, thus belying the appearance of risk.[60]

Reversed results can demonstrate the proposition that exposure to a carcinogen protects against the disease. For example, when General Motors, Ford, and Chrysler paid over fifty million dollars to generate meta-analyses of studies of asbestos-exposed workers,[61] the results indicated that exposure to asbestos-containing brakes actually protected against contracting cancer from asbestos. This occurred because much brake work is performed part-time by "shade tree mechanics," who, when asked, neither would list it as an occupation, nor would think to tell researchers of this part-time work. Aware, however, of their potential numbers and significance, researchers dismissed these part-time exposures, and classified "shade tree mechanic" cancers as occurring in "unexposed" workers. In another type of beneficial misclassification, as defense expert epidemiologist Dr. Wong testified, a lawyer working in an office at a Mobil facility would be classified as exposed, while a contract worker with leukemia who worked cleaning reactor vessels for Mobil would not be categorized as a Mobil worker.[62] Categorizing a full-time office worker who had minimal or no exposures and no disease as an exposed worker reduces the appearance of a cause-effect relationship between exposure and disease.

Corporate-sponsored studies of US refinery workers have employed much the same approach as the automobile industry. The most heavily exposed asbestos or benzene refinery workers are contract workers who clean tanks or install insulation; because they are not regular employees of the refinery, these workers are not included in the count of those exposed. The irrational findings brought about by incorrectly categorizing workers not only counter legitimate science, but also effectively inject further doubt into the whole scientific process—doubt that can then be used to engineer regulatory delays or avoid tort claims.

SCIENCE LAUNDROMATS: BAD SCIENCE GAINS CREDIBILITY

Sometimes corporate consultants are needed to "launder" other consultants' work. Research that is initially discredited can gain "legitimacy" through repeated citation, as was the case for J. C. McDonald's asbestos industry-funded research on the risks of chrysotile asbestos.[63] In 1984, Dr. Crump served as a consultant for the Asbestos Information Association's (AIA's) legal team and testified against OSHA regulations proposed to reduce exposures to asbestos.[64] Almost twenty years later, Crump and co-researcher, Dr. Wayne Berman, received a contract from the EPA to develop a mathematical model to assess the risks of contracting cancer from various forms of asbestos. They concluded that chrysotile asbestos, the type that comprised more than 95 percent of the asbestos used in the United States, probably did not cause mesothelioma—the cancer that is almost uniformly associated with exposure to asbestos.[65]

Remarkably, Crump and Berman based their model on a discredited dose-response analysis that J. C. McDonald had both created and discredited.[66–68] When commenting on the reliability of his dose estimates, McDonald stated, ". . . . the fiber equivalent of this exposure level [the level required to cause asbestos disease] has not been established. Available data suggests that, in Québec, this may be in the region of five fibers per milliliter. It remains doubtful, however, whether conversion to a fiber equivalent can have much epidemiologic validity."[69]

Even though the EPA has not accepted Crump and Berman's model, and the organization's current official policy states that all asbestos fiber types are equally likely to cause cancer, asbestos companies have used the Crump and Berman paper as the basis for dismissing thousands of lawsuits filed by victims.[70] Indeed, asbestos companies being sued by workers who contracted mesothelioma filed a legal motion to have the court adopt Crump and Berman's model as the standard of causation for all asbestos litigation in Texas. Dr. Crump could not testify for the companies in a tort case until the EPA had decided what to do with his model; had he testified for industry sponsors, he would have discredited himself as an impartial scientist. Instead, the companies hired Dr. Laura Green's consulting company, Cambridge Environmental, which describes its litigation services as, "technical strategies for arguing the merits of the client's case and for addressing the likely counter-arguments."[71] Dr. Green gave testimony relying on and affirming the validity of Crump's work.[72] Dr. Green did not disclose that Crump and Berman had based their model on the discredited McDonald dose-response analysis that had been sponsored by the asbestos industry. While such laundering of data through a series of consultant reports cannot change scientific facts, it can change the perception of those facts and influence an unknowing public, that includes judges, juries, regulatory agencies, and the press.

Laundering is not restricted to hired private scientists; sometimes corporations fund government agencies to legitimize bad science. After the EPA cut off Berman and Crump's funding, Dr. Paustenbach suggested that asbestos mine owners and product manufacturers launder money to the EPA to fund a study that would report that chrysotile asbestos did not cause cancer. In this way, the study would have the imprimatur of governmental objectivity, undermine the EPA's regulation of asbestos, and continue to hide the corporate origin of the study's funding. Paustenbach wrote

> I think you guys need to really think about spending the small amount of money it would take to a) finish the Berman and Crump paper through a grant to the EPA that could be passed through to Berman and Crump and others, and b) fill in the rest of that dose-response curve by mining more epidemiology studies and combining it with simulation studies to give exposure components . . . I firmly believe that's the only way this industry will be able to help itself, if those things are done. There's just too much of a tidal wave going the other direction.[73]

ATTACKS ON "OPPOSING" SCIENTISTS

One of the most ethically troubling methods for controlling the scientific debate is the effort by companies to discredit, intimidate, or scandalize opposing scientists. The orchestrated attacks on Dr. Irving Selikoff, the author of several early studies warning about the health effects of asbestos, are a prime example of companies using scare tactics and intimidation for these purposes.

During the 1960s, the asbestos industry continued to deny that asbestos caused cancer among workers. Public relations campaigns and research activities focused on discrediting Selikoff's findings. Public relations professionals pointed to the studies' scientific limitations, which were acknowledged by the authors, and sought to emphasize in the media that the studies were inconclusive. One PR response to Selikoff noted that his research was "based on limited reports relating to a relatively small group of workers who install and/or remove a variety of insulation materials, including some which contain asbestos."[74]

The asbestos companies did not stop with these attacks on the science. Shortly after the landmark October, 1964 Mount Sinai Hospital conference on asbestos health effects—organized by Selikoff, the Asbestos Textile Institute (ATI), via their attorneys at Cadwalader, Wickersham & Taft, sent a threatening letter to Selikoff. It ended with the following paragraph, which includes a veiled threat to sue independent scientists, and suggests the industry's anxiety about economic losses that may result from adverse publicity regarding the dangers of their products:

The Asbestos Textile Institute urges no restraint upon independent medical inquiry or research—indeed it earnestly desires expansion of existing knowledge in this field. Nor does this Association seek in any way to discourage the right to discuss the results of such efforts. But it does urge caution in the discussion of these activities to avoid providing the basis for possibly damaging and misleading news stories. The right to study and to discuss these subjects is clear, of course. But the gravity of the subject matter and the consequences implicitly involved impose upon any who exercise those rights a very high degree of responsibility for their actions.[75]

In order to discredit Selikoff, other asbestos manufacturing companies put him under scrutiny. In November, 1965, Owens-Corning Fiberglass (OCF) personnel worried that Selikoff's activities would hurt sales:

Our present concern is to find some way of preventing Dr. Selikoff from creating problems and affecting sales. A direct approach might be more damaging than helpful and I am only suggesting that we explore, at this time, all avenues open to us.[76]

The OCF staff gathered and reviewed "intelligence" on Selikoff that they believed could be used to discredit him and protect their sales.[77] They discussed his immigrant status and noted that he was licensed as a doctor in the United States through a "broad reciprocal arrangement with a foreign country."[78]

After deciding against the strategy of discrediting Selikoff, the ATI resigned itself to dealing with the persistent problem of Selikoff's findings: Dr. J. L. Goodman, speaking as a member of the ATI Environmental Health Committee, stated that Dr. Selikoff is a "'dangerous' man, and that the asbestos industry is going to have to learn how to combat his tactics! . . ." When asked if something could be done through the American Medical Association to control Dr. Selikoff, Dr. Goodman expressed doubt: "There is a grievance committee of the AMA but was very difficult to get it to act. Thought [sic] that perhaps pressure on the Mount Sinai School of Medicine might be effective."[79]

The attacks on Selikoff did not end with his death in 1992. Thirteen years after he died, a British historian, who also served as an asbestos industry litigation consultant, published a thirty-page article claiming both that Selikoff had fraudulently presented himself as a medical doctor and that he had allegedly never obtained a medical degree.[80, 81] This assertion was untrue, but the history journal that published this slanderous falsehood refused to publish a photograph of Selikoff's medical degree. It was published elsewhere.[82]

CREATING AND INFLUENCING SCIENTIFIC GROUPS
Scientific Advisory Boards

Public relations firms, large law firms, and the companies they represent can work together to control "research" outcomes by establishing scientific advisory boards (SABs). They can further legitimize "bad science" through the creation of SABs that seem independent and unbiased. All too often, SABs are not composed of truly independent advisers but rather scientists on company payrolls who publish industry-favorable research, speak for industry interests at regulatory hearings and to the press, and testify as expert witnesses in tort litigation lawsuits. An SAB can pose as an impartial, authorized scientific body while actually working to further industry goals by generating favorable science and public opinion to avoid liability.[83, 84] Two examples of such SABs include the tobacco companies' Center for Tobacco Research Scientific Advisory Board (CTRSAB), and the beryllium companies' Beryllium Industry Scientific Advisory Committee (BISAC).

The US Gypsum-Hill & Knowlton SAB

In the early 1980s, an asbestos product manufacturer, US Gypsum Corporation (USG), hired a PR firm, Hill & Knowlton (H&K) to develop communications strategies for the express purpose of derailing litigation by public schools that were seeking damages for asbestos removal, discouraging future litigation, and shifting public attitudes about asbestos and individual asbestos companies in the industry's favor. H&K recommended that US Gypsum form a coalition with other asbestos companies to face the threat together. The formation of a scientific advisory board (SAB) was key to the overall strategy. H&K executives proposed the formation of a "third-party panel of independent experts to be available for testimony, commentary, and technical support in appropriate markets and forums."[85] H&K viewed the need for such an "independent" panel to build credibility for a company and industry that was rapidly being discredited:

> [A]sbestos manufacturers, like industry proponents of nuclear energy a few years ago, have little, if any, credibility. Evidence adduced by recognized, independent experts, in tandem with the company's own, could significantly heighten credibility. (This kind of backing could also shore up the wavering school board member who may not be convinced removal is the most efficient or appropriate action).[86]

In addition, the SAB would voice an opinion on asbestos dangers that would support the industry's interests. They were aware that generating controversy over science that did not seem to support the company's interests would help them in a legal setting:

> [T]he scientific evidence supporting the allegation of health hazards posed by these products is ambiguous and can be interpreted different ways. Nevertheless, how the science is read will have a major impact on verdicts. And, the preponderance of the evidence appears to be on the side of the plaintiffs. (The government, presumably a disinterested party, has thrown all its weight behind total removal of asbestos in schools).[87]

While many other SABs kept their industry funding secret, in this case, H&K thought that disclosing industry funding for a supposedly independent panel would in itself be a positive public relations move for the industry:

> [O]ne notable result of the asbestos controversy is the public perception of corporations shunning their social responsibilities. A panel, funded by, but independent of the industry could go a long way in ameliorating that perception . . . As mentioned, the panel should be funded by all the industries cooperating in the coalition. And the coalition should make a public statement that while it is providing funding, conclusions and recommendations are entirely those of the panel. (Two caveats occur here. First, participating companies should make their position clear at the outset, but necessarily, distinguish their position from any arrived at by the panel. Second, to be truly independent, the panel must be balanced—members should be included who in the past may have had questions and concerns about the issue).[88]

The SAB was meant to influence public opinion on a variety of levels and their independent conclusions would be used as a centerpiece for H&K's campaign:

> One important use of this panel could be to request that it review the EPA protocol used in arriving at conclusions. This, then could be incorporated into both legal and public relations strategies . . . [A]n independent panel, like the proposed coalition, could help deflect attention away from affected companies. Technical questions, etc., could be referred to panel members, for example. And, answers would have that much more credibility coming from third-party sources . . . Members of the panel should be available to school boards, on request. They should be available to undertake technical assignment (e.g., review of EPA protocol, etc.) Finally, they should be available to the media and for other forums (speech platforms, etc.) as appropriate."[89]

SABs and "Third-Party Techniques"

Earning the trust of a public skeptical about the veracity of official corporate spokespeople presents big business with a challenge. Corporations have
addressed this problem by hiring seemingly "independent voices" to camouflage
their misrepresentations: "Developing third-party support and validation for the
basic risk messages of the corporation is essential. This support should ideally
come from medical authorities, political leaders, union officials, relevant academics, fire and police officials, environmentalists, regulators."[90] Amanda Little
of the PR firm Burson-Marsteller (BM) explained this to an advertising conference in 1995:

> For the media and the public, the corporation will be one of the least credible
> sources of information, on its own product, environmental, and safety risks.
> Both these audiences will turn to other experts . . . to get an objective view-
> point.[91]

A "third-party technique," which has been defined as putting "your words in
someone else's mouth,"[92] generates public support for a corporate position by
making it seem independent and unbiased. "Third-party techniques" utilize
the media to write industry-favorable studies and include hiring scientists who
appear to be independent, trustworthy experts to lend credibility to industry-
biased "bad science."[93]

In 1976, H&K developed some "third-party techniques" for the vinyl chloride monomer producers group (VCM-PVC) of the Chemical Manufacturers'
Association (CMA). H&K told the VCM-PVC producers group that they needed
"third-party experts" to respond to adverse press coverage of vinyl chloride
workers whose cancer was caused by vinyl chloride exposure:

> As a case in point, this underlines the need for developing third-party experts
> who will come forward and help clarify issues as they develop. We need addi-
> tional third-party candidates for this kind of role, and requested the member-
> ship provide these for future reference.[94]

In 1989, H&K made similar recommendations to Brush Wellman, Inc., the
major manufacturer of beryllium in the United States:

> Third-party scientific and engineering experts from academia and industry,
> NASA for example, should be enlisted to review the Brush Wellman public
> relations materials. The testimonials of these outside experts should be cast as

a foreword in a white paper and liberally referenced in all support materials, such as brochures and video scripts. The review of the material by independent scientists will persuasively verify the scientific inclusions in the public relations materials . . . These third-party experts may also be used to provide objective information that is supportive of Brush Wellman in a variety of forms, such as at congressional hearings to media representatives.[95]

Corporate-sponsored SABs do not produce any science; they are merely PR vehicles through which corporations and industry groups funnel their arguments to limit regulation and avoid liability.

Public Relations Strategies: Organizing Corporate-Sponsored Front Groups, Industry Organizations, Think Tanks, and Media Outreach

Several PR and law firms have notably taken the lead in aiding corporate producers of dangerous goods. These include the law firm of Jones, Day, Reavis, and Pogue (Jones Day) and the PR companies, H&K and Burson-Marsteller. These firms have used similar techniques and strategies for a number of their corporate clients. For example, when courting the beryllium producer, Brush Wellman, H&K assured them that it had conducted campaigns "analogous to the beryllium situation," including the following:

- asbestos and human health
- saccharin and federal regulation
- dioxin and public health
- lead and public health
- vinyl chloride and cancer[96]

Both PR and law firms perform duties for corporations that go well beyond what the general public might consider public relations and legal work. Public relations firms do not limit themselves to planning media outreach. They also contract scientific studies, plan broad-based legal strategies, create "citizens' groups" that support a particular industry or product, and work to discredit scientists seen as opposing the goals of the corporation. Law firms not only work on legal strategy but may also contract scientific studies, formulate scientific defenses, and lobby public officials.

Front Groups

Along with their use of SABs, corporate strategists use "front groups" to provide legitimacy to their science. In their strategy memo to USG, H&K consultants explained how the formation of an industry-wide coalition or "front group" would allow USG to share resources with other companies and counter the public allegations of activists. In addition to serving as an information source and media response mechanism for the industry, a "front group" "could also act to deflect attention away from affected companies," and "take the heat from the press and activist industry critics."[97]

In 1984, the asbestos companies, under the leadership of W. R. Grace & Co., formed a "front group" paradoxically yet strategically named, the "Safe Buildings Alliance" (SBA). The SBA downplayed asbestos hazards to discourage schools and other private and public entities from removing asbestos and suing the companies for removal or repair costs. A court later determined that, "Due to the financial and operational control that the [asbestos manufacturers] exercise over the SBA, the SBA is merely the alter ego of the [asbestos manufacturers]."[98]

In addition, H&K staff intended to use the SBA to influence public opinion through media and sway a range of government and regulatory bodies, school boards, labor unions, medical and scientific professionals, and even "internal" audiences, such as employees, to accept the position that their asbestos was not a hazard.[99]

The "front group" was to do the following:

- Contain problem to schools. Prevent EPA or other governmental entities from yielding to union pressure and pressure from other constituencies to extend mandate to inspect for Monokote (and other brand name [asbestos containing] fireproofing substances) to include commercial buildings
- Minimize the number of cases where removal of the material containing asbestos becomes the option of choice
- Prevent product liability suits
- Prevent or mitigate legislation at all governmental levels that would authorize governmental subsidy to schools for removal of materials, thereby encouraging adoption of the removal option
- Significantly enhance understanding of all target audiences of the health risks associated with removal of the material in question; encourage intelligent assessment of issues affecting options for dealing with presence of material.[100]

While the SBA was an industry-run organization, other "front groups" have been designed to resemble real "grassroots" organizations that appear to be run by and for autonomous citizens' groups.

Burson-Marsteller (BM), a PR firm, has focused on organizing such "front groups." This technique, which is often referred to as the creation of "Astroturf organizations," attempts to capitalize on the moral power of citizens' campaigns to promote private corporate interests. In order to battle the efforts of genuine "grass-roots" groups and provide an air of legitimacy to a company's goals, BM has formed many "grassroots" organizations. Unfortunately, these groups are fraudulent, in the sense that the company organizes and pays for their operation. They are not organic, self-determining organizations that are created through citizen or consumer activism.

One notorious example of an "Astroturf organization" is the National Smokers' Alliance (NSA), developed by BM on behalf of Philip Morris.[101] The NSA sought to portray regulation on smoking in public places as an infringement of basic US freedoms. Backed by millions of dollars of tobacco industry money, BM ran newspaper advertising campaigns, set up a toll-free number, paid canvassers and telemarketers, and published newsletters.[102] By 1995, the NSA, which received less than 1 percent of its funding from members' dues and was headed by BM's vice president, claimed a membership of 3 million individuals.[103] In an attempt to build their membership rolls, the NSA considered drafting Philip Morris employees as members.[104] Some people were counted as members whether or not they paid dues, and at least some were given cigarette lighters in exchange for signing. While the group claimed it aimed to "empower" smokers and make their voices heard, internal memos reflected a cynical concern about this strategy. As one memo expressed: "We don't want to 'empower' them to the point that they'll quit."[105]

Several other examples of BM-generated "front groups" have been cited by Ethical Consumer, a British organization devoted to exposing the environmental record of corporations.[106] These include the following:

- Forestry Alliance of British Columbia, a front for Canadian logging interests[107]
- World Business Council for Sustainable Development (WBCSD), an international big business organization, accused of hijacking the agenda at the 1992 Rio Earth Summit[108]
- Californians for Realistic Vehicle Standards, a front for the auto-industry, opposing pollution regulation[109]
- Coalition for Clean and Renewable Energy, set up to undermine opposition to a controversial dam-building project in Quebec[110]
- Forest Protection Society, lobbying for the Australian timber industry[111]
- Fur Information Council US, a media campaigner on behalf of the fur industry[112]

Corporate-sponsored "front groups" can influence the research and treatment concerns of legitimate, industry-independent science and medical professionals.

Barbara Brenner, the executive director of Breast Cancer Action, has stated that the pharmaceutical corporate sponsorship of "Breast Cancer Awareness" has caused grassroots groups to focus on early detection and treatment (with the sponsors' drugs) and away from "Real prevention [which] . . . means we figure out what is causing illness and we eradicate those causes."[113] In fact, corporate sponsorship has redefined cancer prevention as early detection and treatment rather than avoiding the occurrence of cancer in the first place.

Industry Organizations and Trade Groups: The Asbestos Information Association Example

Industry organizations have served as a vehicle for corporations within a particular industry to develop a common scientific agenda aimed at allaying public and government concerns regarding the dangers of their products. Industry organizations are an efficient way for corporations to lobby—as a group—regulatory agencies. For example, the Asbestos Information Association, formed by the asbestos industry and led by a consortium of many asbestos companies, including Johns-Manville and Union Carbide, successfully weakened OSHA and EPA regulations.

The far-reaching influence of industry organizations is evident from a 1973 AIA recruiting speech to prospective members by Matthew Swetonic, the director of the AIA. He explained the impact of the AIA on regulations:

> I think it is a gauge of the effectiveness of the total industry involvement in this most crucial matter that of eleven main requirements in the [OSHA] standards, the industry position was accepted totally by OSHA on nine of the eleven, about 50 percent on a tenth, and totally rejected on only one. The struggle is far from over. We must not only continue but indeed expand our activities and the various areas of concern.

Among other changes, Swetonic credited AIA's lobbying for OSHA's removal of the signal words "cancer" and "warning" from the product label.[114] He also reviewed the challenges faced by the industry:

> Twenty-five thousand workers exposed to the industries' asbestos-containing products and 5000 of their own manufacturing workers will have died or will eventually die of asbestos-related disease.

He contrasted this "bad news" with the "good news":

> Despite all the negative articles on asbestos-health that have appeared in the press

over the past half-dozen years, very few people have been paying attention.[115]

Think Tanks: The Mercatus Center Example

While not necessarily formed as part of any particular corporation's or industry's strategy to limit regulation and liability, a number of right-wing think tanks share similar goals with corporate actors and funders, and generate research and policy papers to support corporate interests. Their generous corporate funding and intellectual capital make them a powerful force in swaying public opinion and influencing lawmakers. A number of well-known think tanks, including Manhattan, Cato, Heritage, and Mercatus, attempt to both limit corporate liability and curb public health regulation.

Often operating inconspicuously, think tanks can be very effective—sometimes more so than industry groups themselves—at limiting regulation. The Mercatus Center, which is housed at George Mason University but funded primarily by Koch Industries, a privately held chemical company,[116] was described by the *Wall Street Journal* as, "the most important think tank you've never heard of":

> Mercatus analysts sometimes contort themselves to build a case against regulation . . . [They] criticized one EPA rule to reduce surface ozone because the EPA didn't take into account that clearer skies would increase the rate of skin cancer. Later, two other Mercatus scholars blasted a different EPA rule on diesel engines, arguing that it was bad because it would increase surface ozone in some cities. This time they didn't say anything about the cancer-prevention benefits of more smog.[117]

In 2001, the Bush administration, in their first-term year, sought suggestions for government regulations that it could eliminate or modify. Mercatus criticized forty-four regulations and the Bush administration selected 60 percent of those regulations for elimination or modification. In contrast, the National Association of Manufacturers, the largest industrial trade association in the United States, failed to get the administration to abide any of its recommendations for regulatory "reform."[118]

Think tanks can also exert pressure on the media and provide a stream of "experts" on economic, health, and environmental issues. A 2004 survey of think tank citations in the print and electronic media, conducted by Fairness & Accuracy in Reporting (FAIR), found that 50 percent of all press citations in that year were from conservative or center-right think tanks. Only 16 percent of media citations quoted progressive or center-left think tanks; the remaining 33 percent cited centrist think tanks such as the Brookings Institution.[119]

Another conservative think tank, the Manhattan Institute, greatly influenced the Supreme Court decision that granted judges the power to limit the type of "scientific evidence" that could be used to establish cause-effect relationships; as a result, cancer victims' ability to recover medical and other çosts in court has been severely limited. The eventual ninth circuit court Daubert decision cited *Galileo's Revenge*, a book authored by a Manhattan Institute attorney, as authority for the proposition that scientific argument should be limited to peer-reviewed papers.[120] The irony of citing a non-peer-reviewed book written by a lawyer (not a scientist) employed by a libertarian foundation with a political agenda to limit corporate liability was apparently lost on the justices.

Public Relations: Utilizing and Influencing the Media

The triumvirate of corporations–PR firms–and law firms also utilizes a number of secondary actors to carry out key strategies, which have been largely successful in providing scientific alibis for dangerous products and using "bad science" to help companies avoid regulation and liability.

Companies and their PR firms use the popular media to influence public opinion regarding the safety of their products. An extensive media campaign reproduces manipulated science in a popular format. Such a broad-based strategy is meant to influence the public, legislators, regulators, and potential jurors who have the immense power to hold corporations accountable in tort actions.

Hill & Knowlton openly discussed the important ramifications of tort actions and jury decisions for industry: "[O]ne or more adverse jury decisions could alarm the financial community as well as the company's shareholders." Any legal decisions against the company, or other asbestos companies, could "trigger a domino effect," and as litigation continues, "publicity about the suits can bubble up into the national media," leading to "negative consequences for the company as a purveyor of what is popularly thought to be extremely hazardous material."[121]

The PR consultants recognized that popular attitudes toward asbestos, for example, supported by a growing body of medical evidence linking asbestos to lung disease in users of asbestos products, would have a direct relationship to jury attitudes. To avert losses in court and on Wall Street, a company, and the industry as a whole, would have to discredit the science behind the lawsuits and alter public attitudes about their deadly commodity.[122]

Corporate Public Relations Masquerading as Independent Opinion or Journalism

In order to reach potential jurors, who are unlikely to read scientific publications, corporations have developed programs to restrict and coordinate the flow of health information to the media.[123] H&K's asbestos media strategy relied on securing interviews and placing articles—authored by experts "sympathetic to the company's point of view"—in popular media sources. H&K consultants referred to this strategy as "capturing 'share of mind'" on the national level.[124]

To this end, companies also sponsor ghostwritten editorials that advance industry positions without acknowledging their source of origin. As noted above, the asbestos industry used the Safe Buildings Alliance in the 1980s as a conduit for planting favorable ideas in news outlets. Other industries have used similar techniques. For example, the tobacco industry secretly paid a sportswriter to write a biased article that was published in *True* magazine and the *National Enquirer*. The *Wall Street Journal* later exposed this episode and the writer eventually went to work at a PR firm.[125]

More recently, the *Austin Chronicle* exposed the story of a University of Texas at Austin professor of nuclear engineering who submitted to the Chronicle a letter that he himself did not write, supporting the nuclear lobby. The professor confessed to the newspaper that he had merely signed his name on a letter penned by a PR agent from a Washington firm hired by the Nuclear Energy Institute.[126] The reporter searched databases for similar articles and found several editorials with nearly the exact same language under different authors in several other newspapers.[127]

PR firms have also developed a new technique to influence public opinion—using video news releases (VNRs). VNRs, which are often downloadable via satellite, are intended to influence public perceptions by appearing to be actual news segments produced by the broadcast news media. In fact, many VNRs have been aired by broadcast networks without disclosure of their industry source. Public relations firms produce thousands of VNRs every year, many supporting new pharmaceutical products.[128]

Industry's Investment in the Media

With $2 billion spent annually on advertising, the tobacco industry made cigarettes the most heavily advertised product in the United States. While the advertisements themselves sought to shore up the market by reassuring smokers that cigarettes were glamorous and by using images that implied cigarettes were safe, the industry's advertising dollars made the media outlets natural economic allies.[129, 130] A secret memo prepared by tobacco defense lawyers assessed the efficacy of these programs: "Through a studied investment of its advertising dollars, the industry both coerced the print media to avoid coverage of anti-smoking stories and enlisted the media's support in opposition to proposed restrictions on print advertising."[131]

H&K and the Chemical Manufacturers Association (CMA) employed similar techniques to defend vinyl chloride after scientists found that the chemical—used in the formulation of consumer products such as hair spray and plastics—was carcinogenic. The PR techniques, identified in a 1976 memorandum to an industry group, signaled the industry's desire to use the media to allay public concerns about vinyl chloride and cancer.[132] The CMA and H&K retained the services of a number of eminent television and radio journalists to train their personnel in methods to field "volatile" questions from "adversary broadcast and media people."[133]

This type of professional advice calls into question the conflicts of interest of journalists who are paid by the very industries that they might be called upon to cover objectively, especially when fees paid to "high profile" journalists can reach $100,000.[134] For example, Philip Morris USA paid Deborah Norville, a CBS-TV anchor, to run a mock television show at a Philip Morris convention.[135] Five years later, she cohosted a news magazine segment on tobacco taxes that contained factual errors about the effects of cigarette taxes on smuggling and prominently featured (without disclosure) an interview with a paid consultant to the Canadian Tobacco Manufacturers Council.[136]

ABC's John Stossel, a co-anchor/correspondent for *20/20*, produced a segment in 2000 called "The Food You Eat," which misreported research on organic foods.[137] In an apparent conflict of interest, Stossel is also a for-hire speaker through the Agricultural Speakers Network, whose clients include agribusiness companies.[138] For the segment, Stossel argued that organic produce may be more dangerous than conventional produce, with the network's tests showing increased levels of E. coli bacteria in organic sprouts and lettuce. He also maintained that the tests found no pesticide residue in either the conventional or organic produce, thereby removing a key reason for buying organic food.[139] But according to the two scientists that ABC hired, they never tested any of the produce for pesticides; they tested only for bacteria. During the broadcast, Stossel commented: "It's logical to worry about pesticide residues, but in our tests, we found none on either organic or regular produce." The testimony of researchers indicates that Stossel was referring to tests that were not carried out.[140]

Whether or not high fees for speaking engagements influence reporting, journalists violate the ethical standards of their profession when they receive compensation that may "influence coverage." According to the code of ethics of the Radio-Television News Directors Association, journalists have a professional obligation to "present the news with integrity and decency, avoiding real or perceived conflicts of interest."[141] Journalists should not "accept gifts, favors, or compensation from those who might seek to influence coverage."[142] First and foremost journalists "should operate as trustees of the public, seek the truth, report it fairly and with integrity and independence, and stand accountable for their actions."[143]

COUNTERING THE IMPACT OF BAD SCIENCE

Corporations working in concert with law and PR firms have created and used "bad science" to successfully limit both corporate liability and regulation. Currently, the US federal agencies charged with protecting occupational and environmental health are underpowered and underfunded. The Bush administration forged deregulatory policies, carrying on the practice of its predecessors, George H. W. Bush and Ronald Reagan. A similar deregulatory trend is underway worldwide with the globalization of the "free trade" orthodoxy. The resulting corporate profit comes at a great cost—the health and lives of everyday citizens.

Without vigilant oversight by government regulators, a true watchdog press, informed citizen and union participation, and universally enforced ethical standards for scientific research, industries will continue to use "bad science" to maximize profits while minimizing health protections.

To counteract the effects of "bad science" employed by unethical corporations and other parties, concerned health professionals and others should start advisory boards and think tanks and adopt PR and other tactics of their own to protect rather than undermine public health. Scientists must form more effective linkages with unions and authentic grassroots community organizations. We must write genuine editorials and articles for the lay press. And we must testify at congressional and regulatory hearings and in toxic tort litigation. By making ethical use of strategies employed by industry, scientists can help to promote life rather than destroy it. A sharp blade can serve either as a scalpel that removes a cancer or as a murder weapon.

Chapter 3

A BATTLEGROUND— FROM PHENOXYACETIC ACIDS, CHLOROPHENOLS AND DIOXINS TO MOBILE PHONES—CANCER RISKS, GREENWASHING AND VESTED INTERESTS

Lennart Hardell

How do these corporations achieve their stranglehold on our society? When they're not shooting, they're buying. They buy good minds, and tie them to their wagon wheels. They buy students wet from their mothers, and castrate their thought processes. They create false orthodoxies and impose censorship under the sham of political correctness.

John le Carré

INTRODUCTION

It was August 1976, and I was a newly employed physician at the Department of Oncology, University Hospital, Umeå in Sweden. The news media had been intensively reporting the summer spraying in the forests in Northern Sweden with Hormoslyr®, a herbicide of the phenoxyacetic acid class used to protect hardwood; a great deal of opinion had been against spraying.

Despite the claims of the Swedish Environmental Protection Agency (EPA), whose head, Valfrid Paulsson, suggested Hormoslyr® was safe for humans and the environment, many remained unconvinced. In one village in Northern Sweden people chained themselves to tractors in forests to prevent spraying. In another village, several sprayers were reported to have died with cancer. A report from laymen claimed that new diseases were found in animals in sprayed areas of forests, (e g., there was a kind of soft-tissue tumor found among the elk population). In a bizarre act of faith, a forest officer drank Hormoslyr® during a news report on TV; it was later said that he had died of cancer.

After one month's employment on the oncology ward, I met a patient with a particular type of cancer, a soft-tissue sarcoma (STS). He had sprayed phenoxy herbicides in the forests and provoked my further interest in the potential carcinogenicity of this compound of chemicals. STS is a rare malignant disease of the connective tissue comprising less than 1 percent of all malignant diseases in Sweden. In the following couple of months, two more patients with STS and similar chemical exposure appeared at the department. Information on a series of seven patients with STS and exposure to phenoxy herbicides was published by me in my first year at the hospital.[1]

Actually, my interest in this topic had been started some time before—in 1973—when I met a patient with an abdominal tumor living in the county of Norrbotten in Northern Sweden. He was first diagnosed as having liver cancer but at autopsy it turned out to be pancreatic cancer. This sixty-four-year-old man had worked as a forestry foreman. In the 1950s and 1960s, he used a mixture of the herbicides 2,4-dichlorophenoxyacetic acid (2,4-D) and 2,4,5-trichlorophenoxyacetic acid (2,4,5-T) to spray hardwoods. These chemicals were the main constituent parts of Hormoslyr®. He used no protective equipment and his relatives were intuitively of the opinion that his cancer was caused by exposure to the chemicals he sprayed.

The Swedish EPA had issued a report with reassuring conclusions on the safety of the use of phenoxy herbicides in 1974.[2] I received that publication from the agency upon my request for documentation on 2,4-D and 2,4,5-T. This request was prompted by the exposure history of the patient described above. The occurrence of 2,3,7,8-tetrachlorodibenzo-p-dioxin (TCDD) at ppm levels in 2,4,5-T was described in the report. At that time, TCDD was certainly already documented to be a toxic chemical and thus, at least due to its dioxin impurities, TCDD in 2,4,5-T should have come under suspicion of being a toxic substance; eventually TCDD turned out to be *the most* toxic chemical made by man.

These clinical, *bedside* observations prompted further epidemiological studies by our research group on phenoxy herbicides and the related chlorophenols and any association with STS. We reported four case-control studies that showed an increased risk for individuals with such exposure. This was the finding both for occupational and leisure time use of these chlorinated pesticides. I also met some women with STS who had been exposed to Hormoslyr® while washing their husbands' clothes—soaked while spraying in the forests. I was to find out later that this mirrored cancer in relatives of asbestos workers who contracted lung cancer after secondary exposure through outer garment working clothes. Our studies were followed by other investigations in other countries that confirmed our findings;[3,4] however, the purpose of this chapter is not to go back over our findings and those of others, but rather to consider the idea of preventative or precautionary strategies and look briefly at those who have continued to argue that TCDD presents no health problems.

At that time, my opinion as a young researcher was that new cancer risks should be seriously evaluated and prevention considered. My experience over the years has been that this is, in fact, hardly ever the rule. On the contrary, it takes decades until a cancer hazard is recognized and proper prevention is undertaken, if at all. The histories of tobacco, asbestos, and lung cancer are good examples. Sadly and shockingly, my case report in the Swedish Medical Association's paper *Läkartidningen* in 1977 provoked a zoo physiologist to initiate an impudent and irrelevant correspondence attacking my work in one of Sweden's leading newspapers with the title "The Wolf is Coming." The article was, of course, not peer-reviewed and appeared to be based on personal feelings and not facts, without any consideration of the lives of cancer victims.

This was only the beginning of such attacks that have continued on our further research into cancer hazards and prevention. I was initially surprised by the attacks, but over the years I have come to understand this is a kind of standardized procedure from industry and its allied academic experts. The causes are now also quite clear to me, namely money (industrial profit), academic competition for career and research grants, and personal ethical attitude.

This chapter looks at this early work and the attacks on me that it engendered. First, I have described the history and background of this group of chemicals. Following this, I have discussed how proper regulatory attention to these early findings would have resulted in earlier prohibition of some chemicals which would in turn have saved some thousands of lives in Sweden alone.

CHLOROPHENOLS

Chlorinated phenols have been manufactured in large quantities since the 1930s. They are produced by direct chlorination of the appropriate chlorobenzene.

Direct chlorination yields 2,4-di, 2,4,6-tri- and 2,3,4,6-tetrachlorophenol; on the other hand, 2,4,5-trichlorophenol is produced by hydrolysis of chlorobenzene. Pentachlorophenol (PCP) is produced by both methods; 2,4-Di- and 2,4,5-trichlorophenol have mainly been used as starting material for the production of the phenoxyacetic acids 2,4-D and 2,4,5-T. The other chlorophenols have been used as wood preservatives, battery acids, insecticides, and herbicides. PCP is the most-used type, and has also been used to limit growth of slime and algae in water cooling systems and as an antimicrobial agent in many consumer products such as leather and textiles.[5]

The production of PCP for wood preserving began on an experimental basis in the 1930s, and commercial production started in 1936.[6] Technical-grade PCP is contaminated by other chlorinated chemicals such as other chlorophenols, dioxins, dibenzofurans, and hexachlorobenzene.[7] One commercial product of PCP in which the dioxin content was minimized was offered to the market in 1975 but was withdrawn in 1980 due to limited demand, probably because of the higher cost compared with industrial-grade PCP. Since the early 1980s, the purchase and use of PCP has not been available to the US public. Most of the PCP later used in the United States was restricted to the treatment of telegraph and other utility poles and railway sleepers. The use of chlorophenols was banned in Sweden in January 1978.

For this class of chemicals, inhalation and skin contact are the main routes of occupational exposure. The whole population is exposed through the food chain; such chemicals are environmental contaminants and may bioaccumulate.

Chloracne, which involves exposed skin eruptions, is caused only by contact with chlorinated chemicals and is a true chemical disease. The first cases of chloracne among PCP producers were reported in 1951.[8] Ten workers were described with skin eruptions and furunculosis persisting more than one year after discontinuation of contact. Also, other disorders such as heart complaints, disturbances in libido, neuralgic pain, and irritation of eyes and upper respiratory system were reported. In 1957, reports of occupational chloracne caused by exposure to aromatic cyclic ethers were published.[9] Chloracne was found in 7 percent of workers assigned to PCP production at a single plant between 1953–1978.[10] The annual incidence was highest in the 1970s. Also, dioxins and dibenzofurans, by-products of PCP, have been associated with the development of chloracne.[11]

PCP interferes with oxidative phosphorylation, resulting in excessive release of heat. Fatal cases of poisoning among men dipping timber in 3 percent PCP solution were reported by 1952,[12] during manufacture of PCP in 1953,[13] and during use of PCP as weed killer in 1956.[14] Nine deaths within a period of eighteen months occurred among workers in sawmills where PCP was used as wood preservative.[15] Additional cases of intoxication among sawmill workers were reported in 1965.[16] Intoxication of nine neonates exposed to PCP used in laundering of diapers and bed linen was reported in 1969.[17]

PHENOXYACETIC ACIDS

The synthesis of the phenoxy herbicide 2,4-D was first reported in 1941.[18] Scientists involved in biological warfare programs in 1944 became interested in the possibility of using 2,4-D or the related 2,4,5-T for weed control because of their capability to kill selective plants.[19] The US government began field-testing these compounds in 1945 with the goal of using the herbicides to destroy the Japanese rice crop.[20] The war ended before the chemicals could be used. In 1945, a Dow Chemical chemist found that an equal mixture of 2,4-D and 2,4,5-T was more effective than either of the two compounds alone.[21] Phenoxy herbicides were used during the war in Korea in the early 1950s and they were used full-scale for chemical warfare in Vietnam from 1962. Military spraying reached a peak during 1967–1969, but was scaled down in 1970 and finally stopped in 1971.[22] Congenital malformations and genetic damage were feared from Agent Orange, a 1:1 mixture of 2,4-D and 2,4,5-T. It was around that time that the public became aware of dioxins contaminating these herbicides.[23] Agent Orange was also used in the Korean War in the early 1950s, as it was in Laos and Cambodia during the war against the Vietnamese; both sets of facts have been little discussed.

In Sweden, a 2:1 mixture of 2,4-D and 2,4,5-T with the trade name Hormoslyr® was first tested in the late 1940s for control of deciduous forest and was increasingly used from 1950; 2,4,5-T was the most potent phenoxy herbicide for the killing of hardwoods, whereas 2,4,-D and 4-chloro-2-methylphenoxy acetic acid (MCPA) were the most commonly used as weed killers in farming.

Early in the 1950s, while introducing the phenoxyacetic acids, employers claimed that they could be used safely without even protective equipment being necessary.[24] Still, there was concern among some of those who were occupationally exposed. By 1963, a letter regarding the safety of spraying with Hormoslyr® was addressed to one of the manufacturers by representatives of a concerned labor union. In the reply dated March 25, 1963, it was stated that this chemical "cannot in any way be considered to be carcinogenic. The chemical is characterized by low toxicity and no cases of toxic damage of human beings or animals have been reported to us."

The hygiene barrier conditions during spraying were often poor. The sprayers did not regularly wash their hands before eating or taking oral snuff.

The same clothes were used over several days and soiled clothes were later shown to be a significant cause of exposure. Exposure was oral, dermal, and by inhalation.[25]

DIOXINS AND DIBENZOFURANS

Polychlorinated dibenzo-p-dioxins (PCDDs) and dibenzofurans (PCDFs) are tricyclic aromatic compounds with similar chemical and physical properties. They are ubiquitous in the environment and do not occur naturally. There are 75 positional isomers of PCDDs and 135 isomers of PCDFs. TCDD is the most toxic isomer and the estimated toxic risk in humans is calculated in terms of "TCDD equivalents." For example, the toxic effect of different isomers is calculated in terms of the amounts that would cause the same degree of toxicity as TCDD.

Using trichlorophenol for the synthesis of 2,4,5-T gives contamination with dioxins, including TCDD, in 2,4,5-T. The toxicity of these chemicals could—from the beginning—have been predicted with openness and a precautionary approach adopted by the chemical industry. Hexachlorophenol was synthesized from trichlorophenol in 1939, that is, from the same chemical as for 2,4,5-T, at the Givaudan Laboratories, New Jersey, and was patented in 1941.[26] Thereby the same problem with contamination with TCDD occurred as for 2,4,5-T. The first animal testing showed high toxicity.[27] The result was based on testing of only eighteen animals, and inevitably most of these animals were killed by the chemical. The results were never published and no more thorough or pertinent studies of the toxicity were performed.

Due to the high bacteriostatic effect of hexachlorophenol, it was widely used in medical care from the beginning of the 1950s. pHisehex® was one, a trade-named common product in Sweden. Studies of mothers who had used hexachlorophenol in their hospital work and of their malformed children born during 1970–1974 were published in Sweden in the late 1970s.[28, 29] The author received many negative reactions to her observation, which was regarded as "controversial" by both industry and governmental agencies in Sweden. However, during a similar time, an accident in which newborn children were poisoned with hexachlorophenol occurred in France.[30] In total, 206 children fell ill and 36 died. By mistake, a batch of baby powder contained 6.3 percent hexachlorophenol instead of the 0.25–1 percent allowed as maximum. Due to litigation, it took ten years until this accident was known to the public.[31] The producers withdrew pHisehex® from the Swedish market in 1980 and were, of course, well aware of the French accident by that time.

As mentioned previously, chloracne is caused only by contact with chlorinated organic chemicals and has been associated with exposure to

2,4,5-trichlorophenol and 2,4,5-T.[32] In a confidential industry report, TCDD had by 1964 been identified at Dow Chemical, a major producer of these pesticides, as a contaminant in 2,4,5-trichlorophenol and 2,4,5-T.[33] It was identified to be the acnegenic chemical in trichlorophenol. However, it was not until 1970 that the public became aware that 2,4,5-T was contaminated by TCDD, as reported by independent university researchers.[34] The public awareness of dioxins in Agent Orange was an important factor that forced the US military to stop spraying with Agent Orange in Vietnam in 1970.

Thus, in the early 1970s TCDD had been reported to be a contaminant of 2,4,5-T and TCDD had been found to be a toxic chemical. There were, however, no reports of malignant diseases in human beings associated with exposure to phenoxyacetic acids, the chemically related chlorophenols, or TCDD; our studies were the first ones.

Curiously, in this context, it may be mentioned that during the Ukrainian presidential election in 2004, one of the candidates, Viktor Yushchenko, became seriously ill. He was diagnosed with acute pancreatitis, accompanied by interstitial edematous changes, due to a serious viral infection. After the illness, his face became heavily disfigured, grossly jaundiced, bloated, and pockmarked, and he was diagnosed with chloracne. When his blood was tested, it was confirmed that he had been poisoned with TCDD and had more than six thousand times the usual concentration in his body. This was the highest dioxin level ever measured in a human being.

SOFT-TISSUE SARCOMA AND MALIGNANT LYMPHOMA

Soft-tissue sarcoma was the first "signal" type of tumor for cancer risk for persons who had sprayed with phenoxy herbicides or used chlorophenols for conserving wood. However, as it turned out, other tumor types were also related to these types of chemicals. In fact, epidemiological evidence and laboratory studies eventually showed that the dioxin contamination TCDD increased all types of cancer. This led the WHO-linked organization, the International Agency for Research on Cancer (IARC), to classify TCDD as a complete human carcinogen in Group I in 1997.[35] However, until that decision, many things occurred on the troublesome journey to publicly recognizing a clearly harmful and carcinogenic chemical; even today, the decision by the WHO is not accepted by all of industry and its allied experts.

Going back to my own experiences, our research group managed to show that persons who used phenoxyacetic acids and chlorophenols had an increased risk for not only soft-tissue sarcoma but also malignant lymphoma, both Hodgkin's disease and non-Hodgkin lymphoma (NHL). In May 1978, I met a patient with a tumor in his left thigh who was admitted to the Department of Oncology at the University Hospital in Umeå, Sweden. The clinical picture was similar to that of a soft-tissue sarcoma. Furthermore, this male patient reported a massive exposure to phenoxyacetic acids. Histopathological examination showed, however, NHL. All male patients with the same diagnosis admitted to our department during January through September 1978, a total of seventeen cases, were asked about their occupational history. Exposure to phenoxyacetic acids or chlorophenols was reported by eleven patients.[36]

This clinical observation initiated further epidemiological studies on malignant lymphoma by our research group. We performed three major studies, and the overall findings confirmed my early clinical observation. Similar results were found in other studies worldwide, among them on inhabitants in the Seveso area that was contaminated with dioxins in a factory accident in 1976. The aim of this chapter, however, is not to give a scientific review of the evidence for a carcinogenic effect from these chemicals, as such overviews can be found elsewhere, but to show the reaction of industry when honest science exposes toxic dangers.

Immunosuppression is an established risk factor for NHL. Most of the chemicals discussed here have immunosuppressive effects. A very high risk of NHL has been found in patients after organ transplants, and the risk increase is largest during the first years after transplantation. There is also a link between immunosuppression and some viruses; the Epstein-Barr virus (EBV) has been suggested as one explanation.[37] Also, other chemicals with immunosuppressive properties such as polychlorinated biphenyls (PCBs) increase the risk for NHL, especially together with EBV.

Interest in the etiology of NHL was strengthened by an observed substantial increase in the incidence of the disease from the 1960s to the 1980s, reported from most countries with reliable cancer registries. However, this increase clearly leveled off in many countries in the early 1990s, (i.e., in Sweden, Denmark, and the United States). We postulated that the changing incidence may reflect changes in environmental risk factors, such as the ban of use of 2,4,5-T, chlorophenols, and also PCBs.[38] This has been reflected by declining environmental levels, for instance of dioxins and PCBs since the 1980s. However, in recent years there is somewhat increasing incidence of NHL for unknown reasons.[39]

Most of the chemicals discussed here were introduced during or shortly after the Second World War. Exposure to the population increased until restrictions during the 1970s, for example, 2,4,5-T, chlorophenols and PCBs. The highest exposure occurred during the 1970s for persistent organic pollutants such as dioxins, chlorophenols, and PCBs. After that, the concentrations in the environment, and thus also in the food chain, declined although the decline has leveled off since the 1990s.

The Swedish studies on pesticide exposure as a risk factor for NHL were the first epidemiological studies in this area and initiated similar research in other countries. These results have been reviewed in many papers and pesticide exposure is now an established risk factor for NHL.[40, 41] Epidemiologic evidence indicates that TCDD increases the risk for malignant lymphoma and also for all cancers combined. Higher risks are present in several studies for NHL and soft-tissue sarcoma. It is, as concluded by the WHO, unlikely that these findings are due to chance and, as mentioned above, TCDD was classified as a Group I complete human carcinogen by the IARC in 1997.[42]

CONTROVERSY

Our studies have been criticized by different people, including chemical industry employees and the industry's allied experts, all of whom have postulated various *ad hoc* hypotheses as explanations for the results.[43] These *ad hoc* hypotheses could be easily rejected by us with reference to the papers themselves. This is, however, an almost impossible task since it is time-consuming and not all editors are willing to give space to such rebuttals. Thus, such rumors to dismiss the results tend to gain their own lives, propagated by individuals and organizations whose agendas are not disclosed.

THE SWEDISH EPA

The Swedish Environmental Protection Agency (EPA) had defended the use of phenoxyacetic acids in forests, and its opinion was that no health hazards existed.[44] The Swedish decision in 1977 to ban the use of 2,4,5-T and thus Hormoslyr® was in opposition to the opinion of the Swedish EPA, an opinion based also on a symposium arranged and paid for by Produktkontrollbyrån at the Swedish EPA.[45] However, the toxic effects of TCDD contaminating 2,4,5-T had clearly been demonstrated in the report by the Swedish EPA already in 1974.[46]

AGENT ORANGE

The Vietnam War ended in 1975. Large quantities of Agent Orange had been used to defoliate the vegetation in South Vietnam in order to make it easier to find Viet Cong guerillas but also to diminish their food supply. Spraying was mainly done by aircraft and occurred during 1962–1970.[47] Estimates suggest that about 170 kilograms of dioxins were sprayed over South Vietnam.

The use of 2,4,5-T was banned in the United States in the early 1980s, after legal negotiations. Dow Chemical Company defended the product as a representative for industry.[48] Our studies at that time were part of the underlying documents considered in reaching the verdict. At that time, I had my first personal experience that university scientists could be hired by industry to present misleading evidence from published studies to support the industry view that products were not harmful.[49]

In the United States, returning Vietnam veterans reported an unusually high incidence of health problems, such as cancer, diabetes, and birth defects in their children. These reports gave rise to the Agent Orange trial in 1984.[50] With other manufacturers of Agent Orange, Dow Chemical was again one of the defendants. Our studies were used again and the data could not be disqualified. The trial ended with a settlement whereby the chemical companies had to create a fund for compensation of Vietnam veterans with certain diseases, such as STS and malignant lymphoma, diseases that we had associated with exposure to phenoxyacetic acids.[51]

In Australia, an intense debate about health problems among returning Vietnam veterans resulted in the establishment, on May 13, 1983, of a Royal Commission to investigate the issue. The commission presented its report in 1985 and concluded that Agent Orange did not cause any health problems.[52] The concluding statements initiated an intense critique, which increased when it was revealed that volume four of the report on cancer risks from Agent Orange contained manipulated and misinterpreted data from our published studies and other publications. After scrutinizing the commission's report and comparing it with the submission by the chemical company Monsanto,[53] we showed that this part of the report was an almost verbatim copy of the Monsanto submission. Monsanto was one of the largest manufacturers of chlorinated phenols and phenoxyacetic acids, but here also represented other companies. The commission did not acknowledge in the report that the Monsanto submission had been used: this fact was revealed only after comparing the documents.

The commission's views, as provided by Monsanto's counsel, were supported by Professor Richard Doll in a letter to the Commissioner, Justice Evatt:

> [Dr. Hardell's] conclusions cannot be sustained and in my opinion, his work should no longer be cited as scientific evidence. It is clear, too, from your review of the published evidence relating to 2,4-D and 2,4,5-T (the phenoxy herbicides in question) that there is no reason to suppose that they are carcinogenic in laboratory animals and that even TCDD (dioxin), which has been postulated to be a dangerous contaminant of the herbicides, is at the most, only

weakly and inconsistently carcinogenic in animal experiments. I am sorry only that your review has had to be published in book form and not in a scientific journal, as books are so much less readily available to the majority of scientists. I am sure, however, that it will be widely quoted and that it will come to be regarded as the definitive work on the subject.[54]

The late Professor Olav Axelson at the University Hospital in Linköping had been my tutor and much involved in the controversy about the research results. He and I made a summary of the worst falsifications in the Royal Commission's report and sent it to the Governor General of Australia.[55] The Department of Veterans Affairs in Australia admitted in its reply that the commission had erred on several points, for example: in the manipulation of exposure data to suggest no risk increase or lower risk estimates than in the published results.[56] Regarding the manipulation of published data by the Royal Commission, or rather by Monsanto, in order to "demonstrate" so-called observational bias, the Department of Veterans Affairs concluded that "Dr. Hardell's complaint is justified . . . The analysis given in the Report is not correct."[57] Also, a number of other issues were admitted to be wrong in the commission's report.

It was at that time—both surprising and unclear—why the well-known epidemiologist Professor Doll could be so wrong about the carcinogenicity of phenoxyacetic acids and contaminating dioxins, and support a report with almost verbatim enclosure of industry-manipulated scientific data. It was not until later it was revealed[58] that Doll at that time was secretly hired as a consultant for Monsanto with the fee of $1,000 USD per day, later increased to $1,500 USD, as discussed elsewhere in this book.[59-63] Certainly Doll's behavior was not in the interest of protecting public health but to protect industry profits. It was dishonest of him not to reveal his Monsanto consultancy when he wrote his inflammatory letter to the Royal Commission—which was then quoted in countless newspapers. The scientific debate would clearly have been more balanced and truthful had Doll's affiliations been known.

AGENT ORANGE AND ITS ASSOCIATED DIOXINS: ASSESSMENT OF A CONTROVERSY

The advice by Professor Doll that the commission's conclusions should be "readily available" and "widely quoted" was adopted by two of the commission's consultants, A. L. Young and G. M. Reggiani. Dr. Young was involved in the US Air Force's investigation into Agent Orange and dioxin.[64] Dr. Reggiani was a consultant to Hoffman-La Roche in Basel, Switzerland, with particular responsibilities in relation to the company's involvement in the 1976 Seveso dioxin accident.[65]

They edited a book *Agent Orange and its Associated Dioxin: Assessment of a Controversy,* thereby echoing the content of the Royal Commission's report without any critical evaluation of the scientific findings.[66]

Interestingly, Chapter 7 of the book, "Soft Tissue Sarcoma: Law, Science and Logic," was written by Mr. Barry O'Keefe, who had served as attorney for Monsanto in the cross-examinations before the Royal Commission. Mr. O'Keefe reiterated in that chapter Monsanto's manipulated and falsified data from our studies. At that time, he had access to our rebuttal[67] and the reply by the Department of Veterans Affairs in Australia admitting that our complaints were justified.[68]

MEDICINE AT WAR

Some years after the Royal Commission, two Australian professors of history, Brendan O'Keefe and F. B. Smith, wrote a book claiming to give the "true" history of Agent Orange in the Vietnam War.[69] How far this book was from historical truth has been explored in more detail elsewhere by myself and others.[70] The two authors reiterated the data manipulated by Monsanto, mixed results from different studies, and did not critically review the sources. The book is not a historical document but an uncritical defense of a highly ranked and later much-criticized jurist, Justice Phillip Evatt, who had been in charge of the work of the Royal Commission. Instead, a thorough and objective search for different original sources should have been made, and the questionable role of the Royal Commission would have been worth documenting for the future.

In the book, Professor Smith cited Franklin D. Roosevelt: "Repetition does not transform a lie into truth." This is a wise rule, too often forgotten: both O'Keefe and Smith should have adopted it themselves.

THE SWEDISH AFTERMATH

In the fall of 2001, a group of Swedish scientists at the Karolinska Institute (KI), Hans-Olov Adami, Anders Ekbom, Magnus Ingelman-Sundberg, Anders Ahlbom, and one researcher in Lund, Lars Hagmar, initiated an attack in a leading Swedish daily newspaper on other researchers, including myself, who had been reporting on the association between cancer and exposure to various toxic and physical agents (see also chapter 5).[71,72] These *ad hoc* statements on a number of studies of environmental carcinogens, including our studies on pesticides, lacked academic cogency. The article was first published in a leading Swedish newspaper and was rebutted in a peer-reviewed journal,[73] and later discussed in more detail.[74]

Thereafter, one of the authors of the original newspaper article, Professor Hans-Olov Adami, together with Jack Mandel, an epidemiologist working for the US consultancy firm Exponent, Inc.,[75] and Dimitrios Trichopoulos, Professor Emeritus of Epidemiology at Harvard, went to the Dioxin 2001 conference in Korea and gave oral presentations. Together they presented the case for the thesis that dioxins are not associated with cancer in humans. The presentations each gave a "clean bill of health" to dioxin.[76–78] Although no new research was presented, statements casting doubt on the carcinogenicity were made challenging the fact that TCDD had been classified in 1997 as a human carcinogen of Group I by IARC.[79]

Exponent had hired Adami and Trichopoulos and coordinated the presentations on behalf of an unnamed client[80] While Mandel appeared as an employee of Exponent, Adami and Trichopoulos only quoted their academic affiliations, which would infer that they were *independent* researchers rather than consultants hired by Exponent and paid for by some of Exponent's clients. The aim of this remanufacturing of doubt was the ongoing dioxin review process held at the US Environmental Protection Agency.

In another paper by Adami et al.,[81] the authors stated: "There is persuasive evidence that TCDD at low levels is not carcinogenic to human beings and that it may not be carcinogenic even at high levels." This paper was also produced for Exponent. The paper, together with another on other end points, was delivered to be included in the EPA review, for which the vice president of Exponent, Dennis Paustenbach, was on the Science Advisory Board. Exponent's activities on dioxin at the time included a number of other consultants from Exponent giving oral and poster presentations, which again sowed doubt about health effects from dioxins at the Dioxin 2001 conference.[82–87] A couple of years later, a review article was published including some of these authors.[88] They concluded that "The long-term accumulation of negative, weak, and inconsistent findings suggests that TCDD eventually will be recognized as not carcinogenic for humans." This statement was not based on the scientific evidence including the IARC evaluation in 1997 of TCDD as a complete human carcinogen, Group 1.[89]

Litigation on health risks from herbicides in Israel led to a Monsanto website on Roundup (the herbicide glyphosate), see reference[90] that cited Adami. Via a telephone number on this website, an "unpublished reference" in Monsanto's possession was found, in which Adami and his associate Professor Trichopoulos stated regarding the study[91] that "errors in exposure assessment, or chance . . . are likely explanations for the weak glyphosate/NHL association."[92] This statement, posted on the above website, reemerged, as a word-for-word download, without attribution of the source, as a major part of an expert opinion by the chief toxicologist of the Israeli Ministry of Health to the Israeli Supreme Court.[93, 94]

Our study, cited by Adami and Trichopoulos, had been published in the peer-reviewed scientific journal *Cancer*.[95] This was followed by our next study on this topic that showed a statistically significant increased risk for non-Hodg-kin lymphoma associated with exposure to glyphosate as well as phenoxyacetic acids.[96] In March 2015, IARC assessed the carcinogenicity of some pesticides including glyphosate.[97] It was concluded that case-control studies of occupational exposure in the United States,[98] Canada,[99] and Sweden[100] increased the risk for non-Hodgkin lymphoma that persisted after adjustment for exposure to other pesticides. There was sufficient evidence of carcinogenicity in animals and glyphosate was classified as *probably carcinogenic to humans*, Group 2A, by the working group.[101]

The Swedish Cancer Society has for a long time funded Adami's appointment as a cancer researcher. Adami's research team has gained also substantial grants from the society over the years. The main source of this money is the Swedish population. Some of the aims of funds held by the Swedish Cancer Society are *to fund research on different risk factors and improve the possibilities of preventing cancer.* This was especially the situation for Adami's research position paid by the Swedish Cancer Fund for years. His activities, however, seem to have been mainly concerned with casting doubt concerning environmental cancer risks. The Swedish Cancer Society has made no move to require Professor Adami to publicly disclose his potential conflicts of interest.

MOTOROLA, THE SWEDISH RADIATION PROTECTION AGENCY, INTERNATIONAL EPIDEMIOLOGY INSTITUTE, BOICE AND MCLAUGHLIN

Alongside my continuing work on pesticides and dioxins, I and my research group in Sweden moved on to look at the biological effect of mobile and cordless phones. Our research was the first to show a clear association between the use of mobile or cordless phones and brain tumors. These studies were followed by others, by us, and other research groups, and in summary there is consistent evidence of an increased risk for glioma and acoustic neuroma associated with use of wireless phones. Especially worrying in the study from our group, is the finding of highest risk in people whose first use of a mobile phone is before the age of twenty, as well as worse prognosis for the most malignant brain tumor (glioblastoma) among wireless phone users. The current guideline for exposure to microwaves from wireless phones is not safe and needs to be revised.

These results have not been without dispute by certain scientists and some individuals from governmental bodies. In 2002, the Swedish Radiation Protection Authority (SSI; now Swedish Radiation Safety Authority, SSM) hired two US epidemiologists to review published epidemiological studies on the relationship between the use of cellular telephones and cancer risk. They were Dr. John D. Boice, Jr. and Dr. Joseph K. McLaughlin from the private International Epidemiology Institute (IEI). Boice and McLaughlin claimed in their review,[102] that no consistent evidence has been observed for increased risk of brain tumors, including glioma and acoustic neuroma, and mobile phone use. Featuring in their review was a heavily critical appraisal of one of our papers[103] that concluded an association between cellular telephones and certain brain tumors.

However, Boice and McLaughlin were coauthors of some of the studies in their own "independent" review and reserved their most positive words for their own studies, which showed no association between cellular telephones and certain tumor types. Despite the fact that IEI was a cofounder of their studies, cited in the review, Boice and McLaughlin made no statements of any conflict of interest in their report. In fact, the Danish cohort study on mobile users has been evaluated to be inconclusive due to serious methodological problems. For overview and discussion see Söderqvist et al.[104]

The director general of SSI at that time, Lars-Erik Holm, had earlier published several papers with John Boice. Also, it appears that the International Epidemiology Institute (IEI) was—at the time of the SSI review—involved in a cellular phone and brain tumor litigation in the United States on behalf of the defendants, Motorola.[105] The connection was traced by a fax number that appeared on the papers quoting the reviewers' comments to the journal that was considering for publication the Hardell et al. article on cellular telephones and the association with brain tumors. The information that the paper was under review had been communicated to the defendants in a letter from Mr. Tom Watson, defendant lawyer for Motorola, dated January 18, 2002, on referee comments from a fax from International Epidemiology Institute dated 11/19/01,[106] a violation of the confidentiality of the review process. These and other circumstances on this issue have been reviewed by us.[107, 108]

A number of research projects have taken place at the Karolinska Institute, Stockholm, with the participation of Boice and McLaughlin, with at least funding through IEI. One of the studies was published in the *British Medical Journal*,[109] with Hans-Olov Adami as a coauthor. A cohort of Swedish women with breast implants was studied with regard to connective tissue disease. No risk was found. Thanks to strict rules of stating conflicts of interest at that time in the *British Medical Journal*, it was seen that the project was initiated by IEI, and that the funding from IEI was on behalf of Dow Corning Corporation, producer of silicone breast implants. Other examples are studies concerning breast implants and cancer risk.[110, 111]

MOBILE PHONES, BRAIN TUMORS, AND THE INTERPHONE STUDY

The overall results from the Interphone study group on brain tumor risk from use of mobile phones were published with delay in 2010, that is six years after the final inclusion of subjects into the study in 2004.[112] These studies were performed in thirteen countries and used a common protocol. The study center was the International Agency for Research on Cancer (IARC) in Lyon, France, and a substantial amount of the grants came from the telecom industry. Also, according to the contract, the industry had full access to the results one week before publication. Following completion, results from eight of the participating countries were published first and the rest held in abeyance. The period for inclusion of cases was 1999–2004, somewhat varying for different countries, and it is unclear why the final results took several years to publish. Certainly the Interphone study group had a high responsibility to publish its overall results promptly, not least from a public health perspective.

On 31 May, 2011, the International Agency for Research on Cancer (IARC) at WHO categorized radiofrequency (RF) radiation from mobile phones and from other devices that emit similar non-ionizing electromagnetic fields, as a Group 2B (i.e., a "possible" human carcinogen).[113, 114] The IARC decision on mobile phones was based mainly on two sets of human case-control studies on brain tumor risk; our studies from Sweden,[115–117] and the IARC Interphone study.[118–120] Both provided complementary and supportive results on positive associations between two types of brain tumors; glioma and acoustic neuroma, and exposure to RF radiation from wireless phones.

It should be pointed out that in the Swedish part of the Interphone studies, one of the authors, Anders Ahlbom at Karolinska Institute, had stated, even before the study started, that an asserted association between cellular telephones and brain tumors is "biologically bizarre."[121] This statement might preclude him from objectivity in his own investigation and has already been rebutted.[122] Laboratory studies indicated that there are, in fact, biological mechanisms that could link exposure to the development of diseases such as brain tumors. See for example the REFLEX study.[123]

Interestingly, one of the authors of the "opinion" letter (see above "The Swedish Aftermath"), Professor Adami, together with Professor Trichopoulos, both at Harvard, stated in an editorial[124] in the same issue of the *New England Journal of Medicine* that published a US study on mobile phone use and brain tumors by Inskip and coworkers[125] that ... "the use of cellular telephones does not detectably increase the risk of brain tumors" and that "This study allays fears raised by alarmist reports that the use of cellular telephones causes cancer." This statement went far beyond what was scientifically defensible; for example, the longest duration for use of mobile phone was only up to five years and there was no data with ten years latency (time from first use until tumor diagnosis) presented. Maybe this editorial was biased by unreported conflicts of interest among the authors.[126, 127]

Another person who participated in the Swedish part of the Interphone studies, Maria Feychting, also at Karolinska Institute, made a most remarkable comment on our case-control studies, wondering "if the questions really were placed in the same way to cases and controls."[128] This comment seems to cast doubt on Feychting's scientific credibility and the quality of her own research methods. Certainly these circumstances show how economic and other undisclosed interests may influence this research area and preclude objective risk evaluation. Still, these attacks on our research are few in an international perspective and almost exclusively made by a few Swedish researchers with their "not always disclosed" own conflicts of interest.[129] This type of unfounded critique needs to be rebutted. Remarkably, most of this critique is national in Sweden and has not much international bearing.[130–132]

As with Sir Richard Doll, when time goes by, ties to industry creating at least intellectual bias to greenwash cancer risks are often revealed. The moral and ethical questions raised relate to whether or not laypeople should have to pay the price during the silence with impaired health.

THE SWEDISH CANCER SOCIETY, EXPONENT, AND VESTED INTERESTS

It seems as if Hans-Olov Adami has continued his career after the "opinion" letter downplaying the association between pesticide exposure and cancer; he now publishes openly with Exponent and is happy to be sponsored by the chemical industry. Thus, in a review publication on pesticides and prostate cancer the authors state that "Existing evidence does not point to any pesticide as satisfying widely used guidelines for establishing causation." The study was supported by CropLife America and the American Chemistry Council.[133]

In a review on non-Hodgkin lymphoma, sponsored by Syngenta, a firm producing insecticides and fungicides, Adami stated, together with coauthors from Exponent, that "Studies on occupational and environmental exposure (e.g., pesticides, solvents) have produced no consistent pattern of significant associations."[134] Obviously, such statements are not in agreement with the existing literature, but can be used to justify further exposure to people and as a defense in product liability, and are inconsistent with the evaluation at IARC (see above).[135]

Another review by Adami and others concerned atrazine and cancer risk;[136] the authors concluded the following:

> We reviewed the Environmental Protection Agency and Panel reports in the context of all the epidemiologic studies on the specific cancers of interest. A weight-of-evidence approach leads to the conclusion that there is no causal association between atrazine and cancer and that occasional positive results can be attributed to bias or chance. Atrazine appears to be a good candidate for a category of herbicides with a probable absence of cancer risk. Atrazine should be treated for regulatory and public health purposes as an agent unlikely to pose a cancer risk to humans.

Atrazine is suggested to be an endocrine disruptor and it was banned in the European Union in 2004 because of persistent groundwater contamination.

In a review on TCDD and prostate cancer risk[137] it was concluded that "Overall, epidemiologic research offers no consistent or convincing evidence of a causal relationship between exposure to Agent Orange or TCDD and prostate cancer."

Of special interest is the conflict of interest statement:

> Conflict of interest Drs. Chang and Mandel are employed by Exponent, Inc., a for-profit corporation that provides engineering and scientific consulting services. All of the authors have consulted with private and government organizations on the health impacts of environmental and occupational exposures, including Agent Orange and TCDD. This independent scientific review was financially supported by the Dow Chemical Company and Monsanto Company.

Another review relates to perfluorooctanoate (PFOA) and perfluorooctanesulfonate (PFOS).[138] The authors concluded the following:

> Given that occupational exposure to PFOA and PFOS is one to two orders of magnitude higher than environmental exposure, the discrepant positive findings are likely due to chance, confounding, and/or bias. Taken together, the epidemiologic evidence does not support the hypothesis of a causal association between PFOA or PFOS exposure and cancer in humans.

This conclusion is in contrast with a study on tissue concentrations of these substances among prostate cancer cases and population-based controls concluding that: "The analyzed PFAAs (perfluorinated alkyl acids) yielded statistically significant higher ORs (odds ratios) in cases with a first degree relative reporting prostate cancer . . . The results showed a higher risk for prostate cancer in cases with heredity as a risk factor."[139]

According to the Swedish Cancer Register, the age-standardized cancer incidence per 100,000 subjects has increased substantially since 1970.[140] The number of new cancer victims was at an all time-high in 2013, in total 61,297 patients (31,664 men, 29,633 women) compared with 28,497 in 1970. Smoking, diet, and physical activity (i.e., personal risk factors), are usually blamed. Environmental risk factors are downplayed and "no causal association" seems to be the message by Adami and associates. It is a moral and ethical question if the money to Adami by the Swedish Cancer Fund aimed at "fund research on different risk factors and improve the possibilities of preventing cancer" were fully used correctly. In retrospect, the opposite, as exemplified above, seems to be the case.

Among the different diseases associated with dioxin exposure is diabetes mellitus.[141–144] See also review by Institute of Medicine in USA.[145] Adami was coauthor among other persons (e.g., from Exponent), in a recent review on the dioxin type TCDD and the risk of diabetes mellitus.[146] The work was financially supported by the Dow Chemical Company and Monsanto Company and the authors concluded that "the available data do not indicate that increasing TCDD exposure is associated with an increased risk of DM [diabetes mellitus]."[147] Thus, Hans-Olov Adami together with Exponent, the industry, and other allied experts seems to continue to downgrade the risk of potentially toxic agents to humans.

Regarding conflict of interest and Anders Ahlbom at Karolinska Institute, important conflicts were revealed by *Microwave News*[148] a few days before the May 2011 meeting of IARC in Lyon, France.[149, 150] Ahlbom was appointed as chair of the IARC epidemiology group but was then dismissed by the IARC when others disclosed his obvious conflict of interest and his nondisclosure of his engagement on the board of a consulting firm in Brussels working with the telecom industry. Furthermore, curiously enough, he did not state this obvious conflict of interest in a later editorial in the *British Medical Journal* on mobile phones and cancer.[151]

THE PRECAUTIONARY PRINCIPLE

Preventing hazards from known risks is relatively easy (e.g., banning smoking or the use of asbestos). However, it would have needed a precautionary approach to avoid exposure to asbestos in the 1930s to 1950s or tobacco smoke already in the 1930s because evidence of the carcinogenic risks was not sufficient. On the other hand, such precaution would have saved many lives. *Prevention* is justified to restrict exposure to known causes (i.e., an IARC Group I carcinogen), whereas *precaution* is necessary to restrict exposure to suspected or less clear risk factors (i.e., IARC Group 2A or 2B carcinogen).

Vested interests constitute the main reason for ignoring the precautionary principle.[152, 153] Furthermore, in these circumstances, society gets an unbalanced and unfair view of scientific results. Thus, objective information is essential so that people can prudently avoid exposure. To conceal scientific evidence and even denigrate research groups, whose results may be in conflict with corporate or orthodox thinking, makes such personal precautions almost impossible. Furthermore, such behavior makes cancer prevention the privilege of the educated elite who have easier access to information sources and are able to come to their own conclusions.

Research on risk factors for cancer does not have the glamour associated with the development of complicated and profitable new drugs for cancer treatment. But cancer prevention, on the other hand, is cost-effective, and research to identify risk factors should be of equal importance to laboratory studies in molecular biology. As well, while cancer patients are effective pressure groups for better patient care and treatment, individuals avoiding cancer due to preventive measurements are clinically invisible and so have no voice to protest against cancer policy. When we consider the precautionary principle and while planning policy, these cultural, economic, and political factors should be given consideration alongside the scientific facts.

Chapter 4

LOSING THE WAR ON CANCER

Richard Clapp

"Why, sometimes I've believed as many as six impossible things before breakfast."
Lewis Carroll, *Alice in Wonderland*

Global cancer patterns and approaches to the care and treatment of cancer patients are continually changing. Physicians and pharmaceutical companies in relatively wealthy countries now proclaim a new era in which some forms of cancer can be controlled by "personalized care." The claim is that individually targeted chemotherapy can maintain patients with cancer as a chronic, less fatal disease. Only recently, has the cost of this kind of long-term treatment become a public concern. In the United States, Dr. Richard Besser recently reported on *ABC News* that "eleven of the twelve cancer drugs the Food and Drug Administration approved for fighting cancer in 2012 were priced at more than $100,000 per year, double the average annual household income, according to a report by the *Journal of the National Cancer Institute* . . . top-tier cancer drugs cost twice as much in the United States as they do in parts of Europe, China, Canada, and the United Kingdom, where the government sets a limit on pricing."[1]

These claims echo similar overly optimistic projections from thirty-five years ago, during the early years of the "war on cancer." A French documentary film produced in 2006 contains this unusually frank exchange:

Narrator: "The war goes on. Cancer, it seems, could become a chronic illness, with disastrous consequences for public health spending. But there's one thing all generals know. To keep waging war, you need good propaganda."

Robert Weinberg, PhD, Member, Whitehead Institute for Biomedical Research, Professor of Biology, MIT, Cambridge (USA): "Why didn't we tell people in 1980 that we have no idea when these basic discoveries are going to lead to cures? It's very simple. If we would have told people in 1980 that our discoveries would not lead to cures. They would have said 'well, let's shut down this entire enterprise.' And where would we be now in the year 2005? Exactly where we were in 1975. Sometimes one has to tell good stories to keep things going. Do I feel bad that we told a good story in 1980? Absolutely not. It was justified because we realized that people would need to be patient." (From *War on Cancer*, a production of Point du Jour, Les Productions Virage, 2006).

Given these recent trends and rationalizations, the motivation for preventing cancer continues to be the rising global incidence and burden of cancer on families and communities. According to the International Agency for Research on Cancer (IARC), the number of cases of cancer in the world doubled in the thirty years between 1975 and 2005 and is expected to double again in the next twenty-five years.[2] In 2013, IARC estimated there were 14.1 million new cases and 8.2 million deaths due to cancer around the world in the previous year, 2012. This is an increase of 11 percent in new cases and 8 percent in cancer deaths since the previous estimates in 2008. According to the 2013 report, the leading cancer types, excluding non-melanoma skin cancer, were cancers of the lung, breast, and colon/rectum, accounting for more than one-third of the new cases. Breast cancer is rapidly increasing, with 1.7 million new cases diagnosed in 2012, a 20 percent increase over 2008. Lung cancer was the leading cause of cancer death because it is so difficult to treat.

IARC authors also estimated the prevalence of cancer in geographic areas and levels of development and demonstrated large differences in different parts of the world.[3] The highest overall prevalence as a percentage of population is in Australia and New Zealand, Western Europe, and North America. The countries in these areas are also characterized by having a "very high human development index." The cancers that contribute the largest numbers of prevalent cases are breast, prostate, and colorectum, followed by lung and bladder cancers. The countries that are characterized by having a "high human development index," which are primarily in Central and South America and Eastern Europe, have the largest number of prevalent cases from the same three types—breast, prostate, and colorectum—followed by uterine cervix and lung cancers. Countries characterized by having a "medium human development index," which includes most of Africa, South Asia, and Eastern Asia, have the largest number of prevalent cases contributed by breast, uterine cervix, and colorectum cancer, followed by stomach and lung cancer. Because of the large size of the population in these countries, they contribute nearly two-thirds of the total global cancer prevalence.

Finally, in countries characterized by having a "low human development index," which are primarily in sub-Saharan Africa, the largest numbers of prevalent cases are of the uterine cervix, breast, Kaposi sarcoma, and liver cancer, followed by prostate and colorectum cancers.

In 2008, IARC estimated that only about 20 percent of the world population was covered by cancer registries of reasonable quality and completeness. This has changed little in the past five years. As a result, the global cancer patterns must be estimated by extrapolating from areas with fairly accurate cancer incidence data to the rest of the world.

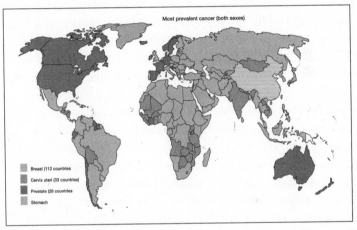

Figure 1: Most prevalent cancer both sexes. Source: Bray F, Ren J-S, Masuyer E., et al.[4]

The picture is only slightly better with respect to cancer death patterns, because high quality cause of death information is available for only about a third of the world's population.

For those regions with reasonably complete cancer incidence data,[5] the following patterns are noteworthy. In the United Kingdom for the years 2003–2007, the age-standardized rate for males was 284.8 per 100,000 and the leading types were prostate cancer (65.0 per 100,000), followed by trachea, bronchus and lung (39.1 per 100,000), and colorectum (35.4 per 100,000). In UK females, the age-standardized rate was 250.3 per 100,000 and the leading types were breast cancer (85.4 per 100,000), followed by trachea, bronchus and lung (23.6 per 100,000), and colorectum (22.7 per 100,000). In the combined data for forty-two US states, the age-standardized rate in males was 362.3 per 100,000 and the leading types were cancer of the prostate (105.0 per 100,000), followed by trachea, bronchus and lung (53.5 per 100,000), and colorectum (34.8 per 100,000). In US females, the age-standardized rate was 283.8 per 100,000 and the leading types were breast cancer (85.3 per 100,000), followed by trachea, bronchus and lung (36.4 per 100,000), and colorectum (25.6 per 100,000). In Western Australia, the age-standardized rate for males was 364.9 per 100,000 and the leading types were prostate cancer (105.9 per 100,000), followed by melanoma of skin (43.6 per 100,000), and trachea, bronchus, and lung (35.7 per 100,000). In Western Australian females, the age-standardized rate was 267.0 per 100,000 and the leading types were breast cancer (81.7 per 100,000), followed by melanoma of skin (29.7 per 100,000) and colorectum (29.1 per 100,000).

In other regions with less complete cancer incidence data, the patterns are quite different. For example, in Costa Rica, the age-standardized rate for males was 182.6 per 100,000 and the leading sites were prostate cancer (53.9 per 100,000), followed by stomach cancer (26.5 per 100,000) and colorectum (14.6 per 100,000). In Costa Rican females, the age-standardized rate was 161.8 per 100,000 and the leading sites were breast cancer (39.6 per 100,000), followed by stomach cancer (15.0 per 100,000), and cancer of the uterine cervix (13.9 per 100,000). In China, the age-standardized rate in Shanghai City males was 202.8 per 100,000 and the leading sites were trachea, bronchus, and lung (40.9 per 100,000), followed by colorectum (27.6 per 100,000) and stomach cancer (26.6 per 100,000). In Shanghai City females, the age-standardized rate was 177.5 per 100,000 and the leading sites were breast cancer (39.2 per 100,000), followed by colorectum (23.1 per 100,000) and trachea, bronchus and lung (18.1 per 100,000). In Uganda, the age-standardized rate for Kyadondo County males was 177.3 per 100,000 and the leading sites were prostate cancer (42.5 per 100,000), followed by Kaposi sarcoma (29.5 per 100,000) and cancer of the oesophagus (15.6 per 100,000). In Kyadondo County females, the age-standardized rate was 212.2 per 100,000 and the leading sites were cancer of the uterine cervix (54.3 per 100,000), followed by breast cancer (32.9 per 100,000), and Kaposi sarcoma (20.2 per 100,000).

GLOBAL TRENDS AND OPPORTUNITIES FOR PREVENTION

With these data limitations and differential patterns, one wonders if it is possible to draw any conclusions about the trends in cancer in the world today. One of the most salient analyses, by Annie Sasco,[6] viewed the changing global pattern of cancer in the context of the globalization trends in the twenty-first century. Sasco implicitly recognizes that we are now in the "planetary phase of civilization,"[7] meaning that we are in a historical transition from a world of a few highly developed consumerist economies, many under-resourced struggling economies, and inequitable distribution of wealth, to a world of increased global connectivity with rapid communication and transportation of goods and people. As a result, the patterns of cancer in many of the intermediate and developing countries are beginning to reflect the patterns observed in the wealthy countries. To the extent that data are available, it appears that overall cancer incidence and mortality are beginning to level off in the past few years in the OECD countries. The exception to this pattern is in some cancers that have occupational and environmental causes, such as kidney cancer and melanoma of the skin, and viral causes, such as liver cancer. In the intermediate and less developed countries, rates of lung cancer in males and breast cancer in females seem to be rising most rapidly.

The following figure summarizes the estimated new cases and deaths worldwide and grouped by broad categories of countries in 2008 (Figure 2):

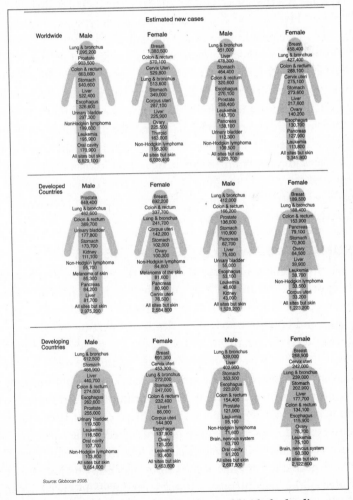

Figure 2. Estimated new cancer cases and deaths worldwide for leading cancer sites by level of economic development, 2008.

Sasco pointed out that the three broad groups of factors that are generally invoked to explain the changing patterns of cancer are genetic factors, "lifestyle" factors, and environmental factors. She notes that in spite of the inordinate attention paid to recent discoveries of mutated and inherited cancer genes, these are responsible for less than 10 percent of all cancers, given the current level of knowledge. Among lifestyle factors, she includes tobacco products and cigarette smoking, which she estimates cause well over 1 million cancer deaths in the world each year, along with alcohol, diet, reproductive factors, obesity, and ultraviolet light exposure as major contributors to cancer. In the group of factors typically referred to as "environmental," she includes chemical, biological, and physical factors, mostly of human origin, that occur in workplaces and communities where people are exposed through the air, water, or contaminated soil. She discusses the difficulty in attributing specific proportions of cancer due to specific factors and, further, states that these proportions will differ in different populations with differing place-time characteristics. At present, however, there are well over one hundred individual substances or conditions of exposure that are known to cause cancer in humans, and hundreds more that probably or possibly cause cancer in humans based on their effects in experimental animals.[8] The challenge is to reduce human exposure to these known causes in all parts of the world, and not subject the developing countries to the same level of exposures that have contributed to the excessive rates of cancer seen in, for example, the OECD countries.

IARC SUMMARY OF WORLD CANCER TRENDS

One of the most ambitious efforts to describe the global trends in cancer mortality, the World Cancer Report, was published by IARC in 2008.[9] This report was based on cancer mortality data in the GLOBOCAN database, with all the uncertainties and limitations of cancer death certification in various countries of the world. Nevertheless, the main features of the trends and projections are as described above, with cancer mortality rates beginning to level off or decline in the high-income countries but continuing to rise in the intermediate to low-income countries in the next twenty years. Furthermore, the report notes that reduction in deaths due to occupationally induced cancers, such as lung cancer in asbestos-exposed workers, seems to have occurred in high-income countries but has not yet occurred in intermediate or low-income countries. This pattern can be expected to continue as hazardous materials and processes formerly concentrated in the high-income countries are shifted to the so-called BRICS countries (Brazil, Russia, India, China, and South Africa) in the coming years.

It is important to note that there has been, and continues to be, strong opposition to policies that would reduce occupational and environmental exposure to carcinogens in both the high-income countries and much of the rest of the world. This has been documented by others,[10] but it deserves mention as we contemplate how to reduce the global cancer burden in the future.

What emerges from the various reviews of cancer incidence and mortality data is that the global burden of illness and economic hardship from this disease is enormous and likely to rise in the next two decades or more. The World Cancer Report estimates that, by 2030, there will be 27 million cases of cancer diagnosed and 17 million cancer deaths occurring each year. Moreover, it is estimated that there will be 75 million people alive and living with cancer in that year. A substantial portion of the burden is due to avoidable causes, including known risk factors such as tobacco products, occupational and environmental exposures to carcinogens, and carcinogenic or tumor-promoting materials in consumer products. These exposures, and the political and economic forces that work to continue producing them, are described in later chapters. What is clear, from the cancer trends currently observable, is that this ongoing human tragedy deserves the highest priority in our public health and advocacy work.

Chapter 5

GREENWASHING: THE SWEDISH EXPERIENCE

Bo Walhjalt

Therefore speak I to them in parables:
because they seeing see not;
and hearing they hear not,
neither do they understand.

Matthew 13:13

Greenwashing is a term adopted for activities that obscure toxic environmental effects of industrial pollutants. Law firms, public relations (PR) companies, university researchers, and journalists are among those involved. Of primary concern are university researchers who are employed by industry but do not disclose that fact and, instead, give opinions and make statements using their university affiliations. The strategy is outlined in this chapter with examples from the chemical industry and academia.

Greenwashing may be divided into two main categories. One is the information emanating from opinion makers, especially in the United States, usually connected to conservative think tanks. The other consists of researchers who consistently defend industry views; usually they are paid to do this. It is the last category that is of interest in this chapter—greenwashers manage active anti-environment and anti-health work. A whole network of organizations is involved in this practice, from law firms to PR companies and universities. One particular concern is the relationship that exists between industry and scientists employed by universities in the evaluation of toxic hazards. Scientists can use the reputation of their universities and the work of other academics to give "a clean bill of health" to an evidently hazardous substance. Seeing the connection between scientists, industry, and academia is the key to the understanding of greenwashing.

Some articles disclosing such connections and meaning to engender a debate about greenwashing have been published in Scandinavia over the last decade.[1-11] A number of articles in the *Journal of the Swedish Medical Association* on the tobacco industry and its allies in academia have attracted particular interest— what kind of mess is hidden beneath this shining surface?

During recent years, following the activities of lobby organizations and industry-linked academics, the principles that the environmental movement stands for have been denigrated. Law firms and PR companies have earned large amounts of money by educating industry to manipulate the media and public opinion while misguiding politicians who advise the regulatory processes.

In reality, however, it is the environmental movement that represents the public interest, the interests of society for several generations into the future. Our planet is continuously being robbed of its resources and polluted while its inhabitants are being impoverished and made unhealthy. The speed of this planetary denigration differs according to geographic location. However, resources are not protected, are not increasing, and our planet is not becoming cleaner. Our heritage becomes less for every new generation and during the recent generations this impairment has accelerated.

Greenwashing means cleaning and polishing the image of pollutants in the environment and entails manipulating data in order to hide the real environmental and health damage produced by industry. The understanding of risks here is negative effects based on both empirical and theoretical grounds.[12]

In the United States, there has been a strong movement in the last couple of years to keep scientific views that don't harmonize with political priorities out from the political process. An editorial in *Science* expresses serious concerns about this development, where industrial interests supporting deregulation weigh more heavily than the public health interests.[13] The scientific question to learn what is worth knowing is thwarted by political ambitions to hide inconvenient knowledge.

During recent years, the issues that the environmental movement stands for have been regarded and treated as something unique for that group of people. Both the group and their objectives have been portrayed by the media as having an adverse effect on industry, and themselves ultimately having an adverse effect on the environment and social progress. It is claimed that these campaigning organizations are dragging us back to medievalism and destroying the progressive industrial and scientific infrastructure.

In February 2002, the verdict was announced in a much-observed environmental lawsuit between the inhabitants of Anniston, Alabama, and the chemical company Monsanto. Monsanto was found guilty. The lawsuit concerned contaminants from a factory that had manufactured polychlorinated biphenyls (PCBs). During the hearings a number of internal documents compromising Monsanto were revealed.[14] From one of these now-official documents, the goal for risk management by Monsanto is clearly explained; this is archetypal crisis management by industry for environmental and health policy in general: the year is 1969.

> ... an "ad hoc" committee was appointed to prepare a resume of the situation concerning the environmental contamination through the manufacture and use of polychlorinated biphenyls (Aroclors). The objective of the committee was to recommend action that will:
>
> - Protect continued sales and profits of Aroclors;
> - Permit continued development of new uses and sales;
> - Protect the image of the organic division and the corporation as members of the business community recognizing their responsibilities to prevent and/or control contamination of the global ecosystem.[15]

That means—business as usual, may it cost what it costs, preferably while sustaining the company image.

In 1980, the Chemical Industry Institute of Technology (CIIT) reported a study on rats exposed to formaldehyde. The CIIT changed its name in 2007 to the Hamner Institutes for Health Sciences.[16] Nasal cancer was found in the rats. For the forest and wood industry this was bad news, and industry does not like bad news. Compact fiberboard was a large industry success and at that time the board was still heavily impregnated with leaking formaldehyde. Kip Howlett,[17] at that time employed by Georgia Pacific, formulated a plan to neutralize the bad news. The goals with the plan were the same as put forward by Monsanto ten years previously—to save business and profit. The plan consisted of four components:

Finance an alternative study carefully designed to minimize the risk for unwanted results.

- Hire a researcher to give independent statements on the safety of formaldehyde.
- Attack every researcher reporting health problems caused by formaldehyde.
- Aggressively direct research on formaldehyde so as to minimize the risks from formaldehyde.[18, 19]

Independent researchers, who are actually greenwashers, give the tools to industry, such as expert statements, testimony and deposition in litigations, overviews and analysis needed for industry to fulfil its plans. Here in the CIIT's plan we again see a pattern, a model, for how industry reacts when profits are at risk.

In an article in the *Swedish Medical Journal* on the tobacco industry, the mechanism of misinformation and the systematic discredit of persons with other views are expressly pointed out: a classical example of *greenwashing*.[20]

Scrutiny of internal tobacco industry documents, now available on the Internet, reveals that Sweden and Finland were classified as "priority 1" areas in which to intensify efforts to resist tobacco control measures. In the late 1980s, Philip Morris increased its activities in Scandinavia in order to counteract penal taxation threats and marketing restrictions. Swedish scientists were engaged by the tobacco industry in the "White Coat" project, a program expected to shed doubt on research linking passive smoking to health risks. The Swedish tobacco company Swedish Match collaborated with Philip Morris in challenging measures to limit tobacco use, including the new, stricter tobacco law proposed in the early 1990s.

The tobacco industry supports a "market of abuse," while the chemical industry reveals information only under compulsion.

The Swedish Society for Nature Conservation says in an advertisement about the chemical industry: "The chemical industry has a unique work method. The test animals (human beings) are not kept in cages."[21] Thus, it may be that pesticides produced in the United States are used in Africa and appear in mother's milk in the Arctic, all illustrations of a massive human experiment.

Of the resources for research and development, 75 percent now come from industry. Industry is the largest funder of researchers with ambitions to grow in influence and power. Unfortunately, the prerequisite for all industry-funded research is to give the market what it wants because that is what has been paid for.

The Swedish minister of education during the early 2000s, Tomas Östros, was an eager advocate of this development.[22] In one issue of *Science*[23] under the heading "Karolinska, Inc," the vision of the former Head, Hans Wigzell, was reported as describing a center for business in science with connecting new companies alongside it. This means business for almost 20 million Swedish Krona. With that vision in mind, Hans-Olov Adami, a cancer epidemiologist at Uppsala University, was recruited to Karolinska, and the institution had shown a substantial growth after the move. It is also this vision that the Minister of Education Tomas Östros saw as the future.

Under the heading "Researchers need to use industry," Hans Wigzell was interviewed in the Swedish newspaper *Dagens Nyheter* (Today's News) of June 7, 2002. He said:

"At several Swedish universities this is not properly done, they have not understood what this is about. They are awaiting the cake from the government to be divided, but most interesting is the new cake to be baked, not the small slices of the old one."[24]

The industry for knowledge has a market, the large knowledge market is run by industry—*Wigzell's cake to be baked.* The small market is in the public domain and should be serving the community—*Wigzell's small slices.* What can an epidemiologist or a toxicologist offer the large market? What can they offer the small market of pieces that are financed by taxes and what can they offer the larger market that gives academic authority to business?

Frankly speaking, the different approaches of these two markets are that the cake market wants a clean bill of health for environmental pollutants, while the pieces market wants to know the risks of industry activities and products to the public and the citizen. The cake market deals with risk management and advocates the criticism of research results that show risk and what is termed *unjustified research alarm.*

Only a small amount of the money spent by industry on research is used for greenwashing issues. Greenwashing deals with PR and virtual information, not the production of new knowledge. Great effort is made in order to prevent research that might result in bad news for industry—the fewer research alarms the better. If it is not possible to prevent such research, it must be neutralized or discredited.

The private cake is growing by the day but the public pieces, ideally independent, are continuing to shrink. Who shall defend the interests of the public?

In September 2002, in the wake of a very public conflict in major Swedish newspapers, when the critical work of Lennart Hardell was attacked, the Swedish medical journal, *Medikament,* published my article "Greenwashing—an introduction."[25] The aim of this article was to illustrate the greenwashing concept related to researchers working with industry on issues concerning the environment and health without revealing their industrial connections. The article explained how these researchers, often prominent in their fields and apparently independent, tend to come up with results that are reassuring to the industry that has secretly hired them. To illustrate the problem, Hans-Olov Adami was chosen as an example. His hidden industrial ties were still not accounted for.

This very public discussion about Adami's work continued into 2003 and beyond, but, despite an increasing number of articles in the Swedish media on the greenwashing theme, there was no public discussion of the problem, despite its obvious importance for public policy. However, there seemed to have been a lot of discussions in the corridors of power. In December 2002, the association of Swedish medical writers had a meeting to which Hans-Olov Adami was invited. The subject of the meeting was: "What happened, Hans-Olov?" The meeting resulted in an article entitled "Adami's inconceivable naivety" by Monika Starendal, features editor of *Dagens Forskning*.[26]

The scene was set in the introductory paragraph:

> At a meeting with the Society of Swedish Medical Journalists shortly before Christmas Adami preferred to talk about "scandal journalism" rather than his unaccounted jobs on the side on behalf of industry. For him it was a new experience after sixteen years of faithful cooperation with Swedish medical writers to meet disturbing questions about his own role as a scientist; it was shocking to meet journalists using the methods of Hell's Angels-like threats, lies, impoliteness, and threatening e-mails.[27]

This meeting was held almost exactly one year after the first article was published, and Adami still refused to account for his industrial ties. Adami's remarks on the methods merit a note.[28] During the meeting, critical questions were few and little was learnt on the issue of conflicts of interest. Perhaps this was because, after years of faithful cooperation, some medical journalists had sunk deeply into the common medical corporatism.[29, 30] The issue of public trust was avoided, and Adami repeatedly stated that only fundamentalists and environmental activists question cooperation between academia and industry.

In 2003, a new head of the International Agency for Research on Cancer (IARC) was to be appointed. The body, governed by the World Health Organization (WHO), produces a monograph series on cancer risks and has a great impact on national regulation policies globally.[31] Throughout the 1990s, the IARC had been seen as independent and free from industry control. In the United States, however, there was a strong movement in the first years of the twenty-first century to keep scientific views that don't harmonize with political priorities out of the political process. An editorial in *Science* expressed serious concerns about this development, where industrial interests weigh more than public health interests.[32] Similar concerns, about undue industrial influence related to the IARC process of appointing its new head, were raised by thirty-one scientists in a letter to the WHO; among the signatories to this was the former head of IARC, the now late Lorenzo Tomatis.[33] Hans-Olov Adami referred to this critique of industrial influence at his meeting with medical journalists, and this was reported in the media:

> He [Adami] contemptuously dismissed the critique from Lorenzo Tomatis . . . as [that of] an "old communist"[34]

This remark actually disguises a much deeper ideological matter that might be addressed—that is, what are the main differences between those who support citizens and consumers and those who support the productive processes and marketing of corporations?

The newspaper *Dagens Forskning* had told the Swedish public about the letter to WHO on the increasing influence of industry within IARC. The same article also explained that it was rumored that Adami was an applicant for the post as head of IARC. He denied being an applicant.[35]

At the Swedish medical journalists' meeting that discussed the new head of IARC, Adami again denied being an applicant for that post. Adami's assertion was true but misleading, for he was the nominee of the Swedish government for that post. Already in the summer of 2002, the Ministry of Health and Welfare asked the Swedish Science Council to try to find a Swedish candidate with broad support in Swedish academic society. There was one such person, but he did not wish to be nominated. The question went one round further, but no name could be found to have general support, so the ministry didn't have anyone to nominate.

Dagens Forskning told this story in one issue.[36] It was said that Adami's name only had support from the dean of Karolinska Institute, but a secretary at the ministry, Cecilia Halle, says in the article that she had received an informal confirmation that the Science Council supported Adami as a candidate. The Dean of Uppsala University, Kjell Öberg, gave the reasons for not supporting the nomination of Adami.

> Hans-Olov Adami is an internationally well-reputed scientist. But he is deeply controversial. He is not a listening person. He slashes down on people and can be unreasonable as a negotiator. This makes him unsuitable as head of such an organization. Furthermore his consultancies for the American chemical industry stand in his way. He has not succeeded in responding to the questions raised, but slipped away. These were the reasons we could not support his candidature.[37]

Apparently the Ministry of Health and Welfare was caught in a legitimacy conflict after this article. The ministry had received a letter from the Karolinska Institute's president at that time, Hans Wigzell, suggesting Adami as a candidate as head of the IARC. Next, Wigzell's wife, Kerstin Wigzell, head of the National

Board of Health and Welfare, and also Swedish representative on the board of WHO, reported to the ministry that she had informally asked representatives of the other Nordic countries if they had any objections against the Swedish nomination of Adami and no objections were raised. The letter to the ministry seems to be a personal letter of recommendation, and the questions in the WHO corridors seemed to have grown from Wigzell's dinner table.

The ministry had a candidate to nominate, although they had little knowledge about Adami's industrial ties before the article on the nomination was published. In spite of these circumstances coming to light, the nomination of Adami was not withdrawn. In the end, it was the IARC that rejected Adami's application, as did the Karolinska Institute in 2004 when a new president was elected. Adami was one of the candidates but again his application was turned down.

The academic's personal route—from the intellectual abstractions of academia to committed support for large-scale industrial science—has not been much studied by sociologists, and the moral, ethical, and conflict issues raised by the journey have gathered like a thickening fog over academia during the last twenty years.[38, 39] Hans-Olov Adami does not consider that his journey from academic epidemiology to defender of the chemical industry has actually covered much ground. He has expressed the view that directly funded industrial research and academic research are likely to become indistinguishable over the next decades.

Medikament shared information with another Swedish science journal, Dagens Forskning, so there was more on the subject, but little that was new.[40, 41] A main theme in the greenwashing article was that industry has a general strategy to implement its goals of expanding markets and deregulation. In some instances, deregulation is in conflict with the precautionary principle safeguarding public health and the environment. The industrial response to such conflicts often takes the form of reversal of the precautionary principle to a precaution of business opportunities and safeguarding of profits on the "free market": free for producers but less so for consumers.

The tobacco industry, the pharmaceutical industry, the chemical industry, the biotechnology industry, and others share all the same game plans. There is nothing odd about this. Industry has a "legitimate" greenwashing interest, having to protect the interests of investors, stockholders, staff, and even in some cases in their eyes, consumers. One might expect elected politicians in democracies to be the safeguards of public interest: those who balance the vested interests of industry and the public. Instead, political interests have increasingly become nested with industrial interests. So we have to ask: who is defending the public interest? The balance of conflicting interests is clearly out of balance, and, possibly, out of control.

A group of Swedish researchers at the Karolinska Institute, Hans-Olov Adami, Anders Ekbom, Magnus Ingelman-Sundberg, Anders Ahlbom, and one researcher in Lund, Lars Hagmar, in the fall of 2001 initiated an attack on some research colleagues investigating the association between the environment and cancer. This critical attack was fairly comprehensive, involving research linking cellular telephones and brain tumors, pollutants in mother's milk and the risk for childhood malignancies, alcohol and dioxins. The article gained interest. The fact that it was the beginning of a campaign went unnoticed in the media.[42]

The focus of the attack was on Professor Lennart Hardell in Örebro, Sweden, a clinical researcher, recognized to be the first to report an association between dioxins and cancer. This enforced the Swedish ban on certain dioxin-contaminated phenoxyacetic acids, (e.g., Hormoslyr). Hardell has been bad news and a thorn in the flesh of industry for three decades. The leader of the gang that attacked Hardell, Hans-Olov Adami, has his own interests to defend in dioxins.

Eager to be both provocative and aggressive, the authors of the article in *Svenska Dagbladet* especially pointed to a study showing a significant association between cellular telephones and brain tumors found at the same side of the brain as is used during mobile phone calls: an absurd finding and biologically not relevant according to the authors. The problem with such articles is that they are full of mischievous, dangerous, and unproven asides.

This particular article carried the assertion that *cancer caused by environmental pollutants is not dose-dependent*. This statement is absurd. Since the distance from the mobile phone is of importance for the exposure to microwaves, it is reasonable to assume that the part of the brain on the same side as used during the phone calls gets higher exposure. In fact, results have shown that this is the fact.

If we are to understand this attack on Lennart Hardell, we should look in some detail at the academic record and employment of Professor Hans-Olov Adami. As with the career and work of the late Sir Richard Doll, Adami presents a perfect case history of an academic working for industry rather than for science.

Adami was on the External Scientific Advisory Committee of CEFIC, the European branch organization for the chemical industry. Adami's activities in this committee have resulted in funding of a project led by Anders Ekbom (in the same department as Adami) on environmental toxins and cryptorchidism and hypospadias.[43] In addition to this information, Adami offered a copy of the review on atrazine.

However, it was dioxin that was at the base of Adami's campaign against Lennart Hardell. This battle has been one of the hardest fought over any chemical, particularly because it is a salient part of many products and processes. The chemical companies of course characterized the reassessment as quixotic and constantly changing, making it look as if the EPA rather than the chemical companies had dragged out the process, and kept moving the goal posts.

Adami's position is determined by his tasks. At the time the newspaper article appeared in Sweden attacking Lennart Hardell, he was the head of the Institute of Medical Epidemiology at the Karolinska Institute. A grant from the Swedish Cancer Fund sponsored that employment. The aim of that grant was to do research on different risk factors and improve the possibilities of preventing cancer.[44]

He was adjunct professor at Harvard Medical School of Public Health. Within that assignment he was commissioned by industry to write "reviews."[45]

Adami was a member of the Nobel Association[46] and had on a couple of occasions been a member of the committee that selected the winner of the Nobel Prize in medicine and physiology.

At Harvard he was the member of the Planning Group, Harvard Center for Cancer Prevention.

Adami was a member of the scientific council for Long Range Research Initiative (LRI), a joint venture between the branch organizations of the European chemical companies (CEFIC), the American chemical companies (ACS), and the Japanese chemical companies (JCIA). One of the tasks has been to give the basis for the long-term industry research.[47–49] He was also undertaking a research project funded by CEFIC.[50]

In 2000, Adami was on the editorial board of the following scientific journals: *Breast; Breast Cancer Research; Cancer Causes & Control; Cancer Epidemiology, Biomarkers and Prevention; Epidemiology; European Journal of Epidemiology; Journal of the National Cancer Institute* and *New England Journal of Medicine.*

Hans-Olov Adami was an influential person.

After the newspaper articles and the criticism from some professional quarters, Adami remained silent. Therefore, I asked Hans Wigzell, President of the Karolinska Institute, a number of questions at that time. The idea was to ascertain Adami's current projects and who was funding them. The section that follows summarizes some of the information that I gained and puts it into context. The information gained from my questions clearly belonged in the public domain, so Wigzell was unable to refuse answers. I put two rounds of questions to Wigzell and after some time all his questions were answered. Wigzell was able to answer these questions because Adami was bound to tell him about his outside commissions. The changing direction of Adami's work had certainly benefited the Karolinska Institute, the preeminent research institute in Sweden, where his Department of Epidemiology increased from a staff of forty in 1997 to well over one hundred by 2004.

One of the major areas of Adami's work was around beryllium; a number of researchers were looking at it in relation to lung cancer. The work is described as preparatory for a study design. A committee was formed at Harvard with four professors from Harvard and one from IARC, to work with the issue. Harvard was where Adami's coworker was at that time. The work was paid for by Brush Wellman, the manufacturer of beryllium. This matter was highly contentious at the time because damage claims were being made in the courts by Brush Wellman workers.

Another highly controversial matter was the role of trichloroethylene in the cause of cancer among dry cleaning workers. It was learned that a study was in preparation by Dr. Elsebeth Lynge, and there was an international committee of four persons to help in the preparations. One was from IARC, one was Dr. Jack Mandel at Emory University with a direct tie to the research company Exponent, and one was the head of the department of epidemiology at the National Cancer Institute. This work was paid for by the Halogenated Solvents Industry Association (HSIA).

At that time, the dry cleaning study was particularly interesting. The participant from the National Cancer Institute was the chief of the occupational epidemiology branch, Dr. Aaron Blair. The participant from IARC who was suggested was Dr. Paolo Boffetta (see chapter 7), who also was adjunct professor in Adami's department. From the information given it seems that HSIA paid for the participation of outside experts and was not involved in the process. Actually HSIA played an active role through Louis Bloemen, an employee of Dow Chemicals, who at least in the early stages acted as the coordinator for the project, a role one would expect Dr. Lynge to have played. Adami seemed uneasy about being involved without a clearly defined position in the work, and expressed his concerns to Mandel.

The herbicide atrazine and its link to prostate cancer at its production facility in Louisiana has been at the base of one of the major arguments between the company's producers and workers. The company claimed that the rising levels of prostate cancer at its facility were due to more specific surveillance and screening—a common rationalization given for all kinds of illnesses and mental states. Others were sure that the increase was caused by elements in atrazine. A document discussing the issue was written in July 2002 at Harvard. Authors were Adami, two professors at Harvard, and Jack Mandel. Later, Adami was asked to help with a study design for investigation of the possible connection between atrazine exposure and prostate cancer. In this new group Adami worked together with Dimitrios Trichopoulos and Harris Pastides. All the work on atrazine was paid for by Syngenta Crop Protection, Inc., the manufacturer of the herbicide.

Trichopoulos also participated in the work on atrazine, as well as Jack Mandel. It's noteworthy that Mandel was presented as an academic with "direct ties" to Exponent, as if he was a professor taking commissions for that firm. Actually Jack Mandel was, at that time, group vice president and a senior consultant at Exponent. The third named participant on the atrazine issue was Harris Pastides. He also participated in the dioxin detoxification campaign, being coauthor of both reviews from Exponent.

Adami gave the following additional comments on the atrazine project in the second response to Wigzell:

> The review of atrazine is interesting both by being representative for the kind of consultancies I have accepted and because it offers an interesting challenge which with good reason can be said to demand an epidemiological competence which rarely is found within the industry itself. In short, the background was that newly discovered prostate cancer was found in excess to what was expected at the plant in question producing atrazine. The basic question was therefore if this was best explained by a carcinogenic effect on the prostate from atrazine or by the fact that all employees were offered free health controls with PSA testing. In a first document these two alternative explanations were explored. In the second phase the aim is to go one step further by performing a formal epidemiological study aiming at quantification of the effect of atrazine and PSA testing respectively on the incidence of prostate cancer. This is proving to be a delicate methodological issue, and my latest "review" on the subject is about these aspects. I attach it as requested by Bo Walhjalt.[51]

In a discursive article, "Lobbyists or Researchers?," Professor Bo Rothstein criticized the image of university research, implying that researchers produce memorials for certain interests, either their own interests or those of employers or customers.[52] He refers to Birgitta Forsman's writing about science and morality that gives a scary picture of what is happening beneath the polished surface.

Necessary regulation is not done in the interests of society and is neglected by politicians. Obviously something is wrong regarding the research business. With some unique exceptions it has nothing to do with the public interests. The greenwashers have been extremely successful. Sweden is not an exception, although it took a longer time for greenwashing to be successful in that country.

Loyalty toward one's colleagues, protection of the reputation of the profession, and concern about careers and personal job security are the forces that support silence and suffering. Civil courage, the ability to disclose and to dare to point at such circumstances is nowadays within most establishments an unwanted and loathsome characteristic; to question is a threat against the status quo.

It has for a long time been legitimate to point mainly at the tobacco industry as a scapegoat. This hides the fact that in relation to greenwashing the tobacco industry is only a part of a pattern introduced by many other industries and corporations. The harmonization of the procedure for risk assessment follows a pattern resulting from cooperation between the tobacco and chemical industries since the end of the 1980s.[53]

In the articles in the *Swedish Medical Journal* on the cynical methods used by the tobacco industry, the thesis that the Swedish tobacco consultants have been naïve and deceived by an industry doing bad business has been suggested. But in the interview in *Aftonbladet*, Adami says, regarding his contacts with the chemical industry: "I am not naïve" and he makes the point that many researchers are working with industry and that the place for research in the future will be within that context.[54]

If the cake model according to Wigzell and the Karolinska Institute is to be the ideal, successful greenwashing will critique the precautionary principle and make good business at the same time as the morality of research is eroded. Greenwashing is a practice that will threaten the confidence of research in general, both the researches in industry and research that is independent of industry. Greenwashing is PR and should be regarded as a disaster for the environment in the scientific culture. The reputation of research is dependent on rules and sustained rules are the instruments to keep a clean record. An open and honest, transparent and independent attitude is necessary for the reputation of research in the long run.

Chapter 6

INDUSTRY INFLUENCES ON CANCER EPIDEMIOLOGY

Neil Pearce

If you hire somebody to look at a paper which has a new discovery, and there have been obvious difficulties in doing the study, and this guy doesn't believe that DES [diethylstilboestrol] causes cancer of the vagina, that there's not enough evidence to implicate tampons with toxic shock, that there's not enough evidence to believe estrogens are related to uterine cancer, has even questioned the cigarette smoking/ lung cancer association. If that's the guy you hire, you don't have to be a genius to figure out where he's going to come down on this issue.

Paul Stolley

This chapter is based on three papers on industry influences on epidemiology that I published in the *International Journal of Epidemiology.*[1–4] Epidemiology is commonly defined as the study of "the distribution and determinants of health related states or events in specified populations."[5] Thus, epidemiology is inherently focused on populations, and epidemiologists recognize that anecdotes about individuals cannot be used to refute evidence about populations. For example, an anecdote about someone who smoked one pack a day and lived to be a hundred, or someone who never smoked and developed lung cancer anyway, does not refute the evidence that people who smoke a pack a day get lung cancer at ten times the rate of non-smokers. Similarly, anecdotes about individual epidemiologists acting ethically or unethically do not confirm or refute evidence about general tendencies.

Thus, I do not intend to comment on specific individuals (with the occasional exception of extreme cases that are too blatant to ignore), but rather to comment on the distribution and determinants of epidemiologic research, particularly the current corporate influences on what cancer research gets done and how the findings are received. This doesn't absolve individuals from the responsibility to act ethically and responsibly, but my main concerns are about the ethical and scientific context in which individuals make such decisions. My focus is particularly on "independent" research based in universities, and the corporate influences on it, rather than on epidemiologic research that is based in corporations. This is partly because I am based in a university and more familiar with research in that situation, but also because I have less concern about corporate-based epidemiology, since in that situation the issues are relatively clear, and in most instances clear guidelines are in place. In contrast, the situation of university-based researchers is often more ambiguous, because they may benefit from their "independent" status while nevertheless receiving corporate funding.

At the outset, I should note that an equally good case could be made for a book that presented "the other side of the coin" (i.e., the political and social pressures) that may lead to epidemiologic evidence being misused in order to wrongly condemn particular chemicals as carcinogenic, or to make sweeping claims on the basis of evidence that is weak and preliminary, or to greatly exaggerate risks that are real but extremely small.[6] In this respect, the two extreme approaches are mirror images of each other,[7] with one denying virtually all occupational and environmental cancer risks, and the other massively over-hyping risks that are (sometimes) real, but (often) extremely small. In this polarized situation, we too easily lapse into collecting policy-based evidence rather than implementing evidence-based policy. Thus, public health and environmental health activists can be every bit as biased and unwilling to accept "inconvenient truths" as the apologists for industry. However, they usually don't have the funding to have as much influence as the corporations do, which is why the current book may play a useful role in redressing this imbalance.

EPIDEMIOLOGY

Why is epidemiological research so often full of controversy? The main reason, perhaps, is that epidemiology deals with hazardous exposures for which it is unethical and impossible to do a randomized trial. Thus, it is impossible to do a perfect study, and epidemiologists must learn to review all of the available evidence rather than attempting to reach a decision on the basis of a single study. For example, the studies linking smoking with lung cancer were bitterly criticized by "conventional" researchers who were not willing to accept evidence from studies where the exposure had not been randomized.[8] However, the preliminary evidence that smoking caused lung cancer[9, 10] was eventually supported by hundreds more studies in other countries. More recently, we have seen similar controversies with regards to the health effects of passive smoking.[11–13]

Perhaps the most legendary critic of epidemiology was the late Alvan Feinstein at Yale University. Before his death in 2001, Feinstein disputed most of the major epidemiological findings in recent decades, including the established causal associations between smoking and lung cancer, between oral contraceptives and thromboembolism, between diethylstilbestrol and vaginal cancer, between aspirin and Reye's syndrome, between tampon use and toxic shock syndrome, and between estrogens and endometrial cancer.[14] In each instance, these controversies were eventually resolved with the vindication of the original studies, but the debates often lasted for many years, and the necessary safety warnings and regulatory procedures were therefore delayed.[15]

It should be stressed that there are also plenty of examples, as in other sciences, where epidemiologists have got it wrong, and the findings of epidemiological studies have been contradicted by subsequent randomized trials. Examples include studies of beta carotene and cardiovascular disease, hormone replacement therapy, vitamin E and vitamin C intake in relation to cardiovascular disease, or fiber intake in relation to colon cancer.[16] However, these examples of "epidemiological failures" primarily involve studies of lifestyle factors (particularly diet). These are notoriously difficult to study, since the "exposed group" (e.g., those with high beta carotene levels in their diets) will often be markedly different from the "non-exposed group" with respect to many different lifestyle factors. Furthermore, the multiple exposures considered in many epidemiological studies mean that such studies frequently produce chance findings that may be widely reported in the press, but which are not replicated in subsequent studies. This has led to some well-justified, and some less-justified, criticisms of epidemiology as being an unreliable science that frequently produces spurious findings.[17, 18] However, these problems with epidemiological studies of lifestyle risk factors can, to some extent, be overcome by requiring replication of study findings, and by adopting a "life course approach," which takes account of the interconnections between different exposures and exposures' contexts.[19] Furthermore, problems of multiple comparisons are not unique to epidemiology and apply to other areas of research, particularly genetic research.

More importantly in the current context, there are some areas of epidemiological research which are less prone to error. Ironically, these are often the areas in which there is the most controversy. In particular, there are usually only relatively minor problems of confounding in occupational epidemiology, since there are usually only minor differences in smoking, diet, etc., between different groups of workers.[20] Such problems can be more serious in environmental health studies, which is why the most valid conclusions can often be reached by study-ing more heavily exposed groups of workers[21] and then interpolating down to estimate the risks from lower levels of exposure in the community.

Thus, there are no universal rules about the reliability of epidemiological studies—it depends on the hypothesis being investigated and the study design being used to address it. Many of the criticisms of epidemiology as being inher-ently unreliable are applicable to studies of lifestyle factors, but are less applicable to pharmacoepidemiology and occupational and environmental epidemiology studies.

INDUSTRY CONSULTANTS

These "natural" tendencies for epidemiological research findings to be regarded with some skepticism are exacerbated by the activities of companies that have produced a chemical that is suspected of causing cancer or some other health problem. The usual approach is for the company concerned to hire epidemi-ologists as consultants to criticize the research publicly, either when it appears in print, or even prior to publication, as well as appearing as expert witnesses once the research has been published[22]. In recent years, these efforts have been further developed and refined with the use of websites and publicity that stigma-tizes unwelcome research findings as "junk science."[23–28] In some instances these activities have gone as far as efforts to block publication.[29] In many instances, academics have accepted industry funding that has not been acknowledged, and only the academic affiliations of the company-funded consultants have been listed. This issue has recently received particular attention because of the con-troversy regarding Sir Richard Doll's undeclared acceptance of consultancy fees from Monsanto during the 1980s, with some condemning this outright,[30] while others have argued that different rules of disclosure prevailed at the time and that, in any case, Doll's opinions are unlikely to have been affected by the acceptance of such fees.[31]

Recent examples include attempts to influence studies on the toxicity of benzene[32] and diesel particulate matter,[33] and the various industry efforts over many years to influence the conduct and interpretation of research into the health effects of dioxin.[34] Perhaps one of the worst such examples has been the industry campaign to undermine an OSHA chromium (VI) standard[35] and corporate infiltration of a panel convened to set standards for chromium (VI) in California.[36] This involved the ghostwriting of an article,[37] which was later retracted by the journal,[38] which claimed that a Chinese scientist had reevaluated his findings and reversed his conclusions on elevated cancer risks in residents of Jinzhou, China, who were exposed to chromium (VI) in water.[39]

Many leading epidemiologists would argue that they are not influenced by industry funding. They study the evidence objectively, and then make their opinions known for the benefit of society, and if they receive some funding along the way, then that is entirely appropriate. In fact, although such consultants are invariably paid well, this is usually not necessarily their main motivation, and the pressures on them are usually more subtle than this. This is typified by remarks from an American lawyer, John C. Shepherd of St. Louis, who was president of the American Bar Association in 1984–85:

> The first thing you need to get along with your expert witness is money. But the hiring and successful use of an expert may not be that easy—a lot of good experts are rich. Although you will eventually be talking about money with your expert, it is wiser to begin on another tack. Tell your expert how justice will be served if he will testify on your side of the case. Remind him how the unfortunate situation in our courts today can be improved if we have people of his caliber to help in the administration of justice. That ploy will impress even the rich expert.[40]

A second line of defense of their activities that is often offered by "modern epidemiologists" involves a relatively crude (and convenient!) interpretation of the (already crude) Popperian philosophy of science.[41] It is argued that "science is about criticism" and that by being critical of colleagues' work corporate-funded epidemiologists are simply doing their duty as scientists—who pays them for it is irrelevant.[42] However, there is substantial evidence that the source of funding strongly influences the conclusions that are reached (e.g., in the cases of tobacco[43] and calcium-channel antagonists[44]). This makes it essential that any sources of funding and potential conflicts of interest are declared. Nevertheless, it has been argued that the declaration of conflicts of interest is "the new McCarthyism in science,"[45] and the requirement that at least one investigator who is independent of any commercial funder should take responsibility for the integrity of the data and the accuracy of the data analysis is "unfair—and absurd."[46]

It should be emphasized that a company clearly has a right to argue against what it believes are weak data or incorrect conclusions, and it is not in the interests of society or the company to withdraw a drug which has been wrongly accused.[47] However, equally clearly, a company has a moral obligation to seek the truth of the matter when obtaining advice from consultants, rather than just preparing the "case for the defense." The latter usually occurs, even if the hired consultants are relatively neutral in the dispute and merely sit on an "expert panel." This is not to imply that deliberate corruption is a common occurrence. However, a company that intends to prepare the "case for the defense" may seek out academics who (usually because of sincerely held beliefs) have been very critical of similar studies in the past. Thus, the shaping of the "case for the defense" usually involves "selection" rather than "coercion" of experts. As Paul Stolley has observed:

> If you hire somebody to look at a paper which has a new discovery, and there have been obvious difficulties in doing the study, and this guy doesn't believe that DES [diethylstilboestrol] causes cancer of the vagina, that there's not enough evidence to implicate tampons with toxic shock, that there's not enough evidence to believe estrogens are related to uterine cancer, has even questioned the cigarette smoking/lung cancer association. If that's the guy you hire, you don't have to be a genius to figure out where he's going to come down on this issue.[48]

It should be stressed that criticism plays an important role in science, and even very biased critics may make important points. However, an overemphasis on criticism can lead to the dismissal of almost any scientific study as being "fatally flawed." At a conference on ethics in epidemiological research, I once presented a satirical set of guidelines for a "corporate epidemiologist" who is asked to review a study:

1. Consider only the specific study that you have been asked to review. Don't consider supporting evidence from other epidemiologic or experimental studies.
2. There are three possible questions you could consider: (1) Is there any chance that the study findings are right? (2) Is there any chance that the study findings are wrong? (3) What is the balance of evidence? Restrict yourself to the second question.
3. Prepare a list of possible biases. Do not comment on the likely direction or magnitude of the biases. Conclude that there are many "fatal flaws" in the study and it is therefore uninterpretable.
4. Decline to comment directly on policy, but insist that further studies must be undertaken that avoid the biases identified in step 3.
5. Go back to step 1.

TWO THOUGHT EXPERIMENTS

To gain a better understanding of the current "system" (scenario 1), perhaps it may be useful to conduct two counterfactual "thought experiments."

The first thought experiment (scenario 2) is to consider what the situation would be if corporate funding was removed from significantly influencing what research gets done and how it is received. This could occur in a number of ways (e.g., if all university-based researchers were not reliant on research grants or consultancy fees for their salaries, and agreed not to, or were not permitted to, accept funding directly from any vested interests—corporate or otherwise). Suppose also that, if a company was concerned about the possible safety of a product, then it was required (or willing) to provide funds through an appropriate public funding agency with no strings attached (and no specification of the exact research to be done, and who would do it). Finally, also suppose that sufficient government funds were available for investigator-initiated research, so that vested interests were not able to set the agenda, even indirectly, with regards to research into issues such as occupational and environmental cancer. Obviously, many current researchers would be attending fewer conferences and would be traveling economy class. Apart from that obvious hardship, what would be the effects on epidemiologic research? Would there be a lessening of debate or criticism of published studies? Certainly not. Epidemiologists love to debate and to criticize each other, at scientific meetings and in the journals, both for the sheer pleasure of it, but also because that is what science is about. The main difference is that there would be a genuinely balanced scientific debate, rather than the "manufactured dissent" that we see too often currently. Of course, the "hired guns" who currently attack published studies on behalf of industry would still be completely free to continue to do this—but it is highly unlikely that they would bother to do so if no one was paying them.

The second thought experiment (scenario 3) is to consider what things would look like if the shoe was on the other foot and various NGOs (Greenpeace, trade unions, community groups, etc.) had millions of dollars to spend on hiring consultants to attack "negative findings" about the potential carcinogenic risks from occupational and environmental exposures, whereas the corporations had none. Would individual epidemiologists change their views about the safety of particular exposures? Would former industry consultants now embrace the precautionary principle[49] and accept funding to attack studies that showed that particular exposures were (relatively) safe? In most cases, probably not. However, the overall debate, and the influences on what research is conducted and how it is interpreted, would certainly change. Once again, funding would set the agenda, but by "selection" rather than "coercion." There would also be, as Sander Greenland notes,[50] an increase in false positives, penalties against innocent parties (although this is primarily a US problem), and misguided public health actions that siphon resources from effective actions.

These two thought experiments (scenarios 2 and 3) make the current situation (scenario 1) clearer, and particularly that the availability of large amounts of corporate funding distorts current scientific debate, and is a determinant of what research is conducted and how the findings are interpreted and received. Of course, there are plenty of individual anecdotes about researchers who are not influenced (or believe that they are not influenced) by their source of funding, but when epidemiologists are considered as a group, if you "follow the money" then you can, most of the time, predict the findings and interpretation of corporate-funded studies. You can also strongly predict the conclusions of consultants who are hired by vested interests to attack published study findings that yield inconvenient truths. This particularly applies to industry consultants who rely on such funding to pay their own salaries, in contrast to, for example, epidemiologists based in public universities whose salaries are state guaranteed.

I should stress that my own experience is that deliberate corruption is very rare. Rather, a company that intends to prepare the "case for the defense" may seek out academics who (usually because of sincerely held beliefs) have been very critical of similar studies in the past. Thus, the shaping of the "case for the defense" usually involves selection rather than coercion of experts.[51] What we have is a system in which almost all of the individuals are acting ethically (or believe that they are) and doing "good science," but the influence of money distorts the process so that it often produces unethical and unscientific results. This can occur even if the funding is given with no strings attached. For example, in some fields of research it is almost impossible to find any leading researchers who have not received funding from industry (with or without strings attached), and the resulting close relationships and networks set the parameters of the debates, albeit by osmosis rather than by coercion.

REGULATORY AUTHORITIES

The selection, by a company with a vested interest, of a few scientists who follow the "guidelines" given above, and are hypercritical of others' work can therefore result in massive pressure on regulatory authorities. This pressure is particularly effective because it seems to come from independent scientists—it would not be taken so seriously if it came directly from the company. In this sense, the company's consultants have the privilege of acting as "lawyers for the defense" while maintaining the image of being an "independent jury."

However, this is not an insurmountable problem provided that regulatory agencies maintain a strict independence from industry (and from other influences), recognize the pressure from industry consultants for what it is, and hire their own independent consultants. Unfortunately, in recent years the threats to the integrity of science have come from government as well as from industry.[52] For example, Clapp et al.,[53] cite a recent report of the US Congress that cited a number of examples of how the current administration has manipulated scientific review procedures, including "inappropriate questioning of prospective members of scientific review committees about their political views; removal of long serving members on the basis of political litmus tests; and blocking research funding and the publications of research results, when these appeared to reflect badly on economic interests supporting the administration." In particular, the recent public-health catastrophe of the licensing of Vioxx, and its continued use after evidence had appeared of its cardiovascular side effects has indicated "lethal weaknesses" in the US Food and Drug Administration.[54, 55] Similar pressures have been exerted on the WHO International Agency for Research on Cancer[56] and its monograph program for the evaluation of carcinogenicity[57–59] and there has been a reluctance of governments and regulatory agencies globally to take prompt and effective action even on established causes of cancer such as asbestos.[60, 61]

WHAT CAN BE DONE?

So what can be done about these pressures from industry, and in some instances from governments, to obstruct or influence the conduct, publication, and policy response to research that shows that particular occupational or environmental exposures may be hazardous?

If you are working in scenario 1 (the current reality), I agree that it is naïve to simply say that no researcher should ever accept any funding from any vested interest. My colleagues have been quick to point out that that would leave the consultancy field open to "hired guns" whose views are very predictable and industries (and other vested interests) that genuinely want to seek independent advice would not be able to do so. Within scenario 1, you can certainly make a case that it is better for independent university-based epidemiologists to engage with vested interests, and to offer them independent advice, with clear rules for ethical behavior and full disclosure. There are some academics who offer good role models for this and have been prepared to testify against their own funders, sometimes at some personal cost. So, within the current reality, a valid argument can be made that it makes sense for academic epidemiologists to engage with vested interests.

The problem is that, despite the integrity and courageous actions of some (but not all) of the individuals involved, in general the current reality isn't working well, and vested interests can massively influence, both directly and indirectly, what research gets done and how it is received. These problems are likely to get worse, as the most hazardous exposures are increasingly located in developing countries, where there is even less regulation of research ethics than there is in industrialized countries.[62, 63]

On the positive side, for the last two decades there has been substantial discussion on ethics in epidemiology,[64–67] partly in response to the unethical conduct of many industry-funded consultants.[68] A number of websites (e.g., www.ucsusa.org/scientific_integrity/ and www.cspinet.org/integrity/) are now devoted to fostering integrity in science, and the International Epidemiological Association has issued a report on "good epidemiological practice."[69] Recently, there have been renewed calls for scientists to engage in processes to assert positive principles of . . . how science should work, and how it should be applied to public policy decisions rather than simply having a list of what not to do. This will require strong pressure from within the scientific community for codes of ethics conduct and financial conflict of interest[70] with the goal, not of restricting what people can do, but of ensuring complete transparency "through full declaration of potential sources of conflicts of interest."[71] For example, Vallance has suggested that full disclosure of conflicts of interests should form the opening sentences of any publication, rather than being buried in small print in the acknowledgment.[72]

So if we wish to mitigate the worst effects of the current reality (scenario 1) while also attempting to move toward a better reality (scenario 2), then talking and writing about these problems is a good start, and this book can play a positive role in this regard. Professional organizations can also play a major role in exposing and mitigating the worst excesses of the current reality, and in moving toward a better reality in which science and the public health come first. This should involve encouraging and supporting epidemiologists to assert positive principles of how science should work, and how it should be applied to public policy decisions, rather than simply having a list of what not to do.

Chapter 7

SERVING INDUSTRY, PROMOTING SKEPTICISM, DISCREDITING EPIDEMIOLOGY

Kathleen Ruff

Washing one's hands of the conflict between the powerful and the powerless means to side with the powerful, not to be neutral.

Paulo Freire

Our lives begin to end the day we become silent about things that matter.

Martin L. King

Scientists and international health agencies, including the World Health Organization (WHO), have expressed alarm over the fact that industries with vested interests—for example, the chemical industry, the oil and gas industry, the fast-food industry—are subverting public health policy and preventing needed action on critical issues, such as climate change, pollution of land, air, and water, and continued use of known harmful products.

Speaking at the 2013 World Health Assembly,[1] WHO Director General Margaret Chan emphasized that, today, efforts to safeguard public health face opposition from a different set of extremely powerful forces. "Many of the risk factors for noncommunicable diseases are amplified by the products and practices of large and economically powerful forces," said Chan. "Market power readily translates into political power. When public health policies cross purposes with vested economic interests, we will face opposition, well-orchestrated opposition, and very well-funded opposition." Chan particularly mentioned industry-funded research "that confuses the evidence and keeps the public in doubt" and, speaking at a conference in Finland, criticized the failure of political will to take on big business.[2]

STRATEGY PIONEERED BY THE TOBACCO INDUSTRY

The tactic of manufacturing doubt was pioneered by the tobacco industry in the 1950s.[3] John Hill, president of the public relations company Hill and Knowlton, advised the industry not to challenge the scientific evidence but instead to seize and control it. A critical element of the strategy, said Hill, was to declare the positive value of scientific skepticism. By claiming to be simply pursuing the search for truth, while funding amenable scientists to deny harm, the tobacco industry could succeed in creating the appearance of scientific controversy. Skepticism, and the truism that there is more to know, were advanced as virtues, but were, in reality, weapons that allowed the tobacco industry for decades to pervert the scientific literature, prevent tobacco control measures and increase sales of its deadly product.

The industry's attack on science was thus two-pronged: on the one hand, it funded scientists to come up with findings relentlessly favorable to the industry and, on the other hand, it endeavored to discredit and promote skepticism toward the work of independent scientists. The strategy proved effective and enabled the industry to delay and sabotage public health regulation of tobacco, resulting in millions of preventable deaths.

The strategy has since been widely adopted by many industries. The strategy is particularly effective when scientists, who have worked for many years at prestigious public health institutions, take on the role of carrying out industry-funded research that manufactures doubt and take on the role of discrediting independent scientific research.

Paolo Boffetta is an example of a prominent scientist who, after working for many years for public health institutions, now carries out industry-funded research that comes up with findings that deny or create doubt about harm caused by the industries' products, and who now seeks to discredit and create skepticism about the work of independent scientists and independent scientific agencies whose research documents harm caused by the industries' products. According to Boffetta, the threat to science today is posed, not by industry influence, as the WHO Director General has warned, but by independent scientists who—motivated by ambition—are biased toward coming up with findings of harm.

Boffetta has an extremely impressive résumé. It runs to one hundred and eleven pages and includes over one thousand scientific articles, reports, editorials, book chapters, and books published since 1987. Boffetta lists eleven scientific journals for which he is an active member of the editorial board, as well as sixty-seven scientific journals for which he has acted as a referee since 2005. His work has been cited more than fifty thousand times.[4]

Currently, Boffetta is the principal investigator for research projects receiving millions of euros/dollars from the European Commission, the French National Cancer Institute, the US Centers for Disease Control, and the US National Institutes for Health. He is a founding member and present member of the executive committee of a number of international scientific consortia. He currently holds prestigious positions—at the Mount Sinai School of Medicine in New York; as associate director for population science of the Tisch Cancer Institute; Charles G. Bluhdorn professor of International Community Medicine; director of the Institute for Translational Epidemiology; and vice-chair, cancer prevention and control, department of oncological sciences. In addition, he holds academic appointments at several universities, including the Harvard School of Public Health.

From 1990 to 2009, Boffetta worked at the World Health Organization's International Agency for Research on Cancer (IARC),[5] rising to become chief of the unit of Environmental Cancer Epidemiology, coordinator of IARC's genetics and epidemiology cluster and director of IARC's training program.

Having achieved significant prestige in the field of public health research, Boffetta in 2008 embarked on a new path that included two components: one was to carry out research, commissioned by chemical, mining, and fast-food industries, that consistently contradicted IARC's findings and denied that the industries' products caused harm to health; and the second was to attack the credibility of independent scientists and scientific bodies, including IARC itself.

A NEW CAREER WORKING FOR TOXIC INDUSTRIES

While still at IARC, in 2008 Boffetta worked with the consulting company Exponent (see chapter 10) to carry out a research project on behalf of the Styrene Information and Research Center (SIRC), a trade organization that defends the interests of the styrene industry. Boffetta was the lead author for the ensuing report *Epidemiological studies of styrene and cancer: a review of the literature,*[6] which relied heavily on industry papers and concluded that: "We found no consistent increased risk of any cancer among workers exposed to styrene."

In a commentary[7] on Boffetta's paper, Peter Infante, formerly director of the office of standards review at the US Occupational Safety and Health Administration (OSHA), and James Huff of the National Institute of Environmental Health Sciences (NIEHS), put forward scientific evidence, ignored by Boffetta, which showed carcinogenic risks to humans posed by styrene. They pointedly made the following recommendation to Boffetta and his coauthors: "In the interests of public and occupational health, we suggest that authors be more cautious in their casual acceptance of industry papers and reviews of epidemiological study results related to occupational exposure to styrene (or other chemicals)."

Boffetta's report was beneficial to SIRC, who immediately used it, identifying Boffetta as lead author and an IARC scientist, to aggressively lobby the National Toxicology Program of NIEHS to classify styrene as a non-carcinogen.[8] IARC's position was that styrene was a potential carcinogen and, in 1994, IARC, with supporting evidence from other relevant data, upgraded styrene to a higher risk category (Group 2A: probably carcinogenic to humans).

It is disturbing that IARC's conflicts of interest rules did not prohibit this conduct. Boffetta says that he carried out this work for Exponent and SIRC pro bono because of the fact that he was, at the time of writing it, an IARC employee. It would be disingenuous to say that this eliminates the issue of conflict of interest. It does not. Boffetta was working for vested interests—a for-profit consulting company and an industry association—to attack the cancer evaluations of IARC and NIEHS, using his IARC position to add weight to the work, which benefited SIRC. Exponent scientists at times carry out work that is very helpful to the interests of particular industries and which they represent as being pro bono,[9] implying that the work was done altruistically to advance the glories of science and the well-being of humanity. In fact, however, these papers, just like the styrene paper, serve industry interests. It would be irresponsibly naive to deny that these papers increase the value of the scientists and the consulting companies in the eyes of industry and thus increase their ability to attract commissions from companies seeking to avoid government regulation of their products and practices, or seeking to avoid paying compensation for harms caused.

Boffetta's relationship with Exponent is significant. While IARC stands for independent science to protect public health, Exponent has earned a reputation for mercenary science that serves industry interests. As David Michaels has documented,[10] Exponent is one of the premier product-defense companies that make a pretense of carrying out scientific research, while salting the literature with studies whose purpose is to manufacture doubt and help toxic industries defeat public health and environmental protections. "This is science for hire, period," states Michaels, "and it is extremely lucrative." Frequently, Exponent's work involves carrying out what they claim is a full and objective survey of the epidemiological literature. Instead, notes Michaels, "It is all a charade." The one overriding purpose is to minimize public health and environmental protection. These surveys distort the evidence so as to come up with biased conclusions that, without fail, suit the interests of the industry paying the bill.

FORMER IARC SCIENTISTS SET UP FOR-PROFIT CONSULTING COMPANY

In 2009, Boffetta left IARC and set up a for-profit consulting company in the same location as IARC in Lyon, France, with the noble name of the International Prevention Research Institute (IPRI). The eight shareholders of the company were all former employees of IARC, with the president of the company, Peter Boyle, having been a former director of IARC from 2004 to 2008. Boyle's candidacy to continue as director of IARC was rejected in 2009, apparently because his views were considered too pro-industry.[11]

While IPRI emphasizes that it is dedicated to preventing disease and serving the impoverished populations of the developing world, it is closely allied to the pharmaceutical industry and is one of the key drivers behind the establishment of "a novel commercial idea" related to drug development, called the Global Action 4 Health Institute Ltd, a consulting company dedicated to serving the interests of Pharma and Biotech companies.[12] In IPRI's major report[13] on the growing cancer crisis in the developing world, IPRI urgently recommends that a multibillion dollar public-private fund be created, led by the pharmaceutical and technology industries.[14] The report was funded by the Roche pharmaceutical company.

Boyle is also a member of the University of Strathclyde's Technology and Innovation Centre's International Advisory Panel. This is "a group of leading industry professionals," including representatives of the pharmaceutical industry, such as Roche, Merck, GlaxoSmithKline, Pfizer, and Global Pharma Consulting. The stated role and remit of the International Advisory Panel is to "advise on the commercial exploitation of research portfolio" and "advise on business model development, sustainability and routes to engagement with industry and health-care stakeholders."[15]

Along with the World Prevention Alliance, IPRI is organizing the first World Prevention Summit.[16] This sounds like a United Nations conference involving key organizations recognized as world leaders in disease prevention in developing countries. No such organizations are, however, involved in the Summit and IPRI has demonstrated no such track record. The World Prevention Alliance (WPA), which is convening the summit and whose name implies a coalition of major civil society organizations, consists apparently of twenty-three founding individuals. Peter Boyle is the founding president and WPA's address is a lawyer's office in Lyon, France. WPA states on its website: "The beneficiaries of the missions and projects financed by the World Prevention Alliance are predominantly the Least Developed Countries (LDCs), and within these, the most vulnerable populations (particularly women and children) and communities.

Special attention is given to countries of sub-Saharan Africa." It provides no information of any projects it has accomplished.[17] The event, by invitation only, was purportedly held at the National Press Club in Washington DC, USA, in November 2014. No report on the conference has been released.

In addition, IPRI seems to be working more for corporate interests than challenging causes of disease in developing countries. For example, the Harvard School of Public Health (HSPH) expresses grave concern over the epidemic of diseases, such as obesity, diabetes, and cancer, being caused by the irresponsible conduct of powerful sweetened drinks corporations, who, just like the tobacco industry, are today aggressively marketing their unhealthy products in developing countries. Research by the HSPH shows that roughly 180,000 deaths worldwide are linked to sugary drink consumption, with 78 percent of these deaths occurring in low- and middle-income countries.[18] In contradiction to its mission to prevent disease, however, IPRI published a review article, funded by Coca Cola, that came up with "reassuring" conclusions for Coca Cola, finding "no link with the consumption of sweetened, carbonated beverages and the risk of cancer overall or individual types of cancer."[19] In stark opposition to the helpful role IPRI is playing for Coca Cola and the sugary drinks industry, the HSPH is calling for government to take regulatory action to stop the unnecessary harm being caused by the irresponsible conduct of the sugary drinks industry. "These products are in a class with tobacco. There's only harm, no benefit," states Walter Willett, Chair of HSPH's Department of Nutrition.[20]

Another major project by IPRI—funded by Johnson & Johnson, a leading seller of mouthwash—was publishing a sixty-eight-page monograph for a special issue of the journal *Oral Diseases*. IPRI stated that "Oral disease is a very common phenomenon globally and it is apparent that use of mouthwash makes a significant contribution to public health." Again, the recommendation in favor of the use of mouthwash hardly seems to address a critical public health issue to help the impoverished populations of the developing world, who have little money to buy mouthwash. Furthermore, the concern expressed over dental disease lacks credibility in light of IPRI's encouraging findings with regard to sweetened, carbonated beverage consumption, which clearly contributes to dental disease.

SCIENTIFIC REVIEWS FINANCED BY TOXIC INDUSTRIES

Since leaving IARC, Boffetta is completely free to accept more commissions from various industries and from Exponent, and he does so, carrying out scientific reviews on products that were judged to be carcinogenic or harmful by reputable scientific authorities, such as IARC. In every case, whether it was the issue of dioxins, acrylamide, beryllium, atrazine, formaldehyde, diesel fumes, vinyl chloride, endocrine disruptors, PCBs, continued exposure to asbestos, or air pollution caused by heavy metals, Boffetta has come up with the findings desired by the industry and stated that he was unable to find evidence that the industry's product caused harm to the populations at risk.

In a study commissioned by the American Chemistry Council, an industry association of chemical companies, for example, Boffetta concluded that there was not consistent evidence to show an increased cancer risk for Vietnam veterans and others exposed to TCDD.[21]

In a study commissioned by Syngenta Crop Protection, Boffetta and his Exponent colleagues recommended use of the company's herbicide atrazine: "Atrazine appears to be a good candidate for a category of herbicides with a probable absence of cancer risk. Atrazine should be treated for regulatory and public health purposes as an agent unlikely to pose a cancer risk to humans."[22] The European Union has banned atrazine. James Huff and Jennifer Sass have written about the role that corporate lobbyists have played in preventing the health risks of atrazine from being fully reviewed by US regulatory agencies.[23]

In another study commissioned by the American Chemistry Council, Boffetta concluded: "At present, there is no consistent or strong epidemiologic evidence that formaldehyde is causally related to any of the LHM (lymphohematopoietic malignancies)."[24] This opinion is contrary to IARC's evaluation.[25]

In a study commissioned by Materion Brush, a company that manufactures beryllium and beryllium metal alloys, Boffetta concluded: "Overall, the available evidence does not support a conclusion that a causal association has been established between occupational exposure to beryllium and the risk of cancer."[26] This opinion is contrary to the deliberations of the IARC working group, which concluded that beryllium and beryllium compounds caused lung cancer in humans.[27]

In a study commissioned by Frito-Lay—a subsidiary company of Pepsi—on acrylamide, a substance that is produced when foods are cooked at a high temperature, Boffetta concluded: "Available studies consistently suggest a lack of an increased risk of most types of cancer from exposure to acrylamide."[28]

Even for substances for which he himself had previously found clear evidence that they caused harm, Boffetta now reversed his views. In 1988, for example, Boffetta published a study that reported an increased risk of lung cancer from diesel exposure with a dose-response effect. In 1989 he published a case-control study titled "Diesel Exhaust Exposure and Lung Cancer Risk" in which he reported increased risks of cancer from diesel exhaust exposure and concluded that a duration-response relationship was suggested. In 2001, while at IARC,

Boffetta authored a report, which concluded: "The results of this study provide evidence of a positive exposure-response relationship between exposure to diesel emissions and lung cancer risk among men."[29] Since Boffetta's 2001 review, two additional studies have been published on diesel exhaust and lung cancer; both demonstrated a dose-response between diesel exhaust and lung cancer.[30, 31]

Yet, in 2012, funded by a coalition of mining companies and engine manufacturers, the Mining Awareness Resource Group, Boffetta came to the opposite conclusion: "In sum, the weight of evidence is considered inadequate to confirm the diesel-lung cancer hypothesis."[32]

In addition to writing articles, funded by the chemical industry, which disputed IARC's findings of harm caused by the industry's chemicals, Boffetta joined with scientists from Exponent and from another industry-allied consulting company, Gradient, to dispute a report on the State of the Science of Endocrine Disrupting Chemicals by the WHO and the UN Environmental Program.[33] Boffetta and his coauthors accused the WHO-UNEP report of being unbalanced, inaccurate, and lacking in objectivity.[34] The authors of the article, the purpose of which was to raise doubt about an issue of extreme importance to the chemical industry—whether environmental chemicals are causing endocrine disruption—declared no conflict of interest and no funding was disclosed. Apparently, this major effort to discredit the WHO-UNEP report was carried out under a Mother Teresa–inspired moment of altruism to serve the cause of humanity. It is difficult not to notice that the article is extremely beneficial to the interests of industries producing environmental chemicals. It is also difficult not to notice that Exponent and Gradient and scientists working for these consulting companies have not won recognition for acts of scientific altruism, but rather for their services to toxic industries.

In a review article with Exponent, Boffetta and his coauthors cast doubt on epidemiologic studies of chronic disease outcomes that used geographic modeling to estimate long-term environmental exposures, particularly with regard to air pollution, magnetic fields, and pesticides, including paraquat. The work was funded by Syngenta. Boffetta is a member of an advisory group to the European Crop Protection Association, which is composed of the world's leading chemical companies, including Syngenta, Bayer, Dow, and Monsanto.

FAILURE TO DISCLOSE CONFLICT OF INTEREST

In September 2011, Boffetta and coauthor Carlo La Vecchia submitted an article[35] to the *European Journal of Cancer Prevention (EJCP)*, which claimed that the scientific literature showed "consistent evidence that for workers occupationally exposed in the distant past, the risk of mesothelioma is not appreciably influenced by subsequent exposures. Further, stopping exposure does not materially modify the risk of mesothelioma over subsequent decades." Italian epidemiologist Dario Mirabelli notes that Boffetta and La Vecchia reviewed a limited number of studies and distorted the results of those they did consider. Mirabelli points out: "For example, they report some results of our most recent article on mortality among workers in the Eternit plant in Casale Monferrato, but they do not cite our main result, which is that mesothelioma mortality is directly proportional to the duration of exposure to asbestos."[36]

Boffetta and La Vecchia stated that the article had been funded by the Italian Association for Cancer Research (AIRC), project No. 10068. Thus the reputation of AIRC was used to add credibility to the article. They also stated that they had no conflicting interests. When questioned, AIRC confirmed, however, that it gave no funding whatsoever for this work.[37] Furthermore, Boffetta and La Vecchia clearly had conflicting interests, which they did not declare. They had been hired as consultants for the Edison and Montefibre companies, which were facing criminal proceedings in regard to deaths of workers from mesothelioma. In July and November 2011, Boffetta and La Vecchia wrote briefs and testified in court on behalf of the companies, putting forward the same arguments that they advanced in the article.

AIRC refused a request that it ask the *EJCP* to publish a correction regarding the false funding information. A corporation, such as Coca-Cola, would not permit such misuse of its name and would take action to stop the misuse. It is disappointing that AIRC chose not to defend the integrity of AIRC's name; it sends a message that, while commercial interests are defended strenuously by corporations, ethical interests, such as the integrity of AIRC's name, are not taken seriously, even by AIRC itself.

Because citizens have placed their trust in AIRC, it receives huge amounts of funds from Italian citizens. It is, in fact, the organization that receives the highest amount of donations under an Italian government donation system and received more than 73 million euros in such donations in 2013. However, this trust has recently been damaged, in a criminal case with striking parallels to the criminal case in which La Vecchia and Boffetta testified. Piero Sierra, President of AIRC for the past nine years and former CEO of the Pirelli tire company, is being tried in court for the crime of manslaughter, along with other former company executives. They are accused of being responsible for the deaths of more than a hundred workers, two-thirds of them from mesothelioma, due to exposure to asbestos in the company's factories in Milan.

While Pirelli states that the company always took action to better protect the health and safety of its employees, Francesco Saia, an employee until 1984, stated in an affidavit that asbestos was on the ground for months with dust flying around and that "There were no masks, gloves were not there, there was nothing."

On May 28, 2014, AIRC elected a new president in place of Sierra. AIRC continues, however, to praise Sierra. In an interview with Alfredo Faieta of the publication *il Fatto*, the general manager of AIRC, Niccolò Contucci, stated: "The association is in a waiting position with respect to this trial. We have a lot of respect for the work done in recent years by President Sierra, a manager with excellent organizational skills that allowed AIRC to continue to grow up to current levels."[38]

Over 160 scientists, health defenders, and organizations signed a letter[39] to editor-in-chief of the *European Journal of Cancer Prevention*, expressing concern over distortions and improprieties in Boffetta's and La Vecchia's article. A complaint was submitted to the Committee for Publication Ethics (COPE) regarding the fact that the publication of the article appears to contravene COPE's code of conduct for editors of scientific journals.

As a consequence of the complaint, Boffetta and La Vecchia were required to publish the following Erratum:

> Role of stopping exposure and recent exposure to asbestos in the risk of mesothelioma: Erratum
>
> *European Journal of Cancer Prevention 2015, 24:68*
>
> The authors would like to bring the reader's attention to the conflicts of interest for their review paper (La Vecchia and Boffetta, 2012), and subsequent correspondence (La Vecchia and Boffetta, 2014). La Vecchia has acted as expert witness for the defendants or the judge in criminal trials involving occasional exposure to asbestos, on behalf of ENEL (Rome, Italy), Edison (Milan, Italy), Pirelli Tyres (Milan, Italy) and the Ordinary Tribunal of Turin (Italy). Boffetta has acted as expert witness for the defendants in a criminal trial involving exposure to asbestos in the manufacture of synthetic polymers and risk of mesothelioma (Edison, Milan, Italy).
>
> This work was not conducted with the contribution of the Italian Association for Cancer Research as stated on page 229 and the authors withdraw this statement on the acknowledgement of funding."[40]

"BIASED AND DELIBERATELY TAILORED, PSEUDO-SCIENTIFIC USE OF DATA"

Boffetta and La Vecchia were hired as consultants by the Riva company, which owns the ILVA steel plant in Southern Italy. The plant, the largest in Europe, has for many years released harmful chemicals from its chimneys, causing what one Italian court has described "an environmental catastrophe." Because of the failure of the company to implement environmental standards, the courts ordered the plant to be put under the authority of an independent administrator until such time as the company took action to stop the harmful pollution and to clean up the contamination.

In June 2013, Boffetta and La Vecchia submitted a forty-four-page report to the special administrator of ILVA, in which they exonerated the ILVA steel plant, saying its emissions had not contributed to the excess cancer and respiratory diseases among the population of Taranto.[41] They did not state on the document that they were consultants for the Riva company. They rejected the findings of the scientists from Italy's National Health Institute, as well as the scientists from the regional environmental authority and the scientists who had provided a report to the court prosecutor, who had all found that the emissions from the steel plant had contributed to excess mortality from lung cancer in the population of Taranto of approximately 30 percent. Boffetta and La Vecchia also disputed the authority of the regional government's environmental regulations, blamed the poor lifestyle of the Taranto residents, and stated that the ILVA steel plant was being subjected to unjust treatment by being held responsible for the harm.

In July 2013, the Italian Epidemiological Association (IEA) issued a press release, which denounced Boffetta's and La Vecchia's report as being "the biased and deliberately tailored, pseudo-scientific use of data in order to invalidate the evidence produced to date from epidemiological studies and to disregard the health impact of ILVA emissions on the population and workers."[42]

The IEA stated that the environmental data showed that the Taranto population was exposed for decades to high levels of different chemicals that have been well documented in the scientific literature to be carcinogenic. The IEA also noted that multicenter epidemiological studies and epidemiological studies of the health impact on populations living in the area have documented that air pollution has led to an increase in mortality and morbidity from heart and respiratory diseases.

The IEA criticized Boffetta's and La Vecchia's report, stating that "it is a matter of concern that in our country a position can be argued, that is clearly opposed to the evidence produced by international studies and accepted by the World Health Organization. This is a pseudo-scientific position, based on the opinion of individual researchers who are in a position of clear conflict of interest [expert witnesses for ILVA]."

BOFFETTA'S INDUSTRY TIES DEFEAT HIS APPOINTMENT AS DIRECTOR OF FRANCE'S LEADING EPIDEMIOLOGY CENTER

In late 2012, Boffetta submitted his candidacy for the position of director of France's Centre for Research in Epidemiology and Public Health (CESP), a position that was to be filled in December 2014. By the end of 2013, Boffetta was the only remaining candidate and was expected to be appointed to the position. An investigative article[43] published by the French newspaper *Le Monde* on December 18, 2013, discussed in detail Boffetta's industry ties and his practice over recent years of denying harm of industry products and denigrating the work of independent scientists. A number of scientists expressed strong opposition to the expected appointment, describing him as a mercenary who in recent years engaged in continuous consulting missions for polluting industries and aided an industry strategy aimed at creating doubt about scientific evidence and at weakening public health protection.

As a condition of the appointment, Boffetta was asked by Jean-Paul Moatti, director of public health at France's National Science & Medical Research Institute, to sever any conflict of interest relationships and private consulting work. Boffetta, therefore, in December 2013, ended his relationship with IPRI. He continued, however, to carry out consulting work; in particular, Boffetta agreed to act as an expert witness for the pharmaceutical company Takeda, in a 2014 US court trial regarding its anti-diabetic drug, Actos.[44]

On January 18, 2014, Moatti wrote[45] to the heads of units that would be affected by the Boffetta appointment, stating that he had spoken with Boffetta and that Boffetta had confirmed his contract with Takeda. Moatti stated that this conduct by Boffetta "leads us to have the strongest doubts about his future aptitude to manage conflicts of interest correctly, as head of a structure such as the CESP."

Boffetta's action was clearly in direct contradiction to the commitment that anyone responsible for public health research should cease all personal relationships with the private, for-profit sector, wrote Moatti. "It should be noted that the Takeda anti-diabetic has been removed from distribution from the French market by a decision by ANSM, following a French pharmaco-epidemiological study of 200,000 patients, which revealed a high statistically significant bladder cancer risk in exposed patients."

Moatti stated he was well aware of the difficulties the termination of Boffetta's candidacy created:

> However, it seems to me, that these difficulties can be overcome [by naming, if necessary, an interim director and the relaunch of an international call for can-

didates] and that these difficulties are less serious than the loss of credibility of
the center and, more widely, of research in public health in the eyes of decision-
makers and society in general, which could have resulted, if the candidature of
P. Boffetta had been continued.

Moatti concluded:

This is why, taking in consideration the recent development described above,
my personal position is that it is desirable that Paolo Boffetta should remove his
candidature as director of CESP and I consider that it is definitely a good thing
that he has just done so himself.

In an interview with *Science*, Boffetta stated that on January 28 he had withdrawn his candidacy for the position of director of CESP.[46]

In March 2014, Boffetta testified on behalf of the Takeda Pharmaceuticals
Corporation and Eli Lilly in support of their argument that their drug Actos had
not caused the bladder cancer of Terrence Allen, a patient who took the drug.
The jury rejected the arguments of Takeda and Eli Lilly and ordered that the
drug companies pay Allen and his wife $1,475,000 for present and future suffer-
ing and medical costs. The jury furthermore ruled that Takeda and Eli Lilly had
acted with wanton and reckless disregard and ordered that they pay nine billion
dollars in punitive damages. This ruling is being appealed and the punitive damages will almost certainly be reduced. However, the extraordinarily high amount
awarded for punitive damages reflects the outrage with which a jury of citizens
judged the companies' conduct.

Boffetta suffered a further repudiation when, on April 1, 2014, IPRI published an announcement stating that "it wishes it to be made known" that the
following articles by Boffetta "were neither IPRI approved studies nor was IPRI
in any way associated with the research grant." These articles by Boffetta were
industry-funded articles on styrene and cancer, TCDD and cancer, beryllium
and cancer risk, atrazine and cancer, diesel exhaust and pancreatic cancer, and
the role of stopping exposure to asbestos and risk of mesothelioma.

DEFENDING INDUSTRY, DISCREDITING INDEPENDENT
SCIENTISTS, AND ATTACKING IARC

While apparently seeing no threat from distortion of scientific evidence by
industry-funded scientists to deny or manufacture doubt about harm caused
by industry products, Boffetta has expressed alarm at what he sees as a serious

threat to science and public policy posed by independent scientists. Boffetta has launched attacks on what he claimed is a major problem of over-interpretation, bias, and erroneous scientific evidence of harm put forward by independent scientists, including IARC itself.

In 2008, while still at IARC, Boffetta published an appeal for action to address what he said was a major problem: the reporting of false positives. Epidemiology is particularly prone to the generation of false-positive results, said Boffetta. "Such erroneous scientific evidence may lead to inappropriate governmental and public health decisions, including the introduction of costly and potentially harmful measures."[47]

"What is needed," said Boffetta, "is greater scientific skepticism and increased humility on the part of epidemiologists. New policies should be adopted so as to institutionalize increased skepticism, such as requiring the prominent listing of study caveats."

Boffetta criticized IARC's Monographs on Acrylonitrile and on 2,3,7,8-tetrachlorodibenzo*para*-dioxin (TCDD) as having relied on insufficient epidemiological evidence. In response, Vincent Cogliano and Kurt Straif pointed out that IARC, for both substances, made use of a much wider body of interdisciplinary research findings than Boffetta acknowledged. It is important not to let preliminary or inconclusive results from one's own discipline outweigh strong findings from another, noted Cogliano and Straif, citing the advice of Sir A Bradford Hill: "All scientific work is incomplete . . . That does not confer upon us a freedom to ignore the knowledge we already have, or to postpone the action it appears to demand at a given time."[48]

In a commentary[49] published in the *International Journal of Epidemiology*, Paolo Vineis noted how the article by Boffetta and his coauthors is the following:

> . . . reminiscent, even in the terminology, of two recent phenomena in science: the plea for skepticism by the sociologist Bjorn Lomborg, who dismisses most of the evidence concerning climate change, species extinction, and other environmental issues; and the claim, by groups related to the corporate industry, that much of the evidence brought (e.g., in front of the court), concerning environmental pollutants (such as secondhand smoke), would be the product of "junk science." This claim has been also extended to the evidence on the health consequences of some dietary habits, such as excess sugar or salt in diet. Claiming that most epidemiological findings are false positives seems to suggest that epidemiology overall is junk science and in this sense echoes the claims of the industry.

Vineis pointed out how "vested interests often invoke high standards and well-founded theories, such as those found in physics, but this leads to a never-ending quest, acceptable on epistemic grounds but not on practical grounds. Epidemiology is at least in part a component of public health, i.e. it has to answer practical questions, as does clinical science when the individual patient is concerned."

The purpose of the IARC Monographs, noted Vineis, is not scientific curiosity but the practical goal of preventing cancer. A consensus process, involving scientists from a variety of disciplines, allows the Monographs to be deeply rooted in science and on independence from vested interests. "Boffetta et al.'s paper seems to describe a naive epidemiological community, unaware of its limits and prone to causal overstatements, a picture that is unfortunately too similar to the vision of some powerful groups with vested interests," stated Vineis.

In response to Vineis, Boffetta, while still at that time working as an IARC scientist, repeated the call for skepticism as intrinsic to the scientific ethos and denigrated IARC's consensus process: "Consensus is, at its core, a political process. Consensus opinion is an attempt to be evidence-based, but often reflects vested interests and various forms of advocacy empty of scientific merit."[50]

Boffetta has also sought to discredit IARC's work in yet another way: by criticizing its policy of choosing, as working group members for IARC Monographs, scientists from a variety of disciplines, who have published significant research related to the carcinogenicity of the agents being reviewed.[51] Boffetta, having now left IARC, stated that many of the IARC working group scientists "have a vested interest in advancing their own research results in the deliberations, if only to increase their prestige and future funding opportunities. The routine inclusion of such self-interested researchers is a clear conflict of interest, and inhibits an open and robust evaluation of the strengths and weaknesses of the studies under examination."

Boffetta et al. recommended that scientists without a professional background in the topic of the working group deliberations "would likely provide a more scientifically open and honest evaluation of the experimental and epidemiologic evidence related to the possible carcinogenicity of the agent being examined."

The tobacco industry exploited to its advantage the truism that, in science, there is always more to learn. It is likewise a truism that sometimes scientists report false-positives and that some scientists are improperly motivated by money and ambition. When this occurs, it should be appropriately dealt with. However, the major threat to science and public health today is posed, not by wrongdoing by independent scientists exaggerating harm caused by industry products, but by the well-documented harassment of scientists by industries in order to suppress evidence of harm; the spending of hundreds of millions of dollars by industries to commission tailored scientific research to advance their interests; the army of lobbyists and front organizations, funded by industries for the purpose of sabotaging public health policy. Boffetta has not seen fit to express concern about these threats to scientific integrity.

The arguments put forward by Boffetta to promote skepticism, to discredit and exclude independent scientific experts as allegedly biased, to isolate expertise so that the cumulative evidence of harm provided by various disciplines is avoided, would serve to undermine IARC's ability to identify carcinogenic substances and would tilt the global balance even further in favor of industry-spun science.

POLITICAL WILL REQUIRED TO STOP EPIDEMICS OF INDUSTRY-CAUSED DISEASE

WHO Director General, Margaret Chan, criticized the failure of governments to show the political will to take on big business.[52] It is regrettable to witness academic institutions and scientific journals, which claim to be dedicated to the defense of science and public health, demonstrate a similar failure to challenge industry subversion of science and public health. The *European Journal of Cancer Prevention* and Harvard University, for example, have turned a blind eye to harassment by Syngenta of scientists who document harm caused by its herbicide atrazine,[53] with the consequent grave discouragement of scientific freedom that conflicts with industry interests. They have likewise turned a blind eye to improper conduct by Syngenta, to prevent the US Environmental Protection Agency (EPA) from taking regulatory action on atrazine, by submitting flawed scientific data and negotiating behind closed doors with the EPA, in violation of the EPA's own regulations.[54]

The *European Journal of Cancer Prevention* had no problem, however, in publishing a Syngenta-funded review by Boffetta and Exponent scientists that encourages use of atrazine, a product that has been banned in Europe. While showing indifference to persecution of US scientists who document harm caused by atrazine, Harvard University is likewise helpful to Syngenta, posting Boffetta's atrazine-promoting article on Harvard's website.[55] Regrettably, the Harvard website fails to post critically important articles exposing the subversion of science by vested industries, such as Syngenta. As noted by LaDou et al.,[56] industry money and influence pervade every aspect of occupational and environmental medicine. Yet Harvard, like other leading universities, turns a blind eye to this issue, which is of imperative importance for the field of science and public health. It is not irrelevant that these universities are increasingly dependent on and entwined with corporate money.

As noted by David Egilman et al., "During the last several decades, researchers in a wide spectrum of fields have documented the direct and purposeful
efforts of corporations to disguise public health concerns and affect government
policies, particularly in the tobacco, alcohol, silica, and asbestos industries, and
more recently, the pharmaceutical, chemical, and ultra-processed food and
drink industries. Corporate-funded 'objective science' leading to the corruption
of scientific literature remains a major problem."[57]

Rob Moodie et al. likewise draw attention to the fact that transnational corporations are major drivers of global epidemics of non-communicable diseases
(NCDs) and that they use sophisticated strategies to undermine public health
policy.[58] The authors note that the term industrial epidemic has been used to
describe health harms related to products such as tobacco, alcohol, vinyl chloride, asbestos, and products of the food and drink industries. The authors point
out that many public health researchers, non-governmental organizations, and
national and international health agencies have financial and institutional relations with these companies and that these conflicts are largely unstudied in public health. The authors conclude that the only evidence-based mechanisms that
can prevent epidemics of disease caused by these industries are public regulation
and market intervention.

The evidence is overwhelming and urgent that the scientific community,
and, in particular, scientific journals and universities, must end their silence and
collusion in the face of epidemics of industry-created harm. They must find the
courage to be true to their mission, to practice what they preach and defend the
integrity of science and public health against documented subversion of public
health policy by powerful industry interests.

Chapter 8

SECRET TIES IN ASBESTOS— DOWNPLAYING AND EFFACING THE RISKS OF A TOXIC MINERAL

Geoffrey Tweedale

"I have a more basic concern, which even goes beyond the asbestos problem. The tendency nowadays for research to follow and be organized by agencies established with private support (whether they be "Institutes" in Boston or "Foundations" in Miami or whatever) means that topics for research will be selected by groups not subject to public control or public scrutiny. The scale and the scope of this new development in science is not derived from the philosophy of Academe."
Dr. Irving Selikoff, letter to Arthur C. Upton, December 20, 1989.
Selikoff Papers, Mount Sinai Hospital, New York.

INTRODUCTION

At the beginning of 2010, a small but significant event took place in the world of asbestos. Quebec Premier Jacques Charest set off on a trade mission to India. He was visiting one of the world's leading consumers of asbestos. The mission had an added piquancy because Canada has traditionally been a major supplier of raw asbestos fiber to India (Canadian asbestos exports to India in 2007 totaled 140,000 metric tons). The visit provoked controversy, both from anti-asbestos campaigners in India and from critics closer to home. In Canada, a letter was sent to Charest calling for an end to the use and export of asbestos. It was signed by more than one hundred scientists from twenty-eight countries, who appealed to Charest, "to respect the overwhelmingly consistent body of scientific evidence and the considered judgment of the World Health Organization (WHO) that all forms of asbestos have been shown to be deadly and that safe use of any form of asbestos has proven impossible anywhere in the world."[1] It highlighted that, according to figures from the Quebec Workers' Compensation Board, 60 percent of occupational deaths in Quebec in 2009 were caused by asbestos. While only three of the scientists who signed that letter were based in Quebec, provincial and national health authorities also became increasingly vocal on the issue. Into this dispute stepped Dr. Abby Lippman, an epidemiologist at McGill University in Montreal. Lippman also sent a letter to Charest, which was cosigned by about a dozen Canadian scientists and activists. The letter protested at the way Charest was ignoring "the overwhelming scientific consensus . . . that the safe use of chrysotile [white asbestos] has proven impossible," and that its use must end.[2]

These exchanges would have seemed unremarkable in any other context. The lethal nature of asbestos has been recognized since the early twentieth century. Subsequent medical research has left no doubt that asbestos causes not only asbestosis (lung scarring) and lung cancer, but also mesothelioma (a virulent and fatal cancer of the lining of the chest or of the abdomen). These health hazards have been extensively publicized on television, in newspapers, and in innumerable articles and books, so that the toxicity of asbestos has been firmly implanted in the public mind. By 2000, most advanced industrial countries had introduced bans on the mineral. The International Labour Organization (ILO) and the WHO have recently stated that asbestos kills at least ninety thousand workers worldwide each year *at present*. According to one report, the asbestos cancer epidemic could take at least 5 million (and possibly as many as 10 million) lives before asbestos is banned worldwide and exposures cease.[3]

However, a layperson on examining the issue further might begin to encounter surprises and entertain doubts. Despite the knowledge of the toxicity of asbestos, the mineral continues to be used in countries in the developing world. World asbestos production has settled at about 2 million tonnes—not much different from the early 1960s. The key producing and consuming countries are Russia, China, Kazakhstan, and Brazil. In some of these countries, particularly China, Kazakhstan, and Pakistan, levels of consumption have increased dramatically in the first years of the twenty-first century.[4]

Another surprise would be found in the medical literature. It is voluminous but contains little mention of corporate negligence or compensation issues. Instead, the layperson would find that the literature is dominated by debates about the health effects of the different types of asbestos fiber, with a heavy emphasis on animal experiments and the amount of fiber retained in the lungs of dead victims. Perhaps the biggest surprise is that, far from urging the banning of asbestos, some of the most influential asbestos scientists have defended the industry—indeed, they have gone further. They have urged that asbestos use should continue and that active efforts should be made to extend the exploitation of the mineral. It was this that made the Lippman letter so remarkable. Asbestos usage has often been actively endorsed, even encouraged, by Canada's leading asbestos scientists, especially those based at McGill University. Lippman's letter was apparently the first time that a McGill scientist had broken ranks to criticize Quebec's production and export of asbestos.

Behind these events lay a complex world of industry influence and funding, in which a web of vested interests and secret ties were (and are) at play. In no other area is it so important to know who wrote a paper and why—and who funded it. Thanks to the writing and campaigning of individuals such as Paul Brodeur,[5] Barry Castleman,[6] David Ozonoff,[7] David Lilienfeld,[8] and David Rosner and Gerald Markowitz,[9] we now know a good deal about how industry and science operated (and sometimes colluded) in the period up to 1960. The picture is one of a highly profitable multinational industry—spanning both asbestos mining and manufacture—which was able to manipulate the scientific debate through a mix of intimidation, suppression of information, corporate sponsorship, and the establishment of trade associations. The use of these strategies since the 1960s, particularly in the developing world, is relatively less well known and forms the subject of this chapter.

INDUSTRY TIES AND THE CHRYSOTILE DEBATE, 1960S–1990S

What transformed the "magic mineral" into a "killer dust" was its ability to cause mesothelioma, which is now (alongside asbestos-induced lung cancer) the leading cause of asbestos-related deaths. Mesothelioma's only known occupational cause is asbestos. In 1960, a landmark study published by South African researchers (which included Dr. Christopher Wagner) showed this linkage between mesothelioma and both occupational and non-occupational exposure to asbestos.[10] It was only in 1964, however, that an American physician—Dr. Irving Selikoff—brought home to the wider public the implications of these findings.[11] His research, which was based on trades union (not industry) records, demonstrated catastrophic cancer mortality among American insulation workers. His findings, which also suggested that non-occupational (i.e., neighborhood/environmental) exposure might cause mesothelioma, were publicized at a conference that he organized in New York City. The horror of mesothelioma was revealed—an incurable cancer that could stay latent for between thirty and sixty years, that could be caused by brief and non-occupational exposure, and that could kill within months.

These events, at the start of the 1960s, began a battle between a multinational industry intent on defending its product (or at least buying time for a staged withdrawal) and public health and regulatory bodies (supported by trade unions and activists) that wanted ultimately to see the use of the mineral ended. In South Africa, government and the industry—although they were unable to prevent the publication of Wagner's research—were able to stifle further research over the next decades. As Jock McCulloch has shown, no further important asbestos research took place in South Africa. Researchers were intimidated and Wagner found his professional interests best served by moving to the United Kingdom.[13] This ensured that crocidolite (blue) production continued in South Africa until the 1990s. Medical men colluded in the cover-up. Dr. Walter Smither, who was physician to Cape Asbestos (the British-based multinational involved in asbestos mining in the region), helped stifle mesothelioma research in the Cape.

Such strategies flourished under apartheid. In the United Kingdom and North America, however, debate was less circumscribed. Here, the industry reacted by forging hidden links with public health physicians and hiring its own consultants. A key strategy was sponsoring research. This research had many strands—such as dust counting, animal inhalation studies, and the pathology of post-mortem lungs—but by far the biggest research question that emerged was related to the toxicity of white asbestos (chrysotile). A crucial fact is that historically the bulk of world trade in asbestos (over 90 percent) has consisted of chrysotile. The South African research had involved blue asbestos mining. If chrysotile could be shown to be "innocent" (a word that would crop up often over the ensuing years), then most of the world's asbestos industry could continue untrammeled.

For the next forty years or more, much of the scientific debate about asbestos would revolve around the question of whether chrysotile could cause mesothelioma. In the early 1960s, this question was of greatest interest in Canada—the home of the world's biggest white asbestos industry. At the heart of this debate was the most famous tie between industry and science in the history of asbestos: that between the Canadian chrysotile mining industry and McGill University in Montreal. At that time, the Canadian asbestos mines employed six thousand workers and exported 1.5m tonnes a year. They were also interlinked with American companies, such as Johns-Manville, which owned many of the major mines. The industry was wealthy and, with government support, was willing to fund lavishly. Its largesse, dispensed through the industry's leading trade body—the Quebec Asbestos Mining Association (QAMA)—settled on McGill University in Montreal. QAMA had since the 1930s fostered links with this university, largely for public relations purposes. In the early 1960s, it revived those McGill links by sponsoring an Institute of Occupational & Environmental Health. It then channeled 2 million dollars into a research project that was designed to explore asbestos-related diseases in the mines. The lead researcher was an English-born epidemiologist, Dr. Corbett McDonald.

McDonald proved to be a dedicated epidemiologist who had the necessary discretion for industry-sponsored work. He never criticized the contemporary asbestos industry and instead blamed "old" conditions. With industry support, he was to research the white asbestos issue for more than thirty years. Over that period, McDonald and other McGill scientists (who, besides his wife, included Drs. Graham Gibbs and Bruce Case) were to become strongly associated with a particular view of chrysotile. In summary, that view argued that chrysotile was an entirely different type of mineral from blue or brown asbestos; that it was not "bio-persistent" in the lungs like blue or brown; that it did not cause high disease rates; and particularly that it did not cause any mesothelioma. Since blue and brown asbestos were known collectively as amphiboles, this view became known as the "amphibole hypothesis"—or alternatively as the "chrysotile defense." That was partly because the McGill research allowed QAMA to re-invoke its old defense: that Canadian working conditions and products were safer than elsewhere and that the dust in the Quebec mines was relatively benign.[14, 15]

It is worth examining how this tie developed. McDonald has apparently never been deposed in legal proceedings and questioned on the link between McGill and QAMA. Canadian state secrecy has also ensured that much of the documentation has never been made available. McDonald, however, has repeatedly suggested that his work was a Canadian government initiative. He told one conference in 1985 that, "We began our work in 1966 at the request of the Canadian Government . . ."[16] However, the truth is more complex. After Selikoff's New York conference in 1964, it was McDonald who approached Johns-Manville and broached the idea of an epidemiological study of Canadian mining, which he argued could "only be done in collaboration with the industry."[17] McDonald had been encouraged in this direction by Dr. John Gilson, Dr. Christopher Wagner, and Dr. John Knox. Gilson was a leading English occupational health physician, who was a head of the government's Pneumoconiosis Research Unit and then later an asbestos industry consultant. Wagner had by now taken up a research post under Gilson. Knox was an industry physician for Turner & Newall. This group had taken the view that Selikoff's research and conference were "alarmist" and that his work should be balanced by evidence from elsewhere. This was also the view of the industry, which soon provided the money for McGill University.

Inevitably, McDonald was to be heavily criticized for the source of his funding and he was dismissed by some as a scientist who simply did the industry's bidding. For example, activist Alan Dalton was critical of McDonald's industry funding and his apparent support in 1977 for an American asbestos factory in Cork, Ireland.[18] However, it was to prove difficult to dismiss the McGill work on that count alone. McDonald had his admirers and he was to retire as an emeritus professor at a leading London medical institution. Even his critics had to contend with the McGill findings, which showed low rates of mesothelioma. It is easy to see, though, how this research had been framed. The choice of Canadian chrysotile mining as a subject for intense epidemiological scrutiny was a singular one. It would have made more sense to further Selikoff's research on asbestos *consuming* industries, where the risks were evidently far greater and where the numbers employed were huge in comparison with the Quebec workforce. Yet these industries (where the fiber was more extensively broken down and therefore arguably more carcinogenic) were largely ignored. Instead, one of the least risky of industries—white asbestos mining, which was often conducted in open-air mines—had been chosen. Thus the conclusions about the benign nature of asbestos were drawn from a highly selective look at an industry.

Even those conclusions needed some clever footwork and epidemiological acrobatics from the McGill group. This was because mesotheliomas (and lung cancers and asbestosis) had been found among chrysotile miners. Eventually, McDonald and his team settled on the explanation that it was due to "contaminants," not chrysotile. The main "contaminant" identified was tremolite—a trace fiber in Canadian chrysotile—that McDonald and the McGill group argued was the main cause of the Canadian mesotheliomas. Carefully mine chrysotile from only non-tremolite asbestos workings—so the argument went—and any potential risk with Canadian chrysotile would be eliminated.[19] All that would be needed for full commercial exploitation was "controlled conditions" (respirators and dust extraction) in the consuming industries.

This argument was so riddled with flaws and ambiguities that it seems extraordinary that it was ever countenanced. Tremolite itself was an asbestos fiber, so regarding it as a contaminant was misleading—especially since epidemiologists had no control over the fiber from the mines and knew perfectly well that Canada never screened its fiber. McDonald and his fellow researchers were similarly aware that Quebec asbestos would never be used in Canada and that it was all destined for developing countries, such as India. So-called controlled conditions had never existed in the West; they were even less likely to be applied in the East. Yet the McGill School proved influential. McDonald's work was to be widely cited worldwide in government inquiries and commissions, where it supported employers' claims about the safety of asbestos. It apparently confirmed all those traditions that Canadian fiber was "safe" and heaped the blame on the amphibole fibers that Canada did not produce. It gave the Canadian government and the Quebec industry the green light it needed to continue exporting asbestos.

The McGill work fed directly into asbestos litigation, where the "chrysotile defense" proved useful to defendant companies. It was also part of a complex web of industry-funded scientific work that was usually conducted through the medium of research organizations and trade associations. The pioneer asbestos research body was the Asbestosis Research Council in the United Kingdom, which was established in 1957 and was funded mainly by Turner & Newall.[20, 21] In 1970, Johns-Manville launched the Asbestos Information Association/North America (AIA/NA). It was followed by the appearance of the Asbestos Institute in Canada in 1984—an extra wing of the mining industry's lobbying effort. In France, the Comité Permanent Amiante (CPA) was another body designed to protect industry interests. Eventually, in 1976, an Asbestos International Association (AIA) was formed. Essentially, these organizations were about product defense and public relations, rather than science. On the other hand, scientists were recruited to run carefully designed (in other words, non-controversial) research projects and also to staff the committees. The ARC recruited first Dr. Peter Elmes, who had succeeded Gilson as head of the Pneumoconiosis Research Unit, and then later Anthony Seaton, another leading physician. In France, Professor Jean Bignon, a leading French chest physician, joined the CPA. What remained hidden were the industry ties that controlled publication. The ARC, for example, had complete right of veto.

While studiously avoiding any criticism of the industry, the McGill group had no scruples about attacking the industry's critics. In 1997, in the pages of an English science journal, McGill scientist (and McDonald collaborator) Doug Liddell wrote one of the most defamatory attacks on a group of scientists ever published in the scientific literature. The target was Selikoff and his group at the Mount Sinai Hospital, New York, whom Liddell accused of being motivated by nothing more than "malice" (in contrast to "honest" scientists elsewhere). The article also proclaimed the "innocence" of chrysotile.[22] The whole exercise was topped off by the endorsement of the editor of the journal, who agreed that the American group had ulterior motives (though their precise nature was not stated). That journal was the *Annals of Occupational Hygiene* and its sponsor was the British Occupational Hygiene Society (BOHS)—an ambiguous group of occupational health physicians that on its formation in 1953 promised industry "the opportunity to influence its policies."[23] Editors of the *Annals*, notably Trevor Ogden, have continued to defend the BOHS's conduct and the research of the McGill School.

It was symptomatic of a medical community that worked with industry, not against it. At a time when scientists should have been ringing the alarm bells, almost all had developed ties with the industry. In the 1980s and 1990s, industry influence penetrated bodies such as International Agency for Research on Cancer (IARC), the WHO, and the ILO, where the agenda was frequently dominated by the industry. For example, after an IARC meeting in Lyon in 1972, Selikoff noted:

> . . . the heavy concentration of asbestos industry personnel and "consultants" with almost half of the participants falling into this class . . . [and] the extraordinary selection of an industry representative to give the only address at the conference dinner (paid for by the asbestos industry!), in which he regretted the fact that some must die in the industrial utilization of asbestos. But, since society needed this valuable material, we had to be brave and accept this unfortunate necessity. This same dinner, incidentally, witnessed the extraordinary decision to exclude Dr. E. Cuyler Hammond, vice president of the American Cancer Society, from attendance. It was only with difficulty, and repeated urging by [trade unions], that place was finally made for Dr. Hammond![24]

The industry had some of the leading epidemiologists on its side. Sir Richard Doll was consultant for UK asbestos giant Turner & Newall. He proved a consistent defender of white asbestos and had little time for that company's critics.[25] In 1989, when the WHO responded to the asbestos industry's lobbying for a meeting, Doll agreed to host a gathering at his Oxford University college. A contingent of industry representatives took part, including Jacques Dunnigan from the Asbestos Institute in Canada. McDonald attended, too. Labor groups were invited, along with Dr. Robert Murray (the Trades Union Congress's ex-senior medical man). The meeting drew on a study that Murray presented as an appendix to the eventual report. The latter was the result of Murray's undisclosed consultancy for the Asbestos International Association. The meeting fully endorsed the Canadian fiber-specific position: that chrysotile use could continue, that more work should be done on "contaminants" and that countries should be educated in controlled use.[26]

Christopher Wagner was potentially one of the industry's most threatening critics. His mesothelioma research had made him one of the big names in asbestos epidemiology (alongside Doll, Selikoff, and McDonald). His early experimental work had highlighted the risk of mesothelioma associated with all types of asbestos, including chrysotile. Yet after the publication in 1986 of a paper that announced the "innocence of chrysotile to humans,"[27] he, too, rapidly reached an accommodation with the industry. By 1997, Wagner could be found in Montreal at an asbestos conference sponsored by the Canadian government. It was a small audience, consisting mostly of those with industry connections or those who had served as expert witnesses at the request of defendant companies. Murray was there; so too was Dunnigan; and Wagner's collaborator was the retired company doctor from Cape Asbestos (the firm that had operated the crocidolite mines in South Africa). The general burden of the conference was purportedly to provide a scientific perspective on asbestos and controlled use, but not surprisingly was oblivious to the fact that most countries had now banned chrysotile.[28] Wagner's bedfellows might have seemed strange ones, given Wagner's troubled dealings with South African asbestos companies: but they would not seem out of place four years later, when it was revealed that Wagner (like Doll) had a secret consultancy and an offshore account with an American multinational.[29] In Wagner's case, the company was US asbestos giant Owens-Illinois, for whom he testified in court and conducted undisclosed scientific work. Wagner collapsed and died almost coincidentally with the exposure of his asbestos consultancy in US litigation.

At the end of the twentieth century, McDonald's support of asbestos use was undiminished. He lamented that it was probably too late to save what he termed chrysotile's "soiled reputation,"[30] but he did what he could to cleanse it. In a letter to an American occupational health journal in 1999, McDonald compared the movement to ban asbestos to the witch craze, Prohibition, and McCarthyism. He stated that, far from banning asbestos, "we should surely be encouraging the search for and exploitation of chrysotile . . ."[31] According to McDonald, the mineral was "remarkably safe." He also accompanied Canada's lawyers to the scientific hearing on Canada's challenge to the French asbestos ban, held at the World Trade Organization (WTO) in Geneva in January 2000. There, in an unusual procedural move made by Canadian lawyers, McDonald testified in support of Canada's position.[32]

ASBESTOS INDUSTRY TIES IN THE NEW MILLENNIUM

Since the Johns-Manville bankruptcy in 1982, the asbestos multinationals have been in flight from the mineral. Slowly asbestos production and manufacture have all but ceased in the advanced industrial countries, with the path punctuated by asbestos bans, litigation, and corporate bankruptcies. Despite the opposition of the Canadians, in 2001 the WTO stated that there is no safe level of asbestos exposure, that all types of asbestos are carcinogenic, and that "controlled" risk in manufacture is unachievable.[33] The passing of asbestos in one part of the world—OECD nations—has left developing countries to embrace chrysotile. Nearly all of that chrysotile goes into the manufacture of asbestos cement sheets and pipes.

Past corporate giants like Manville have been replaced on the asbestos stage by small indigenous companies. However, the debate about asbestos hazards has not changed. Those defending asbestos emphasize, as ever, cost-benefit analysis, the low risks associated with "controlled" conditions, the "safety" of chrysotile, and the unquantified hazards of substitutes. Canada remained an important influence on the industry's science by providing money, a scientific model, and leadership. This has ensured that much asbestos science—or perhaps one should say chrysotile science, since the soiled word "asbestos" has been increasingly elided from the discussion—has continued to be framed by industrial interests.

Industry bodies have remained influential. During the first decade of the twenty-first century, the Chrysotile Institute in Quebec (the word "asbestos" was dropped in 2004) remained a focus around which the new asbestos industry could coalesce. The mingling of industry and science could be seen on the conference circuit. For example, in May 2006 the Chrysotile Institute held a conference in Montreal entitled "Chrysotile at a Turning Point." The conference, which carried the imprimatur of the Chrysotile Institute, the International Chrysotile Association, and the Quebec and Canadian governments, was designed to promote the use of asbestos in developing countries.[34] It featured long-time North American proponents of asbestos, such as conference spokesperson Dr. Jacques Dunnigan, who was joined by speakers and delegates from Russia, Mexico, Brazil, and India. Most of these countries imported Canadian asbestos.

The program was filled with industry consultants. A flavor of the proceedings can be found in the presentation by English toxicologist Dr. John Hoskins, which was entitled "The Great Asbestos Deception." However, according to Hoskins, it was not industry deception that was the culprit, but claims of lawyers, producers of non-asbestos fibers, asbestos waste disposal companies, trade unions, and political parties. What exactly the "turning point" was in asbestos was never made clear, especially since the conference was largely a reiteration of research and ideas that had been around since the 1970s and had long since been either discredited or abandoned. Most of the delegates, such as Nikolai F.

Izmorov from Russia, earnestly stressed the mantras of the standard chrysotile defense: only heavy exposure caused adverse health effects; asbestos was safely bonded into cement products, and any disease was purely due to "past" conditions. Above all, asbestos could be used safely. According to Mexican presenter Luis Cejudo Alva: "Through medical and scientific studies we know chrysotile safe use can exist."

The point was rammed home by the secretary to the minister for natural resources, Christian Paradis, who gave the welcoming address. He told the audience that his government wanted to ensure the safety of exposed workers and that the Chrysotile Institute supported the safe use of asbestos.[35] According to Paradis, Canada had played a leading role in raising awareness of risk and had actively helped developing countries to understand safe use. However, Paradis neglected to tell his audience that Canada, which was the only country to fund the export of asbestos, discouraged its domestic consumption by prohibiting its use in many consumer products and setting stringent limits for the release of asbestos from mines and mills.[36]

Paradis explained that Canada would continue to resist the listing of chrysotile as a hazardous substance under the Rotterdam Convention. That convention is a legally binding multilateral agreement to promote shared responsibilities in relation to the importation of hazardous chemicals. If chrysotile was added to the list, then Canada would have to prepare a document disclosing any restrictions imposed on chrysotile for health and safety reasons. Importing nations could then decide whether to ban it. At a Rotterdam review in 2004, chrysotile satisfied all the criteria for listing. But Canada and Russia, both exporters, organized opposition, which ensured that asbestos was still not listed. At the October 2006 meeting in Geneva, Canada again led a group including Ukraine, Kazakhstan, Iran, Peru, and the Russian Federation in opposing the listing of chrysotile.[37] They argued that a listing would be tantamount to an international ban as it would force tighter domestic regulations on use. Once again the move to list chrysotile under the Rotterdam Convention (favored by over one hundred signatories) failed—thereby severely weakening the convention.

It was part of a broad counterattack. At Canada's prompting, a reinvigorated pro-asbestos movement was soon under way among the chrysotile-using nations. At a conference in Moscow in 2007, interested parties from these countries met again to reiterate their defense of the product. A Chrysotile Association had been spawned in Russia (as part of an International Chrysotile Association)—a group which supposedly had the support of labor through the Chrysotile International Alliance of Trade Unions. Canada, Kazakhstan, Zimbabwe, Ukraine, Uzbekistan, India, Columbia, Brazil, and Mexico sent representatives.

After this event, an "appeal" was made to Margaret Chan, director-general of the WHO, to reconsider the WHO's policy on the elimination of acute respiratory distress syndrome (ARDS). This appeal to Chan—in the form of a fawning letter—had been signed, inter alia, by Corbett McDonald, John Hoskins, David Bernstein, and Dennis J. Paustenbach. The letter argued that asbestos was merely a trade name and that there should be greater recognition of the difference between chrysotile and the amphiboles. It pleaded for yet another review of the evidence. This request was apparently granted in May 2007, when the WHO suddenly included a let-out clause for chrysotile in its document, "Workers' Health: Global Plan of Action," which stated that a "differentiated approach" should be adopted for asbestos regulation.

Most of the signatories to this letter were industry consultants. Paustenbach, for example, has worked almost exclusively for industry through his ChemRisk Company. He has solid academic credentials and a track record of producing studies at the request of companies' intent on defending their product. His research has been prominent in litigation involving asbestos in car friction products (brakes), where he has consulted for companies such as General Motors and Ford. His work, which broadly stresses that asbestos exposures in most jobs are too low to cause disease, shows the circularity of this type of industry-sponsored research, in which a researcher is paid for research, which is then recycled in litigation, often with the researcher appearing later as expert witness.[38]

Paustenbach's allegiances are usually declared in his work. Less apparent was the industry's ties with Dr. David Bernstein. The signatories had suggested that Chan might meet Bernstein for a briefing, as he too lived in Geneva. Bernstein was an American-born "consultant in toxicology," who was a recent publisher in the field of asbestos. His work was an attempt to update the work of the McDonald School, though Bernstein's work contained little that was new; it was based on rat inhalation studies and recycled the old bio-persistence argument that white asbestos is quickly cleared from the lungs without apparent ill-effects. In one report, for example, Bernstein has claimed that "at low exposure pure chrysotile is probably not hazardous . . . [and] . . . the hazard may be low even if high exposures were of short duration."[39] These views, while being rejected by almost all public health bodies, were congenial to asbestos interests, including the Brazilian Chrysotile Institute, who drew on Bernstein's bio-persistence theory to claim that white asbestos was safe to mine and manufacture. His views were also sought by the Canadian government, when Health Canada brought together a group of experts to discuss (yet again) the health effects of chrysotile. The Health Canada report became mired in controversy, because the government blocked its publication. Another dispute arose, too, over Bernstein's involvement. In 2007, at a court hearing in Waxahachie in Texas, Bernstein had been called to testify at the request of a defendant company in an asbestos case. He was questioned by the attorney for the victim's family:

> Q: The chrysotile study that you have been talking about with this jury, those are studies that have been done at the request of Union Carbide, a Brazil chrysotile mining interest, the Asbestos Institute, and the Canadian Government. Is that correct?
>
> A [Bernstein]: That's correct.
>
> Q: So when the lawyers representing Union Carbide helped fund your studies, tell the jury how much money you took from them to do that work that you're relying upon today in court.
>
> A: They asked me to do the scientific evaluation.
>
> Q: How much money did they pay you? I'll take it in francs or dollars.
>
> A: I don't have it in front of me at the moment.
>
> Q: Would it refresh your memory if I showed you Union Carbide's responses . . . where they say they paid you $400,623.20?
>
> [Objections from defendant counsel, followed by an instruction from the court, the Hon. Gen Knize, judge, to Bernstein]
>
> THE COURT: Just, if you can answer that question . . . how much did they pay you?
>
> A: Union Carbide asked me to do these studies in order to . . .
>
> THE COURT: Can you answer my question please? I'm just repeating the question the attorney asked. Can you answer it or can't you answer it?
>
> A: I can answer how much they paid me, but part of what the sum he's referring to was for actually funding the conduct of the study.
>
> THE COURT: Listen. Can you listen? Can you look at me and listen? Read my lips. How much money did Union Carbide, through their attorneys, pay you?
>
> A: I think . . . I don't have the sum in front of me. My recollection is in the order of about a hundred thousand Swiss francs. . . .[40]

None of Bernstein's work appears to carry any disclosure of these conflicts of interest. One Health Canada panelist, Bice Fubini (Italy), complained: "He never disclosed these links."[41]

However, Bernstein and other supporters of asbestos have been quick to complain about the supposed misuse by others of science and scientific bodies. A target of their attention has been the IARC. In 2007, Bernstein was the lead author in an article that complained that the agency did not take into account risk assessment and therefore was eliminating a mineral that could be used safely and bring major benefits to society. The article was published in *Indoor and Built Environment*—a journal that claimed the moral high ground in the asbestos debate.[42] However, recently released documents suggest that the launch of this journal was orchestrated by the tobacco industry as a way of presenting research that questioned the health risks of environmental tobacco smoke.[43] The journal's content came to reflect the outlook of a small coterie of mineralogists, toxicologists, and industry consultants, who supported the continued use of asbestos. Editor John Hoskins consistently supported the Canadian government and its asbestos industry in their quest to extend asbestos manufacture in the developing world. Much the same group of individuals can be found writing in another science journal, *Regulatory Toxicology and Pharmacology*—the official organ of the International Society for Regulatory Toxicology and Pharmacology (ISRTP). In 2008, a whole supplement of one issue was devoted to asbestos, with reference to taconite mining in Duluth, Minnesota.[44] Many of the papers were written by representatives of private consulting firms. The broad burden of the arcane collection of papers was to argue that the environmental risks of asbestos were minimal. Almost all the papers revolved around the fiber type issue and contained little that was controversial. The prominence of industry and private consultants is perhaps not surprising. According to David Michaels, the ISRTP is "really just an association dominated by scientists who work for industry trade groups and consulting firms."[45] Michaels points out that one past president was an attorney who became vice president for a leading product defense group. One editor, Gio B. Gori, was known for his consultancy work for Big Tobacco. The list of advisory editors have included asbestos luminary Dennis Paustenbach.

Industry ties have thrown up some extraordinary characters and pro-asbestos arguments in some unexpected places. In 2001, the lack of asbestos fire-retardants was blamed for the collapse of the World Trade Center (WTC). The argument was advanced by Steven Milloy, a commentator for *Fox News*, only days after the terrorist attacks. In an article entitled "Asbestos Could Have Saved WTC Lives," Milloy wrote that the WTC might have stood longer, preventing many casualties, had the use of asbestos fire-resistant materials not been curtailed.[46] Andrew Schlafly, in an article in a medical journal, attacked what he perceived as the "flawed science" behind the decision to ban asbestos in the WTC. "Litigation-fed hysteria" inspired by Selikoff was supposedly behind the collapse of the WTC, as it was behind the Challenger and Columbia space shuttle disasters (which were also alleged to have been due to the lack of asbestos).[47] Sympathizers with this view now felt able to proclaim the emergence of a "new policy" toward asbestos as a result of the WTC tragedy—one that was based on "actual scientific facts, with less influence from social and political factors."[48]

These views seem less impressive once the credentials of the participants are revealed. Steven Milloy, the apparent originator of this WTC debate, was a paid advocate for tobacco companies Philip Morris and R.J. Reynolds and oil giant Exxon Mobil. Milloy's main claim to fame was as a self-appointed critic of "junk science" and opponent of the idea of global warming. From the 1990s until the end of 2005, he was an adjunct scholar at the "libertarian" Cato Institute, which has a track record of hostility to asbestos litigation. Schlafly was a conservative lawyer and founder of *Conservapedia*, which has been described as the US religious right's version of *Wikipedia*. The publication in which his article appeared, the *Journal of American Physicians and Surgeons*, is not regarded as a valid peer-reviewed journal. The few academic articles that have appeared on this issue were published in *Indoor and Built Environment*.[49]

PERSPECTIVES ON SECRET TIES

Not all of the academy's links with industry were secret, and not every industry-sponsored study was worthless. Landmark articles on asbestos-related lung cancer by Doll in 1955 and the South African research on mesothelioma in 1960 began with industry support, even though the publication of the findings was often fraught. On the other hand, throughout most of this period between the 1960s and the present day, asbestos science appears to have functioned all too often as an extension of an industry agenda that was committed primarily to the defense of its product. The asbestos industry has become yet another case study to join the ranks of numerous other case studies that have flagged the problems of industry influence.[50-55]

It helped the industry enormously that eventually nearly all the biggest names in asbestos research—Richard Doll, Christopher Wagner, Corbett McDonald, John Gilson, and Jean Bignon—were either consultants for the leading companies or involved in studies that relied on the industry for data. Disturbingly, none of these men saw any ethical dilemmas. When he defended his seeking of funds from the Quebec mining industry, McDonald told one critic that, "Coming from a country where scientists are generally considered, and usually are, honorable men, there seemed nothing particularly wrong in this somewhat strange, North American way of doing things. . . ."[56] The only individual to register a protest was Irving Selikoff, who was dismayed at how medicine had become entangled in the "air streams of corporate jets, pound and dollar insignia interwoven."[57] Selikoff complained that the actions of individuals such as Dr. Robert Murray were serving "to cheapen a tradition that so many of us had held valuable. . . ."[58]

The ultimate result of these ties was that, at the very least, they slowed down recognition of the health hazards of asbestos and bought time for the industry.

One of the results can be seen in the striking fact that the bulk of the world's asbestos (some 80 percent) was mined *after* the world was alerted in the early 1960s to the problem of mesothelioma.

The great figures in asbestos epidemiology have now mostly either died or retired. Epidemiology—at least as regards landmark studies—is almost played out. We now know more than enough about the health effects of asbestos. Asbestos has now become a backwater specialty of individuals such as Bernstein—in other words, toxicologists or geologists, who usually have little or no expertise in medicine, occupational hygiene, epidemiology, or pathology. The debate is now more likely to be conducted along narrow lines and in arcane journals, with a heavy emphasis on fiber types, bio-persistence, experiments with rodents and the re-interpretation of old data.

While this article was being completed, in 2012 Canadian asbestos production ceased and the Chrysotile Institute became defunct. However, asbestos lobbying continued through the Chrysotile Association (Russia), the Asbestos Cement Products Manufacturers Association (India), and the Brazilian Chrysotile Institute. When the UN Rotterdam Convention Conference met in Geneva in May 2015, a Russian-led contingent again blocked the listing of chrysotile as a hazardous substance. The Canadian government gave tacit approval to this tactic by declining to support the attempt by a majority of countries to have chrysotile listed. Thus, the issues of secret ties and linkages between medicine, industry, and politics remain very much alive in the developing world, where the scientific battles that were conducted fifty years ago are still being re-enacted.

Chapter 9

KIDDING A KIDDER

Martin J. Walker

It is evident that most scientific inquiry today is dictated not by the thirst for knowledge but by the thirst for profits. Even so, the full extent of the betrayal of the public interest has yet to be appreciated.[1]

Bob Woffinden

On May 1, 1981, eight-year-old Jaime Vaquero died in the ambulance taking him from his home in Torrejón de Ardoz, on the outskirts of Madrid, to the hospital. His illness, which had begun suddenly, signaled the beginning of an environmentally caused epidemic. Over the coming five years, Jaime Vaquero's death was followed by a thousand more—extravagantly reduced by official sources to nearly half their real number—together with around twenty-five thousand admissions to the hospital, in an epidemic that would only begin to decline after three months and would only peter out over four years.

Within weeks of Jaime Vaquero's death, an official epidemiological narrative emerged giving a name, and therefore a cause, to the epidemic.[2] It was to be said by the Spanish government, the Atlanta Centers for Disease Control (CDC), and the World Health Organization (WHO) that the epidemic was caused by rapeseed oil, which was imported and then sold for domestic use. This oil, it was said, had previously been treated with aniline that colored the oil and so protected the Spanish market for pure olive oil. The vendors for this cooking oil, from which the dye had been removed, were said to be salesmen frequenting outdoor markets and door-to-door sales.

Between 1981 and the beginning of the trial of a dock full of oil salesmen that began in 1987, an aggressive but mainly subterranean conflict ensued. Those who did not agree with what they saw as a ludicrous official hypothesis

were harassed, threatened, sacked from public sector jobs, pressurized, burglar-
ized, and accused of emotional instability. It was, in effect, the first mass battle
between corporatism and independent scientists and citizens in the twentieth
century.

Thirty-eight oil sellers and producers suspected of causing the epidemic
were finally tried over four years; the trial became the longest in Spanish history
and the US-backed prosecution proceeded throughout with a complete absence
of scientific evidence. The prosecution called nearly three thousand witnesses
and hundreds of experts, while demanding hundreds of years in jail for the principal defendants.

The defense argued that many individuals had fallen ill who had not consumed oil, while many others who had consumed oil had not fallen ill; corrupted
oil clearly had nothing to do with the epidemic. Circumstantially and epidemiologically, they argued it was almost certain that an organophosphate pesticide
had in fact been responsible.

The most famous witness for the prosecution was Richard Doll, called in to
do an off-the-cuff star turn by a British staffer at the World Health Organization
(WHO). But the man who won the case for corporatism was a US epidemiologist
working for a CDC militarized health section, the Epidemiological Intelligence
Service (EIS), Edwin Kilbourne. Kilbourne was seconded to Madrid under a
military agreement two years into the outbreak.

In retrospect, the official explanations for the epidemic and the trial that
followed had all the signs of a massive mirage created with amazing theatrical
dexterity. While the epidemic itself was very real and happened almost as was
recorded, the finer details of its epidemiology and the most general assumptions
about cause were almost entirely factitious. If we stir into this pot, the Spanish
Syndrome epidemic has all the elements of a classical tale of truth reversal, the
likes of which has become increasingly common in the twenty-first century.[3]

The story has a number of heroes and heroines who are divided into two
groups: (1) those epidemiologists who worked for government or were physicians of one kind or another, (2) a small clutch of journalists, most prominent
among whom, to UK audiences, was Bob Woffinden,[4] who fought the authorities' presentation of the syndrome with exemplary investigative journalism. In a
bizarre fashion, the epidemic was a clear precursor to the global battle over ideas
about HIV- and AIDS-related illnesses that were in 1981 just about to appear on
the horizon.

It was 1985 when Richard Doll was approached by the WHO to add the authority of his name in support of the idea that toxic oil had caused the Spanish

epidemic. In terms of his public profile, he was on a steeply ascending curve. Almost twenty years since his initial research on cigarette smokers, working under Bradford Hill, an apparently freelance consultant epidemiologist, he was becoming better known internationally by the day. At the time he took on the Spanish case, Doll had been approached to carry out a review of polyvinyl chloride (PVC) and brain cancer; facing mounting evidence and a number of court cases, industry wanted to show conclusively that vinyl chloride was not responsible for cancer of the brain in PVC workers.[5]

Doll was awarded this PVC research after being approached by Dr. Brian Bennett, the Medical Adviser to ICI UK. Bennett had asked permission of the US Chemical Industries Association to involve Doll in the research; Doll was welcomed with open arms and given cherry-picked industry data to carry out this research.[6]

The "paper" concluded that PVC production process workers did have brain cancer in higher numbers than the public. Doll claimed that this increase was not statistically significant but an anomaly caused by an unknown factor. The results of this paper were to be repeatedly published by popular news outlets, long after a link between the PVC production process and brain cancer had been commonly accepted.[7]

By the time of his death in 2005, Sir Richard had more or less been "outed" as an industry shill. In the *Daily Telegraph* in 1983 he was quoted expressing a rabid defense of corporatism: "In his 1983 Harveian Oration, Sir Richard Doll warned against environmentalists, who might 'whip up irrational prejudice, unfounded in science.'"[8]

And again, in 1992, writing in the *Daily Mail* at the time of the Rio summit, Doll warned that we may be seeing "a new attitude emerge; an irrational ideology opposed to science, to industry and to progress." Such an attitude, he told us, exists already:

> There is, for example, a large and powerful lobby against pesticides, which they say leave cancer-causing residues in our food. Yet scientific research has shown that those residues are some 1800 times less than the amount of cancer-causing agents naturally present *in the plants*. The lobby does not seem to object to natural carcinogens; only to the infinitesimally small amounts introduced by man.[9]

Knowing what we now know about the way in which crisis PR management works and the perverse intelligence of such articles, it seems unlikely that Doll actually wrote them but simply allowed his name to be put on them. The unbridled alliance of science and industry is transparent in Doll's *Daily Mail* article.

He defended industry on six different occasions in the short article and asked us, not without a dash of desperation, to trust industry and industrialists, science and scientists; these, he said, are the people with the key to the future. He ended the article with a warning that we must stop environmentalists, whom he describes as the "anti-science Mafia," from "hijacking" the Rio summit.[10]

In January 2000, Doll joined the advisory board of the American Council of Science and Health (ACSH), the graveyard for aged corporate science lobbyists: an organization funded by the food, pharmaceutical, and chemical industries that promotes any substance, except tobacco, criticized for its possible toxicity.[11, 12]

Doll was a founder and the first Warden of Green College Oxford. The original intention for it was to be an exclusively medical college. The college was named after Cecil Green, founder of Texas Instruments, who was its main benefactor. The deceptive name disguises the fact that it taught research and epidemiology in the style of Sir Richard—that is, without environmental factors getting in the way.

In the 1970s, Doll was involved in the setting up of the Chemical Industry Institute for Toxicology (CIIT) an antidote to independent university and hospital research departments. The institute claimed to be engaged in "independent research on the effects of chemicals," the results of which were used to give trial evidence on behalf of chemical companies in cases involving civil claimants. In 2007, the CIIT became the Hamner Institutes for Health Sciences.[13]

Throughout the 1980s, 1990s, and later, there were references to the fact that Doll was working to protect industry rather than independently in the name of public health; this contention had been supported by his appearance in a number of court cases in which he gave evidence for industry against civilian claimants. In 2000, he gave a statement to Covington and Burling, ironically the main lawyers for the tobacco industry,[14] acting in defense in Italy and the US of chemical corporations in polyvinyl chloride industry cases.[15]

In both these cases, Doll argued that the industry processes were safe and could not have caused cancer in workers. For the US case, Doll had been paid £12,000, according to Doll as "a donation to a charity" for his work. The charity selected was the Green College at Oxford. The US court found in favor of the claimants, while in the Italian case, the industry, fearful of what would turn up in evidence and concerned at Doll's corporate links disclosed in the US trial, bought out the claimants.

Under pretrial and trial examination in both these cases, Doll's evidence revealed that considerable payments had been made to him in the last decades from a number of toxic industries for work that he had done on their behalf, including a £50,000 payment from Turner & Newall, the asbestos company. To protect himself and ensure that he appeared "clean" of corporate interests, Doll gave the impression—in his statements and under examination—that payments he received were for specifically commissioned studies and, second, that they had in the main been donated to Green College. A number of these payments, however, were not for carefully conducted scientific studies but for opinions and promotional statements on behalf of the toxic industries.

The most venomous of these PR blurbs, for which Doll was paid by the yard, involved a letter to Judge Everett, the presiding judge in the Australian Royal Commission inquiring into the use of Agent Orange in Vietnam.[16]

This slippery letter congratulating Everett on endorsing Monsanto's case at the end of a long hearing, just happened to suggest that some of the work of Lennart Hardell, who had given evidence at the hearing, and whose work with Olav Axelson had been responsible for the Swedish government's banning of dioxin-based herbicides in Sweden, should be struck from the record.

In 2003, it was disclosed that in 1986 Monsanto had renewed a consultancy agreement with Doll, whereby he received $1,500 a day for occasional promotional work he did for them, so raising his consultancy pay by $500 a day.[17] This agreement was brokered by William Gaffey, an industry epidemiologist. Gaffey had been given a place at Monsanto to undermine critical studies of dioxin and draw in epidemiologists to present favorable reports.[18]

However, to talk about payments, or even bias in Doll's epidemiological work, is to miss the point. In the last half of his working life, Doll became an ideological puppet shifted about by corporate interests—a gun for hire, locked into and primed to defend corporate interests at any time.

Written work about Doll when he was alive, or even after his death, has rarely looked at his life from the perspective of whether or not his work sided with toxic industry or the public interest. Although the number of his critics grew, Doll's lack of scientific integrity rarely reached mainstream discussions about epidemiology. Doll lived his life basking in the sun of his first research findings—organized and overseen by Bradford Hill—that doctors who smoked were more likely to die of lung cancer than those who didn't.[19]

Even in his most shallow statements throughout the rest of his career, such as those about obesity and cancer, or "the wrong lifestyle," he never ventured any complaint against industry, leaving the blame for illness hanging over the individual like an ominous cloud. A great deal of his work was, anyway, involved with drug testing for the Imperial Cancer Research Fund—the poorest kind of clinical research paid for directly by vested interest industry, which rarely has long-term parameters and was rarely made public.

In 2002, Chris Beckett, the Archive Cataloguer at the Wellcome Library for the History and Understanding of Medicine, wrote an account of the personal papers that Doll had deposited in the library before his death.[20]

While Beckett did not approach the matter of corporate interests specifically, he looked in some detail at circumstances in which it appeared to him that Doll had "changed his mind" about his conclusions in important pieces of work. The majority of Beckett's account of Doll's work appears to be quietly congratulatory. However, although one of the examples Beckett gives had already been frequently aired his analysis does shed an original light on what might be called Doll's "mercurial methodology."

Primarily, Beckett notes the changes that Doll made to his first paper on asbestos at the behest of the Turner Asbestos directors and then from a more original perspective he discusses the irrational change of mind Doll had in the heat of the controversy. This later account of Beckett's Doll thought so badly represented him that he wrote to the journal making clear that his change of mind had been "scientifically justified." In fact this was far from the case.

Beckett goes no further in his conclusions than suggesting that both examples should make us all aware of "how significant a role is played by the *choice of words in presentation of epidemiological findings.*" It is difficult to tell whether Beckett was writing tongue in cheek, for in the first case, Doll changed the meaning of his conclusions at the behest of T&N executives to such a degree that he was later in thrall to them, becoming a litigation consultant on their behalf.[21]

Doll's evidence in the trial of toxic oil defendants in Spain in 1987 was crucial to the official presentation of the epidemic's cause; in terms of Doll's work record, it was yet another circumstance where Doll got away with acting on behalf of others. Even his official biographer, probably under instruction, excluded, from Doll's life's narrative, any mention of what was, in a public manner Doll's most sensational case.[22] In the second case, his methodological infraction was so severe, turning black to white, that even Doll must have been able to see that he was breaking one of the first rules of epidemiology.

In the 1970s and 1980s, the native olive oil industry in Spain was heavily protected; manufacture was restricted and licensed, with imports banned. To ensure market protection, all oil other than Spanish olive oil, for instance, rapeseed oil used for industrial purposes, was discolored with aniline, a chemical agent used in the manufacture of dyes, drugs, and plastics; it turned the oil blue, signaling its inedibility. However, the official story said, a black market industry had grown up that imported low-quality oil, often rapeseed oil, in which the aniline were not present or had been extracted and the product dressed up to be sold in large plastic bottles at local, usually "traveling," markets, as olive oil.

The outbreak began in Spain in the spring of 1981, with the reporting of a gathering number of adults and children, mainly from Madrid and the surrounding area, attending hospitals' and doctors' surgeries between then and 1985. When the epidemic had concluded, over one thousand people had died and over twenty-five thousand individuals had been damaged, many of them left permanently disabled. It was the biggest incidence of mass "poisoning" in the modern world; it was also a case that could only have been solved if the authorities had wanted it to be with the exact employment of sound epidemiology.

The illness was said by the authorities to be characterized by the symptoms of atypical pneumonia, including coughing, fever, dyspnea, hypoxia, bilateral pulmonary infiltrates, and eosinophilia. One of the many common symptoms, uncommon to pneumonia, which was rarely mentioned by the authorities but frequently alluded to by the dissident camp, was the appearance of lesions on the surface of the body. Some victims of the syndrome recovered quite quickly, while 30 percent went on to experience chronic illnesses that included neuropathy, myopathy, sclerodermiform skin changes, joint contractures, sicca syndrome, pulmonary hypertension, persistent eosinophilia, and death.

Although various etiologies were informally hypothesized, initially the epidemic went unexplained to the public until June 1981. Rumors and unverified theories were allowed to develop without any overarching epidemiological research. Dr. Juan Tabuenca Oliver, who appeared to propound the first official theory, found that, on being questioned,[23] all of the children admitted to the Hospital Niño Jesús in Madrid with this syndrome had recently consumed an unlabeled oil, sold for use as a food in 5-litre containers by itinerant salesmen. Only 6 percent of children admitted to the hospital with different complaints had consumed such oil.

As in a wayward police inquiry in which one detective adduces guilt without proof prior to serious investigation, toxic oil became embedded from the beginning in the minds of first the authorities and then the public as the cause of the epidemic. To what extent this was spontaneous or engineered at these beginning stages is unknown.

After what appeared to be some initial hesitation, the government adopted the oil theory as the official theory. On June 10, just a month after the first death, an official announcement was made on late-night television, informing the public that the epidemic was caused by contaminated cooking oil. As with many of the public statements claiming that illicit oil was responsible, the parameters of Dr. Juan Tabuenca Oliver's off-the-cuff research with children varied as time went by. In another offhand study done the following day, Rigau and others[24] compared "case" households in the town of Navas del Marqués, Avila province, with randomly chosen and size-matched "control" households from the town. Suspect oil had been consumed in all of the case households, but in only thirty-two (24 percent) of the randomly chosen and size-matched control households.

However, there were from the beginning amazing anomalies in the data, which should have realigned the epidemiological course of events: the simplest of these was that many who had consumed oil did not fall ill and many who did fall ill had not consumed the oil. Secondly, it was never possible, given the erratic beginning of the epidemic and the slow response of the authorities, to equate the general pattern of the illness with any particular type of oil. This absence of toxicity was strengthened, in the minds of many scientists, by the fact that animal tests, using illicitly manufactured oil tested on a wide range of animals, caused no illness of any kind but only increased the health of those animals.

Dr. Vettorazzi,[25] a WHO official and staunch supporter of a proposed organophosphate cause of the epidemic, was the only scientist of note to make the point that Nemacur, the pesticide suspected, had in previous research in 1974 been shown to have different and more toxic effects on humans than on animals, something that the oil argument promoters might have grasped at when it proved that rats only grew healthier. All the common sense arguments, let alone the scientific ones, were inadequate to prove the case, so much so that one of the most senior actors in the story, Dr. Vettorazzi, was led to say "there is absolutely no possibility that oil was responsible for this epidemic."

However, with cause apparently substantiated, in the official and public mind, clear evidence had to be found, involvement and blame apportioned. The WHO proposed the name "toxic oil syndrome" (TOS) for the disease. The supposedly implicated oil was traced to its source, a distributing company whose principal office was located near Madrid. The company was closed and its oil was seized. To remove any remaining suspect oil from domestic use, the Spanish government offered pure olive oil to owners in exchange for it.

No attempt was ever made, using standard epidemiological research techniques, to lock the theory down to one specific make of oil. In fact, the story that developed was not founded on epidemiology. Any "official" epidemiology that was carried out, as time went by, was set out to bolster this narrative rather than to test its basic assumptions. On the other hand, the common sense and even epidemiological arguments against this narrative were many and almost all destructive of the official theory.

In choosing the oil, its "manufacturers" and distributors, as the culprit for the epidemic, the government and the medical establishment had chosen a fringe, black economy group mainly made up of itinerant "gypsies" and other indigenous Spaniards that Karl Marx might have called the *lumpen proletariat,* those outside the organized labor movement—such people were easily suspected.

As both the epidemic and the official explanation unfolded, there was immense cynicism among doctors, scientists, and public health officials about the official explanation. The principal medical hero of the "alternative" cause of the epidemic became Dr. Antonio Muro y Fernández-Cavada (Dr. Muro), the director of the children's wards in La Paz hospital, Madrid, to which the first cases of the illness traveled. Muro immediately began doing the things that a good epidemiologist should do. For instance, he brought together the relatives of those afflicted and began asking a series of rigorous questions about the foods that they had eaten. Quite early in his inquiries he found that salad was a more important factor in their meals than the oil with which some of them garnished these salads.[26]

Muro collected oil from the houses of those afflicted before the authorities decided that this might be a good idea. He sent the oil samples to a private laboratory and had results back from analysis by June. As he had expected and as with the official samples, none of the oil sent to the laboratory had any recordable toxic ingredients. These results helped Muro and his colleagues commit themselves against the oil etiology argument. However, when Muro made the first results of his ongoing research public, he was immediately and unaccountably sacked from La Paz hospital.

While Muro had handled his oil samples from sufferers' households with care, the belated government-backed exchange program—that took place three weeks after the official announcement that it was oil that had caused the epidemic—was hopelessly mismanaged. Few usable records were kept of who was exchanging what, or most importantly, whether the oil came from affected or unaffected households. As an inducement, families who handed oil in were given expensive pure olive oil in exchange. With such a guarantee, many people simply handed in any oil they could find, even motor oil. Consequently much of the oil that supposedly caused the epidemic was never available for subsequent scientific analysis.

Over the coming months and indeed years, until he died in 1988, Muro continued with colleagues or ex-colleagues at La Paz to carry out a classic epidemiological investigation. Eventually Muro and colleagues carried out interviews with over four thousand individuals,[27] tracing the route of tomatoes, the one ingredient of the salad that the great majority of the victims seemed to have eaten.

Another part of Muro's epidemiology was to try to link the symptomatic picture presented by the *afectados* (those affected) with the substance that could be at the heart of the epidemic. Very quickly Muro and his colleagues matched the symptomatic picture of the *afectados* generally to an organophosphate chemical and specifically to a pesticide named Nemacur, produced by Bayer and frequently used on tomatoes grown in Almería, where vegetables were force-raised. The instructions for this pesticide were accompanied by a skull and crossbones within a triangle, beneath which was the word "veneno" (poison).

Most specifically, this organophosphate pesticide on its ingestion produced the same lesions that Muro and his colleagues had witnessed in a great number of victims of the epidemic. Throughout the epidemic, those in Muro's circle stuck to the fact that the epidemic had been caused by the release of tomatoes onto the market while they still had pesticide on them.

Alongside this explanation, a number of other critics of the official version drew attention to the fact that an unexplained explosion had occurred at a US base in the town of Torrejón de Ardoz, in the province of Madrid, in the first quarter of 1981. This base, they said, had stock piles of bio-weapons. From the beginning, both Bayer and the US government denied the "alternative" theories, but both narratives grew in the vacuum created by the un-evidenced official version of the cause of the epidemic.

One of Muro's colleagues had in May, at the start of the outbreak, speculated that Nemacur might be the cause of the epidemic. Dr. Angel Peralta, the head of the endocrinology department at La Paz hospital, interviewed for a newspaper article, commented that the symptoms they were observing were very similar to those of organophosphate poisoning. The next day, Peralta received a telephone call from the Ministry of Health ordering him to say nothing more about organophosphorus poisoning to the media.[28]

Behind the scenes, the WHO and US public health agencies very quickly got involved in arguing the case in favor of the theory. In 1983, an international conference was convened in Madrid under the auspices of the WHO, and despite the reservations of many scientists present, the epidemic was officially named Toxic Oil Syndrome (TOS). However, no further epidemiological evidence was substantiated at or after this meeting.

By 1984, with people still dying by the day, the battle to explain the epidemic and to treat the *afectados* had become bogged down; many of the indigenous Spanish scientists and public health officials were opposed to the idea that toxic oil had caused the epidemic. Dissenters, however, found themselves ranged against an implacable opposition composed of the US health vigilantes, the WHO, and an authoritarian Spanish government.

The WHO took an early interest in the illness outbreak. Dr. Roy Goulding, an Englishman, selected internally as Chair of a WHO steering committee on the epidemic, seemed to be charged with making the case for the WHO that toxic oil was responsible. Goulding was then at the Toxicology Unit at Guy's Hospital in London. He trained initially in agriculture and acted as an adviser on food production during the Second World War and afterwards developed an interest in toxicology. After working as a lecturer at Guy's Dental School, he became an adviser to the Ministry of Health in 1956, with special responsibility for matters relating to pharmacology and toxicology.

Goulding had a special place in the history of pesticide regulation in Britain. In 1963, with others he founded the National Poisons Information Service at Guy's Hospital and was Director of the evolving organization until 1980. This, together with its laboratory, was for a long time called the Poisons Unit and is now the Medical Toxicology Unit, Guy's and St. Thomas' Hospital Trust. For many years Goulding was a member, and later chairman, of the Scientific Sub-Committee of the Advisory Committee on Pesticides, the committee that approves all pesticides for use in the United Kingdom. The Poisons Unit and its later incarnations were in more recent times held as highly suspect by many activists and claimants involved in pesticide cases.[29]

Goulding traveled to Madrid in August 1981, at the behest of the WHO. At this early time in the epidemic, Goulding seems to have had an open mind about its cause. In his first report he suggested, "The pathology seems to correspond to multiple toxic agents, since none of the known ones could explain all the aspects that the disease shows . . ." he pointed out "We should not keep on looking for anilines and start looking for herbicides and insecticides, as well as toxic agents used for industrial purposes which cause intoxication with other of the observed symptoms. . . ."

However, it appears that Goulding was either not then familiar with his brief, or alternatively he was saying only what would keep the doctors he met in Spain happy. Very soon after returning to London, he wrote a ten-page report for the WHO, describing the nature of the disease and the epidemic without a mention of pesticides or herbicides.

Two years on, in March 1983, when no real advance had been made in the science or cause of the epidemic, Goulding was again in Madrid but now whole-heartedly pushing the hypothesis. When the Epidemiological Working Group submitted its report, it failed to mention Dr. Muro's work and stated baldly, after looking at the case for oil, "No convincing alternative view has been submitted."[30] In fact, this was far from the truth.

Dr. Muro had supposedly been invited to this March meeting, but when he arrived, laden with two cases full of his research and accompanied by a former WHO chief epidemiologist, Dr. Francisco Martin Samos, he was forbidden entry into the meeting. The following day, he was allowed to talk to a small private meeting of WHO working group members at the Ministry of Health. After a short description of his findings, he was dismissed from the meeting and sent home, not being allowed access to any other meetings or levels of the WHO group.[31]

The epidemic and the official review of cause, together with the epidemiology, had descended into a state of stale and obdurate reflection that simply repeated toxic oil like a mantra. Dr. Vettorazzi at the WHO, who had become implacably opposed to Goulding's overseeing of the epidemic, was scathing about the failure of the WHO-organized initiative to find the cause of the epidemic. Vettorazzi, a convinced believer in the organophosphate pesticide theory, suggested that the first WHO-organized report from the committee in Madrid should not be taken seriously and amounted to nothing more than the authors' "personal opinions." About the fact that over three and a half years had passed without a solution, Vettorazzi said in an interview with *Cambio16*: "How can it be that after three and a half years, when mankind has been able to land on the moon we still don't know the cause of the Spanish syndrome."

Clearly, something had to be done to move the analysis of the epidemic forward, not least of course, so that the "affected" could be seen to be receiving suitable treatment. On August 29, 1984, Goulding wrote to Sir Richard Doll, who was then Warden of Green College Oxford, asking him to review the epidemiological evidence.

At this time, three years into the epidemic, Goulding was complaining that there had been little progress, because although most people associated with the WHO and its collegiate agencies were "convinced" of a "strong statistical association between the disease and the *illicit oil*, there were elements, *certain, vociferous movements and individuals* in Spain who argue otherwise." (My italics)[32] Being a dissident was becoming a blameworthy position.

Doll received what epidemiological data there was, all neatly presented to him by Goulding, just before he began work on his study of the production of PVC and workers' cancers. He accepted the "corporate," or "establishment" data relating to the study without question just as he received the data in the PVC study from the industry body asking for the research. In the Spanish case, this data was even more manipulated that the pre-prepared PVC data. Doll was given none of Dr. Muro's data nor indeed any data that disagreed with the government and corporate picture of the epidemic, nor was he put in touch with Dr. Muro or any of the dissident doctors.

However, even Doll revolted in the first instance against this exploitation of his authority as a world-renowned epidemiologist. Initially he was cautious, after all he was being consulted about an epidemiological situation which had its origins four years previously, and at first sight he, like any other epidemiologist, could see the terrible inadequacies of the work that had been done to support the hypothesis that one particular oil was responsible for an epidemic that was on its way to killing around one thousand people in diverse parts of Spain.

Over the next year Doll exchanged letters with Goulding informing him of his progress.[33] At this stage, Doll seemed to be concerned about the disastrous moves made by the Spanish government and others to promote their hypothesis. Beckett says that in May 1985 Doll was concerned:

> ... to discover that the Spanish government had provided incentives to case-reporting in the form of promised compensation and free medical care, and that the available epidemiological data, much of which seemed to have been gathered in haste, may not have been free from bias.[34]

Of course, Doll had a good point here, but the bottom line was that biased or free from bias, all the epidemiological studies—conducted in haste or otherwise—failed to link the oil with any type of illness, let alone the epidemic.

By 1985, Doll was able to present an interim report to the July meeting of the Steering Committee that had been set up in Madrid by Goulding with the authority of the WHO.[35] In the report he refused to draw any kind of conclusion, waiting, he said, until he had met with "dissident scientists" in Spain. But there was more to this than an ethical position; it must have been clear to him that in accepting the task from the WHO he had bought a pig in a poke and the view that he was supposed to espouse was insupportable.

At this time, Doll made one definite statement that should at a later date have contributed to him leaving or being sacked from his consultancy and his work erased from the research record. He said: "If it could be shown that *even one person* [author's italics] who developed the disease could not have had exposure to [the oil], that would provide good grounds for exculpating the oil altogether."[36]

While Doll was not about to change his spots overnight and support an "alternative hypothesis," or even examine any of its data, he was clearly unable to reason his way through the discrepancies in the data that actually completely collapsed the theory, or the failure of the animal tests to show any toxicity with a series of different illicit oils. In his first report he stated the following:

Laboratory studies have . . . failed to demonstrate toxicity in any of the samples that were recovered, no specific chemical that might have caused the disease has been identified and the conclusion that the oil was responsible rests primarily on the epidemiological evidence.[37]

While this is of course true in the most general sense, it failed to point out that the epidemiological evidence was next to useless because there were no control data of any kind useful for discriminating between the various foodstuffs consumed by victims at the same time as the oil. In fact, it would be true to say that there was no epidemiological *evidence* at all, only the suggestion of an association.

At the Madrid WHO-organized meeting, Doll presented his report and met with two of the dissenting scientists, Dr. Clavera Ortiz and Dr. Martínez Ruiz, a husband and wife team from Barcelona. In December, two months after the meeting, he wrote to Goulding that he did not find the "alternative suggestion . . . at all impressive."[38] In this letter to Goulding, Doll departs—as he often did and all corporate lobbyists do—from science, to give his impression of the psychological state of the dissidents: "they were now emotionally concerned with disproving the oil hypothesis."[39]

In fact, Clavera and Martínez had not been "emotionally concerned" to settle on a theory, but had become dissidents on the basis of good epidemiological principles. In the beginning they "absolutely believed the oil was to blame," they said. "We thought the only problem was that the information was disorganized and the research inadequate."[40]

They set about a rigorous examination of the official information. The results shocked them. Martínez looked at the pattern of admissions to hospitals and realized that the epidemic had peaked at the end of May. The incidence curve went down at least ten days before the government's June 10 broadcast, and about a month before the withdrawal of any oil. In fact, the official announcement that oil was to blame had had no effect on the course of the epidemic. If this was the case, then the "official" warnings about the cause of the epidemic had failed the people and the public health considerably.

Meanwhile, Clavera had examined the patterns of distribution of the suspect oil, which it was claimed had come across the border from France. She realized that vast quantities of the oil were sold in regions (notably Catalonia) where there had not been a single case of illness. Subsequently, they learned that the government was already fully aware of this. The powerful, indeed irrefutable, evidence that the suspect oil was sold throughout parts of Spain where not a single case of illness resulted could be coupled with equally clear evidence of the converse: individuals who could not have been exposed to any illegal oil, fell victim to the epidemic. Martínez and Clavera were fired from their public sector jobs and, as such sackings did not entirely prevent the possibility of the commission reaching inconvenient conclusions, it was soon closed down. Other public servants suffered in a similar manner.

At the time of the epidemic, the government created a new post, at cabinet level, of secretary of state for consumer affairs. Chosen for this appointment was a rising lawyer and economist, Enrique Martínez de Genique. Genique himself had drawn up maps of the distribution of the oil and the pattern of illness. He quickly realized that there was no correlation between the two and, accordingly, that the oil was not the cause of the epidemic. After presenting his findings to the health ministry, he was immediately sacked from his government post, and soon decided to retire from politics altogether. He was to emphasize later that he had never regretted what he did: "I had very grave doubts [about the government's stance on the epidemic] and I was morally and ethically obliged to voice them."

Thirty years after the Spanish epidemic, the American epidemiologist Edwin Kilbourne took complete and singular credit for "solving the Spanish crisis."[41]

Who was Kilbourne and how did he manage single-handedly to "solve the Spanish crisis," a problem which had alluded many?

Kilbourne and the new data that he authored was apparently to change Doll's entire professional and public opinion about the epidemic. Kilbourne's consultancy credentials include his being an accomplished, internationally experienced clinician, scientific investigator, and program manager/developer in the areas of epidemiology, public health surveillance, environmental hazards, medical toxicology, WMD-based terrorism, and WMD non-proliferation.[42]

WHO WAS EDWIN KILBOURNE?

The theorists were sailing in very stormy seas and the pressure was now on them to find ways of strengthening their story. Although Doll's first report was anything but certain, his principles in the WHO wanted no more investigation into the "improbable" alternative hypotheses. In November 1985, Doll received a communication from Kilbourne, who was introduced to him by Goulding at the WHO. Kilbourne was, it appeared, an American working for the Centers for Disease Control and Prevention (CDC).

Doll received Kilbourne and Goulding in Oxford and at this meeting the two visitors exhorted him to provide his stamp of approval to the oil theory. Kilbourne now asked Doll to make "a more specific conclusion on the likelihood of the oil hypothesis,"[43] suggesting that it would be easier on everyone all round if Doll was to get off the fence. Doll wrote back to Kilbourne suggesting "that the case of the oil might come to be regarded as proven out" if some more research was carried out such as Doll suggested in his report.[44]

Kilbourne, who came from a medical research family—his father Edwin was famous for having worked on the first flu vaccine—was actually part of a secretive militarized organization inside the CDC grandly titled the Epidemiological Intelligence Service (EIS). In Kilbourne's time, the EIS wore military uniforms and could be ordered anywhere in the world by the use of "inter-governmental bilateral or other agreements." Kilbourne, who had worked for the WHO before for the International Program for Chemical Safety (IPCS) and the World Bank, was seconded to Spain for a period between 1985 and 1987.

Kilbourne was, in some respects, an odd public health investigator; both before and after the Spanish epidemic, his specialty was chemical toxins and germ warfare weapons.[45] Kilbourne retired as a commissioned officer in the uniformed Public Health Service in July 2005 with the rank of captain after twenty-four years of service.

The EIS had and presumably still has a deeply political agenda. A troubleshooting organization, it sends personnel round the world to public health "hotspots." Its interests are particularly with incidents that might have begun with military or political intervention or which have been caused by industrial toxicity, or incidents, the reverberations of which might have serious consequences for the perception of governments, corporations, or the medical establishment.

Although there was no EIS or its equivalent in Britain, Doll occupied a very similar position to that of Kilbourne and their careers, especially in relation to the pharmaceutical industry and the State showed similar traits. In his work as an expert witness for the nuclear industry, for instance, Doll was very close to the British State, involved in the same work as Kilbourne, dampening down fear and creating spurious reports of causation.

Doll worked for years for the Imperial Cancer Research Fund[46] not just testing cancer drugs but on all kinds of pharmaceuticals. Kilbourne also worked with the pharmaceutical industry.

There can be little doubt that at the time of Kilbourne's secondment to Spain, the US and their major corporate power bases imagined that Doll and Kilbourne would get on and cooperate in resolving the corporate conundrum that was injuring thousands.

Unfortunately, it seems that the two men, although both in thrall to the United States and United Kingdom corporate state, were imbued with national characteristics that hampered camaraderie. Doll was a product of the English university system in his education, his teaching, and his work; though he was drawn into duplicitous maneuver, it appears that he still held firm to a view of himself as an independent and ethical worker, working in the long-term interests of the people. On the other hand, Kilbourne worked for and on behalf of a cold state-determined organization that had little moral understanding of truth or ethics.

However, as epidemiologists Doll and Kilbourne were capable of disastrous and immense stupidities and deceptions. Kilbourne was, for instance, capable of underestimating the number of *afectados*—while he quotes "twenty thousand cases and three hundred deaths," others quote around one thousand deaths and at least forty thousand people damaged—while Doll was capable of saying on one occasion, if one person who has not had the oil falls ill, the whole model fails, but later giving evidence in favor of the theory, despite hundreds of conflicts.

However, even Kilbourne, given the task of turning attention away from corporate damage, has a real problem in presenting a plausible argument. He has to admit that there is no real etiology to the illness because no agent has been found within or around the oil that could have caused the illnesses. In 2009, the journal *Chest* reprinted Kilbourne's 1985 paper "Toxic-Oil Syndrome Epidemic with an Elusive Etiology."[47]

Coincidentally, this paper was first printed in the Scandinavian journal that published Doll's highly questionable paper on PVC manufacture and cancer, which concluded that PVC production did not cause cancer in its workers. This route for publication, without peer review, of a paper that had been guided through the academic hoops by Gaffey at Monsanto, was suggested to Doll by the medical advisor at ICI.[48]

Epidemiology is a complex science; however, good and bad epidemiology have certain distinctive features. The good epidemiologist will want to get as close to those affected as possible, to examine them, their habitat, and their stories. The good epidemiologist will want, in Alice Stewart's brilliant and remarkably modern phrase, to "record the background noise."[49]

Rarely are the answers to epidemiology simple and it is always the anomalies that can confound the science. It is not until such apparent anomalies are encompassed in any study that it can be said to be concluded. The bad epidemiologist, or the epidemiologist who purposefully wants to present easy answers for vested interests, will stay well away from the people or those victimized, will use data passed on by others, will shut out the background noise, and fudge anomalies.

Kilbourne, during his time in Madrid, came up with studies that solved the problem of the Spanish Syndrome. Faced with this *fait accompli* at the trial, and who knows what other inducements, he surrendered his epidemiological integrity to the North Americans and hidden corporations.

Throughout this life, Kilbourne, much like Doll, gained critical praise, and it is easy to see the imprint that the *invisibles* in powerful social sectors wanted to leave in the minds of the public. Kilbourne's accolades didn't quite reach the heights awarded Doll as "The Man who saved 100 Million lives"[50] but they were very flattering.

Despite the fact that Doll was to become the chief and most authoritative witness for the prosecution, in the case of the Spanish ~~Toxic Oil~~ he still expressed private doubts to Goulding. In April of 1987, on receiving news about Kilbourne's *new* research, he suggested that the evidence was strongly "in support of association"—anyone who knows anything about epidemiology and the English language will understand that "in support of association" means next to nothing in epidemiological terms and misses that necessary word "proves."

Just before the trial, Kilbourne showed himself more than capable of providing the new evidence having magically produced two pieces of classic epidemiology which, though written two years after the event, might have flowed from the quill of a contemporary John Snow as he sat among the dying in the center of Madrid. In June 1987, only weeks before giving evidence in the trial, over July 6 to 7, 1987, on the basis of Kilbourne's further studies, Doll wrote an addendum to his first report that confirmed a categorical link between "the" oil and the illness, "with the addition of this new evidence, *I conclude that adulterated oil was the cause of the toxic syndrome.*"[51] If not linguistically, scientifically this judgment *completely* reversed the conclusions of his earlier report.

The apparently most important epidemiological evidence, presented by Kilbourne, was, he said, a "classic study" carried out under his authority of a *closed order convent* in which it was said that, while nuns had used illicit oil, visitors had been given pure olive oil; reportedly, this had resulted in illnesses among the nuns but no illnesses among visitors.

This time, however, as against other times when Doll had "rigorously" changed his mind, the incidence of his forced advice left a bad taste in his mouth. After all, while acting for industry, Doll had done his best to hang onto an image of an analytical scientist and an English gentleman. So manipulated did Doll feel, that he expressed serious discontent with Dr. Kilbourne, the pushy American responsible for the "study" of nuns that was supposed to present an answer to one of the biggest and most dangerous epidemics of the twentieth century and give Doll a way out.

Doll was concerned about the way in which his less subtle colleagues had acted and he wrote to Roy Goulding after accepting the "new evidence," saying that he was far from happy with Kilbourne, "I remain most disturbed that Kilbourne should have allowed himself to be used in this way."[52]

In another area of the problem, however, even Kilbourne was unable to produce anything close to definitive evidence. Having said that no toxic elements of any kind could be found in any of the oil seized and that no animals responded to being administered the oil in high quantities and by different routes, Kilbourne comes out with an epidemiological classic, worthy of Doll at his greatest. Perhaps, says Kilbourne, "The etiologic agent in the oil may have become inactive over time." By "time" Kilbourne is talking of a couple of months. "These observations are consistent with what one might see when a toxin with a limited lifespan declines in concentration over time." It also could bring to an ignominious end the discipline of epidemiology. After all, perhaps all unknown substances responsible for epidemics can disappear from the body in weeks. This, of course, would make the toxin one of the most sought-after poisons in the world, something that destroyed human life but leaves not a single trace within days or weeks of being administered.

The months prior to the trial of oil distributors saw an expansion in the illegal information gathering, as well as attempts to threaten and bribe those who believed in the pesticide case, involving Spanish Security Agencies, local police, multinationals, and various lawyers.

It was said that Bayer had paid over 72,000,000 into the Plan Nacional del Síndrome Tóxico, the organization set up by the WHO and the Spanish government.[53] The alternative understanding of the cause of the epidemic suffered from a continuing news blackout. Not only did Bayer refuse to give information to the alternative press, investigators, and writers, but whole events were hidden from public view.

Just before the beginning of the trial, a group of patients suffering from the epidemic staged a twelve-day hunger strike, consuming only sugared water and the toxic oil said to have made them ill. The hunger strike was almost completely ignored by the media.

The apartment shared by the two dissident scientists who took part in the WHO Epidemiology Committee was burgled. The intruder cared nothing for valuables but took their most important records and papers. Such burglaries had gone on before the trial date was announced: in 1985, one of the lawyers for the company said to be responsible for starting the epidemic found that all his case papers and records had vanished from his office.

One of the strongest patient support groups was organized in Fuenlabrada, a Madrid satellite town. Feelings against the WHO-organized whitewash was so strong there that sufferers continued to publicly use the stored oil, without any ill effect. The association in Fuenlabrada, unlike hundreds of others across Spain, received no grant funding from the government. Coming up to the time of the trial, their offices had been broken into on five occasions. On the sixth occasion, however, Fuentox officers and members caught the thieves in the act, only to find to their astonishment that the burglars were two municipal policemen and the local government head of public health.

Burglaries and thefts of papers continued right up to the trial, even involving premises allocated to the defense counsel in the Casa de Campo Park where the trial was held. Not long after the trial began, the laboratory of Dr. Frontela, a scientist who had been charged by the court to carry out research on monkeys to find the effects of both the oil and organophosphate pesticides, were broken into by four young men armed with knives on four occasions in one week. The most successful trespass was only halted when a security guard fired shots into the air.

A previous piece of Frontela's research had been scuppered: while he was attending meetings in Switzerland, the university stopped feeding over four hundred rats allocated to his research.

The main paper that carried the most supportive of alternative stories suggesting that the Bayer product was responsible, Cambio16, was sued by Bayer for printing the alternative narrative and the editor was immediately fired. The case was settled out of court with an apparent reversal of the usual legal maneuver, when Bayer paid money to Cambio16.

Journalists who carried out research in 1987 for Spanish national television, concluding that the oil had not been responsible, were immediately sacked.

By the time the trial of forty oil producers and distributors began in 1987, 627 people had died, and twenty to twenty-five thousand had been affected, according to disputed official figures. The trial began on Monday March 29, 1987, in the auditorium of the Casa de Campo Park on the northern edge of Madrid. The defendants, two of whom were absent—having fled the country—were separated from the public and their lawyers in the courtroom by bulletproof glass.

The charges against them ranged from manslaughter to fraud. Prosecutors asked for sentences totaling more than one hundred thousand years for each of the eight main defendants, despite the maximum possible jail sentence in Spain at that time being thirty years. For the first time in Spanish legal history, the trial, expected initially to last from four to six months, was recorded on videotape.

The prosecution case was simply that those standing trial had been responsible for tampering with oil, which had then been distributed and had caused the

Spanish Syndrome epidemic. The defense argued what had ostensibly been Dr. Muro's case prior to his death. Drs. Clavera and Martínez reported Muro's case in this way:

> The toxic syndrome epidemic of the spring of 1981 was caused by organophosphate pesticides or toxic substances, and carried by tomatoes, many of which came from the same place and were distributed through alternative ways of commercialization, among which open air markets and traveling sellers have an important role.[54]

Leading expert witness Dr. Luis Frontela, Professor of Legal Medicine at the University of Seville, while leading the opposition to the toxic oil theory, was unable to persuade the court of the pesticide theory. Judges dismissed claims by defense lawyers that the true cause was either tomatoes laced with combined effect of two pesticides—Nemacur and Oftanol—or an accident involving biological weapons at a United States airbase at Torrejón.

Although all the evidence supporting the case for tomatoes being the vector of the epidemic was epidemiological, there was circumstantial clinical evidence that showed clearly that OP pesticides caused identical symptomatic presentations to those of the victims of the epidemic.

The idea that pesticides had been used in the south of Spain in an unregulated and cavalier fashion was also incidentally supported by evidence called by the defense and given by representatives of Bayer. It was said by these witnesses that field trials that had been held with organophosphate pesticides in Almeria were ended with the subject tomatoes being sent out to markets. Production of tomatoes and other crops in Almeria came under intense scrutiny during the trial, and it was notably recorded that many immigrant farmers and workers and their families, who had come to Spain from North Africa, were illiterate and often unable to read the instructions on pesticides that the agrochemical companies were selling to them by the ton.

The prosecution, as it stood at the start of the trial, had nothing to support their case except a very rough association between some incidents of oil use and the dispersed outbreaks of the illness. There was no epidemiological or clinical connection between these two phenomena and, most pointedly, the prosecution had been completely unable to proffer an iota of scientific evidence that there was any toxic effect of any oil that might result in any illness of any kind.

The defense, although involved in an uphill struggle, had both epidemiological and toxicity evidence that supported their case. On the one hand, Muro's detailed epidemiology linked outlying areas of the epidemic not covered by the oil theory with the distribution of tomatoes and, on the other hand, the symptomatic clinical picture shown by those who had fallen ill fitted the unusual effects of organophosphate poisoning.

As Doll had pointed out to Kilbourne and Goulding after his first report, unless there was good epidemiological evidence that cemented together an oil with the illnesses, all that could be said was that there appeared to be an association between the two things—of course, there would have been if any number of those affected had risen each morning at exactly the same time.

Kilbourne's new study of nuns and visitors, apparently given two types of oil, for the first time added gusto to the prosecution case. Disputing the "new" evidence entered by Kilbourne and agreed by Doll, the defense called the nuns of the convent that had been the subject of the research. Bob Woffinden, who steadfastly covered the epidemic and the whole of the trial for British television, saves some of his most scathing comments for this new piece of epidemiology:

> Even more amazing was the study concerning a convent outside Madrid. According to this, forty-two out of forty-three nuns fell ill after using the oil, while visitors whose food was prepared in a different oil did not fall ill. From an official perspective, the beauty of this epidemiology was not just that it provided game, set, and match for the oil theory, but that no one could afterwards check the veracity of the paper. This was a closed convent. The nuns had no routine contact with members of the public, and they certainly didn't talk to the media. In the event, senior nuns from the convent did give evidence at the trial. Their testimony flatly contradicted what was written in the study. Of course, all the food was prepared in the same way and cooked in the same oil. In fact, only very few nuns (about eight or nine) suffered any illness. The epidemiological report was a fabrication.[55]

As Beckett points out, after stating the case that the oil had caused the epidemic, Doll stuck to this view. In Madrid, Doll was feted by relatives of victims of the epidemic as a savior, although, of course, they could not have had the faintest idea in whose interests he was working. It is easy to imagine that as for some backwater dictatorial potentate, the crowds, the handshaking, the glad-handing outside the court could well have been organized.

The trial ended, after two years, in May 1989, by which time deaths were recorded at around seven hundred. The transcript of the hearing stretched to thirty-thousand pages, while three thousand witnesses had been called, along with hundreds of experts. The judges themselves stressed that the toxin in the oil was "still unknown." This somewhat fundamental difficulty did not prevent them from handing down long prison terms to the oil merchants who were convicted, in effect, of causing the epidemic.

> At the end of the hearing . . . amid angry protests from a crowded courtroom, three Spanish judges dismissed murder charges today against distributors of an adulterated cooking oil that was found to have caused almost seven hundred deaths since a mass poisoning disaster occurred here in 1981.
>
> The judges were forced to suspend the final session of the longest trial in Spanish history after an uproar followed their announcement that none of the thirty-seven accused had intended to provoke death or injuries and that only two would serve lengthy prison terms. Outside the courthouse, relatives of victims and some of the twenty-five people who survived the poisoning with lifelong injuries continued their protests, shouting, "We want justice." Heavily armed police called to restore order fired at least one teargas canister into the crowd.

Prosecutors had asked for sentences of more than sixty thousand years for eight of the accused, although Spanish law limits prison terms to thirty years. Instead, the judges sentenced one man to twenty years, another to twelve years and several others to suspended sentences of between six months and ten years, while twenty-four were acquitted.[56]

Judges also ordered payment of compensation of the equivalent of $125,000 to relatives of each person who died of poisoning and sums ranging from $1,250 to $750,000 to survivors.

The majority of relatives of those affected were utterly convinced by the blanket corporate media reporting of the epidemic and the trial.[57]

As has been the case in a number of such situations, the rewriting of history after a good lapse of time, solves, for the record at least, the hardest scientific problems. By 2015, however, the sanitized history of the Epidemic Intelligence Service (EIS) on the CDC site, presents—in a very short section—the alarming news that by 1995, the EIS had identified, "a number of other toxins found in victims"; "more than twenty-five new compounds that *are associated* with ~~TOS~~," or as it should be said, "were found to be associated with" the victims of what came to be called ~~TOS~~. Oddly, these now included Dioxin, PCB, and chlorinated hydrocarbon pesticide exposure.[58] The very toxins that many had argued were responsible for the deaths and illnesses.

CONCLUSIONS

Beckett's "case study" of Doll's involvement in the Spanish toxicity epidemic of 1981 only scratched the surface of Doll's weakness and duplicity as a man and an epidemiologist. Beckett's use of this example disturbed Doll enough to make him write to the editors of *Medical History* attempting to justify his change of opinion.

In his letter, Doll appears to be concerned that because Beckett did not go deeply enough into "the new evidence," readers might think that he had succumbed to "pressure from the Spanish authorities."

In fact, an influential part of this "new evidence" came from the US Centers for Disease Control and was nothing to do with the Spanish Epidemic, *but was suddenly exposed details of a "sharp dose-response relationship between the risk of developing the disease and the amount of contamination . . . of aniline."*[59]

Like Doll's last-minute intervention in the Royal Commission on Agent Orange, his perverse involvement in the Spanish syndrome was odd to say the least. In 1984, Spain was a modern country working its way out of the Franco Era; it was also a country with a considerable US military presence that continued after Franco under the organization of NATO. Why was Doll's presence in Spain to solve the case of the deaths necessary? Why did the WHO invite him in, and why the massive US involvement in the case? After all, neither Doll nor Kilbourne were there at the get-go assembling evidence and epidemiological data. In effect, especially Doll had nothing to contribute to the epidemiological arguments.

When the trial ended, the debate was ostensibly over and the public who had suffered, having followed everything through the media, appeared convinced that the official version of the epidemic represented the true and immutable story of the Spanish ~~Toxic Oil~~ Syndrome.[60]

THE CORPORATE AND SCIENTIFIC SPECTACLE AND THE ROLE OF THE MEDIA

Bob Woffinden, the British journalist who covered the tragedy from beginning to end, says that his role in the conflict over ~~TOS~~ was mainly governed by the fact that at this time he was allowed by his funders and employers to stay in Spain for three months covering the epidemic. Writing in 2001 he said the following:

> A decade later (ten years after the trial concluded), it is now inconceivable that journalistic investigations on such a scale would be supported. In future, without even the remote possibility of a bunch of journalists turning up years later to ask inconvenient questions, it will be even easier for international science to organize its cover-ups.[61]

In his book *Flat Earth News*, about the decline of classic journalism and the work of media,[62] Nick Davis says more or less the same thing, citing the long-running investigations carried out by the *Sunday Times* into Kim Philby and the "Cambridge spies" and then Thalidomide, investigations undertaken prior to 1981 when the *Sunday Times* was taken over by Rupert Murdoch. Davis makes the following points.

> The paper in those days made a healthy profit and, with the support of Lord Thompson's managers, much of the money was recycled back onto the editorial floor. Harry Evans was able to hire talented reporters as he saw fit. Some of these staff went weeks without getting anything into print or indeed being seen in the office. But the impact on the paper's journalism generally was powerfully good: reporters filed far more stories than were needed . . . so the best could be picked; and Evans was able to put together ad hoc teams not only for hard-nosed investigations but for all kinds of special projects. *Sunday Times* reporters could spend whatever time and money they needed in order to get their story . . . a second factor behind the paper's ability to land an (investigative) story . . . was the attitude of Lord Thompson and Harry Evans to government. Neither of them considered it his business to make the government feel happy.[63]

On the cusp of the twenty-first century, it has almost become commonplace to suggest that the corporate or state explanation of a reality is one entirely created as it were "virtually," by falsehoods, semantic, and digital mirages. In the majority of cases, the disputed reality lies at the heart of the explanation of who was responsible. Although public disputes continue for years, the official view usually settles, if uncomfortably, into the miasma of modern history.

Developed society appears to be passing through a phase during which an alternative reality is turned on, much like a high-definition television screen. We are in the period now when the screen flickers as the different reality is shown us. Although these different realities are labeled as the product of conspiracy theories, there can be no doubt that we are entering a period of new but distorted realities—where public health and public order, political stability, and a hierarchy of scientific experts set the agenda and do battle with the affected.

Gradually, global history begins to echo the information on the back of a cornflakes packet rather than the research of competent and ethical historical writers; we have entered belatedly the much-trumpeted era of *1984*. If those in power can now create false realities of massive proportions, we no longer live in a world that can be unified or ever return to any semblance of democracy.

For some writers, filmmakers, and investigators, the Spanish ~~Toxic Oil~~ Syndrome definitely plays a part in this history of illusion. Their inability to make their voices heard with truth, however, signals a consequence of this theatrical history: the bigger and more realistic the spectacle, the greater the impossibility of publicly proving its most obvious contradictions.

In the understanding of the twentieth and twenty-first century *theatre of political illusion*, the commentary of the oil traders' trial in Spain, given by Bob Woffinden, is trailblazing. He peels back the screen that formed the false reality of TOS and tries to articulate how such a trick was performed. Of the whole TOS scandal, he says the following:

> The worldwide deception continues, automatically recycled by a compliant media. The enduring feature of the TOS saga is that it provided a blueprint for the international scientific community. If even a theory as palpably bogus as the "toxic oil" syndrome can be sustained internationally, then suppressing the truth must be remarkably straightforward. All it takes is a series of epidemiological reports, accredited by scientists of a similar persuasion and then published in reputable scientific journals. There are, as Disraeli might have said, lies, damned lies and peer-reviewed scientific papers . . . Given increasing privacy constraints, the media can never independently verify the data, and just have to report whatever they are told . . . It was the prototype contemporary scientific fraud . . . It marked the first time that multinational interests successfully contrived a major cover-up in international science . . . It is also increasingly understood that scientific research is now hardly ever conducted in a spirit of disinterested inquiry. Usually, it is funded by global companies whose concerns are anything but disinterested. Even when research is financed by government agencies, those, too, will want to call the tune.[64]

AFTERWORD

I have written about the late Sir Richard Doll since the 1980s, when the late Teddy Goldsmith gave me the files that he had collected on Doll's work. Letters from campaigning groups covered most of the areas where Doll had obstructed citizens' campaigns to right the wrongs of toxic effects, illnesses, and death.

There was, anyway, from an earlier date than this, some evidence that Doll worked for toxic corporations, although little of this was specific, detailed, or referenced and most of it seems to have avoided mentioning possible state or government involvement.

After Doll's death, it became known that he had donated "personal" papers covering certain subjects to the Wellcome Institute Library. When I scrutinized the index to these papers, I saw two things: first that the papers might contain proof that Doll had been under contract to Monsanto, and second that there was a good deal of material on the Spanish Toxic Oil Syndrome, a subject that I had not got around to covering and which some people had "warned" me off covering. The Wellcome Institute itself did a good job of safeguarding its material from visitors—one clause in their agreement stipulates that readers and viewers should take away nothing which might damage the reputation of the papers' initiators.

I published the information about Doll and his contractual relationship with Monsanto in an essay in 1989. I was later criticized by some for not getting this broadly publicized in the media. When those with this opinion did this very thing with my work, it resulted in a number of reports and statements justifying Doll's work at the beck and call of industry. Of course, it is not possible, as society drifts toward corporatism, to raise problems with reality in the corporate media.

What, however, I found of great interest in Doll's papers deposited at the Wellcome was the amount of material on the Spanish ~~Toxic Oil~~ Syndrome. In some respects, over the years in investigating Doll, I had come to respect certain aspects of his behavior—a kind of Stockholm syndrome reflection on my part. He was a very canny and strategically intelligent man, who unlike the US Quackbusters, for instance, didn't sound off against people with great personal insults. When he was pulled up about things, he would more than likely admit that there were other sides to the argument; he could even back down completely, knowing that the work he had done for corporations would always remain authoritative and cast in stone, like the Ten Commandments. He was most typically English in his evident desire to politely smooth out the ruffles of "personal" disagreements.

But the information on the Spanish ~~Toxic Oil~~ Syndrome was breathtakingly different. My attention was drawn to Doll's official biography, which had not one word on his involvement in the biggest toxic epidemic ever in Europe. This could only be the case if Doll had given definite instructions to his biographer. His correspondence and reports in relation to ~~TOS~~, revealed a situation in which Doll had been heavily pressured. The principle pressurizer had been the US uniformed public health officer, Kilbourne, who seemingly acted on behalf of the US corporate state.

Doll went ahead with his research and his evidence, but his Englishness, his gentlemanly demeanor, even what integrity he had, revolted against the pushy American, and even perhaps against the whole concept of railroading itinerant oil salesmen for killing over a thousand fellow citizens.

Doll kept the case from his biography but deposited important papers, full of clues in the Wellcome. I can't say for certain that Doll laid this paper trial to be followed by an anti-corporate researcher. It's actually more probable that

Doll's actions were personal; having been slighted and demeaned by Kilbourne, Doll wanted to get his own back.

Although I believe that most of Doll's work, apart from his involvement in the smoking studies, should be struck from the record and never again presented as examples of ethical epidemiology, I can't help but feel a sneaking respect for a villain who leaves clues against those whom he considers even greater villains for the investigators who come after his death. With regards to Doll's life, the Spanish ~~Toxic Oil~~ Tragedy echoes the most interesting postmodern detective fiction.

Chapter 10

ESCAPING ELECTROSENSITIVITY

Christian Blom

I'm working on a dream
Though sometimes it feels so far away
I'm working on a dream
And I know it will be mine someday

Rain pourin' down, I swing my hammer
My hands are rough from working on a dream
I'm working on a dream

Let's go!

Bruce Springsteen 2009

I am electrosensitive, a condition that everyone in our present society should learn about.

What I call electrosensitivity struck me fourteen years ago. It has been possible to demonstrate this as a clinical pattern of reactions and symptoms, which have tended to repeat themselves during a fourteen-year period.

It was during the midsummer of 2003. The outbreak was clear and at the same time so violent that I ended up with something classified as very serious electrohypersensitivity (EHS). Not only that, but the symptoms continued to get worse during the first year. After that, though, there was a delicate balance in my health, which allowed me to continue living my life. Maybe it was not the hypersensitivity that came into balance but that I started to find ways of dealing with it.

I am now sixty-eight and I have retired "for real," although I lost much of my pension since 2003 when I was never again able to return to my work. I failed to get compensation because I failed, at numerous hearings, to get my disease classified as an occupational injury or even a disease possible to diagnose.

The EHS turned into aggressive cancer in my neck and throat in 2009. The treatment, equally aggressive, including six weeks of chemotherapy (Cisplatin) and thirty-five sessions of radiotherapy treatment, successfully yielded complete remission of the cancer and it has not returned since then. After the cancer treatment, I lived in uncertainty, wondering how the electrosensitivity would manifest itself.

It might even be gone? But it wasn't, although some changes in its appearance were noticeable. After the cancer, I was able to move more freely among people, socialize, and do things such as go to the theatre. But the EHS is still there. It has been trying new "pathways" in my body and my neural system, and it has become "duller" and more unpredictable in its nature. It appears now more as a chronic pain in my muscles and joints, and I have indisputably become much more sensitive to various weather conditions: incoming rain, fog, charged air before a thunderstorm, low pressure that is left circulating in the air: it all causes almost unbearable states of cramp and aching.

I react very strongly to solar flares. I have kept a diary of symptoms for several years and compared the data with the statistics for solar flares. I learned to find statistics on various Internet sites, mostly on spaceweather[1] and on the Finnish site Auroras Now.[2] I have found my own tolerance values for space and atmosphere magnetic and radioactive radiation. If the speed of the solar wind during a solar flare exceeds 400 kilometers per second, or atmosphere magnetic radiation exceeds 30 to 40 nanotesla, I become very ill.

My tolerance limit for microwave radiation, that is cell phone radiation, is about 10 to 20 microwatts per square meter. For me to be able to sleep, the level should be around 0 to 5 microwatts. In Helsinki, where I live in the wintertime, the microwave levels in the street vary between a few microwatts and ten thousands of microwatts. Inside our apartment, we have a narrow sector where the microwave level is always around 500 microwatts, sometimes even higher. Otherwise, the radiation value in our apartment is between 1 and 100 microwatts.

My tolerance limits for low-radiation electromagnetism (around 50 hertz) are harder to define. It is more about what kind of disturbances in the fields that are present or how "choppy" the fields are—or how well the appliances are grounded. I react most strongly to the new energy-saving bulbs and all sorts of transformers and dimmers. Many common household appliances emit a complex combination of various electric, magnetic, and microwave fields. When I also react especially strongly to various compressors or the sound of compressors, for example in the presence of freezers, my reaction pattern gets complicated. It often ends with me having to turn off the main power switch to be able to carry on. In 2004, we were forced to keep the refrigerator and the freezer closed all winter. The balcony served as a fridge and freezer on those days that were cold enough.

THE ONSET OF MY ELECTROSENSITIVITY

My electrosensitivity started in the midsummer of 2003. What then happened was so concrete and tangible that I constantly seem to return to these events whenever I try to tell others about my condition. Despite the fact that I, on that occasion, was treated by several doctors, the specific onset was more or less undocumented. I am sure that the doctors during those critical days would have been able to measure strongly deviant values regarding my health—values that might have been both an important guide in defining the onset of my electrosensitivity and of great help in explaining it to others.

The first onset set in by midsummer, but it had begun by the end of March 2003; a definitive and permanent change in my health condition had occurred. First I want to tell you about the midsummer of 2003.

We were to spend the midsummer in Viitasaari, in a cottage belonging to my wife's family. I was driving the 450 kilometers from our own summer house in the Esbo archipelago to the cottage. In the car were also my wife, two children, and our cat. The day at home had been very hot and dry. The sun was strong; the UV index was probably reaching 6 or 7.

I had been raking dry grass in the garden before we left, and had eaten something earlier that I might even have had a slight reaction to. After only half an hour of driving north, with the strong midsummer sun shining in my face, I was fiery red and blotchy on my face and on my chest. But I had been used to that earlier in the spring and I knew that the attack, whatever it was, usually wears off, at sunset at the latest. On the E4 highway, my situation became rapidly worse. The flaring persisted.

Just as I realized that I needed help, a hospital sign appeared adjacent to the highway, and I swiftly turned into the entrance and followed the signs to the center of the hospital.

At the hospital, I collapsed and was taken in for emergency care. Everything pointed to a severe allergic shock and I received treatment for that: adrenaline, cortisone, antihistamine intravenously, and fluid therapy. Just before the collapse, I had felt a sensation that something was trickling from my mucous membranes and almost "running" down into my lungs.

The doctors left me to make the choice, either staying for observation at the hospital or leaving. We chose to leave and get to the cottage that was waiting for us. During the remaining drive to central Finland, I became very sensitive to certain smells, such as vehicle exhaust, the smoke from houses as we passed, and newly laid asphalt on parts of the road.

Somehow, we arrived at the cottage, and I was stuck in bed for the first few days, without daring to move or leave the house. The smell of grass from outside felt like burning gas through my respiratory organs. It felt like a combination of infernal asthma and allergy, and sometimes it was sufficient just to look at something smelly to feel my lungs burning. I was unable to eat. But the acute feeling of panic slowly subsided and I could get up and walk into other rooms in the cottage.

Late in the evening on the second day, we decided to watch a film and turned on the TV. Even though I was standing three to four meters from the TV, my whole upper body and my lungs started to tremble, vibrate, and burn. I intuitively turned off the TV, and the feverish, trembling feeling slowly subsided. We turned the TV back on and the same thing happened. We repeated this about ten times, each time with the same result.

I guessed what this was all about. In May, earlier in the same year, I had visited a doctor who treated me with antioxidants, and the doctor then asked me if I was sensitive to electricity. The suggestion sounded irrational, but the thought was planted in my mind and grew in my imagination as a nightmare. The following day, I found that I could no longer stay in a big store, being unable to stand the fluorescent lights or the sound of the freezers for a second.

That time, we stayed for three weeks in the cottage in Viitasaari and the situation grew steadily worse every day. Every day I encountered new obstacles to my existence. At this stage I was still using a mobile phone—I did not understand that the mobile phone also emitted electromagnetic radiation. I finally stopped using my mobile phone in late January 2004. But I will tell you about that later on, because that event was almost as dramatic as what happened during the drive to Viitasaari.

MARCH–JUNE 2003: STEADILY INCREASING ALLERGIES

I had become electrosensitive: there was no doubt about that anymore. And the onset came after an allergic shock reaction to something. The most central organs to react had been the lungs, the mucous membranes, and the bronchi. Still today, I remember the horrifying feeling of something glowing and running down the lungs.

The only thing strongly abnormal, which could later be detected during my examinations at the Allergy Hospital in Helsinki, was significantly elevated values of nitric oxide in my exhaled air. But these values also slowly subsided and reverted to normal during the fall of 2003, despite the fact that my allergy and my hypersensitivity only worsened. A permanent change had occurred in my mucous membranes, pharynx, and bronchi, and that was why I was to feel the deterioration in my health during the following months precisely in those organs: the pharynx, the bronchi, the lungs, and all muscles surrounding those organs around my shoulder blades and my chest.

Twice, in the fall of 2003 and winter of 2004, I was to feel once again how my lungs and my chest were "struck by lightning." The first occasion was in late October 2003, when the worst solar flare in centuries occurred, the so-called *Halloween Storm*. As a result, a herpes-like inflammation spread in my pharynx and my bronchi.[3] The second time was January 31, 2004, when the GSM-Edge-signal was turned on in the mobile network of Helsinki. The first strong, digital, and intricately modulated mobile broadcasting caused me a similar reaction to the one around midsummer in 2003, when my electrosensitivity started. Only this time, I could not turn off the signal. It is still now turned on (2016) and additionally supplemented with 3G and 4G transmissions and quite a few other broadband digital transmissions in the mobile network.

My electrosensitivity, then, started full-strength in the midsummer of 2003. But all through the winter and spring of 2003, my allergies had continuously grown stronger and I became allergic and hypersensitive to more and more things. I had been allergic and suffered from asthma since early childhood. I had strong reactions to chemicals, too, at a very early school age. Several times in primary school, I fainted during handicraft lessons when someone used varnish or solvents.

I have been told that my asthma started at two years of age, when we spent the summers in an industrial city called Jakobstad. When the wind blew from the northwest, gases and smoke from a cellulose factory chimney came to us from a distance of about one kilometer. That was in the early 1950s and the smoke was probably not cleaned and filtered in those days. I suffered from severe asthma and allergy attacks throughout my childhood.

Since the late 1990s I had been working as an educational director of a cultural program in a college outside Helsinki. The buildings in which we worked were severely water damaged and moldy. The same year, I was starting to use a mobile phone more frequently (analogue NMT phones and later digital phones in GSM network) and new computers were regularly brought to the college. I always felt the smell from the new computers, as well as the smell from the big constantly used copying machines. At home we started using wireless DECT telephones in the early 1990s.

Summer and fall of 2002 were the warmest in Europe in decades. The smoke from constant forest fires in Russia and in Eastern Europe had been tormenting me throughout the late summer of 2002. My reactions to the mold in my workplace were intensifying. The winter and spring of 2003 in Helsinki were bone dry; the street dust was thick. Then in March came the pollen grains.

We spent the last March weekend in our cottage in the Esbo archipelago, near Helsinki, and I did a lot of gardening. That weekend something happened to my lungs. The asthma, which I had felt frequently during the last months, did not disappear, even though I had taken all the medication available at that time. The nature of the asthma also changed and became more frightening.

The muscles in my chest swelled. I visited a respiratory physician hardly a week later and she told me I could not go back to work due to the mold I had told her about. During April and May, the new kind of asthma was almost permanently active. My allergies increased and the allergic reactions also changed their nature. I had seizures, during which I was fiery red on my chest, on my neck, and in the face.

The seizures came more frequently and I could not find any pattern in the way they occurred. I also reacted to almost any food that I ate. I had to avoid spices, everything with gluten, and fried food. In two months I lost twenty kilograms. My mucous membranes were permanently inflamed. My breathing was affected by more substances in the air—not only pollen and street dust but also ordinary dust and all smells. Eventually, I could not take a single breath inside the buildings at our college.

My lectures were held on the lawn outside the school. If I had to make copies of the lecture material, I held my breath, then rushed into the building, set the copying machine, turned it on and quickly ran out again, without taking a single breath inside the building. My worst symptoms were always connected to the copying machine.

Much later, when I was examined at the Allergy Hospital, we tried without success to figure out what was the reason for the total collapse of the breathing. The lung function was rather ordinary, but the breathing was paralyzed.

Then it was no longer possible for me to stay in our own summer cottage in Esbo. After May 14, 2003, I could no longer breathe in the main building there. I tested all possible respiratory protection, even with a chemical filter, but nothing worked. We have not slept one night in our summer house since May 14, 2003—almost fourteen years.

Now—fourteen years later—however, I am sitting in the house again writing on my laptop. We have removed the mold contamination as much as we could, but the air is still not good. I can be here about one hour every day and use the kitchen, the bathroom, and the computer. From the summer of 2003, I noticed that the smell in our cottage changed significantly if the electricity from the main switch was turned off. The smell of mold more or less disappeared. The smell of paint, varnish, and other things also changed when the electricity was gone.

Constantly, I began wondering: is there a radical change happening in me and in my sensory organs when the electric current is turned off, or is the electricity affecting micro particles flying in the air, or is their charge affected—or something similar? Professor Tari Haahtela at the Allergy Hospital once told me, when my examinations were ongoing at his clinic, that researchers have found that mold spores and their toxins in certain cases can change "behavior" if the basic conditions for their growth are suddenly changed. Probably, electromagnetic radiation could change their natural conditions, make the toxins more "wild" and aggressive, as Dr. Haahtela put it.

In the year 2000, we had built a little log cabin on the plot of our summer cottage, about thirty-five square meters, including a sauna. There was no electricity in the building. We moved to this cabin in May 2003. The smell of turpentine from the fresh timber had decreased significantly and my lungs accepted the air in the building: I was able to breathe there. But during the first months, we could not heat the large wood-fired oven because I reacted strongly to the smell of burning wood and the smell from the mortar when the oven was heated. The summer was warm, though, and we could live there until midsummer approached and we were to go to the family cottage in Viitasaari for a couple of weeks.

THE FALL OF 2003

Even after our stay in Viitasaari, where the fully fledged onset of my electrosensitivity finally occurred, I could continue my stay in the log cabin on our own plot in the Esbo archipelago. In fact, fourteen years later, my wife and I still, today, spend almost six months a year in the cabin without electricity. The main building, with certain mold damage, is still left on the plot, but nowadays I can stay there for several hours a day. I do not remember when I once again started to learn how to breathe in this building. Presumably it occurred gradually during late summer and fall of 2003, after the first repairs.

Thinking that I was improving, I tried to go back to work in the fall of 2003 after five months' sick leave. My office was moved to another building where there were no acute mold problems. But my sensitivity had become extreme: the smallest change in air quality started a crowd of symptoms. In the fall of 2003, it came home to me that electromagnetic radiation had an impact on me.

In practice, it meant that I had to stop using one device after another. I could no longer use the copying machine. All computer use had to stop. What I tried to avoid the most was the mold. Still, throughout the fall I used my mobile phone, without realizing that it radiated as much as the computers.

Our college moved to the center of Helsinki in October 2003. All the furniture and the books were moved as well, and my reactions in the new location continued as dramatically as before. Only this time, I also saw the effects of the mobile phones. Along the streets by our school, there were several base stations for the mobile network. My reactions immediately got worse. The radiation from the base stations felt like knives within me. My lectures were often spoiled by students using their mobile phones during class.

In early November, I was once more forced to take sick leave, and this time we had also moved back from our summer house to the apartment in the center of Helsinki. My hypersensitivity reached a totally new level. I realized that the mold meant less than the mobile radiation.

Simultaneously, the solar activity cycle went into a more active phase: the sun flares in the fall of 2003 were to become the strongest ones in over fifty years. And I had also started cleaning up my many amalgam fillings in a hurry. My condition deteriorated quickly, and I was once more forced to take sick leave. Now, the struggle for income-related sickness or possibly occupational injury compensation entered a new phase: disability pension was looming in my mind.

The process began. But it would prove to be infinitely difficult and lengthy, and in the end, just wishful thinking. I would push my case twice to the highest insurance court, only to lose both times. I got my disability pension in 2008, at the age of sixty, based on a legal clause that did not require the establishment of a diagnosis. That EHS and mold hypersensitivity were to be mentioned in my medical certificates was only to aggravate this torturous process.

MY FIRST DISEASE DIAGNOSIS

In the winter of 2003, most of my doctors' appointments concerned finding out why my allergies suddenly increased so drastically. I was convinced that it all started with the mold. And then, eventually, hypersensitivity to other substances added to the picture and also very strong hypersensitivity reactions to chemicals. My intention had been to surface-treat the new log cabin with tar and paints. I could still breathe in the smell of pure tar, but when I diluted the tar with turpentine and linseed, my lungs reacted very strongly.

I began to name my asthma attacks "chemical asthma," since the muscles around my chest and my lungs swelled, and then they stayed swollen for days or even weeks. No medication helped. And, as I said before, the connection with magnetic fields was still unknown to me in the spring of 2003.

We had a good health service at my college and I was immediately taken care of by specialists: pulmonologists, allergists, and general practitioners. I also started to see Karin Munsterhjelm, a doctor at the Helsinki Antioxidant Clinic. She, together with several others, was to become my doctor for over ten years. She was one of few doctors in Finland who recognized electrosensitivity, and she tried to treat it with antioxidants but also other good care advice. Without her support I would hardly have made it through the process in which I was about to become embroiled.

I went to doctors and specialists who worked at the staff health center, while also visiting specialists. Privately, I consulted Dr. Munsterhjelm and several other doctors. In June, I got a referral to the Allergy Hospital, which is under the central hospital of Helsinki University. During the following five years, I regularly visited the Allergy Hospital, where I was supported by the Medical Director, Dr. Tari Haahtela; unfortunately my own doctor at the hospital was not so supportive.

At the same time, I also got a referral to the State Institute for Occupational Health (Työterveyslaitos), to investigate whether my mold hypersensitivity had been caused by the mold spores at my workplace. When I was first interviewed, I made a fatal mistake: I told them about a burnout at work, which I had suffered almost thirty years earlier. Thereafter, the doctors constantly came back to this issue, and the issue of my exposure to mold, electromagnetic fields, or possible chemicals was deliberately ending up in the background. My health continued to worsen and I had no strength left to fight against the doctors' diagnoses or decisions.

Professor Haahtela at the Allergy Hospital took my story seriously, and at various clinics within the University Central Hospital I went through a lot of examinations. I told them about my symptoms and many different specialists examined me. The doctors in neurology and psychiatry diagnosed both neuropathy and fibromyalgia. I also got a referral to a psychiatric examination, and since it took a long time to do the examination, I really was in a bad shape. During my last visits to the psychiatrist, I was seriously afraid—in the worst instance—of being forcibly detained. But the psychiatrist could not establish any specific psychiatric diagnosis in particular for me. Much later, Professor Haahtela did give me a moderate depression diagnosis in an attempt to help me get my disability pension. All in all, in the years of 2003 and 2004, I was diagnosed with multiple allergy, asthma, neuropathy, fibromyalgia, and balance disorders in the central nervous system, among other things.

FIVE YEARS OF PSYCHOTHERAPY

Ultimately, my doctor visits were of no help to me; on the contrary, I felt more dejected after each examination at each appointment. In connection to my psychiatric examinations, I had been recommended several different psychotropic drugs, which I never used. I was not given a referral to a psychotherapist through the public health system, but through my own private health insurance I could begin prolonged psychotherapy treatment.

For five and a half years I went to psychotherapy once a week. Why? To cope with the situation I had been forced into: no longer to be able to work, go to the theater or the cinema, not even walk around freely in the city. I suffered from panic, fear of mobile phone base stations, and antenna masts. I knew exactly on which roofs there were mobile transmitters—at that time I was so extremely sensitive that my body found each and every transmitter. The psychotherapy did not help me to reduce my fear of the masts or the transmitters, but it helped me to survive, to stay with my family, and somehow establish a new life in the middle of my new desperate situation, when I could no longer stay among people, watch TV programs, nor hardly even listen to the radio.

At the same time, I went against the flow compared to other electrosensitives in Finland. In Finland, the electrosensitive (EHS) association had made recommendations from the start to keep EHS as a disease "of non-mental nature." Psychotherapy was more or less forbidden in our circles. Despite that, I met more and more electrosensitive people who told me they had taken medications, for instance against panic disorder, depression, and psychosis for years.

Several EHS patients had been treated at hospitals because of the trauma they experienced as a result of electrosensitivity. The psychotherapy treatment was also problematic because the authorities and the Finnish Medical Association constantly recommended cognitive therapy as a treatment for the EHS patients. Today, fourteen years later, I am still convinced that falling ill with EHS is tremendously psychologically traumatizing for the patients. During my fourteen years' electrosensitivity, I have been in contact with several hundreds of EHS patients in Finland and have become increasingly convinced of the severity of this trauma.

In the spring of 2009, it appeared that I suffered from aggressive cancer in my neck and throat—mostly on the right side of my neck, where my mobile phones had been more or less attached since 1993. The cancer treatment started in the spring of 2009, and after the treatment—in late 2009—I ceased to go to psychotherapy. A major cause was that I was not able to speak for many months after the cancer treatment.

THE THROAT CANCER DIAGNOSIS IN 2009

Ever since the onset of my electrosensitivity, I had experienced some especially harsh pain in and around my right ear in connection with my mobile phone use. I told my doctors about these symptoms in 2004; however, they denied my pain experience and stressed that mobile phone radiation cannot cause pain.

As I have already said, I still used my mobile phone to a small degree until late January 2004. Then a dramatic deterioration in my health occurred in one single evening. We were living in our apartment in Helsinki, in a part of the city called Skatudden, which is close to the South Harbor (Södra Hamnen), the harbor of the Swedish ferries.

On the evening of January 31, 2004, I suddenly experienced similar symptoms to those I had in midsummer 2003, except that this time I had no TV on. I was just sitting in our almost totally dark apartment. All the muscles around my chest started to vibrate and tremble. I panicked and searched for a cause inside the apartment without finding anything. Outside, the cold was intense but I needed to get out into the fresh air.

I went out onto the harbor and for many hours I walked around Skatudden, continuously with the same feeling of panic in my body, the same vibrating feeling in my lungs and around my chest. No relief anywhere—until eventually I went behind a big port warehouse and suddenly the cramps and the body vibrations eased. I walked out into the street again and instantly I was affected by the same horrible feeling—and then again into the shadow of the warehouse where my feelings came to a halt. After several hours behind the warehouse, I walked back home, able to calm down and go to sleep.

The following day, I called all phone operators in Helsinki, and also the port authorities and the national defense, to find out what change had occurred the night before. It turned out that the largest telephone operators had started a new mobile network, GSM-Edge, or 2.5G as they also called it, the previous evening. The first digital broadband transmission was on.

Since that evening, I could no longer use my mobile phone without feeling enormous pain in my head and all my upper body. If I, in case of emergency, used the cell phone just very quickly, I felt as if a nail had been hit in my right ear. This story is documented after several doctors' visits to the Allergy Hospital. In the fall of 2008, I made my last visit to the Allergy Hospital. They could not keep a patient only under observation for more than five years, and for administrative convenience I was declared healthy by the doctors.

The same autumn, I began to suffer from toothache on the right side of my jaw. My teeth were treated several times, and root canals were renewed, but the pain continued. In February 2009, I suffered from mysterious neck influenza with neck pain, an almost herpes-like pain in the mucous membranes. My wife remembers me complaining about the feeling of having a fish bone stuck in my throat.

One April day, I saw how the glands under my right lower jaw were swollen and felt hard. I went back to my dentist, who instead urged me to see a throat doctor. The same day I got an appointment with a throat specialist and he gave me an acute referral to the Ear Nose and Throat (ENT) Clinic at the University Central Hospital. Already at my first visit the doctors told me I had a tumor in my pharynx. Then it all accelerated.

On May 1, 2009, the MRI of the neck area was done, and one week later samples of the tumor were taken under anesthesia. The surgeon, who had examined me, told me loudly, lying there in the recovery room—in front of the other patients—that the examination went well, and that yes, they found a big tumor, probably cancer. One week later, the surgeon called me at home and confirmed the cancer diagnosis.

The primary tumor was in my throat and metastases had spread to all glands in the right side of the neck, later also to the left side. I was diagnosed with cancer; in Latin *C10.0 Ca epidermoides valleculae dx cum metastasibus colli T2N2bM0, stage IV A*. The tumor was located at the root of the tongue, but all the glands on the right side of my neck were pathologically affected with metastases. The area was exactly where I had pressed my mobile phones or DECT phones against my ear for more than ten years.

One day at the end of May, I was sitting in the surgeon's consulting room at the hospital and she was showing me the computer pictures of how the cancer was spread over my neck region. Everything flashed red. She told me that a medical team recommended chemotherapy for six weeks and then thirty-five sessions of radiotherapy—the maximum amount of radiation possible. I approved the treatment, but I also asked if the mobile phones could have caused my cancer, as it appeared in the same spot where I had felt pain by cell phone use since 2003. The surgeon answered: "We do not discuss that question here at the Helsinki University Central Hospital. Do you approve the treatment or not?"

I was silent, looked at my wife and my oldest son who were present at the doctor's appointment, and said, "Yes, I approve the treatment and I shall not ask questions about cancer and mobile phone use again."

About one month later, I sat in front of my radiotherapist at the Cancer Clinic, and we were discussing my treatment. "Oh, you are an EHS patient," the doctor said. "Then I will tell you that you will now receive more radiation than you ever have done before in your life." But I did not feel that he said it out of malice. Later it was confirmed that I had received the following amount of radiation during my treatment: 50 Gy in the form of 2 Gy fractions, and later additionally, as a boost in the tumor area, up to 70 Gy.

Then the cancer treatment started. Two weeks later, I was unable to swallow or talk anymore. In my diary, I have documented every single day of the thirty-five sessions of radiotherapy, and I cannot describe in a few words here what I went through. But the cancer was beaten and shrank by late fall 2009. In November 2009, I was able to swallow food again and to speak.

I spoke my first coherent sentences in front of the Finnish Parliament Communication Committee, where I was heard as an expert in connection with the new so-called EU Telecom Directive, which was then incorporated into the Finnish telecommunications law. I warned of what the increased mobile phone radiation, which would be caused by the new legislation, would bring in terms of health risks.

Again, I draw on my diary for this period in June 2014. Writing these sentences, at night between the 23rd and 24th of June 2014, I knew that the cancer had kept away, but during the spring of 2014, certain cancer markers in my blood had increased, and new examinations at the University Central Hospital ENT Clinic had to be undertaken.

Once again on June 24, 2014, at the ENT Clinic, I am meeting my doctor Mari Markkanen-Leppänen, the same doctor who five years ago diagnosed my cancer. She now examines my throat once more and says I am finally declared healthy from the original cancer. She tells me that today, a new factor that often is behind throat cancer has been found—wart virus.

Then I tell her the same thing as I did five years ago, that I know that my cancer derives from my frequent use of the mobile phone. Five years ago, I was forbidden from discussing this issue. Now she says that it is impossible to prove the causal relationship between mobile phone radiation and cancer.

She also tells me that the type of cancer that I had does not show through cancer markers in the blood. But the most important thing she says is that I am now healthy. She continues, saying that if I am afraid of getting a new tumor, I should visit a doctor and ask for an examination. "But here at the ENT clinic, we only treat cancer in the neck and head area."

I am walking out in the street in Helsinki again in the gentle summer rain. The cancer marker Ca 19-9 whirls in my blood, but that is for some other clinic to take care of. Maybe I am happy now?

I am sitting in the car driving home, with the same strong reactions as every time I drive. Now it is once again the time before midsummer, as in 2003. And once again, Finland has got a new prime minister, as in 2003. A prime minister who never has given us—the electrosensitive—a straight answer to our request for actions from the authorities to reduce the mobile phone radiation.

On the contrary—the new prime minister, Alexander Stubb, declares in his first press releases that the project of building another large nuclear power station in Pyhäjoki together with the Russian company Rosatom is to be taken to the parliament to be decided as soon as possible. The parliament is also in the final state of considering a comprehensive new package of laws covering most questions regarding the information society.

This code means, in plain language, that all legislation in relation to telephony, Internet, telecom in the broader sense, and more in this area, is gathered in one big package of laws. The package of laws will make it easier for the IT industry and the phone operators to get their products and services in use. For one thing, the property owners will no longer be able to, as they have until now, slow down the telephone operators' attempts to install mobile phone transmitters everywhere outside or inside buildings.

Helsinki is infinitely beautiful this day, with low drifting rain clouds, slowly moving in an indefinite direction, now and then precipitating slight showers of rain. I leave the city behind me and soon I reach the cottage in the archipelago, with an average mobile phone radiation of only 1 to 3 microwatts per square meter. Here, I can start my computer and write about my visit to the cancer physician.

PROFESSOR OSMO HÄNNINEN'S RADIATION EXPOSURE SURVEYS

The Finnish EHS association was founded in the late 1990s, and in the early 2000s they initiated collaboration with Physiology Professor Osmo Hänninen at the University of Eastern Finland. The cooperation continues today even though Hänninen is now retired. Osmo Hänninen at that time conducted research in the Medical Faculty at Kuopio University (today the University of Eastern Finland, or UEF.fi), and he started a comprehensive project at his faculty, which was about trying to prove how microwaves and mobile phone radiation affect people physiologically and biologically.

Hänninen built a so-called "Faraday cage" at the university, and there he tested a total of one hundred electrosensitive patients and registered their reactions to radiation during the years 2004 to 2008. I participated myself several times in examinations made in Kuopio, and we even did experiments at my home in Helsinki with similar devices. The patients were exposed to radiation inside the cage, and we were to tell the researchers about our subjective reactions, and simultaneously there was a device measuring our blood pressure and heart rate. The measurement results were then interpreted by a program developed by the Russian Academy of Sciences. Professor Hämminen's assistant was Dr. Sergei Kolmakoff, who also cooperated with the universities in Moscow and St. Petersburg.

Despite big technical issues with the Faraday cage and with the specified mobile phone signal, the researchers could see very strong correlations between the patients' physiological reactions and the mobile phone transmissions. When my reactions were measured, the measuring program warned about too strong and dangerous reactions in my body.

The test methods were developed through the years, but simultaneously a witch hunt against Professor Hänninen was initiated. He was compelled to shut down experiments and was eventually fired from the university, as were all the members of his research team. Hänninen presented a scientific report in the fall of 2004 on the basis of his research at a seminar that WHO arranged in Budapest, with the focus on the possible health risks of electromagnetic radiation. He also presented his results to the Finnish parliament at a hearing some years later.

It had been found that the experiments in Kuopio were difficult to implement for a number of reasons. One thing was that the patients were in a bad shape after having traveled to Kuopio from various parts of Finland. They should perhaps have been "acclimatized" some time before to the environment where the tests were conducted. Another thing was the measurement surroundings and the measuring instruments should have been more highly developed; however, we were given no opportunities. The resistance to his experiments was solid. But the clear and unambiguous measuring results showed that we were on the right track.

CONCLUSIONS OF A KIND

I realize that in this chapter I have primarily tried to find words and concepts for *my* electrosensitivity. Electrosensitivity is often described schematically, with a few standard reactions as its expression, while in reality it appears as a wide spectrum of feelings, sensations, and physical reactions.

The term electrosensitivity is itself "evasive": a medical diagnosis that lacks adequate directions. Electrosensitivity exists both psychologically and physically. It is sometimes infinitely alert, and the reactions appear at the slightest change in the surroundings—and sometimes more "tardy" and the reactions are "lagging," then they appear in the wrong order, contrary to the most common way.

The biggest conflict with this pattern is that the chain of reactions is triggered sometimes by mold, sometimes by street dust, sometimes by the sun, sounds, smells, or vibrations, and most frequently by mobile phone use. Often, reactions are also triggered by low pressure, rain, thunderstorms, or sun flares, and also by mental sensations. Often, these various factors interact, but sometimes one factor is enough to start the electrosensitivity process. One such factor is the sound or the radiation from certain compressors—mainly refrigerators. This sound gives me a feeling of a key pulling up something inside me, something is strapped to the limit until the compressor motor stops and my nerve and muscle tension starts to decrease. But after a complicated process, the situation calms down, the sensations scale down, and a delightful sense of balance, equilibrium, and well-being arises.

Professor Osmo Hänninen has it all described in a short sentence: Electrosensitivity is all about a serious disturbance of the autonomic nervous system.

Throughout my whole time as an electrosensitive, I have kept a diary. Up to now, I have about fifty diaries of documentation of what I have been through and experienced day by day. Many times, I have tried to make a list of which reactions I experience when I am exposed to radiation. The list becomes endless. Instead, I have tried to divide the symptoms into groups, or group them after what I believe caused the symptom. The groups and the underlying factors have become numerous, and I am still struck by how often I am surprised by the symptoms, how they constantly change their characters, and how they are always so frightening.

Also, there is the fact that I cannot always find the word for a feeling. Riggert Munsterhjelm, doctor of biology and an artist, arranged a course in 2007 that was about how to describe the symptoms of fibromyalgia or electrosensitivity, symptoms that people experience in relation to "invisible diseases," as he called them. I participated in the course, and the participants managed to come up with hundreds of new words and concepts for our feelings and reactions. It felt good and meaningful, and we got a grip on the elusive feelings we almost always experience as electrosensitive patients.

Eventually, after all these years, I have learnt to recognize the most important variations of the symptoms, some of them recurrent patterns.

All symptoms seem to be related; they emanate in some way "from myself," from what has always been me and my way of reacting with my body. Various environmental factors also constantly play their part regarding what triggers the symptoms within me: the beginning could be an overdose of mold spores or street dust and then I know it will be followed by stronger reactions to electricity, microwaves, sound waves, light waves, heat waves, and air pressure, etc. Everything is related and follows one after the other, and finally it leads to interactions.

Furthermore, the symptoms vary, depending on my general condition and the condition of my immune system. If I am catching a cold or have some inflammation, I know that the symptoms will come more frequently, more violently, and often be more appalling. Usually the symptoms follow a pattern; they are triggered by something, develop, and find their way down through my body, and then fade away. Sometimes very dramatic reactions can disappear in an hour or by the next morning at the latest. If not, something worse is going on.

I have created certain pictures to describe some symptoms for myself. An example is when it feels as if I am hung up on a hook attached to my back above the shoulder blades, I know that a strong solar flare is on its way. The feeling is horrifying and it makes me almost lose my breath, but I also know that pulses from solar flares come in relatively short waves, often only lasting for two to three hours.

Very often, my feelings are connected to something that I have named "the meridian of my left side." That concerns neural pathways that start in the big toe on my left foot and continue up through my leg, left groin, and through the left chest area, through my throat, my left side neck, and behind my left ear. An activated cell phone that is just connecting the signal to the network near me causes strong pulsations along these nerves. The most frightening feeling is when it occurs around my heart. If it tingles and feels almost electric in the nerve near my toes, I know there is dense fog outside.

The reactions often come in forms of vibrations within me: vibrations and a feeling of pressure. Certain cell phones cause a hard, stinging pain somewhere locally.

A combination of strong sunlight and certain smells (grass, mold, or something I have eaten) can cause a violent "flush," which causes the chest and the face to be red and hot in seconds. During my first years of electrosensitivity, this flush was often only on one side, more frequently on my left side. In that case, I recognized the feeling and I felt "secure." It was harder if it occurred on the right side, because then I had been exposed to something of which I did not know.

During the worst periods of fall 2003 and winter 2004, the mucous membranes in my mouth and throat would be burned, very quickly, by something unknown.

General muscle cramps and other very strong cramps have been common throughout all these years. Particularly in the city, where the radiation level around the clock is higher, I suffer from daily pain in all my body. That, in turn, has led to chronic sleep problems—but mostly in town. Coming to a new environment with low radiation, my sleep gets much better.

I have chosen not to encapsulate our apartment with protection fabrics and nets. Throughout the years, I tried various kinds of nets, but I often reacted to the smells or the poor air quality under the net. Instead, I have learned to be where there is lower radiation, partly with the help from a radiation meter, but mostly in relation to what my body tells me. In practice, I live in turns in Helsinki, the cottage in Esbo, or the cottage in the wilderness of Viitasaari. I feel the best in the electro-less log cabin in Esbo archipelago. The symptoms and reactions might keep quiet for a day there but then return for various reasons.

Often, my symptoms are "self-inflicted"—if I feel healthy for a day, I might go to the theater at night, and the reaction comes later. Initially, the reactions were immediate and I was forced away from the exposure as soon as possible. Six or seven years went by without watching TV or using a computer. Today, I watch TV sometimes and I regularly use the computer, always with wired Internet, with various reactions following. One often raised question is whether my cancer was "self-inflicted"—since I did not sleep under a canopy or protect myself enough. It is hard to say. Professor Tari Haahtela at the Allergy Hospital always told me to try to "harden" myself against the things I was hypersensitive to. I do not think that I hardened myself.

This is more about the limits to what you can stand, to what extent you can live totally separated from society. I was secluded for the first years when there were no alternatives. Since then I have gradually returned to society, often for social reasons. But lastly my most important dream is to find a timber house somewhere in Finland, where I could live permanently, as good as free from electronics, mold, and chemicals. But to realize a choice like that demands power and strength, and also that my wife retires from her work at the theater.

My current feeling is that our society is sliding into a really *mobile phase*, and even more things are integrated in the wireless network. The word "smart" is used as a description. Everything gets more and more "electrified," while we simultaneously try to save energy and make organic solutions. This is a way of bypassing "Shannon's law" in physics, which suggests that the amount of information that can be conveyed wirelessly is limited. Shannon's law can be bypassed; for instance, if Bluetooth is used at short distances, the amount of radiation source increases but the transmitting power decreases.

The same frequency can be shared by many more users. The major carrying waves (GSM, 3G, 4G) are filled with smart technology, so that they do not transmit full radiation for just a few users, as happened before. With smart technology, the radiation power can be modified in relation to the customers' demands for "fields." It is also possible to define the occasional space in a carrying wave, and use that "undercapacity" space more efficiently. This means more passive radiation. Simply, all frequencies available will be more used than before. The mobile carrying waves will no longer "let the fire go up the chimney." The transmission power can be decreased in case of few users, and increased at greater demand, by fully using all frequencies available. The use of satellites for wireless transmissions will also increase significantly. "Radio shadow" will be an expensive luxury in the future.

In Internet technology, our society is heading toward the new M2M technique—machine-to-machine communication over the Internet. That means that most common household appliances are starting to communicate with each other, and with the producer, deliverer, or service company, wirelessly over the Internet.[4]

For this to succeed, there must be a constantly connected WLAN network everywhere. In the near future, the WLAN network will merge with the new mobile phone 5G technology. Wireless microwave radiation in 5G will reach all corners of society—no "radio shadow" will ever be permitted again.

But this is not just about the increase of radiation closeness and near radiation. We are starting to abandon all previous "analogical," physical, and "organic" society. The "paper newspapers" disappear and move into cyberspace; a big change occurs in people's lives and their experiences of the world. Different kinds of news are read on the Internet. We read less background information and less deep analyses. What is read is read through wireless terminals. This is about our right to find knowledge developed by journalists. And it is about our right to disconnect this information from the Internet, take it in our hands, without too much exposure to microwave radiation, and reflect on it. Additional information is always to be found on the Internet. I often get a feeling that our society is not, despite all the digitizing happening now, developing in a more democratic direction.

When I became electrosensitive in 2003, I got on quite well with the surrounding society. People still believed in my reactions and they respected me and my demands. All of my friends turned off their cell phones when I was present. Today, almost nobody does that anymore. Nobody cares about what I say. Nobody is any longer interested in electrosensitivity or if microwave radiation might lead to cancer. The tidal wave of microwave radiation is incoming. Society will be totally inundated with this radiation in the future. And all this reality is camouflaged behind the "smart" concept.

To me and to several others, it is all about recreating an "analogue" and "organic" world, where we are able to live without constantly sitting in a radiation fog of so many milliwatts per square meter—or without constantly living in the modulated radio waves, which move along the digital and wireless broadband on the same wavelength as our human bodies function deep down: at 8 to 10 hertz. Our goal must be something more than just regions of low radiation. We must conquer the whole diversity of life, beyond the cyberspace of microwave fields.

Chapter 11

IGNORING CHRONIC ILLNESS CAUSED BY NEW CHEMICALS AND TECHNOLOGY

Gunni Nordström

The chronically ill people who have been affected by modern technology are thrown out into the cold.

Sweden once had the world's best Law of Occupational Injury. It was passed in 1976, during the late Swedish Prime Minister Olof Palme's time. Today this law is gone. The occupational injury insurance has been integrated into a general social security code.

Today, those who became ill or had an accident before 2011 have their cases judged by the old law. But the Law of Occupational Injury gradually went through a series of reductions during the time it was used, and in practice became more constrained.

Today, it is difficult to imagine that there once was a legal text presenting the idea that the person who became ill at work should not suffer as a consequence of imperfect science. However, that was how the original law worked. If there was no more evidence against than in favor of a connection between the illness and the work, the judgment should be in favor of the employee. Today, all Swedes know that it is virtually impossible to get a disease classified as an occupational injury, unless there is an almost complete consensus between physicians and scientists—such occasions are rare. Sweden is perhaps going to have a list of sicknesses allowed for compensation, like in other countries in the world.

Accidents at work, on the other hand, are harder to deny or whitewash. In these circumstances, the insurance policy does work. However, anyone who gets a disease at work due to exposure to any detrimental factor can expect a protracted lawsuit and mostly a final rejection. First, it must be established that the detrimental factor actually is pathogenic, and second, a connection between the detrimental, claimed causal factor and the disease must be proven.

For people claiming that they have become ill due to environmental factors, such as chemicals or any form of radiation, there is little hope. Regarding these kinds of so-called *new* or *undiagnosed* diseases, authorities refer to no current consensus in the research field, or no research whatsoever. The latter is often the case, since alarming reductions even in Occupational Safety and Health (OSH) research have occurred in Sweden during the last few years.

When in the 1980s it was clear that the electronics industry, particularly the microelectronics industry, had by far the highest rate of occupational diseases in California, United States, the statistics of occupational diseases were restructured. From then on, it became harder to get an idea of the rate of known diseases like cancer or other disorders in the workplace. Also, such industries were hurriedly moved by the Americans to countries with weak trade unions and often corrupt authorities.

It is also difficult in Sweden, a country very proud of its statistics, to get an idea of new illnesses arising at work. But the obstacles are more subtle than in the United States. Both the authorities and the medical profession have shown great ingenuity in finding new and evasive names for a range of symptoms that are often labeled as "syndromes."

The WHO has coined the term Idiopathic Environmental Intolerance (IEI). The essence of this term is that it has to do with unspecific symptoms with no basis in reality. Generally, IEI is perceived as a paraphrase for underlying psychiatric illnesses. Under this umbrella term several symptom groups have been gathered, such as Multiple Chemical Sensitivity (MCS); Electrohypersensitivity (EHS); and Chronic Fatigue Syndrome or ME, an abbreviation for Myalgic Encephalomyelitis or Myalgic Encephalopathies. Sometimes, the abbreviation ME/CFS can be seen.

Swedish authorities willingly refer to the WHO term Idiopathic Environmental Intolerance, but together with the medical profession they also let their imagination run riot finding different Swedish names for these conditions. Sometimes a summary such as "Lack of Confidence Disease,"—probably relating to the patients' lack of confidence in both WHO and in the medical profession—is used. Another disguising name is "Culture Diseases." Furthermore, there are new names for subgroups. In Sweden, the term MCS, or Multiple

Chemical Sensitivity, is seldom used, while it is a generally known term in the United States. Swedes, who often use euphemisms, speak of "Fragrance Disease" when referring to chemical scents. Such a defining label has delayed the insight that new chemicals of any description in our environment mainly mean a danger to health.

The most adequate term to use in all cases of sensitivity beyond allergy might be the overall expression "other hypersensitivity." These words describe a condition where no regular allergy is involved, even if the symptoms are often similar to allergic symptoms. A common denominator for all named innovations in this field is that the illnesses they describe and their subject sufferers are usually not eligible for sick leave or for work injury compensation.

Anyone who wants to find out how widespread these syndromes are at work will find it hard to get an overview. Due to the variety of designations, statistics are a rather vague source of knowledge.

GULF WAR ILLNESS IS ESTABLISHED

Gulf War Illness belonged for a long time to the Idiopathic Environmental Intolerance group and was assumed to be mainly a group of stress-related mental symptoms. The term "Gulf War Illness" was coined after the Gulf War in Kuwait in 1990 to 1991, when about two hundred thousand of the seven hundred thousand American soldiers participating in the war fell protractedly ill, experiencing, among other things, memory and concentration difficulties, chronic headaches, light sensitivity, and general body aches.

These symptoms have a striking similarity to the descriptive symptoms of the other syndromes mentioned above. Also, during the Balkan War, soldiers fell ill with the same kind of symptoms. Advanced modern technology was a characteristic feature for both wars. The soldiers were exposed not only to radiation, but also to a great number of biocides and immunizations.

Maybe the combination of microwaves and chemicals could explain the soldiers' illnesses and chronic symptoms. The suspicion was there. Scientists from the US Air Force hurried to Lund, a small university town in the south of Sweden, to take note of the research done there. Namely, in the 1990s, Leif Salford, Bertil Persson, and Arne Brun, three professors from Lund University, drew public attention to the fact that microwave radiation of the same frequency as used in mobile phones caused the blood/brain barrier in rats to be disrupted and leak albumin. This meant that the protein in the bloodstream of a rat could enter its brain. Furthermore, the proteins could be carriers of substances that are not meant to reach the brain. Could the same thing happen to human brains? This is a question that it is more difficult to answer in humans for ethical reasons.

In 2008, a US Congressional report was published, which established that Gulf War Illness is an organic state of illness that involves disorders of the brain, the autonomic nervous system, and disorders of immunological and neuroendocrine functions.[1] It was also noted that the syndrome could not be characterized with the methods of examination usually available at hospitals.

The same year in December, a Swedish professor of social medicine, Robert Ohlin, wrote an article published in the Swedish medical journal *Läkartidningen*. He claimed that the results referred to in the US Congressional report ought to be instructive for those in Sweden who were still using the term "Cultural Illnesses."

> A thorough biomedical investigation may show that many diffuse diagnoses actually have provable organic explanations.

Unfortunately, the contribution to the debate from Robert Ohlin came too late. No debate was started. In Sweden, there had already been an epidemic of disorders, to some extent comparable to Gulf War Illness or maybe even more comparable to Silicon Valley Syndrome. However, the people who had possibly realized this had managed to repress it altogether.

SILICON VALLEY SYNDROME

The first time I heard of Silicon Valley Syndrome was in 1986. A man called Joe LaDou came to Stockholm. He was a doctor at the California University School of Medicine in San Francisco. He had been following some peculiar disease symptoms for twenty years, among the semi-conductor industry employees in Silicon Valley, a cradle of IT technology.

Employees had become ill despite working in so-called clean rooms, laboratories as carefully made as rooms for surgery in a hospital, avoiding access of dust and pollutants. This was done to protect the fragile components, which were dipped in different chemicals. However, what the employees could not be protected from were toxic gases from acids and solvents, which spread, for instance, through the laboratory return air system. In work processes, also, different kinds of radiation were used, primarily UV and microwave radiation.

My journalist colleague, Carl von Schéele, got an opportunity to interview LaDou. When I read his article, I was struck by the similarity between the symptoms of the employees in the Silicon Valley clean rooms and the symptoms that we had been writing about in the TCO Paper over the last year. The paper was owned by the Swedish Confederation of Professional Employees, and since the fall of 1985, we had received phone calls from many members of the different

TCO unions, telling us about different symptoms that they suffered from when working in front of the cathode ray tube computer screens existing at that time.

In Sweden at that time, there was a lively debate about electromagnetic fields from data equipment. Clusters of increased frequency of miscarriages were reported among pregnant women both in Sweden and other countries, but also a range of symptoms, like skin rashes, ophthalmia, respiratory problems, severe fatigue, headache, light sensitivity, and peculiar forms of hypersensitivity. Computers were the main reason mentioned among those affected. Many people asked themselves how low-frequency electromagnetic fields alone could accomplish this range of symptoms.

Other possible causal factors close at hand were chemical substances. At this time, Joe LaDou presented a similar cluster of symptoms in factories where people worked with new technology. I read in the interview with him, written by Carl von Schéele, how one of the Silicon Valley women, after working four and a half years in the chip industry, found her immune system impaired. Her disease looked similar to AIDS, but instead of a virus, chemicals had ruined her immune system. She could not even go to the supermarket anymore without getting headaches and nosebleeds. She was hypersensitive to everything. Even tap water made her sick.

Joe LaDou explained that dozens of the substances used in this industry were known carcinogens. Many of the substances had effects in extremely low concentrations. Nobody knew which synergy effects there could be from various aerosols and gases combined in room air. LaDou also pointed out that there was a serious concern for the synergies that could emerge when these substances were combined with microwaves and other radiation occurring in the laboratories. Also, he mentioned chemicals that could react to light in the lithographic processes where UV radiation was used.

LaDou was very pessimistic. To answer all the questions, extensive and expensive research efforts would be necessary in the United States, Europe, and Asia. But the industry did not want to let researchers enter the workplaces, and no authorities were interested in taking actions that might obstruct technical development.

Trials of claimants against IBM, among other companies, took place later in the United States, since the employees affected by various diseases sued the company. One of the expert witnesses for the claimants was Richard Clapp, an environmental chemistry professor at Boston University. (See chapter 4) He had gained access to some secret IBM statistics on the causes of death among almost thirty-two thousand employees during the period from 1969 to 2001. It appeared that the frequency of death from cancer, among both male and female employees, was significantly above average for the American population. The risks of multiple myeloma, a rare type of malignant disease in the plasma cells, as well as brain tumors and breast cancer, were especially elevated. Moreover, the deaths had occurred in younger age groups than expected. Even the frequency of neurological diseases like MS and Parkinson's disease was elevated.

Both in the United States and in Europe, powerful forces did what they could to hide Clapp's information. IBM defeated the claims, but in several cases, the company made financial settlements out of court with the victims. Swedish media failed to report this, or Joe LaDou's visit to Sweden. The TCO Paper article about the backlash of the technological development in Silicon Valley was the only one. Still, Joe LaDou met the labor minister of that time, Anna-Greta Leijon, and several government representatives responsible for environmental issues. People seemed to think that this had little to do with Sweden, since we had no chip industry to talk about; moreover, the opinion was that Swedish work environments were surely the safest in the world.

CHEMICALS IN APPLIANCES

Four years after LaDou's visit to Sweden, previously secret measurement reports were published, showing that IBM monitors emitted a lot of chemical substances into domestic air during ordinary use. Swedish newspapers noticed the news but it had no impact. Also, the US trials against IBM had not yet reached the Swedish novelty threshold.

Probably the world's chemical industries were pleased to note that the debate on illness among the Swedish display users was focused on the radiation aspect. Several more years would pass before chemical industries had any reason to fear the Swedish chemists.

The Swedish authority representatives, whom Joe LaDou had visited, drew no parallels between what they had heard from him on the one hand and the ongoing epidemic among Swedish office employees on the other hand. A chemist from the now-closed National Swedish Safety Board of Occupational Health did visit Silicon Valley after LaDou's visit to Sweden, but he only wrote a short article in the house magazine about the "odd" chemicals present in the production.

Even if there are no obvious parallels between working conditions in the Silicon Valley laboratories and working conditions in Swedish office environments, the fact is that uncured residues of various substances remain in finished electronic products and are spread in room air. Today, it is difficult to know the amounts of substances in the appliances that gave thousands of Swedes problems during the 1980s and 1990s. Those appliances are long gone, either to waste dumps or ground down by recyclers.

At this time, recycling companies became problematic workplaces. Blood concentrations of chemicals among employees who handled electronics scrap—considered as hazardous waste—could be measured, and so it was understood that there could be health risks both in the production stage and in the scrapping stage. One Swedish recycling company noticed that employees got skin disorders when being close to a machine that crushed printed circuit boards. Thanks to cooperation with Åke Bergman, a Stockholm University professor of chemistry, safety measures were developed at the company, and requirements for better work environments in companies like this became general in Sweden. Nobody knows, however, what happened to the immigrants and the unemployed who early on were put to work with electronic scrapping without adequate safeguards.

INFORMAL DISCUSSIONS
An internal, informal discussion was ongoing among Swedish chemists regarding the peculiar symptoms among the employees who had been working with the first generation display screens. The chemists talked about the "Office Disease." They thought there was too little focus on the chemical content in both computer equipment and other electronics in those environments where a real epidemic of occupational diseases raged among officials, even among highly skilled technicians, such as engineers.

For example, in Gothenburg, at the Swedish Institute of Production Engineering Research, later named Swerea, a great deal of knowledge was accumulated about plastic covers and entrails in the modern appliances. In 1995, an interesting Institute report was published, titled: "Waste from electrical and electronic products—a survey of the contents of materials and hazardous substances in electric and electronic products." This report, written by Per Hedemalm, was ordered and paid for by a joint Nordic project for cleaner technology, initiated by the Nordic Council of Ministers. I succeeded later in getting a copy of the report, which again definitely failed to reach the novelty threshold in the media.

Per Hedemalm and a colleague from Swerea applied for governmental funding in 1991 to study the degradation of flame retardants in printed circuit boards and possible interaction with other factors. Their idea was to find an explanation for the ongoing illness epidemic among monitor users. They particularly referred to the measured emissions from IBM monitors. The earlier mentioned National Swedish Safety Board of Occupational Health advised against funding, writing that chemical emissions were "unsubstantiated claims" and the reference to IBM "speculative." No funding was received.

There was also no funding to the chemists of the National Swedish Institute of Working Life (long since closed), who—in 1997 by accident—discovered emissions of organic phosphate compounds from the plastic around monitors. The compounds appeared as noise spikes in laboratory gas chromatography analysis of outdoor air. One scientist, Associate Professor Conny Östman, said that initially they could not understand where the compounds came from until they realized that they existed in the laboratory air. The scientists found it interesting and carried out experiments at offices, showing that triphenyl phosphate escaped from monitors in normal use. Triphenyl phosphate was used, among other chemicals, as a flame retardant in electronics. It was known as allergenic but could also affect the blood counts in humans. Several organic phosphate esters could react with acetylcholinesterase, a signaling enzyme in the body, regulating nerve impulses to the muscles and even to the brain in the memory and learning processes. Acetylcholinesterase affects the autonomic nervous system. This chemical group includes the nerve gas sarin.

These scientists took measurements in offices without computers, then with computers that were not turned on, and finally with computers in use. They found that triphenyl phosphate undoubtedly came from the computer equipment, and also that the levels in the screen covers, for instance, could be between eight and ten percent. Conny Östman and his colleagues were surprised to notice that the researchers funded by the government, who did their research on the health of display users, only focused on electromagnetic fields and did not show any interest in chemical emissions. Still, the fact that the temperature inside a monitor could reach 120 degrees Celsius was known, and this made it likely that triphenyl phosphate and other chemical gases would be emitted.

Conny Östman told me once when I interviewed him that "We would have been interested in a partnership with the radiation researchers, but we realized that the chemical aspect of these problems was not considered to be important, although a large part of the population is continuously exposed to these kind of substances, both at the workplaces and in their homes."

Östman and his colleagues later moved to Stockholm University to form a unit for Work Environment Chemistry. Their expectations of money for partnership projects with toxicologists, to find out what health effects could be caused by chemical emissions from electronic equipment, were not realized. As soon as words like "Office Disease" or "electrohypersensitivity" were mentioned, no authority granted research funds.

CHEMICALS A NON-ISSUE

But let's go back to 1985, when the Swedish debate on the "Monitor Disease" among office employees really began. More particularly, it was in October that year, when Björn Lagerholm, associate professor, histopathologist, and physician at the department of dermatology, Karolinska Hospital, hit the headlines in Swedish newspapers.

Lagerholm had signed a medical certificate, attesting that a female bank manager in Stockholm had gotten skin lesions during her monitor work. He explained that the skin lesions were similar to the ones usually seen in relation to UV radiation or Bucky (wavelength between X-rays and UV radiation) treatment. The bank manager, who became a pilot case for Monitor Disease, claimed occupational injury, and got her case approved at the first level.

Superior authorities, however, reacted immediately, and the decision was appealed. A ten-year-long lawsuit, which ended with a rejection in 1994, began. Nobody denied that the bank manager had skin lesions similar to the ones seen especially in relation to UV radiation. Nor was the competence of Dr. Björn Lagerholm questioned. But it was asserted that displays could not emit so much radiation that such damage could be caused.

While that pilot case had been dealt with in different jurisdictions, a large number of similar work injury reports were submitted to insurance offices around the country and had been put on ice in anticipation of a precedent-setting ruling. After the judgment, several thousand monitor users, who had submitted work injury reports, lost hope. Media interest was extinct. The debate died. But the victims were still there; their chronic symptoms stayed with them.

Björn Lagerholm had received more and more patients, from the early 1980s, with skin lesions in combinations that surprised him. When I interviewed him, he described noticing under the microscope clumped elastic fibers, or even the absence of fibers, as the lesion "Elastosis solaris," also called "Elastosis senilis," in samples taken from young people. He explained that the skin of people who have spent a lifetime at sea or at least outdoors usually looked like that. He had started by asking these patients what their work was like, and it turned out that they all had been working with monitors; he related their problems to this.

Björn Lagerholm was not the only dermatologist in the country who had had these kinds of patients from the early 1980s, but he was unique in that he took skin biopsies, which were later microscopically analyzed. Dermatologists around the country contented themselves with what they could see with their naked eyes, patients with swollen and flushed faces, expanded blood vessels and vesicles in their faces. Usually they were diagnosed with rosacea and were prescribed cortisone ointment.

Björn Lagerholm, though, did not think much of the rosacea diagnoses, instead he wanted to call the symptoms "rosacea-like," since there are different kinds of rosacea, but none exactly corresponding to what he found under the microscope. His perhaps most important discovery was that most patients in this group had unusually high levels of mast cells in their skin, which in turn might have explained the patients' symptoms. The question was: Why did they get these mast cells?

In the fall of 1987, another associate professor, Olle Johansson at the Karolinska Institute, became interested in the debate about the Monitor Disease. He was listening to a radio program in which a woman, active in the trade union, called for research assistance for various types of analyses concerning injured monitor users. Olle Johansson called the union woman to explain that he was willing to help with microscope analyses. He was interested in peptides in particular, kinds of messengers in nerve fibers.

An interview with Johansson was published in the TCO Paper 1988. There, he said, he had done a pilot study, which was so interesting that he wanted to continue doing a major survey, studying skin from these patients; such research would, he suggested, cost at least a million Swedish crowns. During the following years, Johansson made studies that, in his own opinion, verified what Björn Lagerholm had seen. His findings made headlines but were never completed due to various conflicts. The biopsies that he was studying, together with dermatologists, during a few years in the early 1990s, were thrown away during a relocation at the Karolinska Institute in the 2000s. Olle Johansson stated, when I inquired, that the biopsies were too old to be relevant as an object of study anymore. Consequently, there are no concrete documents left regarding biopsies from his observations, but there are some articles in various journals. Björn Lagerholm has been dead for many years. No other researchers or skin doctors have done studies under the microscope of these patients today calling themselves electrohypersensitive, because they became sensitive to all types of electrical devices and often also to normal light.

BROMINATED FLAME RETARDANTS

The woman who became a pilot case for Screen Dermatitis had provided the court with all the contemporary information available on chemicals inside electronics, but the courts were not interested. In 1996, the news arrived that Professor Åke Bergman at Stockholm University was able to measure brominated flame retardants in human blood for the first time. However, the woman's preceding ruling was already a fact at that time. It would be impossible to bring up similar cases or to point out that the same kind of chemicals existed in computer equipment available at this time.

The chemicals Åke Bergman found in human blood were polybrominated diphenyl ethers (PBDEs), abundantly existing in all electronics. Now, the news spread that these chemicals were endocrine disruptors and might have significant health effects. Many of those who had become sick from their computer work contacted Åke Bergman, but this did not lead to any real studies of the chemical concentrations in the blood of the victims. Single measurements, however, showed that there could possibly be high levels of various chemicals in their blood. The patient group had already in 1987 formed an association to pursue their interests.

The ruling from 1994—concerning the pilot case—overshadowed the whole issue. It was a precedent-setting ruling, in a case that was classified by the authorities as very important to calm down. A few thousand work injury reports, similar to the pilot case, were put on ice, to become completely forgotten over time.

As a journalist, I noticed that no news about chemicals had any impact on the debate. A common reaction was: "Why chemicals? It has been all about radiation." The word radiation had been in the air ever since Sweden had been reached by the international debate about the risks for miscarriages among pregnant women working in front of monitors. Earlier, the TCO ombudsman, Per-Erik Boivie, had started a cooperation that would lead to TCO's monitor labeling, the internationally renowned TCO Label, which would adorn millions of screens all over the world in the 1990s.

Realizing that the authorities did not want to tackle the issue, Per-Erik Boivie got the idea that the unions could have an influence on manufacturers and suppliers to develop harmless products. So, a very unusual trade union campaign was initiated. In the beginning, the campaign was only about decreasing the monitors' electromagnetic fields, but during the 1990s, the parameters were expanded to apply to chemicals, primarily brominated flame retardants inside the plastic covers of the screens and inside the appliances. The suggestions of requirements for chemical limits came primarily from the Swedish Society for Nature Conservation, but also from Per-Erik Boivie.

An important contributing factor was that the number of people with electrohypersensitivity (EHS) was increasing during the 1980s and the 1990s. The victims said that they no longer tolerated either fluorescent lamps or other electrical devices. They coined the "Electrohypersensitivity" expression, which contributed to the skepticism from the medical profession.

THE "SVENSKA FLÄKT SYNDROME" IN SWEDEN

Many researchers and technicians thought that this was some kind of mass psychosis induced by media, maybe particularly by the trade union press. I must admit that I myself, as a journalist, many times stood helpless before the implausible reality I witnessed, interviewing victims, experts, and scientists. The patients were trustworthy in describing their symptoms, while the experts figuratively tore their hair out to find explanations. So did the journalists for many years, until most of them lost interest when no definite news or explanations were presented.

Quite early, in an interview I did with the dermatologist Professor Berndt Stenberg at the Norrland University Hospital in Umeå, Sweden, he mentioned that he had seen a cluster of symptoms similar to the one he was to see in patients exposed to monitors. He did not claim that the phenomenon was the same, but his story evoked associations.

He told me about 76 out of 127 workers on the shop floor in a factory outside Umeå, Svenska Fläkt, who, beginning in 1979, reported initial skin and eye troubles, disorders that later proved to be chronic for many of them. The skin disorders were described as a tingling, burning, and tightness feeling in the face, and there were also rashes and edema. Eventually, light sensitivity occurred. The victims could not stand artificial light from unshielded fluorescent light or halogen lamps, not even from bulbs. Some people became so seriously light sensitive that they could not stand common daylight. They also started to react to smells and fragrances, and their symptoms were accelerating with temperature changes like heat, cold, or wind. When I did an interview with some of the victims from the factory in the late 1990s, it was obvious that they still had difficulties watching television or staying in a room with fluorescent light.

My first reaction when I heard of this was that, except for minor variations, these symptoms were similar to those described in relation to Monitor Disease. Regarding the factory workers, there was an explanation to be found, reported in the *Lancet* in 1983.[2] In spaces adjacent to the shop floor, there had been painting going on, painting with a color powder containing epoxy and polyester. The heat had caused photoactive substances to spread through the ventilation systems. When the powder paint passed through the hot surfaces of an air heater on its way back, the binders in the paint had disintegrated. Air samples were collected and seven workers with light sensitivity and one control subject were tested. Tests showed that the sick persons reacted to some of the disintegration products, those that reacted with light. The strongest reactions from the subjects came from the products created by the highest heat, when all the machines were running and the light was on.

There were suspicions that phototoxic effects were involved, a reaction between some substance and light, and the suspicions were strengthened in conjunction with a follow-up of the victims ten years later.[3] What happened in this factory was nothing unique. At the same time, clusters of similar symptoms were present at the SAAB factory in Linköping, Sweden, and single cases were reported now and then.

While the epidemic in the factory outside Umeå broke out, the American researchers H. Allen and K. Kaidbey reported an outbreak of light sensitivity among eight plumbers, who had been exposed to steam from heated epoxy.[4] They had symptoms on the body parts that had been exposed to the steam and there they experienced reddening of the skin, edema, and so-called papules, inflammatory acne. Four men responded positively to a patch test for epoxy resin. All of the plumbers responded positively to 4,4 isopropylidenediphenol, an ingredient in bisphenol A, which in turn is part of the epoxy.

Two months after the plumbers' acute exposure to heated epoxy, all eight men suffered from a tingling and burning skin rash about ten to fifteen minutes after exposure to either direct sunlight or light filtered through the windows. Two men had similar symptoms when sitting next to a fluorescent table lamp. The symptoms persisted for all eight men, at least as long as they were followed by the researchers. One year after the exposure, they were still forced to stay indoors in the daytime.

The researchers Allen and Kaidbey first suspected contact allergy, but they also put forward a hypothesis that there was an interaction with light. They referred to the American dermatologist Albert Kligman, who had written that when the skin was exposed to molecules of certain substances, they could stay in the skin and interact with light. Professor Albert Kligman, professor of dermatology at the University of Pennsylvania, should know about the effect of chemicals, after his infamous experiments at the Holmesburg Prison, where he exposed the prisoners, most of them black, to dioxins, among other things.[5]

If the temperature inside a monitor could reach 120 degrees Celsius, and we know that most circuit boards and other components at this time contained epoxy, was it not possible that something similar to the incident on the factory shop floor had happened to the monitor users? The monitors' printed circuit boards were often based on epoxy. Moreover, how many other chemicals react with light? When I heard about both Swedish and foreign cases of phototoxic reactions, I remembered that Björn Lagerholm at some point mentioned so-called PUVA treatment for psoriatic patients. This treatment is based on the same principle: a so-called psoralen is combined with UV light. Lagerholm stated that the time of the exposure was a critical moment, since the treatment was connected with significantly increased risk for cancer.

CHEMICAL STRESS

Today, probably all of the old cathode ray tubes have been disposed of. But modern laptops and other electronic equipment contain chemicals that also get hot. And recently, some dermatologists at the Stockholm Karolinska Hospital alerted about laptops causing heat symptoms when held against the skin. According to the doctors, the skin temperature could reach 43 to 47 degrees Celsius, and young people in particular are fond of placing their laptops on their laps. That is not enough to cause heat damage, but can cause vasodilation and inflammation. This disease was known hundreds of years ago as "ab igne," which means "from fire." Abroad, it already has the name "laptop dermatitis." But nobody mentions the chemical emissions that are probably triggered from heat, even in these new appliances.

The early victims of Monitor Disease were not tested, except for a few people, to find out what chemicals were in their bodies. Not until 2008 was the first and only study of chemical concentrations in the blood from such patients presented. The study included people claiming to suffer from symptoms similar to electrohypersensitivity, in most cases appearing after work in front of a monitor. The study was published in the journal *Electromagnetic Biology and Medicine* and was conducted by a research group at the Örebro University in Sweden, led by Professor Lennart Hardell.[6] It covered thirteen subjects with claimed electrohypersensitivity and twenty-one control subjects without these symptoms. Since there is no existing clinical diagnosis for electrohypersensitivity, the subjects had to answer a number of questions, such as types of symptoms and when they first appeared. Their disease onset was found to be between one and nineteen years back in time. Most of them had experienced their first symptoms in front of computer screens and/or fluorescent lights. The blood samples for the study were taken, on average, eleven years after the disease onset.

The subjects were tested for polychlorinated biphenyls (PCBs), DDE (a long-lived degradation product from DDT; high levels still exist in human blood and mother's milk), hexachlorobenzene, chlordanes, and brominated flame retardants of the PBDE type, which are polybrominated diphenyl ethers. The statistical calculations were adjusted for age and body mass index, factors that might affect the concentrations of the chemicals.

The concentration of environmental toxins was higher in the group of electrohypersensitive persons than in the control group. That was the case for example PCBs if the different varieties of the substance were summarized. The levels of PCB 153, a separate variety, were higher in the patient group. PCB was earlier used in carbon paper and as a flame retardant in office appliances. Furthermore, PCB has been used in various kinds of transformers, condensers, glue, and solvents. The substance has also been used as a plasticizer in making polyvinyl chloride (PVC). PCB is related to PBDE, an endocrine disruptor, which has been shown to affect the hormone thyroxine. The research group found significantly elevated levels of PBDE-47 in the patient group.

According to Lennart Hardell, there are no firm conclusions to be drawn from this study, as to if the chemicals were the trigger of the symptoms of the patients. He believes, though, that this study could form the basis for a larger and more detailed study, which among other things might demonstrate the interaction between chemicals and electromagnetic fields.

Professor Bert van Bavel, a colleague of Lennart Hardell, says that PBDEs in humans are recently starting to level off, especially in European countries that have introduced bans, but he says that BDE-47, BDE-99 and BDE-153 still can be found. He is concerned, though, that relatively unknown brominated substances are beginning to be detected, and that these substances, with similar properties, probably would replace PBDE.

There are reasons to remember that mainly younger women of childbearing age were put to work in front of the first cathode ray tubes. Those screens issued both chlorinated and brominated flame retardants, endocrine disruptors whose effects today on future generations worry scientists worldwide. The women were themselves freed from some of their chemical burden when breastfeeding their babies. But complaints of acute symptoms were often explained away as being in their own imagination.

Already in September 1998, Lennart Hardell, together with three Umeå University researchers, wrote a debate article in *Dagens Nyheter* (Swedish for *Today's News*), Sweden's largest daily newspaper. They warned of emissions of the brominated flame retardant PBDE, from appliances like computers and TVs, as these substances have chemical and toxicological similarities to environmental toxins, such as PCBs and DDT. The writers referred to a Swedish study from Uppsala University showing neurological developmental disorders in newborn mice and pointed to the fact that similar effects have been observed in American children with a high intake of PCBs via breastfeeding. At this time, every five years a doubling of PBDE in Swedish mother's milk was observed, a rate of increase that later leveled off, but not for all brominated substances.

The same year, researchers produced their own studies showing that the subjects with the highest levels of PBDEs ran a tripled risk of getting malignant lymphoma compared to the group with the lowest levels of these kinds of flame retardants in their fat tissues. This research group had earlier shown that other environmental toxins, such as dioxins and PCBs, increase the risk of malignant lymphoma. In their debate article in *Dagens Nyheter*, they wrote that the probable common denominator was that the environmental toxins weakened the immune system. These researchers were among the first Swedish researchers who demanded a ban on brominated substances. Thanks to the Danish-born researcher at Stockholm University, Sören Jensen, PCBs were already banned in Sweden since the 1970s. He was the one to discover that PCBs were already spread in the environment.

Regarding Lennart Hardell, some findings he published caused him an unprecedented persecution in the form of anonymous letters from a Swede with a good knowledge about the debate and the allocation of research funds in Sweden. The persecution was intensified when Lennart Hardell presented a research result about an association between brain tumors and microwave radiation from cell phones and cordless phones. At that time, an anonymous letter, containing slander against his research, was sent to a senior manager at the Karolinska Institute in Stockholm. This letter was spread widely underground and was also taken up by a Swedish newspaper where Lennart Hardell was accused for being a master of sending out alarms on cancer risks. In fact, these "alarms" were confirmed by other research groups over time and also contributed to classification of certain agents as human carcinogens.

SWEDEN TODAY

Reality is, therefore, different from the image of Sweden as portrayed by various activists. Regarding electrohypersensitivity, a variety of untrue claims flourish, unfortunately partly spread by Olle Johansson at the Karolinska University in Stockholm. In articles and lectures, he has made himself a spokesman for this patient group worldwide, and he tells them that their symptoms are fully recognized as a disability in Sweden, which is often interpreted as if the electrohypersensitivity is recognized as a disease diagnosis by Swedish authorities. Certain activists, such as Dafna Tachover from Israel, have stated that there are hundreds of thousands of electrohypersensitive patients in Sweden receiving state grants for their disabilities.

The truth is that the Swedish health authorities do not recognize electrohypersensitivity as a diagnosis. On the other hand, the patient organization has around three thousand members, and is part of a central association, the Disability Federation (Swedish "Handikappförbunden"), which is a non-governmental organization (NGO), representing a total of four hundred thousand people with various kinds of disabilities.

All affiliates, including the patient organization for electrohypersensitive persons, receive government funding for their activities, but some money is earmarked for the umbrella organization to bring various Swedish disability groups' actions against the parliament, the government, and the towns. The state agency that distributes money to the patient organization has accepted that the electrohypersensitive members suffer from a disability. But to go from this to spreading information about Sweden as the promised land for all suffering from this disease is irresponsible and has caused great disappointment to those victims from different parts of the world who have turned to Sweden for help.

DAMAGE "SIMILAR TO RADIATION"

Some patient descriptions will illustrate the history described above. Closest at hand is to start with the so-called pilot case, the female bank manager—let us call her B. She is no longer alive. A few years ago she died from cancer.

Before 1979, she had never had any skin problems, except for light sun sensitivity. At that time, she started to work on a word processing project in a Stockholm bank. At first, she was sitting at an IBM 80, a word processing machine without a screen, but after that she began working at a Xerox 850 and 860 with a screen. Initially, her right shoulder, the one most facing the screen, started aching. She then started to experience dizziness, dyspnea, and palpitations. In early 1983, she got something like eczema on the right side of her neck. It was twinging, burning, and then spread all over the face and to her breast and her back. She felt numbness in her right cheek and in her mouth. Eventually, she reacted to all kinds of electric appliances. After having been on sick leave for some time, she tried to return to the bank, but she could no longer stand the work environment at all.

Fortunately, B became a patient of Björn Lagerholm, who as a histopathologist took biopsies. He noted skin changes that were not normal for her age—she was forty-eight at that time—and not normal considering her caution in exposing herself to the sun. He wrote a medical certificate for B, and she—together with the bank—made an occupational injury notification, which was upheld by the Stockholm Social Insurance Agency but was later appealed against by a nationwide authority, at that time called the Swedish National Social Insurance Board.

To keep her sickness benefit, the Social Insurance Agency required her to undergo a psychiatric examination. She saw that as an insulting proposal and desired to hire the best existing expertise. Therefore, she consulted a professor of forensic psychiatry and an associate professor of forensic psychology. The professor wrote that she was "a mentally stable and robust woman with a nuanced picture of her problems and their origins." The associate professor of forensic psychology had her undergo extensive testing, and then wrote an appreciative certificate on her abilities to analyze and find solutions to her problems. The latter really came to be confirmed during the following ten years when her occupational injury case was taken through different legal authorities. Even though two lawyers from TCO brought her action, she herself mobilized the latest research and compilations of knowledge on electromagnetic radiation and chemicals.

The judgment of the court (the National Superior Social Insurance Court, at that time), in the fall of 1994, contained a wide range of opinions from prominent Swedish experts, invoked by B herself but also by the National Social Insurance Board (Swedish RFV). Professor Kerstin Hall, at the Karolinska Hospital Endocrine Clinic in Stockholm, was one of the experts. She wrote a certificate in March 1992 where she mentioned that she had repeatedly observed, since 1985, that her patient B got erythema over her face after the lighting of a fluorescent light in the examination room. She continued:

> The redness on her face, throat and breast looked similar to the erythema as can be seen in the release of neurotransmitters from tumors emanating from the gastrointestinal tract. These neurotransmitters from tumors of polypeptide nature are usually found in the gastrointestinal tract, but also in the brain and in the skin. Several of these were originally detected in frog skin, where they play a crucial role in the frog's adaptation to the environment. When methods for determining neurotransmitters were developed, blood samples were taken. At the first time of testing, B had an increased plasma level of neuropeptide-K, which, however, was not found in subsequent tests. B also had significantly increased levels of a signal peptide called pancreatic peptide (PP). During the following years she has had significantly increased blood levels—two to ten times increased fasting levels—of this substance. At the sampling on December 13, 1991, she was free from symptoms since her home had been cleaned up from electricity during the fall of 1991, and her medical values were normal. To exclude the presence of a small tumor causing the increased PP values, a CT scan was done, with normal result. The increased PP levels in her blood do not prove that this neurotransmitter causes her skin problems, but it can be used as a marker of her symptoms.
>
> Pancreatic polypeptide was used as a marker in a test on May 16, 1990, when she was subjected to a self-selected provocation in front of a television screen. Care was taken to reduce the radiation in the patient's room where she was located before the test. After the provocation she had several times increased blood levels of PP. This test was not a double blind test, since placebo test was not possible to implement. In connection with the provocation, a skin biopsy was taken before and after the outburst of erythema. These biopsies were examined with immunohistochemical technique by Associate Professor Johansson, and obvious changes were observed, as evidenced by his certificate.

Unfortunately, there are no biopsies of B's provocation tests left. They were part of a biopsy collection from electrohypersensitive persons, which was thrown away when Associate Professor Olle Johansson was forced to change rooms within the Karolinska Institute in the late 2000s, since no actual research had been going on in his laboratory since the early 1990s.

Professor Kjell Hansson Mild at the Umeå University in Northern Sweden also made a contributing certificate to this pilot case. He referred to a questionnaire study that he had carried out in 1989 through 1990. It covered about six thousand office employees in the Swedish Västerbotten County, and was followed by two reference studies, one concerning the Sick Building Syndrome and another one concerning skin diseases among monitor users. The material from the questionnaire study revealed that the risk of developing facial skin diseases was increasing with increased amount of monitor work. But technically, he found an increased risk only in connection with the picture of repetitive magnetic fields. He wrote in his certificate that factors like temperature, humidity, electrostatic body potential, and the display surface potential did not seem to contribute to the risk of developing skin diseases.

What is striking in the observations cited in the court decision is that the certificate from Björn Lagerholm about B's skin damages "similar to damage by radiation" never was questioned. On the contrary, it was emphasized by the National Social Insurance Board expert that the only explanation for her skin lesions must be either from ultraviolet radiation or X-rays. But all experts agreed on the fact that X-rays were not possible from a screen and that the level of UV radiation from screens was too insignificant to be harmful to B. The remaining suggestion was to refer to B's skin as type II, which meant a certain sensitivity to the sun, and it was pointed out that she had been working in a room with large windows, which let in plenty of sunlight.

Flame retardants in computers were mentioned generally. An expert from the Swedish Chemicals Agency, Lena Petreus, outlined the dominant substances in computers, which are polybrominated diphenyl ethers, or PBDEs, and tetrabromobisphenol A. According to Petreus, the latter might only have slight effects on the skin and eyes. But she mentioned that PBDEs have the potential of forming dibenzodioxins and dibenzofurans when heated or combusted.

According to Lena Petreus, low levels of polybrominated dibenzofurans had been measured in room air in office buildings with various numbers of computers. Also PBDE had been measured in one experiment. A citation from the court text, which refers to Petreus is as follows:

> Dust samples from the same rooms contained low ppb-levels of polybrominated dibenzofurans and high ppb-levels of polybrominated diphenyl ethers. The compounds mentioned might cause a skin disease similar to acne. The

problems regarding brominated flame retardants have been noted mainly because of their ability to form dioxins and furans when heated or combusted.

This important report by Lena Petreus did not evoke any response, since it was never followed up by the pilot case union lawyers, who should have seen one of the greatest working environment hazards in the modern office in general and should have understood that this was an essential factor that could be invoked not only in the case of B, but also in a number of other cases that were current at the time. There had been alarming reports from Germany already in the 1980s about chemicals in TVs and computers.

The highest instance at this time, National Superior Social Insurance Court, simply found that although there were studies to support the suspicion that monitors might through electric or magnetic fields or "otherwise" cause skin diseases, sufficient scientific evidence was missing to prove that monitor work can cause skin diseases. The judgment stated that B could not in the legal sense be considered to have been exposed to harmful agents.

Something that was not discussed at that time, and hardly has been taken seriously later on, is the fact that the UV radiation could have been an indirect part of the interaction between chemicals—despite the fact that there is ancient knowledge of how UV radiation together with both endogenous and exogenous substances might cause phototoxic or photo allergic reactions. All halogenated bisphenols, that is phenols based on the elements fluorine, chlorine, and bromine, but also other phenols, are considered to be able to cause light sensitivity.

I called Björn Lagerholm some years before his death to ask him if he thought that chemicals in interaction with light might have been the cause of the changes in several layers of the skin that he observed with the monitor patients. "That is an interesting question, but I am not a chemist, so I cannot give you an answer," was his comment.

THE ELECTROSENSITIVE TECHNICIANS AT ERICSSON

Per Segerbäck is one of almost seventy technicians who in the mid-1980s began to get symptoms when working at their computers at Ellemtel, an Ericsson subsidiary in Stockholm. He had been hired by the company in 1977 and he became a team leader of about fifteen engineers who were developing some of the company's most commercial products. Segerbäck was known to be a workaholic and he worked a lot of overtime. Sometimes he went on business trips to the United States and Britain to keep abreast of developments and capture the latest knowledge.

In the workrooms at Ellemtel, there were plenty of displays and Per Segerbäck had three computers. Many people have testified that the rooms smelt badly of chemicals. Often, circuit boards were soldered, and at that time the emissions were especially noticeable. Per Segerbäck did a lot of circuit board soldering in the late 1970s and in the early 1980s. He did not, at this time, use any special devices like masks during these operations. The ventilation was poor and there was no extractor over his desk.

When the problems at the Ericsson Company started to become general in the mid-1980s, the company registered forty-nine affected persons, but the number was constantly increasing. The symptoms were a burning sensation in the face and on other body parts, nausea, dizziness, and also light sensitivity. Already in 1985, Per Segerbäck noticed a gritty feeling in his eyes and began to use antistatic spray on the screen. During the years 1988 and 1989, his symptoms worsened. The end of the work week was the worst, but during the weekend the symptoms were alleviated. He used to like having all fluorescent lights on but he noticed that he could no longer tolerate them because he quickly became nauseous. Almost all of his team colleagues were affected to a greater or lesser extent.

In January 1990, Per Segerbäck experienced a dramatic deterioration. He now got symptoms from electrical appliances in general and from the electric system in his car. His light sensitivity was so severe that he got a reaction from the street lighting outside his house. At work, he did not only get symptoms from the fluorescent lights in the ceiling above him, but also from the luminaire in the floor below. Later, in an account of the crisis in Ellemtel, it was stated that the luminaires delivered ten times stronger electromagnetic radiation than the displays.

Per Segerbäck was now on sick leave, but he could not stay in his house because it was heated by electricity. Now and then he slept in his car, despite the fact that it was winter and about minus 10 degrees Celsius. As a first emergency measure from Ellemtel, he got a caravan placed in his garden. Then, Professor Yngve Hamnerius at Chalmers University of Technology was contacted to design electricity decontamination (electro-sanitation) in the Ellemtel premises and in the house of Per Segerbäck. In a book called *Hypersensitivity in Work Life*, published by the Ericsson Company in 1993, this stage was called the internal project. All costs at this stage were paid by the company. This internal project during 1990 and 1991 cost the company 4 million Swedish crowns. "It was well worth the cost," to cite the book.

> All the victims were back at work, even though at this point, not everyone could return to their regular duties. Only one employee at this time was still on sick leave, and only for 25 percent of his service.

Per Segerbäck was found to be among those who could return to work. At first, he worked in an electricity-decontaminated barracks outside the Ellemtel house, and later in a well-screened module inside the house. Aluminum plates had been used as insulation to suppress the magnetic fields. But because all types of fields in the electronic environment were to be mitigated, also two layers of one millimeter transformer plate and a five millimeter aluminum plate were used to line the walls, floors, and ceiling in the modules where the most sensitive employees were to be placed. An indoor transformer that delivered strong magnetic fields was isolated with two millimeter copper plate. It's obvious that these changes made it possible for Ellemtel to keep their technically professional staff.

Per Segerbäck was given an LCD screen with a lightbulb as backlight. He had actually been one of the constructors of this equipment, which later went into series production. All around Per Segerbäck now had colleagues in other electricity-decontaminated (electrosanitized) modules. He himself was not free from symptoms, but he could work. This is how it is described in the book:

> The thirty-seven-year-old expert on integrated circuits (ICs) is electrosensitive. But he is working, and he is an important resource in a large development project.

After this first phase, a new project was launched at the Ericsson company Ellemtel. At this time, a special Government Work Environment Fund had been set up, and the company sought a grant from this fund. They got 8,875,000 Swedish crowns and launched project number two, called the ALF project, now with money from the taxpayers. A consultant was commissioned to lead the project. This consultant soon gained referral right into the financing fund, which meant that all other companies seeking money for similar projects would be judged by the Ellemtel consultant. At this time, many Swedish companies had the same problems. The Ericsson Group now gained influence and insight into what happened in the area.

The state money was used for several research projects that did not give any interesting results. The projects were about acupuncture and stress measurement. One million Swedish crowns were used for a skin provocation examination, where subjects were exposed to electromagnetic fields but no skin biopsies were taken. Researchers who believed that stress was the main reason for the problems, and rejected all other explanations, also got their share of the state money through Ellemtel. It was pointed out from several sources that it was unsuitable for a private company to influence research grants. I called the Ericsson consultant several times to learn if there were any projects on chemicals going on, but I always got the same negative response. When the projects were finished, the consultant announced that he had not been able to find a suitable chemist in time. Thus, this state-funded project did not answer the question of whether chemicals might be activated by various types of radiation.

Many employees at Ellemtel were severely affected and their problems could not be completely solved. The destiny of Per Segerbäck became disastrous. When a base station for mobile phones was placed two hundred meters from his home, his symptoms became once again acute and he was forced to flee his home. He was occasionally living in a caravan in a protected location close to Drottningholm outside Stockholm. The spreading of wireless technology had made it more difficult for him to travel to and from his workplace but he continued working from his isolated settlement.

The new managers within the Ericsson Group did not show the same understanding of electrical hypersensitivity as the earlier managers did. It was declared within the company that all problems had been solved. Per Segerbäck disturbed the image of the company, especially since his trade union suggested that he could use a protective overall on his way to and from work to avoid microwaves. This kind of overall was also used in Germany and in the United States. It had also been used earlier in Sweden, when employees at the Ericsson Company had tested the electronics used in the JAS airplane at SAAB in Linköping. Segerbäck's employer refused to pay for the overall, which would cost 19,000 Swedish krona. It was instead paid by the Insurance Fund—that is, the Swedish taxpayers.

It was obvious that Per Segerbäck would mean bad publicity for Ericsson mobile phones. In the spring of 2000, he was dismissed after twenty-three years' employment at the Ericsson Company. His trade union stood up for him and they reported the dismissal to the Swedish Labor Court. At the trial the Ericsson lawyer spoke plainly:

> A totally unacceptable and risky situation would occur for the company in relation to the employees, customers, and other outsiders, if one of the company's employees would wear protective clothes because of the assumed health risks related to the technology field and the company's products.

The trade union relied on Swedish labor law to claim that the dismissal was illegal, but the Ericsson lawyer managed to convince the court that Per Segerbäck would not be able to do any work from the croft where he was now staying. The trade union pointed out that the Ericsson Company actually was expert on modern technology, which should make it possible for him to work from home.

Nothing helped. The Swedish Labor Court ruled that Ericsson had the right to dismiss Per Segerbäck.

VAPOR FROM PLASTIC HEATED TO 400 DEGREES CELSIUS

S is a radio and telecom technician and he was also an elite athlete when he was hired by a company that would ruin his health. At first, he was working at an offset printing press but soon he advanced to become a printer. I am now quoting from his own story:

> The printing press and the thermoplastic grouting machinery were placed in the same room as the butter packaging production. The plastics were heated to 400 degrees Celsius before thermoforming. The ovens where the plastics were heated did not have any direct extraction. In case of a machine breakdown, the plastic burnt in the ovens, and developed plastic smoke. When cleaning the pressure rollers, color mixing plate, and worktable, I used thinner, which later was substituted by ethyl acetate. Two vacuum pumps were placed less than one meter from my feet. They let out oil mist, which then stayed in the air that we were working in. I was starting to detect this by nasal congestion and breathing problems.

An ENT (Ear, Nose and Throat) clinic found adenoid formations in the nose of S, something he'd never had before. During the period 1982 through 2000, he underwent fifteen operations for adenoid formations, after several years of daily exposure to emissions from various chemicals heated to high temperatures. In his environment, among other substances, were polyvinyl chloride (PVC), polyester, polypropylene, and epoxy. PVC was strongly questioned in Sweden, but the company exported their products to Britain, a country less scrupulous on the use.

Since PVC contains chloride, high temperatures create not only chlorine-containing substances but also dioxins. It is not far-fetched to believe that the exposure to chemicals caused S's nose mucous problems. Due to all the surgery, he lost sensitivity in the left part of his upper lip. His last surgery was done to move his nasal septum, but to no avail. He was prescribed nasal spray for the rest of his life, but it made his nasal mucous membranes bleed.

Despite his difficulties, he continued working and became a quality engineer, with independent responsibility for quality and hygiene controls. In addition to his serious nose problems, S also got chronic hypersensitivity symptoms, which were similar to those described by people suffering from electrohypersensitivity.

That might have decided his destiny. Neither the company, nor the insurance fund—Occupational Medicine—nor the trade union bothered to see the big picture. As an electrosensitive person, he was easily dismissed, as this was the prevailing practice at that time. All instances washed their hands.

S worked for six years in the laboratory where he first began to feel his electrohypersensitivity close to measuring equipment called a Shadowgraph, a kind of microscope with transformer. He had two halogen lamps with transformers beside him, one of them directly under his feet, and the other one twenty centimeters in front of him at table height. He was exposed to both UVA and electromagnetic fields from the lamps. Furthermore, he was exposed to fields from the transformers and from a fan. A large substation to power the machines was located in an adjoining room.

Already in 1999, S had been complaining about heat sensation, numbness, pricking, and tingling on the back of the lower legs and under the soles of his feet. At first, he thought it was due to some ergonomically incorrect posture, but when the symptoms occurred in front of the TV or the computer, and when later he could not stay near fluorescent lighting or electrical appliances, he got seriously worried. Among the symptoms were also headache and dizziness.

When he consulted an occupational medicine clinic, they took common blood samples and suggested that S should see a psychologist. He declined. He claimed to have no psychological problems whatsoever. A trade union ombudsman came to know of S's feet problems, and said that that was strange, since the electrohypersensitive people usually have problems with their face. The union lawyer refused to take on his worker's compensation case, but S himself tried to pursue the case. The insurance fund and the legal authorities claimed that there were no harmful factors in his workplace. After this, S gave up.

This is the situation in Sweden today. The cover-up of what happened earlier has made today's technological development possible, without interference of demands for alternative solutions to avoid health risks.

The trade union no longer exerts pressure for better product control before launching new technology or new products. TCO is no longer a central organization dealing with occupational and environmental issues; these questions are left to the member unions.

But the affiliated member unions hardly have the resources that a powerful central organization with employed experts would have had.

The chronically ill people who have been affected by modern technology are, in other words, thrown out into the cold.

Chapter 12

A TALE OF TWO SCIENTISTS: DOCTOR ALICE STEWART AND SIR RICHARD DOLL[1]

Gayle Greene

Why we couldn't have been working together all those years, I don't know, since we shared a common goal, to understand the causes of cancer.

Alice Stewart

As the world watched the Fukushima reactors spew incalculable quantities of radionuclides into the sea and air and wondered what effect this would have on our health and that of generations to come, the warnings of Dr. Alice Stewart about low-dose radiation risk assumed a terrible timeliness. As industry, governments, and the media attempted to quiet the alarms, assuring us that radioactive releases will dilute and disperse and become too miniscule to matter, the reassurances of Sir Richard Doll, foremost among Stewart's detractors, also became relevant. It is clear, as proponents and opponents of nuclear energy thrash it out, that there is not much more scientific consensus about the hazards of low-dose radiation exposure today than there was half a century ago, when these pioneer radiation epidemiologists locked into opposition. Their arguments are reiterated as mainstream radiation scientists invoke the Hiroshima studies to assuage fears about Fukushima, while critics cite Chernobyl as a warning.

Stewart's career trajectory reads like a cautionary tale to anyone considering challenging received opinion in such a high-stakes, highly politicized area as radiation science. Though she began with honors that came to few women of her time, the first woman under forty and the ninth ever to be elected to the Royal College of Physicians (in 1946), once she discovered that fetal X-rays double the risk of a childhood cancer, she never again received major funding in the United Kingdom. Her findings—published in the *Lancet*[2] and expanded in the *British Medical Journal*[3]—were not welcomed: the arms race was ratcheting up, the governments of the United States and United Kingdom were promoting "the friendly atom," and nobody wanted to hear that "a tiny fraction" of a radiation dose "known" to be safe could kill a child. Studies of the Hiroshima and Nagasaki survivors, the basis of radiation safety standards throughout the world, assured that risk diminished as dose decreased until it disappeared altogether. Stewart was suggesting there was no threshold beneath which radiation ceased to be dangerous.

First to launch a study to discredit her was Dr. Richard Doll, and later, Sir Richard. They moved in the same circles, sat on the same committees and editorial boards; their lives were so intertwined that Stewart taught medicine to the woman Doll later married. Stewart was born in 1906, received her medical degree from Cambridge in 1936, and worked more than twenty years at Oxford; Doll, born in 1912, received his degree from St. Thomas Hospital Medical School in 1937 and was appointed Regius Professor at Oxford in 1969. They both started out with left-wing ideals and an interest in the environmental causes and prevention of disease, both taking part in the Socialist Medical Association that campaigned for the National Health Service after the war, he moving further left than she, joining the Communist Party. But for his demonstration of the link between lung cancer and smoking in the 1950s, he was made Regius Professor, knighted, and had a building named after him that became home to Oxford's Cancer Research UK Epidemiology Unit and the Clinical Trial Service Unit, both of which he helped found. He spent the latter part of his career at Oxford's prestigious Imperial Cancer Research Center, becoming, in his own words, ever "more of the establishment"—"about as establishment as the Bank of England," a colleague quipped[4]—while Stewart became more oppositional. Drawn into international controversy by her 1970s studies of the Hanford nuclear workers— which found a greater risk to low-dose radiation than was being claimed—she testified on behalf of workers, veterans, and down winders, while Doll testified against them.

Stewart died in relative obscurity, in 2002, with only a handful of radiation scientists appreciating the importance of her contributions, while Doll went out, three years later, on a cloud of hyperbole, hailed as "the world's most distinguished medical epidemiologist," as "the greatest epidemiologist of our time."[5, 6] But a year after his death, a front-page *Guardian* headline rocked the world of radiation science: "World-famous British scientist failed to disclose that he held a paid consultancy with a chemical company for more than twenty years while investigating cancer risks in the industry."[7] A letter from a Monsanto epidemiologist was found among Doll's papers at the Wellcome Institute, renewing his contract as consultant, at the rate of £1,000 a day (in 1986, when this letter was dated, that would have earned him in a week what a worker made in a year); only the year before, he had taken part in a review of Monsanto's Agent Orange that cleared dioxin as "only weakly and inconsistently carcinogenic."[8] Evidence was also found that he received £15,000 from the Chemical Manufacturers Association and Imperial Chemical Industries, the largest producer of vinyl chloride, even as he was exonerating vinyl chloride.

These disclosures inspired a flood of detractions and defenses. But Doll's reputation has survived unscathed, to be enshrined in Conrad Keating's *Smoking Kills: The Revolutionary Life of Richard Doll*.[9] The "Authorized Biography," commissioned by the prestigious Wellcome Institute, depicts Doll as "the quintessence of the scientific ideal," "the ultimate in dedication, perseverance, and integrity,[10]" and portrays Stewart as a confused, "embittered" woman whose scientific work was tainted by political sympathies. This is the reputation she had in mainstream radiation circles, the reputation Doll did his best to perpetuate when he wrote her entry in the *Oxford Dictionary of National Biography* after she died, describing her as having damaged her "reputation as a serious scientist."

Stewart would not have been surprised by his disapproval—he made no secret of it—though it did mystify her: "Why we couldn't have been working together all those years, I don't know, since we shared a common goal, to understand the causes of cancer," she said to me. I didn't know either, and the long interview I had with Doll at Oxford in 1998 gave me no deeper insight into their vexed relationship. I could only conclude this part of my biography, *The Woman Who Knew Too Much: Alice Stewart and the Secrets of Radiation*,[11] with a series of questions: was it a difference of opinion about radiation risk that motivated his antipathy, or personal dislike, or sexism, or rivalry?

But information has come to light since their deaths that makes me see their relationship in a new light. More than a conflict between two striking figures who took contrary courses in their lives and work, which is how I read it in 1999, I now see a story about the making and breaking of reputations and the power of reputation to shape scientific "knowledge." Doll was a man with "the instincts of a politician," as his biographer writes. With his backward sweep of white hair, his highbrow, patrician profile, and "notoriously elegant dress,"[12] he could have been sent by Central Casting to play the role of Distinguished Scientist, and he played the part brilliantly, using his status, position, and the podiums afforded him to project an image that had considerable influence on scientific opinion and public policy. From early in his career, he had a knack for producing radiation risk estimates pleasing to the powerful.

When Prime Minister Anthony Eden sought a go-ahead for nuclear testing, Doll produced a report that concluded, "The present and foreseeable hazards from external radiation due to fall-out from the test explosions of nuclear weapons . . . are negligible"—thereby giving the okay to the H-bomb trials that took place in the Pacific in 1957 and 1958.[13] His complacency was not shared by the more than nine thousand scientists who signed Linus Pauling's petition warning that weapons testing would produce millions of cancers and birth defects, a petition that helped bring about the 1963 moratorium on aboveground testing. But Doll's reassurances about low-dose radiation have helped create the climate of complacency about radiation risk that has enabled the nuclear industry to win public endorsement and move forward, resurrecting itself from its ruins at the end of the last century, when it crumbled under its costs, inefficiencies, and catastrophes.

In 1943, Stewart was invited by Oxford Regius Professor John Ryle to help build a department of Social Medicine, a new area that focused on the social and environmental causes and prevention of disease. When Ryle died in 1950, Social Medicine was demoted from a department to a "unit," leaving Stewart a lowly reader with tenure but no staff or funding. Having won a grant of £1,000, she set out to investigate rising rates of childhood leukemia. She devised a questionnaire for mothers who had lost children to cancer and mothers who had not (which gave her a control group), a questionnaire that cast a wide net, asking about exposure to automobiles, aerosols, hens, rabbits, dogs, colored sweets, fish, and chips—and, "had you had an obstetric X-ray?" It was a revolutionary idea, "asking the mums," but Stewart, a mother herself, thought they might remember something the doctors did not. She included the question about X-rays because it was common practice in the 1940s and 1950s for doctors to X-ray pregnant women in the third trimester, to ascertain the position of the fetus. Within the first thirty-five questionnaires, the answer leapt out: the children whose mothers had been X-rayed were running three to one with cancer—not just leukemia, but all kinds of cancers.

Doll countered with a study, coauthored by William Court-Brown, that found no association of fetal X-rays with leukemia.[14] His findings were consistent with the Hiroshima studies, which found no excess of cancer in children exposed in utero to the blasts. Doll later admitted that his study was "not very good"[15, 16]; it lacked a control group, looking only at children who'd been X-rayed; it looked only at leukemia rather than all childhood cancers and it did not follow subjects long enough for the effects of the radiation to become apparent. "But it didn't matter, the damage had been done," as Stewart said; "After the Court-Brown Doll study, we never got support from Britain again. If funding hadn't come through from America, we'd have been finished."

The Court-Brown-Doll study enabled doctors to go on X-raying pregnant women for the next two decades. Stewart spent those decades testing and retesting her hypothesis and expanding her database, until it included information about prenatal exposures to infections and inoculations, parental age, occupation, social class, smoking, and, later, ultrasound. With the instinct for inclusiveness that was a signature of her science, she developed a monumental set of data, the Oxford Survey of Childhood Cancer, the world's largest and longest-running study of childhood cancer, producing evidence so compelling that, in the 1970s, official bodies recommended against fetal X-rays.

She next found herself on a collision course with Doll when he came to Oxford as Regius Professor in 1969. He announced, in an interview with Georgina Ferry, that "there was little [at Oxford] in the way of epidemiology research," which enabled him "to bring several people with [him]," including his protégé and subsequent collaborator, Richard Peto.[17] He set about building his department, conferring research budgets, distributing chairs, and "scouring the academic field all around the world" for talent.[18] Julian Peto, Richard Peto's brother and, like him, a statistician who worked with Doll, commented: "It was odd that [Stewart] wasn't given a chair really because she was quite eminent and was a real founding father of the science. But . . . Richard created a new chair—social and preventive medicine and gave it to Martin Vessey—and that was a bit peculiar . . . it just seemed so natural that she should have it. . . .Martin . . . didn't have an outstanding reputation, and for him to be given that chair at thirty-seven years old, over her, was the most extraordinary affront, and it really was a bit of power politics."[19]

Stewart, in her sixties, was easily brushed aside. She had been immersed in her research, scrambling around for funding, and she had raised two children (on her own); after her son's death, she had helped care for his children—which left her little time to do the kind of networking that creates allies. Made unwelcome at Oxford, she accepted a position at Birmingham. But then came the question, what to do with the Oxford Survey, which by this time consisted of twenty-three thousand manila envelopes. "Since my office in Birmingham was a trailer, a sort of hut, and the records were prodigious, it became a real problem." She offered to leave the files at Oxford, feeling that the survey ought to continue: "We were building a database that would have allowed us to test several hypotheses about cancer. It ought to have been put on an on-going basis. That's what you have to do if you're going to find the cause for cancer." But Doll had no use for the files— even though he would, several years later, launch his own study of childhood cancer, with great fanfare and £6 million funding (some from the nuclear industry), announced in 1992 by the UK Co-coordinating Committee on Cancer Research,[20] as a "new" and "unique nationwide investigation into the causes of cancer in children," "the largest and most wide-ranging study" of its kind "to be carried out anywhere in the world."

"It's as though we'd never existed," Stewart said, "though it was hard to see the difference between his study and ours. . . . It's hard to describe, like a current I was swimming against. When the Medical Research Council put together a committee on epidemiology, Doll was made chairman, which gave him enormous influence. [He directed the MRC's Statistical Research Unit from 1961 to 1969.] After that, every department in the country was called in to consult— except us. We never got invited to official meetings, never got asked to give our point of view." She was thus excluded from the processes, decisions, reviews, commentaries that shaped medical research in the United Kingdom, all the while she was developing an international reputation as an authority on radiation risk and receiving invitations to speak and consult from researchers throughout the world.

Omissions are difficult to document, but here's one that leaps out. Doll, reminiscing (in "conversation" with Sarah Darby in 2003[21]) about the early days of epidemiology, describes how he and several young men (all men) gathered around "those few senior people such as Professor Ryle at Oxford who were interested in developing the subject." He makes no mention of Stewart, though she was one of those young scientists: in fact, she is the one Ryle chose, when he was made Regius Professor at Oxford in 1945, to help launch his program in Social Medicine—which set her on the path to epidemiology. Doll simply writes her out of the story.

In 1974, Stewart, having found a trailer in Birmingham where she could store the Oxford Survey, was in the process of packing up to leave Oxford, when she got a phone call from Thomas Mancuso, a professor at the School of Public Health at the University of Pittsburgh. Mancuso, an epidemiologist expert in industrial medicine, had been commissioned by the Atomic Energy Commission (AEC) to do a study of the health of nuclear workers at Hanford, the vast weapons complex in Eastern Washington that had produced plutonium for the Trinity and Nagasaki bombs. Since workers' exposure to radiation was well within the limit "known" to be safe, as determined by the Hiroshima studies, it was assumed that such an investigation would turn up nothing incriminating.

Mancuso had been looking at workers' health records for several years and had found no evidence of increased cancer. The AEC was urging him to publish, but he wanted another opinion, so he called in Stewart. She and her statistician George Kneale took the long trek to the United States. After several days studying the data, she declared, "I believe this industry is a good deal more dangerous than you are being told." The government terminated the study, going so far as to break in to Mancuso's office, attempting to seize his work. Stewart absconded with what data she had, taking them back to England, and continued to study them, with Kneale and Mancuso, for the rest of her life—consistently finding a ten to twenty times higher cancer risk than was being claimed.[22] These findings were dismissed, as the fetal X-ray findings had been, on the grounds that "exposures were too low" to produce a cancer effect— "too low" as determined by the Hiroshima findings.[23]

The Mancuso scandal inspired the efforts of antinuclear activists to pry radiation data loose from government control and open it to the scrutiny of independent scientists. In the last years of the 1980s, amid breaking scandals throughout the nuclear weapons complex and the growing furor of citizens' groups, Stewart was much in demand as a speaker and expert witness. Though in her eighties, she was often the only respected scientist to respond to activists' calls. She made dozens of appearances: on a given trip to the States she would lecture at Yale, the University of Chicago, and in Fork River, Idaho, to a group of activists. "Audiences loved her," recalls Diane Quigley. "Her humor . . . her folksy expressions and tales, her obvious compassion, were irresistible. . . . She was equally at ease with all types of people, never talked down to them; her presentations were complex and ambitious, assuming her listeners' intelligence."[24]

Finally, after two congressional hearings and several Freedom of Information Act requests, activists succeeded in getting the Department of Energy to open the nuclear worker health records to independent scrutiny. In 1992, Stewart and Kneale took possession of approximately one-third of the health records of workers employed by the US nuclear industry since it began in 1942, records not only from Hanford but from Los Alamos, Oak Ridge, Rocky Flats, Savannah River, and other nuclear facilities. It was a landmark victory, hailed by Keith Schneider on the front page of the New York Times as a blow for scientific freedom.[25, 26]

"It helps, in this area, to be long-lived," as she commented.

She lived to see another victory announced in a front-page New York Times headline, nearly a decade later: "US Acknowledges Radiation Killed Weapons Workers, Ends Decades of Denials: Compensation Is Possible for Survivors of Cancer Victims Who Worked on Bombs."[27] This happened a few weeks after my biography went to press, too late to include it. It was clear that her story was not over.

The Oxford Survey brought Stewart into conflict with the medical profession, but the Hanford studies brought her up against more formidable authorities: the nuclear industry, the governments supporting the industry, the international regulatory commissions that set standards for radiation risk—and, ultimately, the Hiroshima studies on which these standards are based. Turning her attention to these studies, she was amazed at what she found.

The Atomic Bomb Casualty Commission, as it was originally called, began its studies of the Hiroshima and Nagasaki survivors in 1950, five years after the blasts. (The name was changed to "Radiation Effects Research Foundation" in 1975 to get the "atomic bomb" out, around the same time the "Atomic Energy Commission" was changed to the "Department of Energy.") According to its calculations, the death rate from all causes except cancer had returned to "normal" by 1950, and the cancer deaths were too few to cause alarm: all those expected to die from radiation effects had already died, and no further radiation-related effects were expected.

Stewart's experience as a physician and researcher told her it would not be possible for a population to return to "normal" a mere five years after so devastating a holocaust. This was not a normal or representative population that could yield reliable information about the health effects of radiation exposure: it was a survivor population made up of the heartiest. The Oxford Survey had found that children incubating cancer became three hundred times more infection sensitive than normal children.[28] Children so immune-compromised would not have survived the harsh winters that followed the bombings, when food and water were contaminated, medical services at a halt, antibiotics scarce; but these deaths would not have been recorded as cancer deaths. The survivors' studies were also problematic on account of the guesswork that went into estimating radiation exposure; the radiation the bombs gave off was calculated according to tests done in the Nevada desert and was recalculated several times in subsequent decades. Most importantly, the extreme, high-dose radiation this population was exposed to could tell you nothing about the effects of chronic, low-dose radiation over time, the kind of exposure received by nuclear workers and people living in the vicinity of reactors or accidents.

"Radiation risk estimates based on A-bomb survivors would be substantially underestimating the cancer risk from protracted low-level exposure to radiation," Stewart maintained, and criticized the "outdated emphasis on evidence about radiation health effects based on studies of A-bomb survivors," which have been "used as a lens through which studies of radiation-exposed . . .

populations are viewed."[29] The data were "skewed," and calculations based on them were no better than "Bible arithmetic."

But there were powerful incentives to downplay radiation risk. The first Western scientists and doctors allowed into the devastated cities, in late 1945, were with the US Armed Forces, under military escort. The Japanese scientists and physicians who had been on the scene told horrific stories of people who had seemed unharmed but then began bleeding from ears, nose, and throat, hair falling out by the handful, bluish spots appearing on the skin, muscles contracting, leaving limbs and hands deformed, many dying from some unidentified "atomic plague"—but their accounts were ignored or suppressed. When Tokyo Radio announced that people who entered the cities after the bombings were also dying of mysterious causes, American officials dismissed the allegations as propaganda intended to imply that the United States had used an "inhumane" weapon. As State Department attorney William H. Taft asserted, the "mistaken impression" that low-level radiation is hazardous has the "potential to be seriously damaging to every aspect of the Department of Defense's nuclear weapons and nuclear propulsion programs. . . . it could impact the civilian nuclear industry . . . and it could raise questions regarding the use of radioactive substances in medical diagnosis and treatment."[30] A pamphlet issued by the Atomic Energy Commission in 1953 insisted that low-level exposure to radiation "can be continued indefinitely without any detectable bodily change."[31] The Atomic Energy Commission was paying the salaries of the Atomic Bomb Casualty Commission (ABCC) scientists and "monitoring" them "closely—some felt too closely."[32]

Doll was among the first "non-military foreign scientists" invited to Hiroshima, in 1957, to evaluate the Atomic Bomb Commission's work.[33] He told me he had been "satisfied with the Commission's procedures and conclusions"—which I had no reason (then) to doubt.

When Doll was knighted in 1971, two years after he came to Oxford, some of his left-wing friends found it an oddly incongruous honor for "Red Richard."[34] "To suddenly become Sir Richard Doll, the most powerful person in medical academia, was an extraordinary change," comments Julian Peto: "He had real power and he used it, and Alice Stewart was an early victim."[35] He had welcomed the Regius Professorship, since he "questioned whether he would ever conduct original research again," and became absorbed in university administration.

He cut a fine figure, sporting around Oxford in an open MGB Roadster, wearing elegant suits, the details of which were overseen by his wife, who played the Oxford grand dame in their splendid Victorian house. "We have a communist who lives in great luxury . . . who's got original paintings of the sort that most communists would feel were the things that only the rich should have," was a view expressed by critics.[36] Whatever the processes that transformed "Red Richard" to Sir Richard, he emerged in 1981, with the highly influential monograph *The Causes of Cancer*,[37] as a powerful spokesman for industry.

In 1978, Joseph Califano, Secretary of Health, Education, and Welfare under President Jimmy Carter, published an "Estimate Report" that gave a figure for workplace cancer of around 20 percent, unsettlingly high. Richard Peto was invited by the US Office of Technology Assessment to provide a more "judicious" assessment. The report he and Doll produced, *The Causes of Cancer*,[38] attributed the majority of cancers to individual lifestyle choices, claiming that roughly 65 percent of US cancer deaths were caused by diet and smoking, with only 4 percent of cancers due to occupational influences and a mere 2 percent to industrial pollution.

There were reputable scientists—Richard Clapp,[39] Irving Selikoff,[40] Devra Lee Davis,[41] Samuel Epstein[42]—who took issue with these figures, pointing out that Doll and Peto had excluded African Americans and people over sixty-five. (African Americans suffer high rates of cancer and are the most likely to be exposed to toxins, since they have the highest-risk jobs and live in the poorest neighborhoods.) But the claims were welcomed by those who maintained that "cleaning up the environment" is not going to make much difference in cancer rates.[43] The report was embraced by the Office of Technology Assessment and the National Cancer Institute, and praised by the *New York Times* for bringing about "a less alarming view of the danger from carcinogenic pollutants."[44] It enabled the Reagan Administration, come to power in 1981, to weaken the Environmental Protection Agency, dismantle environmental, health, safety, and occupational legislation, and reduce by about 70 percent the number of cases against polluters referred to the justice department.[45] It allowed Margaret Thatcher to move forward with an aggressive expansion of the nuclear industry. Doll was called as expert witness in dozens of court cases and official inquiries on UK facilities; he testified against plaintiffs suing British Nuclear Fuels Limited (in the Sellafield cancer case, as the media called it), against workers and veterans. He saved governments and industry untold millions in compensation and regulatory efforts.

"One of the biggest myths in recent years is that there is a cancer epidemic caused by exposure to radiation, pollution, pesticides, and food additives. These factors have very little to do with the majority of cancers," Doll announced.[46] In a puzzling reversal, the researcher who had declared in 1967 that "an 'immense' number of substances were known to cause cancer . . . besides cigarette smoking, exposure to nickel, asbestos, tarry products in gas production, and radioactivity, were major causes of cancer," now virtually dismissed environmental pollution as a cause of cancer and lashed out at those who saw such a link as "irrational" and unscientific.[47] He warned, in the Harveian Oration, that "environmentalists" might "whip up irrational prejudice, unfound in science."[48] He cautioned, in a letter to the *Daily Mail*, that environmentalists represented "an irrational ideology opposed to science, to industry, and to progress."[49] He urged the public "to trust industry and industrialists, science and scientists"—these are "the people with the key to the future"—and ignore warnings by the powerful "anti-science Mafia."[50]

Doll began to display what an observer described as a "penchant for splenetic and patronizing attacks on those who published findings running counter to his assertions."[51] When asked why he had not considered an assessment of vinyl chloride by the International Agency for Research on Cancer in Lyon, which had found a link between vinyl chloride and brain cancer—as well as lung cancer, leukemia, and lymphoma—he called the investigators "incompetent."[52] Of the Swedish cancer researcher Lennart Hardell,[53] who had testified against dioxin in the 1985 court case, Doll wrote an unsolicited letter to the judge, claiming that "many of his published statements were exaggerated or not supportable . . . [and] should no longer be cited as scientific evidence."[54] Hardell termed Doll's science *epidemonology*.[55] Of the work of Devra Lee Davis, a leading analyst of environmental toxins and cancer, he used the terms "uninteresting," "uninformative," "boring," "old junk."[56] It is difficult to square this with the claim made by his biographer, in a 2009 podcast, that he was "always supporting of other scientists."

Most of Doll's criticisms of Alice Stewart were behind the scenes or after her death, but in 1996, he lit out at her in a Channel 4 British television documentary, "Sex and the Scientist,"[57] dismissing her methods as "a bit slapdash." "She was very enthusiastic. She got a great deal of cooperation throughout the country, but she tended to accept results at their face value without detailed checking to test their accuracy." *Slapdash* is an odd term for a researcher who took twenty years corroborating the fetal X-ray findings and the rest of her life studying the Hanford data, and who published more than four hundred studies in refereed journals—no mean feat, given the unpopularity of her findings.

But Doll, to a nationwide television audience, described the Hanford work as "barmy . . . yes, it just wasn't a scientific analysis" (though it was a crucial part of the case that persuaded the US government to grant nuclear workers compensation for cancer). When asked, in this documentary, how he perceived Stewart, Doll said, "Well, I don't really perceive her frankly. I mean I think that's . . . except when it's . . . except when I have to." And yet he did "perceive her" long enough to write that damning epitaph in the *Oxford Dictionary of National Biography*, to fix her reputation for all time.

Doll's version of Alice Stewart is the version his biographer gives us. Keating[58] portrays Stewart as embittered by her failure to achieve status and recognition, "antagonistic," "adversarial," "abrasive," "rude," "caustic," "paranoid," and without humor. This is the reputation barrister Stephen Sedley was familiar with when he decided not to call her to testify in a case against British Nuclear Fuels, owner of the Sellafield nuclear facility, "because of the way in which the establishment had branded her an eccentric . . . slightly nutty, loose cannon—because she wouldn't accept the conventional wisdom, *and now I gather she has turned out to be more right than wrong*" (emphasis added).[59] This is the reputation Klarissa Nienhuys, a scientist from the Netherlands, encountered at a seminar at Groningen University, when a speaker implied "that this scientist had more or less flipped out and now these two crackpots, Stewart and Mancuso, had found each other." However, when Nienhuys met Stewart, she found her "friendly, warm, and human," "stimulating and nourishing me as an intellectual as hardly anyone ever had before."[60] Steve Wing, a young epidemiologist who dreaded meeting Stewart on account of the things he had heard about her, was "totally taken" by the woman he met: "she is so wonderfully unassuming and down to earth and goes to such lengths to make you comfortable, to behave in a way that denies the inequalities of society."[61]

How well did Keating know her? He does not say, though he slips easily onto a first-name basis, referring to her as "Alice" (Doll is always "Doll"). In the five years I spent writing my book, I got to know her well, and the person I knew bears no resemblance to the character Keating describes. Over the years, I spent several weeks with her, tagging along with her to her work in Birmingham, traveling to Wales and Bristol to meet her family; I heard her lecture at a conference in New York and watched her consult on a legal case at Rocky Flats and talked with her late into the night, many nights, at her cottage near Oxford—and I can tell you, she was excellent company, had a splendid sense of humor, and an extended network of friends, colleagues, and fellow scientists who were there for her in her old age. "Belligerence," says Keating, "was, as often as not, her first emotional response" when she met with resistance.[62]

But as the third of eight children, five of whom were male, tact was more likely to be her first response. Far from being "allergic to decision-making process," as Keating describes her,[63] she was legendary for the way she inspired assistants to do their best for her, mobilizing student volunteers and health officers to give their all—it was how she kept her projects going on such slender means (she often paid staff from her own salary). "The way she could motivate so many people to help her carry out her work . . . was extraordinary," says a Birmingham colleague Tom Sorahan. The way she inspired me to take on her biography, when I was writing another book and teaching full-time in California, was extraordinary, too.

Keating hints darkly and repeatedly at her quest for "status," but she was not ambitious for honors. She was pleased to receive the Right Livelihood Prize in 1986, the Alternative Nobel, as it's called, conferred in the Swedish Parliament the day before the Nobel to honor those who have made contributions to the betterment of society. She was happy to be awarded the Ramazzini Prize in 1991, the leading prize in Italy for epidemiology. But she had none of the status anxiety one associates with Oxbridge, and so little drive for self-promotion that more than one friend commented on it. "She was not prepared to go to the right places and be nice to the right people," observed Molly Newhouse, a lifelong friend and occupational health expert herself. "She could always think of something more interesting to do than to go to a vice-chancellor's garden party where you had to dress up and be nice to people."[64]

Doll, on the other hand, was, in his biographer's words, "a high-status person" accustomed to being "treated in a deferential manner," "a natural patrician."[65] David Weatherall describes him as "a superior kind of person and used to getting his own way."[66] "Few people, even his closest colleagues, had a personal relationship with him," observes Julian Peto.[67] "He emanated intimidation," says Marie Kidd, who worked with him on a lung cancer study.[68] The words *detached* and *detachment* recur in his biography; I find no mention of a sibling. When asked if he was a "family man," Joan (his wife) replied, "No. Richard likes his family, but he's very busy with his work." His daughter Cathy "did not think that he was a real dad to her."[69] Stewart, meanwhile, was changing diapers and incurring disapproval when she took time away from family to do her research. (She loved children, and, as I had occasion to see, was good with them.)

Michael Dunnill, who had helped bring Doll to Oxford in 1969, was one of many people watching that 1996 Channel 4 documentary[70] who was shocked by Doll's insults: "He absolutely destroyed Alice Stewart on television. He said that her work was 'slapdash.' Doll can be ruthless. He destroyed her really."[71] But he did not destroy her. I was with her, watching that documentary, and I heard what she said: "I really—I'm really quite shocked! I knew he didn't approve of me, but that he'd say this! It explains a lot—the cold shoulders, the lack of offers or invitations. I see that I haven't made it up." Far from being devastated by Doll's remarks, she was relieved that the undercurrent of disapproval and dislike was out in the open for the world to see.

What she envied Doll for was not status or recognition—it was the support he had, the teams of researchers, "the best in Britain," as she said, statisticians like the Peto brothers, whom she admired. She has been much criticized for choosing George Kneale as her statistician, a man of enormous intelligence but painfully awkward personality, whose communication skills have never been up to clarifying or defending the unconventional methods he uses. But she never had Doll's resources to "scour . . . the world" for talent. I wonder what she might have accomplished if she had. She died with many theories untested.

"It is very difficult for the Alice Stewarts of the world to survive," said Sheldon Samuels, presenting her with the Ramazzini Prize. It's "a struggle not only to be independent but to find the support—social, intellectual, and material—that a scientist needs."

"The wounds and scars received by advocates of unpopular opinion, and by persons publishing reports of adverse effects that are 'inconvenient' . . . are real but rarely presented in scientific journals," writes Morris Greenberg.[72] "It hasn't been easy for Alice. . . . Yet she carried on, making her case in a sensible, unhysterical manner. She is a polite, gentle soul who doesn't express herself aggressively, just firmly. I respect also that she doesn't complain."[73].

She put up with slights, snubs, rebuffs, and rudeness that take the breath away, eyes rolled, eyebrows raised, and glances exchanged. She was called "senile," "barmy," "gone round the bend" as far back as the 1950s. Keating professes "compassion" for the confused, benighted Alice, while characterizing her as "angry," "humorless," "belligerent," "campaigning" (he calls my biography—"The Woman Who Knew Too Much"— "tendentiously titled."[74] These are familiar stereotypes, stock terms used by insiders for outsiders who are challenging their positions, who can easily look contentious and tendentious, since they are challenging accepted opinion.

But "embittered" Stewart was not. I came across "embittered" scientists while writing my book, independents more badly scarred than she. Thomas Mancuso, whose career and reputation were destroyed by the US government, felt so hard done-by that he refused to speak to me, and then, when my book came out, complained to Bob Tredici that I hadn't interviewed him. But Stewart always said she was "extraordinarily lucky"—lucky to have a steady income, lucky to have bought a cottage in the Cotswolds when cottages could be afforded, blessed with a physical and psychological robustness that enabled her to carry on. She had a marvelous capacity to "make the best of it." She felt that being a woman had worked to her advantage: "If I'd been a man, I'd never have stood it—the pay was too low, the prospects too bad. As a woman . . . I was left to go my own ways." She even felt that being marginalized "was just right for me personally," and that her work was better for the opposition: "Since no one accepted our position, we had to dig in and prove that it was so." And since she had no full-time staff or department, she could take stands: "I speak out because there are not a lot of people who can. I have nothing to lose. A lot of people do."

None of the above tells us about the relative merits of Doll's or Stewart's science, but it does point to the distortions in the Doll-Keating version of her personality. Doll found it "unacceptable," says Keating, that Stewart "was making a political campaign out of the work she was doing": he saw this as "incompatible" with being "a serious scientist,"[75] implying that her objectivity had been compromised by her sympathies with the activists. Doll was himself, according to his biographer, a "neutral, dispassionate scientist" who kept aloof from "campaigning"[76]; as though writing letters to the national press and denouncing opponents in public forums were not a form of "campaigning"—as though accepting large sums of money from industries while assessing the cancer risk of chemicals produced by those industries incurred no taint.

Actually, it could be argued that Stewart was the one innocent in the whole agenda-driven fray: she blundered into it, as surprised as everyone else when her investigations turned up so lethal an effect from X-rays. She was never the banner-waving "campaigner" Doll and Keating make her out to be but a scrupulous scientist who made every effort to keep her work untainted by sympathies. "I'm very sympathetic with the activist point of view," she said, "but I'm not an activist, and I'm determined that this sympathy not influence my interpretation of the data. You must hear what the data are telling you, see what the numbers say": this was the first principle of her work.

It could be argued it was Doll's work that was slanted—toward the interests of "the ruling class," says Robert Park[77] of the National Institute of Occupational Safety and Health. "Doll's dealings with occupational issues were almost always with individuals from the management side; the data he analyzed was usually collected, described, and documented by the management class. His deliberations in interpreting findings were within that same social context." Relying on company data provided him by Turner and Newall, Ltd., makers of asbestos products, for example, Doll found much lower rates of asbestos-related disease in the asbestos insulation industry than did Irving Selikoff, who looked at medical records provided by trade unions, records of workers who had daily contact with asbestos.[78] "Learning about the nature of industrial process exposures by listening to the architects and managers of the system rather than those who must function, succeed and survive within the lower reaches of it, cannot help but color one's fundamental perspective," Park points out. "The closest he came to most workers . . . was from a podium."

Stewart did not, truth be told, think well of Doll's epidemiology. She faulted him for following trodden paths (such as the Hiroshima data). She would have been astonished to hear him described as *revolutionary*, the word Keating uses in his subtitle. Even joining the Communist Party, though no doubt courageous and sincere, was something British intellectuals were doing in the 1930s and indicated, perhaps (as Stewart commented), that he was not averse to "party lines."

She criticized Doll for not carrying his studies out for the length of time radiation studies require, for not casting a sufficiently wide net: "you have to include the noise rather than try to shut it out in the interest of time or tidiness." Doll, she said, was always in a hurry: "He has been heard to say that no survey that hasn't been completed within five years is worth its salt. This has had a very dampening influence on the whole field. You can't do it that way . . . you can't tidy it up like this. It needs a long time; it's got to have untidy edges. Doll admitted, of a study of ankylosing spondylitis he did with Court-Brown, that "we were rather keen to get it completed quickly as we knew the Americans were writing a report as well and we wanted to get ours out before theirs."[79] The exclusion of African Americans and people over sixty-five from the 1981 *Causes of Cancer*[80] cut out a lot of "noise." Similarly, in the vinyl chloride study, "older, highly exposed workers were left out, as were entire plants."[81]

In an interesting twist to their long, complex relationship, Doll has twice admitted publicly that Stewart was right, and elsewhere stated positions that agreed with hers but that he did not publicize. First, was his admission that she had been right about fetal X-rays, and that his own study was "not very good." He also told me, "it looks like Alice will be proved right on this—the A-Bomb studies are turning up effects other than cancer." (By 1998, when he said this, more radiation-related health effects had indeed turned up in the survivors;[82–84] the longer these studies go on, the more effects they turn up, as Stewart predicted.)

Years later, I found, in a box in my basement that I'd not sent to the Wellcome Institute along with Alice's papers, a confidential memo that had fallen my way by chance written by Doll and Court-Brown to the Medical Research Council (MRC), after Doll had visited Hiroshima: "It must be presumed that many of those killed in Hiroshima would have developed leukemia if they had survived so that the surviving population is a selected one . . . and this would have introduced a bias into subsequent incidence of various types of leukemia."[85] Here was Doll admitting that the population being studied was "selected," not representative—that is, comprised of healthy survivors, exactly as Alice maintained. It seems that Doll, too, suspected a "bias," but did not wish to go public with his suspicion; the memo was marked "confidential."

Most interesting was a paper he wrote that was accepted by the *Journal of Radiological Protection* in 1955 but not published until 1996,[86] which states, "there is *no threshold* dose below which no effect is produced" (my emphasis).

Why had he not published this in 1955? It seems that Sir Harold Himsworth, the Secretary of the MRC, advised him not to: "Look, I think this is so speculative, I wouldn't publish this if I were you, it will only damage your reputation as a scientist." And where did Himsworth get the idea that the paper would damage his reputation? The Atomic Energy Commission (AEC) had "advised Himsworth that it really wasn't reliable and shouldn't be published."[87] It's easy to see why the AEC would not want a scientist who had visited Hiroshima suggesting there is no threshold beneath which radiation ceases to be dangerous. Nor would it be pleased to hear that "the time which has elapsed since the explosion of the bombs is short in comparison with the induction time usually observed in human cancer, and it is probable that the total number of cases attributable to the explosions will eventually be considerably increased"—as Doll states in his 1955/96 paper.[88]

So the AEC warned Himsworth who warned Doll against publication on the grounds that this paper might damage his reputation, and Doll withdrew the paper from publication. He only published it in 1996 because it was cited in a legal case. "So I said to our lawyers, 'Look, I've got to get hold of a copy of that paper.' And, of course, they were able to get hold of a copy because the other side had cited it. I got the paper, I read it, and I thought, 'This is bloody good.' The estimate really wasn't far from what we would make nowadays, and to cut a long story short I published it forty years later," he told Cook,[89] seeming oblivious that there was anything odd or off-putting about his failure to publish it in the first place.

By 1996, official estimates of low-dose radiation risk had moved in Stewart's direction, with reports from the Biological Effects of Ionizing Radiation[90] and the National Radiological Protection Board acknowledging that there is probably no threshold beneath which radiation ceases to have an effect.[91] As low-dose radiation was acknowledged to be more dangerous than previously assumed, Doll's unpublished estimate came closer to "what we would make nowadays," and he took credit for knowing the risks all along—as it seems he did. Yet it was Stewart who went public with the warning—and paid the price—and Doll who was first on the scene to launch a study to discredit her and last on the scene to write a damning epitaph.

Yet he came to her funeral. At a country church not far from Oxford, a small group of family and close friends had assembled, when in walked an aged man with a patrician air. A murmur ran through the gathering—Who's that? Can that be? He came late, left early, and, to my knowledge, spoke to no one.

"What had been that stubborn, vain old man's thoughts, as he mouthed the words of the hymns?" writes Margaret Drabble, who found the situation so intriguing that she put it in her novel, *The Sea Lady*.[92] "Had he repented of his attempts to block the woman's research, or had he attended the funeral in a spirit of triumph? In order, finally, to see her off, and to make sure that she had gone to earth for good. Rivalry endures until death, and after. . . ."[93] Some said it was conscience, most saw it as a political show. But a show for what, for whom?

We all have a story or stories of our lives that make sense of who we are and how we came to be. Here is how Doll tells the story of the lung cancer discovery: "after the war the mortality [from lung cancer] had gone on going up and . . .the MRC had a conference to discuss it.[94] And the conference concluded—this is back in 1947 . . . that really we ought to try to find out to see if you could find any cause for [the increase]. . . . And, in fact, it was left to Bradford Hill and he asked me to help him. And we said, 'Well, we'll interview patients attending hospitals for lung cancer.'"[95]

In fact, Doll was assigned to a committee that was commissioned to look specifically at links between lung cancer and smoking—as this summary of the MRC meeting indicates: "At this meeting it was agreed that Professor Kenneway, Dr. Percy Stocks, and Professor Bradford Hill should be asked to draw up a preliminary plan for a large scale statistical *study of the past smoking habits* and other characteristics of persons with cancer of the lung" (emphasis added). "Doll was a young man put on a committee," says Stewart, who was present at the meeting: "Once you got in there, it was big as a house. You couldn't miss it." There were actually five papers on the dangers of smoking published the year Doll and Hill published theirs, 1950;[96] in fact, cigarettes had been suggested as a cause of lung cancer as far back as the 1920s.[97]

You can see, in Doll's account, an exaggeration of his role in the discovery. John Lilburne[98] describes Doll as given to "telling Just-So" stories about how he came upon the smoking–lung cancer link, a tendency "to confabulate his own narratives, perhaps unknowingly . . . Almost all major scientists restructure their own narratives of discovery after they become famous, as one can see by examining the lab notes of Nobel prizewinners and comparing them with the subsequent autobiographical story. There is not necessarily anything very harmful about this very human trait, unless it obscures the contribution of others or misleads young scientists about how great work is done." Lilburne notes that major recognition usually "comes relatively late in a scientist's career, and is therefore unlikely to have a major impact on his or her research. When it comes early, or the scientist remains active for decades, perhaps as the head of a research institute, such innocent confabulation can provide a sense of infal- libility or invulnerability." Recognition did come early to Doll, and he remained active for decades.

Geoffrey Tweedale[99] comments: "He eventually constructed, perhaps unconsciously, his own narratives of his early tobacco work and the reaction of the tobacco companies. He dismissed pioneering work in other countries as unimportant and flawed, whilst mythologizing the roots of his own research, perhaps under the welter of adulation."[100] And "a welter of adulation" there was. Take this obituary by David Simpson:[101] "Days before he entered hospital, he attended the Green College summer dinner, a fine figure in a white tuxedo, charming friends young and old, and enthusing about the new building that bears his name. He drew envious glances from men, who told each other they would be happy to be half as active at seventy, never mind ninety, and admir- ing glances from women, some joking with each other that given the chance, they would leave home for him. Sir Richard Doll used to say that he wanted to die young as old as possible. That is exactly what he did; and thanks to his life's work, millions of others have the chance of doing the same."[102] A dazzling description and a bit bedazzled, too.

Even the feisty, outspoken environmental scientist Devra Lee Davis[103] comes under the spell: "One evening, after a symposium in Lyon, France, I was thrilled to find myself having drinks with none other than Sir Richard Doll. His entry in *Who's Who* listed conversation as one of his hobbies, and sure enough, he was a captivating, engaging and scintillating man to talk with. Doll assured me that he was taking the time to speak with me because he wanted to help. I was honored by the attention. . . . I was flabbergasted and flattered. I had spent an evening with the great Sir Richard."[104] You can see how a person might get a bit puffed up by all this adoration. "On a personal level," writes Tweedale,[105] "Doll was a charming and approachable man: but he also had a highly developed sense of his own importance that was later tinged with dogmatism and a belief in his own infallibility."[106]

I think he had a story he told himself, a story he told to the national press, to an admiring biographer, to the many audiences his position provided him, a story of a scientist dedicated to truth and the betterment of humanity, a story he believed—and that was in part true. Though the self-image had, perhaps, slipped a little out of alignment over the years, what with compromises made, positions taken, leaving him a little too convinced of his own rectitude, that only made him a more persuasive teller of the tale. "Man ends by fully believing the story he has told so many times and continues to tell, polishing and retouching here and there the details," writes Primo Levi:[107] the "transition to self-deception is useful" since the self-deceived are more convincing narrators, "more easily believed by the judge, the historian, the reader."[108]

"I've done nothing but try to help her," Doll said to me, said it more than once, seeming keen to convince me he had behaved honorably toward her. The Doll I met was a man of formidable charm—witty, winning, every bit the gentleman—though I could tell, as we chatted, that I was being sized up by a shrewd observer, and I felt my questions bounce off a hard, polished surface. I came away thinking, this is a man well versed in the art of public relations (an impression I doubt anybody ever got of Alice Stewart), adept at the presentation of self to create effect, a master craftsman, and enormously persuasive: a Channel 4 "Power List" program on October 31, 1998, listed him as 122 among the most powerful (or influential) people in Britain.

And he left a dynasty. "A high proportion of the scientists who were to dominate the field passed through the doors of his department," boasts Keating.[109] Many who leapt to his defense after the 2006 revelations were people who had worked with him or under him. With such a flock of followers, his reputation is assured.

So secure is Doll's reputation that the 2006 revelations bounced off it like Teflon—as I discovered, in 2008, when I came across Richard Horton's review of Davis's *Secret History of the War on Cancer* in the *New York Review of Books*.[110] Horton's review was very peculiar. It started out sounding sympathetic to Davis's arguments about the "misplaced emphasis on treatment over prevention" and about the strategy of "doubt promotion," whereby aspersion is cast on scientists who dare to suggest that environmental pollution has a role in cancer causation. But then Horton spun about-face, put off by the "vitriol and innuendo" in Davis's discussion of Doll, concluding that her book was a tissue of "vague exhortations," and that the real reason cancer was on the rise is not environmental but that people smoke and eat too much—and how dare she say such things about this revered scientist?

This hit a nerve. My biography of Stewart had been turned down by Verso Press on account of a reader who had this same kind of apoplectic response to Stewart's criticisms of Doll. But that was in the 1990s, when Doll's name was sterling—how could his reputation be so untarnished, two years after those conflicts of interest had been revealed?

I wrote to the *New York Review of Books*, saying that if Horton was shocked by what Davis said about Doll, he should hear what I learned about Doll while writing *The Woman Who Knew Too Much*.[111] To my amazement, the *Review* published my letter—usually Doll's detractors get listservs and email and blogs to air their opinions, while his defenders get the *London Times*. I received a flood of mail, all of it anti-Doll. Horton wrote no response to my letter, though it is the *Review*'s policy to give authors the opportunity to reply.

The Woman Who Knew Too Much[112] was never published in England on account of what we said about Doll. Not only did Verso turn the book down, but later, the Women's Press, which accepted it for UK publication, withdrew their offer when their legal department warned of libel issues. I never took it to another British publisher. "I know of no one who has had critical things published about Doll whose work has not been thoroughly obstructed by lawyers," writes Martin Walker, who himself received a warning from Doll's solicitors after the critique he wrote in *The Ecologist* in 1998.[113] In Britain, where many journalists are "frightened off by legal matters, there has been next to no serious debate inside or outside science about these matters."

That's what a "Mafia" looks like, not the little band of outsiders nipping at Doll's heels.

Thus has the esteemed Sir Richard Doll constructed the story of his life and been in a position to make it stick. And so is the "Authorized Biography," which is receiving laudatory reviews in mainstream journals,[114–116] on its way to becoming the official story. It was inevitable that this biography be commissioned, given Doll's iconographic status—but that Stewart's story was written was pure chance. I just happened to interview her for a book I was writing on cancer and the environment, and I just happened to be able to find the time her story required—though it was time carved out of teaching responsibilities half a world away and from leaves paid for by myself.

A year after Doll died, when the media were publicizing his industry ties, the MRC issued a press release in the *Sunday Times*, signed by the head of the MRC and other luminaries: "It is with dismay that we now hear allegations against him that he cannot rebut for himself."[117] But Doll himself showed no reservations about speaking ill of the dead when he wrote that damning entry on Stewart in the *Oxford Dictionary of National Biography*, and nobody from the MRC or the Wellcome Institute came to her defense. Far from defending her, The Wellcome Library (which houses her papers as well as his) commissioned a biography that gave Doll the last word.

I'm afraid it mattered that Doll looked like a grandee and Stewart looked like a granny. She dressed like a woman who had other things on her mind, never gave a thought to what she wore, and had not a shred of image-consciousness. And she was the bearer of bad news—"In the old days they killed the messenger who brought bad news, these days they just cut off your funding," as she'd say—whereas Doll dispensed bromides. "We are, for the most part, winning the fight against cancer" was another of his reassurances.[118]

Those who have power have access to venues that enable them to secure more power. Stewart existed so far outside institutional structures that she had no such venues, whereas Doll dominated British epidemiology for the last half of the twentieth century, defining who was in, who was out, who was scientifically respectable, and who was fringe, and effectively silencing his critics. He shaped cancer research in the United States and the United Kingdom, assuring that occupational cancer remains a low priority and putting a virtual end to inquiry into the environmental causes of cancer. The Imperial Cancer Research Fund that he represented has never, as Martin Walker[119] observes, carried out research on "the possible carcinogenic effects of exposure to . . . environmental factors."[120] "His contribution on occupational and environmental cancer has been a disaster," says Rory O'Neil.

Keating[121] asserts that "millions of people are alive today who would otherwise be dead had Richard Doll not made his enduring contribution to medical science."[122] Perhaps. But Chris Talbot[123] points out that it may have been a draw between the lives he saved and the lives he cost: on account of positions Doll took on Agent Orange, vinyl chloride, and radiation, people were denied compensation, endured further exposure, suffered, and died. His defense of dioxin enabled the United Kingdom to refuse its ex-servicemen compensation, even as Australia, New Zealand, and the United States were granting compensation to theirs. Richard Stott, in a blistering article in the *Sunday Mirror*,[124] denounced Doll as among those responsible for Britain's heartless refusal to acknowledge the damage the bomb tests had done its servicemen: they "should hang their heads in shame for the misery, torment, crippling disease they have caused."

Stewart saved lives, too: putting an end to the X-raying of pregnant women, she spared the human race untold numbers of malignancies and mutations. But with her, there's no negative side to the ledger.

The confusion sown by Doll and those who have accepted his reassurances about low-dose radiation has enabled proponents of the nuclear industry to proceed as though the risks were understood and under control, to pass off as "clean" this energy source that has polluted half the globe. The Chernobyl catastrophe released hundreds of times the radioactivity released by the Hiroshima and Nagasaki bombs combined: 57 percent of it spread outside the former USSR, contaminating more than 40 percent of Europe and the entire Northern Hemisphere.[125]

As technicians struggle to contain the Fukushima reactors, and as experts disagree about radiation released and new cover-ups come daily to light, the Hiroshima studies are invoked by way of reassurance. "The risk of cancer is quite low, lower than what the public might expect," a researcher from the Radiation Effects Research Foundation informs the *New York Times*, explaining that the Hiroshima studies show that "at very low doses, the risk was also very low."[126] The Department of Energy assures us that the "miniscule quantities" of radiation in the radioactive plume spreading across the United States pose "no health hazard."[127] British journalist George Monbiot[128] cites the Hiroshima studies as evidence that low-dose radiation produces low rates of cancer and no genetic effects, pointing to these as "scientific consensus." In a shrill, much publicized debate with Helen Caldicott, on television and in the *Guardian*, he chides, "You have to go with the scientific consensus, rather than with a few outlier papers," and calls Caldicott "unscientific" (Doll's term for opponents)—though she is a physician and he is a journalist.

As Fukushima is upgraded to a "level 7" disaster, on a par with Chernobyl, the public looks for information about Chernobyl, only to find in mainstream media, human interest stories, denials, and evasions. "There is no evidence of a major public health impact attributable to radiation exposure two decades after the accident at Chernobyl," announced the *New York Times*, a few days after the Fukushima reactors began to destabilize.[129] So says a World Health Organization study that found "minimal health effects" and estimated that only four thousand deaths "will probably be attributable to the accident ultimately," a report the *New York Times* had publicized in 2005, quoting an expert who explained that the worst effect of the accident was a "paralyzing fatalism" that leads people to "drug and alcohol use, and unprotected sex and unemployment"—the "lifestyle" causes invoked by Doll and Peto.[130]

The *Times* did not mention two other studies that came out in 2006, "The Other Report on Chernobyl"[131] and "The Chernobyl Catastrophe" by Greenpeace,[132] both of which gave much higher casualty estimates than the 2005 report. Nor did it mention *Chernobyl: Consequences of the Catastrophe for People and the Environment*,[133] translated into English and published by the New York Academy of Sciences in 2009—which estimates casualties at 985,000, orders of magnitude higher than the 2005 report. Drawing on "data generated by many thousands of scientists, doctors, and other experts who directly observed the suffering of millions affected by radioactive fallout in Belarus, Ukraine, and Russia," this report incorporates more than 5,000 studies, mostly in Slavic languages (as compared with the 350 mentioned in the 2005 report, most of which were in English). The authors are Dr. Alexey Yablokov, environmental advisor to Yeltsin and Gorbachev, and Dr. Vassili Nesterenko, former director of the Institute of Nuclear Energy in Belarus, who flew over the burning reactor, giving us the only measurement of the radionuclides released. Nesterenko, together with Andrei

Sakharov, founded the independent Belarusian Institute of Radiation Safety (BELRAD), which treats and studies Chernobyl children; when he died, in 2008, as a result of radiation exposure, his son Dr. Alexey Nesterenko—third author on this study—took over as director and senior scientist at BELRAD. Dr. Janette Sherman, translator and contributing editor, is a physician and toxicologist.

Comparing contaminated areas of Belarus, Ukraine, and Russia with the so-called "clean areas," the studies find significant increases in morbidity and mortality in contaminated regions: not only more cancer, especially thyroid cancer, but a wide array of non-cancer effects (as Stewart predicted there would be)—ulcers, chronic pulmonary diseases, diabetes mellitus, eye problems, mental retardation, and a higher incidence and greater severity of infectious and viral diseases. In fact, every system in the body is adversely affected: cardiovascular, reproductive, neurological, hormonal, respiratory, gastrointestinal, musculoskeletal, and immune systems. The children are particularly damaged: "Prior to 1985 more than 80 percent of children in the Chernobyl territories of Belarus, Ukraine, and European Russia were healthy; today fewer than 20 percent are well."[134] In the animals, too, there are "significant increases in morbidity and mortality . . . increased occurrence of tumor and immunodeficiencies, decreased life expectancy, early aging, changes in blood and the circulatory system, malformations."[135]

Parallels between Chernobyl and Hiroshima are striking: data collection was delayed, information withheld, reports of on-the-spot observers were discounted, and independent scientists denied access. Yablokov and colleagues[136] note that "The USSR authorities officially forbade doctors from connecting diseases with radiation and, like the Japanese experience, all data were classified;" and "the official secrecy that the USSR imposed on Chernobyl's public health data the first days after the meltdown . . . continued for more than three years," during which time "secrecy was the norm not only in the USSR, but in other countries as well."[137]

But the parallels are more political than biological, for the Hiroshima data have proven to be an "outdated" and inapplicable model, as Stewart said, for predicting health effects from low-dose, chronic radiation exposure over time. Thyroid cancer, for example, increased "exponentially" in the years after Chernobyl, appearing earlier and more virulently than in Hiroshima (a three-year as opposed to a ten-year latency). Doll—among others— denied that this could be a radiation effect since doses were too low—"too low" as determined by the Hiroshima data—yet epidemiological studies kept turning up a link with radiation. Finally, in 2005, a case-control study headed by Elisabeth Cardis confirmed "a very strong dose-response relationship" between thyroid cancer and radiation exposure, at doses "not thought to be sufficiently high" to produce this effect.[138]

The Hiroshima studies find little genetic damage in the survivors, yet, "Wherever there was Chernobyl radioactive contamination, there was an increase in the number of children with hereditary anomalies and congenital malformations. These included previously rare multiple structural impairments of the limbs, head, and body."[139] Such anomalies and malformations are especially pronounced in the children of the "liquidators," the men and women called in to put out the fire, decommission the reactor, and clean up the site— 15 percent of whom were dead by 2005 (these were young, healthy men and women). The correlation with radioactive exposure is so striking as to be "no longer an assumption, but . . . proven," write Yablokov et al.,[140] and the damage will go on for "at least seven generations."[141] As in humans, so in other species, "gene pools of living creatures are actively transforming, with unpredictable consequences . . . It appears that [Chernobyl's irradiation] has awakened genes that have been silent over a long evolutionary time."[142]

The inescapable conclusion is that "there is no threshold for ionizing radiation's impact on health. . . . Even the smallest excess of radiation over that of natural background will statistically . . . affect the health of exposed individuals or their descendants, sooner or later."[143] Radioactive contamination does not "dilute and dissipate": as Stewart warned, it becomes part of what we breathe and eat, adding, over time, to cancers and genetic damage throughout the world. "Even more than the cancer threat is the genetic damage," she cautioned: "that's what you ought to be really afraid of, the possibility of sowing bad seeds into the human gene pool."

As low-dose radiation is demonstrated to have health effects beyond those predicted by current theoretical frameworks, the discrepancy between the models and the evidence becomes glaring. Rudi Nussbaum,[144] professor emeritus of nuclear physics, Portland State University, describes an increasing "dissonance between evidence and existing assumptions about . . . radiation risk," a gap between new information and the "widely adopted presuppositions about radiation health effects."[145] The mechanisms by which low-dose radiation does its damage are not well understood, however. Stewart hypothesized that rather than killing the cell outright, as a high dose of radiation does, radiation at low dose allows it to attempt repair, and it's the attempt that produces the mutations leading to cancer and genetic aberrations. There are "many different complex cellular interaction scenarios [that] can be hypothesized," write David Brenner and Rainer Sachs,[146] that may lead to an understanding at the molecular level. A 2004 report of the Committee Examining Radiation Risks of Internal Emitters

(CERRIE) suggests that internal emitters from radiation ingested or inhaled have been insufficiently taken into account or understood, and points to newly discovered biological effects of radiation, "genomic instability (on-going, long-term increase in mutations within cells and their offspring), bystander effects (cells next to those that were irradiated can also be damaged) and minisatellite mutations (inherited germline DNA changes)"—which "need further research."[147]

"The Chernobyl accident created a unique possibility for specialists in radiobiology and radiation protection for examination of their hypotheses and theories," writes Michael Malko,[148] a researcher at the Joint Institute of Power and Nuclear Research in Belarus. But rather than using this evidence to expand their knowledge of radiation effects, experts invoke the old studies to dismiss new evidence. Chernobyl is a better predictor of the consequences of Fukushima than Hiroshima is, but Yablokov's book has met, as he said in a press conference in Washington, DC, in 2011,[149] "mostly with silence"—while the Hiroshima studies continue to be cited.

I keep hearing Doll's words, "it looks as though Alice will be proved right. . . ." But it's clear, from the way scientists cling to the old model, how strong their desire is to believe the industry-sanctioned and government sanctioned reassurances of Sir Richard Doll.

Chapter 13

THE CORPORATE HIJACKING OF THE UK VACCINE PROGRAM

Martin J. Walker, MA

The real political task in a society such as ours is to criticize the workings of institutions that appear to be both neutral and independent.

—Michel Foucault

The first task of the doctor is . . . political: the struggle against disease must begin with a war against bad government.

—Michel Foucault

In July 2014, Dr. Brian Hooker, a biochemist and father of an autistic child, published a paper[3] that showed that the analysis of data presented in a paper published in February 2004 by the Centers for Disease Control and Prevention (CDC) had been incorrect.[4] The analysis had disguised an effect of the MMR vaccine on onset of regressive autism in black male children.

There are a number of important factors that the uncovering of this "science bending" brings into focus. Perhaps the most important matter the new information brought to light was the fact that thousands of African American children have disproportionately acquired autism spectrum disorders, having been prescribed the MMR vaccination.

With the ensuing controversy, conflicts of interests within the CDC, described as a federal agency managed by the US Department of Health and Human Services, have been brought to the surface.

In danger of receding into the historical twilight is the fact that the CDC's original findings vindicated, to some extent, the work of the British doctor Andrew Wakefield, who published a twelve-child case review paper in 1998, which suggested further research was needed into a link between regressive autism and MMR.[5] Wakefield was pursued, harassed, accused of fraud, and stripped of his professional qualifications by the British government, medical establishment, the pharmaceutical companies, and dark, cynically prejudiced forces linked to the Skeptic movement and the Murdoch media.

When the brouhaha is over, however, the most important question remains unanswered: in a society which is gradually being taken over by corporations, especially in the field of drugs and health, how are we able to retain a sense of independent truth in the area of public health research and how might we sanction criminal behavior which puts profit before health and threatens the lives of—in this case—thousands of children? How is it possible for civil servants, doctors, regulators, and corporate shills who pose as guardians of the public health, to slip away into the shadows without even being confronted with their lack of accountability? Finally, how do we erect a critique which can be used to stop the continuation of this aberrant behavior? What are its component parts?

This chapter is unable to answer these questions, but in outlining the particular circumstance in which the United Kingdom vaccine regulatory body, the Joint Committee on Vaccination and Immunisation (JCVI), like the US CDC, is driven and affected by obvious vested interests, it hopes to make readers aware of the immense problems that stand in the way of promoting firstly, social debate and secondly, independent and honestly promoted science in the field of vaccination.

CORPORATE CHAOS IN THE UNITED KINGDOM

The system of regulatory and oversight bodies in the hands of the pharmaceutical-funded individuals, organizations, and corporations is virtually the same in the United Kingdom and the United States, and, although there have been constant criticisms over the years of conflicts of interests such conflicts are now entrenched and their distortions of power most pronounced.

The UK Joint Committee on Vaccination and Immunisation (JCVI), the body which makes a final decision to sanction or reject vaccines, is defined as an "independent advisory expert committee of the United Kingdom Department of Health." The committee submits recommendations to the government regarding vaccination schedules and safety. The committee operates under the leadership of the Medicines and Healthcare Products Regulatory Agency (MHRA), an agency attached to the Department of Health, which is almost *completely* funded by pharmaceutical companies.

The JCVI was set up with other committees in the 1960s in a push to democratize drug regulation in the wake of the thalidomide crimes. This committee along with others is said to be "independent" (i.e., free from outside control, not subject to another's authority). However, the committee has made some appalling decisions, mainly on industry's behalf and at the expense of the people.

In 1987 and 1988, the committee agreed the licensing and promotion of the Urabe-based MMR vaccine, despite having information from Canada and Japan that the vaccine had been found to be seriously damaging.[6] In Canada, the vaccine was withdrawn even before its licensing in Britain was accepted. In Canada, Japan, and Britain the vaccine damaged thousands of children with meningitis and other adverse effects.

After Urabe, MMR was withdrawn following four years' use in Britain, remaining stocks were sold to developing countries, and British researchers traveled to these countries to observe this ongoing child-damaging experiment.[7] In the wake of the withdrawal, accompanied by claims that meningitis wasn't after all that serious a childhood illness, the most elaborate conspiracy was practiced to protect those who had been a part of the committee in 1987 and 1988 and ensure that no one was brought to account.[8]

No one who was part of the JCVI when the Urabe strain MMR was passed as safe has taken responsibility for the damage done by it. Rather, those who were responsible put their shoulder to the wheel to divert public attention and destroy the work and standing of the completely innocent Dr. Wakefield, who drew attention to certain adverse reactions caused by MMR.

In order to ensure that no such compromising event occurred again, instead of democratizing, opening up, and making honest the regulatory system, the pharmaceutical corporations in Britain began to erect a whole new guarding edifice of deeply vested interests around the regulatory structure.

AN INTRODUCTION TO PROFESSOR ANDREW POLLARD

Professor Andrew Pollard took over the chair of the JCVI in October 2013. By 2014, he had become the principal agent, strategist, and presenter of the duplicitous re-democratization of the JCVI under a June 2013 new code of practice. This code of practice, which includes details on conflicts of interests appears to rewrite a new and extensive, more liberal code of practice for members of the JCVI.

Professor Pollard works part of his time at the Jenner Vaccine Foundation, where Professor Salisbury, who oversaw the UK MMR campaign, now has an office after his retirement from his senior position in the UK Department of Health (DoH). Salisbury presided from beginning to end over the Urabe vaccine scandal in Britain and was director of immunization at the DoH and medical advisor to the JCVI throughout the period of propaganda attacks on Dr. Wakefield. Salisbury now heads up his own vaccine consultancy business.

The Jenner Vaccine Foundation is a massively rich organization with a bogus charitable status, partly funded by the UK Department of Health and the Bill and Melinda Gates Foundation together with major US vaccine research organizations.

Pollard, apparently plucked out of nowhere as a shoo-in for the chairmanship of the JCVI for the vaccine industry, now chairs both the JCVI and the European Medicines Agency Scientific Advisory Group on Vaccines, which is based in London. In Oxford Pollard runs one of the largest research groups in the United Kingdom, with seventy staff, that undertakes clinical vaccine trials with children and adults.

The foundation funds the Jenner Institute, which is partnered by the University of Oxford and the Pirbright Institute. Professor Pollard is a trustee of the Jenner Vaccine Institute, for which he is also a Jenner Investigator in one of the largest vaccine development organizations in the western world. He is professor of pediatric infection and immunity at the University of Oxford and director of the Oxford Vaccine Group.

The Pirbright Institute, the third party to the vaccine research conglomerate, like the Jenner Vaccine Foundation, is funded by the Biotechnology and Biological Sciences Research Council (BBSRC), one of seven research councils funded by the government's department for Business, Innovation and Skills (BIS) (i.e., the British public, to the tune of millions of pounds). The Pirbright's total annual coffers recently amounted to £467M; it also retains funding from various corporate sources and supports 1,600 scientists and 2,000 research students in universities and institutes across the United Kingdom.

Apart from proselytizing vaccines and many other science-based roles, the Jenner Vaccine Foundation runs vaccine trials assessing vaccine safety prior to them being put before the JCVI; such a system is in fact very similar to the US CDC system.

In May 2014, the European Medicines Agency's Public Declaration of Interests and the interests of their scientific committee members and experts changed. In June 2013, under "other interest or facts," Pollard had written "N/A" (Not Applicable). In the May 31, 2014 version he now included

"Chairman of the Department of Health's Joint Committee on Vaccination and Immunisation" and alongside he noted, "I am not planning to take on any new grants for clinical trials with vaccine manufacturers."

But was this declaration real or just an artifact which simply disguised his deep-seated involvement with the pharmaceutical cartels? Included in Pollard's EMA declaration is his record as a current "principal investigator" at Okairos,[9] the Swiss vaccine developer acquired by GSK for $325 million. Professor Pollard's project is funded by the Okairos Company and sponsored by Oxford University, where Pollard is the director of the Oxford Vaccine Group. Pollard also has involvements in Pfizer and Novartis pharmaceutical companies and as an investigator in one case, involving Pfizer. No date is available for when these affiliations will end.

Other slightly stranger organizational filigree have occurred since 2013 that are just as dangerous in undermining the accountability of the JVCI but perhaps less noticeable to the lay eye. The measuring of regulatory ethics and account-ability in any organization is almost completely dependent upon the regular nature of its composition.

One of the ways in which the JCVI has since 2013 constantly muddied the waters in relation to conflicts of interests is by moving committee members and non-committee attendees around in the hope of obscuring links between attend-ees and vested interests. At the meeting of February 6, 2013, for example, the chairman announced that it would be the last meeting for Dr. Anthony Harden and Dr. Syed Ahmed, a Glasgow-based consultant in public health medicine and immunization coordinator, along with Professors Ray Borrow and Jon Friedland who had completed two terms on the committee.[10]

Membership, under the code of practice issued by the commissioner for public appointments, is only permitted for a total period of ten years. All four members were appointed between February and October 2006. A further term of three years' duration initiated in June 2014 would put them beyond the per-mitted ten years. The duration of a term in office is a maximum of three years.

However, by June 2013, only four months after leaving the Committee for good, Ray Borrow was back as an "invited contributor on bacteriology" for a meeting, along with the suddenly appearing "invited contributor"—not yet then Chair—Andy Pollard. Dr. Syed Ahmed was back for no reason in particular, while Dr. Anthony Harden returned as a "General Practitioner member." This entirely ad hoc approach to Committee membership never introduces lay mem-bers or the parents of vaccine-damaged children.

Entering 2014, not only does the Committee begin to play fast and loose with statements of conflicting interest, but Committee members are swapped about like players in a third division football team looking at relegation in their last match of the season. In the June 2014 meeting, the Chairman explains two of the kaleidoscope substitutions in this summary way: "The Committee noted that Dr. Anthony Harden had returned for this meeting as an ex-officio member, and that Prof. Ray Borrow had returned as an invited expert."

Despite the announcement that Dr. Harden would be retiring from the JCVI in February 2013, he subsequently reappears at each meeting as: "a JCVI member," a "general practitioner member" and an "ex officio member." Ray Borrow meanwhile reappears initially only for the meeting in June 2013 as an "invited expert contributor," moving on to June when he appears as an invited expert on bacteriology for that meeting. He continues at the February and June 2014 meetings as an "invited expert." Dr. Ahmed returned to the JCVI Committee by June 2013 despite the announcement that his final meeting was in February 2013.

Entering the twenty-first century, with corporations becoming stronger and creating deeper attachments to civil organizations, the rules on conflicts of interest and vested interests must have begun to appear like annoying impediments to the pharmaceutical companies and the researchers to whom they trusted the licensing of their medicines. The years between 2012 and 2014 became the years of regressive revolution for the regulating committee. Under the guise of a new beginning, with stress placed on public accountability, the opposite was happening.

Pollard seemed experienced in the ways of committees and vested interests. In fact, he was no stranger to the JCVI before he was wafted into the Chair of its main committee. For some years, he had been a member of the Meningococcal sub-committee. It looks very much as if Pollard was initially shooed into the JCVI to pursue the licensing of two contentious vaccines, Pandemrix and Bexsero, the research for which he had been deeply involved.

PANDEMRIX

Although Pandemrix sounds like a bake-at-home cake mix, it is actually an influenza vaccine specifically for use in influenza pandemics. The vaccine was developed by GlaxoSmithKline in September 2006.

The vaccine is one of the H1N1 vaccines approved for use by the European Commission in September 2009 on the recommendations of the European Medicines Agency (EMA). The vaccine can only be used when an H1N1 influenza pandemic has been officially declared by the World Health Organization (WHO) or the European Union (EU).

Pandemrix was initially licensed for use with subjects aged eighteen to sixty years on account of the fact that there was a lack of data outside of this age range.

It was then made available to children in the United Kingdom over the age of six months and up to the age of five, following an announcement by the Cabinet Secretary for Health and Wellbeing on November 19, 2009, at the height of the swine flu pandemic propaganda.[11] Simultaneously, in 2009, all EU countries that used pandemic vaccines indemnified the companies that supplied them,[12] meaning that if the vaccine did harm to people taking it, the government and not the producing company could be sued.

Millions of doses of the vaccines were distributed, with Pandemrix having by far the lion's share of the market. However, in August 2010, the Swedish Medical Products Agency (MPA) and the Finnish National Institute for Health and Welfare (THL) launched investigations regarding the acquirement of narcolepsy as a possible side effect to the Pandemrix vaccination in children. They found a minimum 6.6-fold increased risk among children and youths, resulting in a minimum of 3.6 additional cases of narcolepsy per one hundred thousand vaccinated subjects.[13]

Professor David Salisbury at that time still head of immunisation at the UK Department of Health, was a great supporter of Pandemrix, saying that vaccines with adjuvants offer good protection even if the virus changes over time. He commented wisely, "One of the advantages with adjuvanted vaccines is their ability to protect against drifted (mutated) strains. It opens the door for a whole new strategy in dealing with flu."[14]

Pandemrix contains thiomersal (thimerosal), which is added as a preservative and about which there have been blazing rows between corporate scientists and the parents of those damaged by vaccines. Being manufactured in chicken eggs, it also contains trace amounts of egg proteins. Additional important non-medicinal ingredients are formaldehyde, sodium deoxycholate, and sucrose.

Professor Pollard has participated in clinical trials in respect of GSK products, earning himself the title of "study director" in a 2009 trial to study the effects of both Celvapan (Baxter) and Pandemrix (GSK) in children. The sponsor for this experiment was the University of Oxford.[15]

In July 2009, the Daily Mail reported on how GSK were planning to charge £6 per dose of swine flu vaccine, when it cost only £1 to manufacture, and predicted how their sales were set to be "boosted by up to £2bn" when supplies of the vaccine began.[16] This spurred some members of parliament (MPs) into inquiring how much "the people" had paid for the vaccine. Paul Flynn, the Labour MP for Newport West, was respectfully told that neither he nor the British public had a right to know how much of their money had been spent on the vaccine.

Paul Flynn: To ask the Secretary of State for Health what the monetary value is of the NHS stock of swine influenza vaccine.

Gillian Merron: As of January 3, 2010, the total amount of vaccine delivered to the United Kingdom was 23.9 million doses of the GlaxoSmithKline vaccine, Pandemrix, and 5.0 million doses of the Baxter vaccine, Celvapan.

The Department is unable to divulge the monetary value of this stock as it would violate confidentiality clauses in the contracts with the manufacturers.[17]

Sadly for its victims, the clinical trials undertaken prior to licensing, despite acknowledging the vaccine to be more reactogenic (i.e., capable of causing an immunological reaction) failed to detect any correlation between the vaccine and the life-restricting and highly dangerous condition of narcolepsy.

In July 2011, the WHO issued a statement advising that there had been an "unexpected increase of cases of juvenile narcolepsy following immunization with Pandemrix."[18]

On July 21, 2011, the European Medicine Agency's Committee for Medicinal Products for Human Use (CHMP) published its conclusion following a review of findings on Pandemrix and narcolepsy from Finland and Sweden. The EMA, on a precautionary basis, recommended restricting use of Pandemrix in persons under twenty years of age but indicated that overall the benefit-risk of the vaccine remained positive.

Things had come full circle, with the indications for the use of Pandemrix virtually reverting back to the position in 2008, when it was restricted to use in over-eighteens, having damaged a significant number of children.

In 2013, the British government admitted that they had found a causal association between narcolepsy and swine flu vaccination.

The Department for Work and Pensions (DWP) said that after new information provided by the Department of Health they would pay damages to some individuals who were treated with the Pandemrix vaccine before August 31, 2010.[19]

An Irish study published in May 2014 identified a far greater risk of narcolepsy in children and adolescents vaccinated with Pandemrix compared with the unvaccinated: "Our study found a significant, 13.9-fold higher, risk of narcolepsy in children/adolescents vaccinated in Ireland with Pandemrix compared with unvaccinated children/adolescents."[20]

Legal action is being pursued by those affected but because of the Indemnity, claims will be brought against the government and not GSK.[21] So, in fact, the people pay twice for the mistakes and cover-ups of regulatory academics and scientists. Some of them pay with their health while others pay through taxes, from themselves and their fellow citizens.

Was it the case that Pollard and his colleagues missed a causal link between Pandemrix and narcolepsy in the trials he conducted?

BEXSERO

Meningitis B is a rare but aggressive disease that can kill or cause serious lifelong disability within twenty-four hours of onset.[22] About one in ten of those with the disease will die despite appropriate treatment. Bacterial meningitis occurs in about three people per one hundred thousand annually in developed countries but is much more prevalent in developing countries, specifically in South America and North Africa.

In July 2013, the Bexsero vaccine was turned down by the JCVI in the United Kingdom. Professor Andrew Pollard, three months before becoming chair of the JCVI, discussed this rejection in the Blog newsletter linked to Southampton University Hospital.

> The BBC reported yesterday that the Bexsero Meningitis B vaccine has been rejected for use in the UK because it is not cost-effective. This has caused some derision from charities such as Meningitis UK, the pharma industry (Novartis) and me! We have run clinical trials testing Bexsero in Southampton, and it is a crying shame that our hard work seems to be undermined by financial concerns.

After the rejection by the JCVI, Bexsero "Men B" vaccine became the subject of much hand wringing in the United Kingdom. By October 25, 2013, and Pollard's first meeting as Chair on October 2, however, the JCVI had published an "update on the outcome of consultation about use of Bexsero Meningococcal B vaccine in the UK."[23]

Under item IV "Meningococcal B Immunisation," the minutes of the October 2 meeting record that "The Chair took declarations of interest from members and invited contributors." No declarations were attached to the minutes of JCVI meetings after June 2013, so it is impossible to know what, if any, were declared. One thing is clear, however, from Professor Pollard's EMA declaration: he was working as principal investigator from October 2012 for Novartis Men B and OMV NZ (Bexsero) vaccine, a trial which is still described as "current."

Professor Pollard's disclosure also includes the fact that, as well as having a current involvement with the Bexsero vaccine, he was principal investigator for two previous trials between 2008 and 2012 involving this vaccine.

In respect of Bexsero, the meningococcal group B vaccine that contains parts of the bacterium *Neisseria meningitidis* group B, Pollard was doubly conflicted. Not only did he have financial ties to the manufacturer of this vaccine, but he himself has led the clinical trials and compiled the results, which presumably were later presented to the JCVI supporting the safety and efficiency of the vaccine. In the same way that Pollard can diminish or absolve himself of financial affiliation with the industry by not accepting monies directly, he will probably achieve similar "distancing" if his clinical trial work is presented to the committee by the manufacturer. In time-honored tradition, the JCVI probably got around the problem—that their chairman is actually the individual who has compiled the data in the safety trials under consideration by the committee—by ensuring that they are tabled with a Novartis logo on the corner.

The October 2 meeting of the JCVI, which reopened the Bexsero case, was Pollard's first meeting as chair of the JCVI. And in March 2014, after a new discussion from which Professor Pollard does not appear to have absented himself, the JCVI recommended the inclusion of the Bexsero in the UK National Immunisation Program (NIP) for the routine use in infants from two months of age. Following this decision in the United Kingdom, the United States FDA gave the vaccine a Breakthrough Therapy designation.[24]

Unfortunately, the conflict of interest described above is, as far as Professor Pollard is concerned, only the tip of the iceberg. Pollard is currently listed as Principal Investigator for a trial "investigating the Immune Response to 4CMenB in Infants,"[25] due to end in January 2016 with a start date of May 2014 (and processed by the Clinical Trials Register on March 11, 2014), the same month his EMA declaration of interest advised that he was "not planning to take on any new grants for clinical trials with vaccine manufacturers" and eight months after he was appointed Chairman of the JCVI.

An Internet search identifies Pollard as "chief investigator" in a trial for an improved meningococcal vaccine,[26] which according to the text is also named Bexsero (Novartis), but not presently available for use in the United Kingdom. This trial will not be completed until January 2016.[27]

Pollard's apparent grand gesture in not taking on new grants for clinical trials with vaccine manufacturers falls flat when one considers that when he said it he knew he would not be completely free from obligations until the beginning of 2016. This will be nearly two years after his appointment as Chairman of the JCVI and twenty months after his undertaking in his EMA declaration not to enter into new agreements.

GlaxoSmithKline (GSK) is the company that was not only involved in the MMR scandal in the United Kingdom but was also preparing a strategy for avoiding damage claims for the 1970s whooping cough vaccine damage cases. The road to monopoly is not always a straight one and, in the case of Bexsero, the lines of profit ready to be snorted by the owning corporations were anything but clear.

At the time that Bexsero was being discussed by the JCVI, negotiations between Novartis and GSK around the Novartis vaccine business were unresolved. Should the negotiations prove fruitful, it will not be Novartis who will benefit from the contract, but GSK. In April 2014, a month after the JCVI recommended Bexsero for infants in the United Kingdom, GSK and Novartis entered into a "swap." In return for selling its vaccine business to GSK for up to $7.05bn, Novartis would receive GSK's oncology portfolio for $16bn.

Novartis will exit vaccines, selling all its non-influenza interests, including its meningitis B shot Bexsero,[28] to GSK for an initial cash consideration of $5.25bn with subsequent potential milestone payments of up to $1.8bn and ongoing royalties.[29]

CONCLUSIONS: THE BIGGER QUESTIONS

Since the Second World War, a large number of institutions in Britain have been critically analyzed and questioned as to their independent decision making. The critical voice has usually pointed to a prevailing force or network that has skewed, particularly at the top, policy making, and at the bottom, everyday workings. While institutions like the police service, general practice doctors, and civil servants have to some degree been forced into some, albeit weak, accountability, the government, the pharmaceutical industry, and the regulatory agencies have escaped almost entirely accountability to their subjects.

In the 1960s, in the wake of thalidomide, faced with a wave of criticism and exposure, the medical establishment and nascent corporations in the United Kingdom were forced to compromise on democratizing government structures in relation to pharmaceuticals. By the mid-1970s, however, faced with constant economic crisis, although ideas of democratization and accountability appeared to still be on the table, the industry began resolving a defense against democratic regulation.

In the United Kingdom, many of the drug companies joined together to become some of the most highly capitalized corporations in the world. They fought consistently to avoid accountability through law, by collapsing, for instance, the thousand-year right of the citizen to claim for civil damages,[30] or they passed on responsibility for damage to the government by signing indemnity agreements. They waged massive propaganda campaigns to defend sometimes deadly drugs and vaccines from bad publicity, while attacking alternative treatments and remedies.

In the contemporary period, with the drug cartels' profits on specific drugs diminishing in the face of generic production, vaccines have become one of the most stable and profitable medicines on the market. In Britain and in the United States, vaccines are sold to satisfy the nebulous needs of public health profiteers, distributed through government agencies and dispensed in the arena of "socialized medicine," to schools, hospitals, and general practitioners.

Vaccines are constantly redesigned and reintegrated into the vaccine programs over lower and lower age ranges and greater multiplicity. In the United States, where the pro profit, pro vaccine wisdom is that a child's immune system can take up to ten thousand viral strains in one shot,[31] the future for vaccines represents a Valhalla of profitability for the pharmaceutical corporations. Those state and federal agencies that regulate and test the safety of vaccines and which field criticism have become the most important performers in the pharmaceutical three-ring circus.

We live in a society in which, often, the projected reality from government and its agencies is little more than an edifice of lies. While the corporations paint the pictures, we view them and then hang them on our walls.

The US childhood immunization schedule specifies twenty-six vaccine doses for infants aged less than one year—the most in the world.[32] Over the last sixty years, the vaccination rate in the United States has gone from sixteen doses of four vaccines between two months and age six, to forty-nine doses of fourteen vaccines between day of birth and age six, and sixty-nine doses of sixteen vaccines by the age of eighteen.[33] In the United Kingdom, between two months and fourteen years, the British child is expected to have twenty shots.[34]

When the British drug regulatory system is paid for by the pharmaceutical industry, and while it influences the choice of committee members who are also utterly tied to the industry, all chance of democracy, independent scientific discourse, or lay opinion flies out of the window. Jamie Deckoff-Jones, MD, summed up the lack of basic reasoning in relation to vaccines in her article: "The fox guarding the hen house: the CDC & vaccine safety."[35]

> This work (of the CDC) isn't science. It is religion. There is no room for the precautionary principle here. Vaccines are good. Necessary. Period. No need to discriminate which babies might be at greater risk for complications, because we need our herd immunity. The needs of the many outweigh the needs of the few. Only it isn't just a few anymore.[36]

Regardless of the bigger questions, it is, of course, still valuable to pick at the much smaller questions. But we shouldn't believe that we can build a fair and independent system on concerns about small conflicts of interest.

For years the debate has centered on "conflict of interest," but this is, however, a weak and sterile debate which hinges on immeasurable quantities, such as the ability of academics to make independent scientific assessments, the values of which are claimed to be quite separate from the rest of their lives, to perform with personal ethics while being open and vulnerable to all the economic, social, and moral pressures of the surrounding society, and the ability of regulators to think outside the box and decide initially whether or not a vaccine is the best solution to a public health problem. The question of conflict of interest is seemingly redundant in a society that runs mainly on the profit motive and is driven by massively capitalized corporations.

The fact that a number of publications coauthored by Pollard contain declarations advising that he does not receive "personal payment" from vaccine manufacturers and that his "industry sourced Honoraria" are paid to a fund at the Department of Paediatrics at the University of Oxford does not absolve him from his responsibilities as chairman of the JCVI to refrain from having "interests which might conflict with the issues under consideration" or enhance his suitability for the post.

It seems worth saying at some point, that there appears to be very little possibility that someone who dedicates his whole life to researching the production and licensing of novel vaccines, whose interests are massively extended into the world of pharmaceuticals and apparently philanthropic vaccine providers, could ever be considered "independent" in the real sense of the word.

While Pollard functions as investigator on behalf of Oxford University in clinical trials funded by vaccine manufacturers, his livelihood and his professional career path are both supported and financed by the vaccine industry; the assumption that vaccines are clearly without risk and the best "cure" for dangerous diseases is obviously part of his life's mantra. The fact that he is not receiving what is being termed "personal payment" from vaccine manufacturers is meaningless since his monthly salary paid by his place of work is coming ultimately from that source.

It should be borne in mind that the difference between a Yes and a No vote by the JCVI in respect of a vaccine can be the difference of millions of pounds to a manufacturer. A JCVI-endorsed vaccine presented to the Minister virtually guarantees contracts to supply by the manufacturers when they are introduced into the UK immunization program.

A No vote, such as that suffered by Bexsero first time around, must have been devastating for a manufacturer eager to snap up lucrative contracts before the opposition arrived before the committee. But the decision to turn down

Bexsero at the 2013 meeting also brings to the surface a number of important questions. With Meningitis B affecting only three in one hundred thousand individuals in the United Kingdom, this is not the first vaccine that many clinicians would have elected to research. In fact, many clinicians might have suggested that research funding should have been ploughed into treatment protocols and information campaigns addressing the problem with parents.

As in the case of every vaccine, fundamental priority questions should be asked about the nature of the illness and what singles out those children who contract it. As well, money should be ploughed into research which gets to the bottom of idiosyncratic adverse responses to vaccines, so that they can be given discriminately rather than with total inclusion in national vaccine programs. On all these levels, it is clear that the first response of the JCVI, suggesting that Bexsero was not cost-effective, was perhaps one of the few vaccine decisions which was eminently sane.

But in the case of Bexsero the vaccines manufacturers had other, greater plans in mind that needed the consent of the JCVI. As with many illnesses and diseases, their prevalence and effect are more marked in Africa and other developing continents and countries. It is here that the vast trail of money-making diseases can really profit the pharmaceutical cartels. A first prerequisite, however, for a sales pitch in Africa or Latin America is the acceptance of a vaccine or a drug in Europe or North America.

The pharmaceutical industry, working through the MHRA, in the United Kingdom, is responsible for considerable tragedy. In our present society, however, they appear immune to all critique and punishments. Despite the fact that in the pharmaceutical universe many people die consequent upon bad medicines, there is only praise for the "philanthropic" pharmaceutical companies.

While the building industry, the automobile industry, the construction industry and the air transport industry, to name but a few, are logically and rationally liable to have punitive damage claims leveled against them and even government action, the pharmaceutical industry, in the United Kingdom at least, escapes entirely following any damage done by its products.

There is now a considerable amount of research that concludes that researchers with vested interests or who are corporately funded tend to come to conclusions favorable to corporate products.[38] The CDC whistle-blowers' revelations that the non-Urabe form of MMR, MMR II were responsible for causing regressive autism, particularly among black children, comes at the end of a long campaign organized against Dr. Andrew Wakefield, who first observed regressive autism following vaccination with MMR.[39]

The recent case in the United States exposed the fact that CDC researchers hid for fourteen years research results that showed that the MMR vaccination could produce regressive autism, especially in black boys. That case seems to mirror the Urabe mumps strain MMR and the JCVI case in Britain, showing clearly that regulatory agencies that have close ties with pharmaceutical companies and governments are incapable of independent decision making on behalf of the public.

The pharmaceutical companies run the program for public health, from the first decision of what diseases are prevalent, to what novel vaccines are necessary, through the trial stages into licensing and marketing. They know now that whatever they do wrong there will be no enforceable comeback; however many children or adults they damage, they can rest easily on their academic laurels, owing their secure and well insulated lives to the industry.

It is, of course, always the argument of corporately tied academics and researchers that they adopt an independent approach to their research and their results are uninfluenced by funding. However, much deeper and more fundamental questions have to be asked to ensure independence. It is of considerable importance that the United Kingdom vaccine program is not industry-led but develops expeditiously directly from the real needs of the people and their public health environment.

So, we have to ask whether or not, rather than skirting the issue with questions about "minor" conflicts of interest, we shouldn't be asking more basic questions about vaccinations, about how necessary they are, who gains from their productive growth, and who ultimately profits from their distribution—questions about the long-term effect of vaccines, about their overall efficacy, about the industry choices to produce vaccines for an increasing number of illnesses, and, obviously, questions about the human immune system and its natural capacity to overcome illness. All that is necessary for the vaccine industry to lighten its guilt is that it puts adequate funding back into researching which children are affected adversely in the short and long-term by each vaccine.

It is not simply "independent" vaccine researchers that are needed, but a continuing long-term debate about a health system, independent from industry—questions about who runs our lives and those of our children, whether it's the government we vote in or the corporations who entwine themselves with governments.

Chapter 14

EXPONENT AND DIOXIN IN SWEDEN IN THE EARLY 2000s

Bo Walhjalt and Martin J. Walker

What I have done is absolutely uncontroversial.
I'm following the path of Science and Truth.
If something else is demanded from me, I decline.

Hans-Olov Adami.[1]

An article, critical of Lennart Hardell and his colleagues that appeared in September 2001 in *Svenska Dagbladet*,[2] seemed to suggest that *some* environmental health research, such as that critical of mobile phones, aspartame, and the presence of dioxins in breast milk should not be considered seriously. In fact, the article hinted it might be better altogether if there were a moratorium on such research—studies which, in the opinion of the authors, "lacked both professionalism and judgment" and could be "biologically bizarre" and "scientifically feeble."

Greenwashers depend upon their attacks, promoted by PR companies, not entering the academic arena or being discussed scientifically. In public attacks, they skip lightly over the science of the studies they disagree with, while making unscientific and ad hominem attacks on their authors. In December 2001, the most widely distributed Swedish daily, *Aftonbladet,* carried a full-page article, in rebuttal to the September article, revealing Hans-Olov Adami's hidden industrial ties.[3] The article was met with complete silence. This silence represents another major strategy of corporate interests; they refuse to be involved in actual scientific debate, especially in public.

The work of Hardell and colleagues has covered a number of areas, including: risks associated with mobile phones, the health dangers to workers with dioxins in herbicides, high levels of dioxin in breast milk, the carcinogenicity of vinyl chlorides, and the risk of non-Hodgkin lymphoma from exposure to pesticides.[4] Hardell and Axelson's early work on dioxin in herbicides had spectacular results in Sweden. In 1977, Hardell publicized the first cases of patients with an unusual connective-tissue tumor (sarcoma) among men who had sprayed the same herbicides as present in Agent Orange in the forests of Northern Sweden.[5] This resulted in a larger study, published in 1979.[6]

In 2001, Professor Hans-Olov Adami went to the Dioxin Conference in Korea and gave an oral presentation a few weeks after the anti-Hardell article had appeared in *Svenska Dagbladet*.[7] Adami's presentation was reported in the Swedish news media *Aftonbladet*[8] and the attacks on the research of Hardell were repeated, this time with special reference to dioxins. According to other participants at the conference, the appearance of Adami was a surprise and he was asked about the reason for his attendance. He answered that he had been employed to attend, but he did not disclose his employer.

Adami appeared together with Jack Mandel and Dimitrios Trichopoulos.[9] Together, they presented the same variation of one message: Dioxins are not associated with any health problems. It was reported in the Swedish media that the large American consulting firm Exponent had coordinated the presentations. Mandel himself appeared as an employee of Exponent—Adami and Trichopoulos, with their academic affiliations, as *independent* researchers. However, Exponent had paid for all of them and gained three presentations, two by "independent researchers." No new research was presented, in spite of that being the aim of the session, and all three men gave the same message. It was enough for the employer to create uncertainty.

In the case of dioxins, much is at stake for industry. There has been a continuous battle in the United States at the Environmental Protection Agency (EPA) since the 1970s about risk assessments of these chemicals. Reports have been presented both for and against health damage.

Dioxins[10] come from two main sources: they are a part of some pesticides and defoliants and other chemical products, and are produced when some materials are burnt. Dioxins have been a major environmental issue since the end of the US war against the Vietnamese. During the war, the US army dropped tons of it as a defoliant on Vietnamese villages.[11] As a consequence, many US and Australian personnel returned home with chemically induced illnesses.

The generational consequences of exposure to mutagenic effects of Agent Orange were felt for decades in Vietnam. After the war, Monsanto, one of the manufacturers of Agent Orange, worked hard to stop independent evidence about dioxins becoming public.[12]

Dioxins are also produced when waste is burnt and during the manufacture of chemicals containing chlorine, such as pesticides, vinyl chloride plastics, and paper products. There are over two hundred toxic waste incinerators operating in the United States; some are actually cement kilns and lightweight aggregate kilns, which burn waste like tires. These kilns are major sources of highly poisonous, persistent, bioaccumulative toxins, including dioxin.[13]

With Exponent's heavy commitment to the public relations problems of half of the two hundred toxic waste incinerators operating in the United States, while also acting for companies that produce chlorine-based chemicals, it is hardly surprising that the company has taken a continuous interest in dioxin.

The US Environmental Protection Agency (EPA) completed its first health assessment of dioxin in 1985. It found that the cancer risk to humans from dioxin exposure in North America was by far the highest defined for any chemical by any government agency anywhere in the world. The regulated industries immediately protested that this risk estimate was too high. As part of its efforts to convince the EPA of its position, the Chlorine Institute (later Chlorine Chemistry Council) convened a scientific conference on dioxin. In 1991, seemingly swayed by the conference, the EPA announced a new reassessment of the health effects of dioxin.[14]

Hardell and his colleagues in 1979 had found a clear connection between pesticides of this kind and sarcomas.[15] Their scientific report, however, was soon attacked in the Swedish daily *Svenska Dagbladet*[16] by Jonas Müntzing, a zoo physiologist from Lund, under the heading *Researcher or Doomsday Prophet*. These allegations were not scientifically based and easy to refute. In fact, over time several reports confirmed the initial findings, and in 1997, the World Health Organization (WHO) established that there was a clear link between the dioxins found in Agent Orange (TCDD) and cancer.[17]

Greenwashers, however, like elephants, have long memories and at the Dioxin fest on September 13, 2001, in one all-morning session entitled *Use of Agent Orange in Vietnam: Assessment of Impact on Veterans*, chaired by Mandel, all three epidemiologists, apparently independent but linked to Exponent, spoke about Agent Orange, manufactured by Monsanto.

The presentations by Mandel[18] and Adami[19] criticized the size and the methodology of studies that concluded that Vietnam veterans developed cancer after contact with Agent Orange. Adami used the opportunity of his paper to criticize

Hardell and his work.[20] Trichopoulos's paper concluded that there was "No evidence that dioxin is a human carcinogen."[21]

In the Exponent review *Dioxin and cancer*,[22] Adami et al. discuss case-control studies showing increased risk for cancer from exposure to dioxins. In a response to *Dagens Forskning*, Adami refers to this review because he is co-author of one of these studies. He wrote the following:

> The uncertainty about dioxin arises from the indisputable carcinogenic effect in animal trials, while the epidemiological support for a similar effect in humans has been classified as "limited" by the IARC. Also it has been remarkably hard to confirm among other things the positive findings of Swedish researchers in international epidemiological studies. Therefore I have accepted a commission to review the methodology of the Swedish studies - a commission with elements of self-criticism since I'm co-author of an early study limited to soft tissue sarcomas. My conclusion is that these studies because of methodological shortcomings do not allow conclusions about a causal relationship between dioxin and cancer.[23]

In *Dioxin and cancer*[24] there is only a short dismissal of the positive Swedish studies. It reads:

> Case-control studies of pesticide applicators have focused on soft-tissue sarcoma and malignant lymphoma. Studies on soft-tissue sarcoma may be divided into those done by Hardell and those done by others. Studies by Hardell reported very high relative risks, with the exception of the study co-authored by Adami. Even this study needs careful interpretation due to small numbers (low statistical power), multiple comparisons and possible differential misclassification of exposure.

and:

> The single case-control exception is again a study by Hardell that reported statistically significantly elevated five-fold risks.[25]

In the study coauthored by Adami, there was also an instance of five-fold elevation of risk.[26] The exception on risk elevations when Adami is involved thus seems overstated.

In the case of exposure to dioxin, the agenda is to refute cancer risks in hindsight of research already done. Then 237 cases compared to 237 controls are too few to give enough statistical power, according to the Exponent review (this is the number of cases in the study where Adami is coauthor!). Adami goes so far as to say his conclusion is that the study gives no guidance on the issue of causality.

While Exponent describes itself as the biggest and best independent research organization that resolves corporate problems as they occur in the path of globalization, it might more accurately be described as a hired gun for corporate science which attacks and hopefully knocks out any science that hampers its clients "global spread—practical solutions to problems that affect our clients' ability to conduct business with toxic products globally."

Originally called "The Failure Group"—an unbelievable start-up name for a crisis management company—it changed its name in 1998 to Exponent. From then on, its growth has been considerable through 2002 and 2005, when it opened offices in China, to the present day when Exponent offers more than ninety different disciplines through a network of over twenty US and five international locations.[27]

According to their website, their staff totals over nine hundred and includes more than 425 PhDs and MDs. What the Exponent website does not say is that the basic tenet of its work in the field of health is always from the corporation's perspective and the information of health damage or toxicity which is being refuted, from the perspective of workers or citizens.

Exponent, a company deeply involved in producing good news studies about dioxin, was—at the turn of the century—one of a new brand of companies that tried to manipulate the public perception of social and environmental problems encountered by big corporations. While older industries founded "Foundations" or "Institutes" set up by PR companies,[28] which laundered information and research data for their parent industry, Exponent, superficially unrelated to any particular industry, retains experts, commissions research, and works with lobby groups, solving problems of public perception of confidence-losing products and industries.

In its publicity, Exponent cites its early problem-solving and PR work in relation to the grounding of the Exxon Valdez (1989) and its massive oil spillage. Exponent was then a middle-sized company with annual revenue of around $100 million. The directors of Exponent, still a relatively cohesive group, had interests in systems analysis, PR, management consultancy, investment and software systems, genome research, and business failure analysis.

Exponent got lucky in 1998, when it acquired a lucrative contract to solve battlefield communications problems for the US army. The outcome of this was the "Land Warrior" system, which led to new technological assessment contracts for the US army. Obtaining these contracts might have been helped by Company Director Leslie G. Denend, who served as a special assistant to the president for National Security Affairs and was an advisor to the Chairman of the Joint Chiefs of Staff before joining Exponent. In the area of major PR for the chemical companies, an involvement with the US government is, if not obligatory, extremely useful.[29]

Exponent has been particularly involved in the technological, regulatory, and PR aspects of hazardous waste production management, assisting clients, both technically and with image and regulatory management, on almost half of the two hundred–odd incinerator sites in America. The waste industry is intimately linked to problems with dioxins which are a by-product of burning waste and which have stirred the ire of many local communities in the United States.[30, 31]

Besides toxic exposure and risk assessment, the company also gives support when client companies become the subject of toxic tort, class action, and general litigation from consumers, campaigns, or environmental organizations.

Exponent is involved in all the post-industrial areas of health risk, such as organophosphate pesticides and PCBs. To make sure that it was on top of endocrine-disrupting chemicals,[32] it formed an Endocrine Disruptor Focus Group, which has ensured its ability to lobby the Endocrine Disruption Screening and Testing Advisory Committee (EDSTAC) set up by the EPA. The chemical companies have always panicked over this issue, touching as it does on more than eighty-six thousand chemicals used by industry.

Dr. Mandel joined Exponent in 1999 from the University of Minnesota, where he had been a faculty member for almost twenty-five years. From 1999 to 2002, he was a Group Vice President at Exponent, directing operations in Health and Epidemiology, and Environmental Science Practices. He rejoined Exponent in 2010 after a university break.[33] During his tenure at the University, in the Division of Environmental and Occupational Health, Mandel served as a consultant to industry, professional associations, and governmental agencies.

One aspect of Mandel's work at Exponent is illustrated by the company's intervention at National Semiconductor in Greenock, Scotland, in the 1990s. Following complaints of serious ill health among women "cleanroom" workers, an energetic campaign, PHASE II (People for Health and Safety in Electronics), begun by trade unionist Jim McCourt, managed to attract a Health and Safety Executive (HSE) team to Scotland.

The HSE report, which looked only at cases of cancer rather than the wider range of serious illnesses, was not able to rule out the possibility of work-related causes of some cancers at the plant. The report found that the incidence of certain types of cancer was higher than in the general population, including eleven cases of lung cancer in women, more than twice as many as expected; three cases of stomach cancer in women, four to five times as many as expected; and three deaths from brain cancer among men, about four times the expected level.

As part of their strategy to defeat PHASE II, National Semiconductor called in Exponent, who sent Mandel to Scotland.[34] The company trumpeted Mandel's off-the-cuff analysis as complementing the report carried out by the HSE:

> The company employed a renowned epidemiologist to carry out a parallel study to the HSE report. Dr. Jack Mandel looked at the cases of eleven women who had developed lung cancer. Dr. Mandel made the observation that two of the women had developed the tumor within ten years of commencing work at NSUK in Greenock. Given that the latency in tumors of this kind is typically fifteen to twenty years, he suggests that this indicates the cancer was not related to the workplace at NSUK.[35]

Jim McCourt, angered by Exponent's public relations exercise, pointed out, on behalf of the women workers, that Mandel's "study" had concluded that because two women with cancer had possibly not contracted cancer while working at the plant, there was no problem there with working conditions and ill-health at the plant.

Exponent, representing a range of groups, organizations and companies and their hired epidemiologists, give evidence—always in favor—about a variety of suspected carcinogens besides dioxins. The Halogenated Solvents Industry Alliance, Inc. (HSIA), an Exponent client, supported by four main industrial groups including Dow Chemicals, "sponsors" the chemical trichloroethylene. Through Exponent, the HSIA commissioned Hans-Olov Adami, Dimitrios Trichopoulos and Jack Mandel to present research on trichloroethylene.

Both the Report on Voluntary Children's Chemical Evaluation Program (VCCEP),[36] set up in 1999 and the Report on Carcinogens 2001, an annual publication by the National Toxicology Program, have taken evidence on trichloroethylene (TCE), which is mainly used as a degreaser for metal parts and a solvent component in adhesives, lubricants, paints and varnishes, etc.[37]

There can be no doubt about the HSIA view of the carcinogenicity of trichloroethylene. In a White Paper published in 1995, they draw the following conclusions, having referred to (but not referenced) only three pieces of research. "The substance has been demonstrated by well controlled epidemiological studies not to be associated with any increased risk of cancer in exposed humans."

One group concerned about procedural bias in VCCEP, *EPA Stop Stalling*,[38] published its own paper on trichloroethylene, using citations from the Hazardous Substances Data Bank. The paper cited hundreds of peer-reviewed studies, human voluntary experiments and autopsy findings that record a formidable range of damages to the human system from short, medium and long-term exposure.

The "Report on Carcinogens" (RoC) is published by the National Toxicology Program, a US government agency based in Research Triangle Park. The report, previously called the "Annual Report on Carcinogens," is prepared as a legal obligation. In the "Ninth Report on Carcinogens,"[39] compiled by the National Toxicology Program, trichloroethylene is listed for the first time under the category of "Reasonably anticipated to be a human carcinogen," and cited as being associated with cancer of the liver and biliary tract, with non-Hodgkin lymphoma and cancer of the kidneys.

The HSIA agreed in 2001 to sponsor the scientific research, including toxicity testing and tests on rodents,[40] on trichloroethylene for the VCCEP. The fact that papers on different chemicals were to be presented for peer review was heralded at a move toward independent evaluation. The EPA used a private organization, Toxicology Excellence for Risk Assessment (TERA), to gather the peer reviewers together and allot them papers. The pool of 108 peer reviewers contains no less than five officers of Exponent.

Adami and Trichopoulos's evidence to the RoC, in favor of trichloroethylene, is in the form of a three-page letter. Five documents are cited, two of them authored by Mandel and one of them by Paul Dugard, of the HSIA. Adami and Trichopoulos's review of eight recent occupational cohort studies, carried out over the previous decade, concludes that there is no evidence that TCE causes kidney cancer.

The 1994 Public Review Draft on Dioxin, released by the EPA in 1994, again concluded that dioxin posed a serious cancer risk and that the average American had a level of dioxin in their body that could cause adverse health effects.[41] The massive community campaigning by parents led to the review being followed by a 150-day comment period and eleven public meetings around the country to receive oral and written comments. In addition to this public review, each document was reviewed by EPA's Science Advisory Board (SAB).

Dioxin-generating companies launched an aggressive campaign to stall the release of the latest report. The attack began with a peer-reviewed report, led by industry scientists who rejected several chapters in the draft document, forcing the agency to rewrite them and delaying the process of finalizing the report.[42]

In June 2000, when the EPA did finally publish its 1994 reassessment, it found even stronger links between exposure to dioxin and adverse impacts on human health. One of the EPA's key findings was that the risk of getting cancer from dioxin exposure was ten times higher than reported in 1994.[43] From June 2000, the industry intensified its efforts still further to challenge and discredit the scientific findings in the report and to further stall its release.

The EPA scheduled the publication of its final dioxin reassessment for early in 2001. By mid-2001, however, the reassessment had not been finished. In May 2001, a panel of scientists urged the EPA to release the long-awaited report. Environmental groups, angry that the draft report had been unfinished for ten years, suggested that the process had been constantly delayed by industry groups.[44]

At one of the last meetings before the release of the report, the EPA's Science Advisory Board (SAB) dioxin review subcommittee met in November 2000 to review the EPA's dioxin reassessment—members of the SAB are presumed to be neutral scientific experts and are subject to US government Conflict of Interest (COI) regulations. The statutes governing these regulations are "aimed at preventing individuals from (knowingly or unknowingly) bringing inappropriate influence to bear on Agency decisions which might affect the financial interests of those individuals, their family members, and/or the organizations which employ them."[45]

SAB members and consultants are required to reveal: Research conducted on the matter. Previous pronouncements made on the matter. Interests of the employer in the matter. Any other financial interests they might have in the matter. Other links such as research grants from parties—including the EPA—that would be affected by the matter. None of the disclosure statements of the November meeting panel members included the above information. Research done by the Center for Health, Environment, and Justice's *Stop Dioxin Exposure Campaign (CHEJ)* showed, however, that members of this panel were strongly tied to dioxin-generating companies: in fact a third of the committee had received funding from ninety-one dioxin-polluting corporations.[46]

Exponent was represented by Dennis Paustenbach, a vice president of the company. Exponent prepared comments on the latest draft of the dioxin reassessment on behalf of Chemical Land Holdings, Inc. and Occidental Chemical Corporation. The document essentially repeated the chemical industry's arguments on the lack of linkage between dioxin and cancer and other adverse health effects. These comments were sent to the subcommittee well in advance of the November review meeting.[47] Paustenbach however failed to mention Exponent's actions.

The chemical companies of course characterized the reassessment as quixotic and constantly changing, making it look as if the EPA, rather than the chemical companies, had dragged out the process and kept moving the goal posts.

In October 2000, Jack Mandel spoke at a one-day International Society of Regulatory Toxicology and Pharmacology (ISRTP) Conference entitled *EPA'S Characterization of Dioxin Risks: Background Dioxin Exposures Pose a Human Health Threat?* Mandel's talk was entitled *Dioxin and Cancer.* ISRTP is an organization wholly supported by chemical companies and the American Chemistry Council. The Conference was supported by the Chlorine Chemistry Council, an Exponent client and the leading player in the battle against EPA regulations of dioxin. The closed talks were later published in the *Journal of Regulatory Toxicology and Pharmacology*, which the ISRTP refers to as their "peer-reviewed" journal.

In his talk, Mandel made the case for dioxin as a benign chemical and took the opportunity to personally attack Lennart Hardell. The attack echoed the one mounted by Sir Richard Doll a decade earlier:[48]

> The early studies (case-control studies of soft tissue sarcoma) by Hardell found very high risk estimates which have never been replicated. These studies, however, had significant methodological problems. They violated almost every principle of good epidemiological methods.

This statement went far beyond scientific evidence and clearly showed the lack of understanding of epidemiological practice. In contrast, the Institute of Medicine in the United States in a review of health effects of Agent Orange used in Vietnam concluded, regarding the Hardell group studies, the following:

> Although these studies have been criticized, the committee feels that there is insufficient justification to discount the consistent pattern of elevated risks, and the clearly described and sound methods employed.[49]

Other speakers at the conference included Rory B. Conolly, at that time a senior scientist at the then called CIIT, an industry-based institute;[50] Michael Gough, PhD, current vice president of the International Society of Regulatory Toxicology and Pharmacology; Clifford T. "Kip" Howlett Jr., vice president of the American Chemistry Council (ACC) and executive director of its Chlorine Chemistry Council (CCC).

Companies like Exponent are the face of the future—large companies whose sole objective is the strategic defense of corporation profits. Wherever they are able they crowd out and diminish the voice of independent researchers. They consolidate corporate interests in the presentation of science, PR, and what are essentially illusions and tricks involved in publicizing only partial information.

Chapter 15

BURYING THE EVIDENCE— THE ROLE OF BRITAIN'S HEALTH AND SAFETY EXECUTIVE IN PROLONGING THE OCCUPATIONAL CANCER EPIDEMIC

Rory O'Neill, Simon Pickvance, Andrew Watterson

If the various preventive measures outlined were effectively applied, it is likely that an appreciable degree of preventive control of numerous occupational cancer hazards might be obtained.

—William Hueper

This chapter will explore how and why authorities and industries are failing to acknowledge or deal effectively with an epidemic of work-related cancers in the United Kingdom. Industrial and commercial companies and governmental agencies have sometimes either ignored or covered up this major public health catastrophe. The chapter uses a number of case studies, for example from the chemicals, metals, and electronics industries, to explore how this has happened, at what human cost, and how workers themselves have been able to expose the failings of employers, politicians, researchers, and the civil service to protect them. Government has underestimated and continues to underestimate the exposed population, the risks faced as a result of those exposures, and the potential for prevention. Social inequalities in occupational cancer risk have been downplayed, as manual workers and lower employment grades are most affected.

There is also a greater likelihood these groups will experience multiple exposures to work-related carcinogens. The largely uninvestigated and non-prioritized risk to women workers has been neglected and the Health and Safety Executive (HSE) currently has neither a requirement nor a strategy for reducing the numbers and volumes of cancer-causing substances, processes, and environments at work. The result is that the United Kingdom faces at least twenty thousand, and possibly in excess of forty thousand, new cases of work-related cancer every year, leading to thousands of deaths and an annual cost to the economy of between £29.5bn and £59bn. This paper outlines key flaws in the HSE's approach and makes recommendations to address effectively the United Kingdom's occupational cancer crisis.

The UK government's workplace safety agency, the Health and Safety Executive, greatly underestimates the number of workers exposed to a workplace cancer risk and the numbers developing occupational cancer, while seriously underestimating the attributable fraction of cancers due to several cancers when compared with other countries such as France.[1] Although the HSE has organized closed seminars and workshops recently on occupational cancer and is exploring policy options, it still presents findings of a 1981 US study as "the best overall estimate available."[2] This is the basis of its estimate of just six thousand occupational cancer deaths each year. Yet the cost of one occupational cancer death has been put at £2.46m (US$5million). Even with the HSE estimate of just six thousand occupational cancer deaths a year, this amounts to a total annual cost of almost £15bn (approximately US$30bn). Estimates included in this paper suggest the real toll and financial cost in Great Britain could be at least double this.[3] Preventing just one hundred of these occupational cancer deaths each year would more than offset the entire HSE annual budget.

The findings of HSE's preferred source, the 1981 Doll/Peto report,[4] have been disputed[5] and described as "discredited," with authors criticizing both errors in methodology that led to a substantial underestimate of the true incidence[6] and the pro-industry leanings of the lead author.[7] Recent analyses suggest the real number of work-related cancer deaths in Great Britain each year is at least twelve thousand cases and could be as high as twenty-four thousand.[8] New figures from the International Labor Organization support claims that the occupational cancer rate in developed nations is substantially higher than HSE's estimate.[9] Basing official policies on Doll/Peto estimates has resulted in a chronic failure to secure either the resources or the priority required for meaningful preventive action.

Exposure to a workplace cancer risk is not a minor concern affecting few people. The European Union's CAREX database of occupational exposures to carcinogens concluded the following: "According to the preliminary estimates, there were circa five million workers (22 percent of the employed) exposed to the agents covered by CAREX in Great Britain in 1990 to 1993. The number of exposures was circa seven million."[10] Other recent studies have suggested the number of workers at risk may in fact be increasing. Even by the CAREX estimate, over a fifth of the UK workforce has been exposed to possible human carcinogens and for these workers most of the resultant cancers will emerge only in a couple of decades or more.

Where HSE acknowledges there is a risk, its new estimates of the at-risk working population seem designed to downplay the problem. In the case of cancer-causing beryllium, for example, HSE in 2003 said 250 workers in the United Kingdom were estimated to be continuously exposed and one thousand workers occasionally exposed to "very low concentrations of beryllium or beryllium oxide." Its 2007 estimates say there are fewer than one thousand exposed in fewer than one hundred workplaces yet acknowledges that beryllium use is increasing. HSE also ignores exposures to beryllium in the scrap metal and recycling industries. Even collectors of old radio sets take a more concerned stance, flagging up risks of beryllium exposures when dismantling radio sets.

HSE's under-resourced inspectorate is not capable of ensuring adequate safety oversight of Britain's workplaces. This was highlighted by the recent "world's largest" outbreak of extrinsic allergic alveolitis and occupational asthma, in which over one hundred workers at Powertrain in Birmingham developed serious and chronic occupational lung diseases, despite the risks being well-established over a decade earlier.[11] The poorly controlled agent responsible, metalworking fluid, is also an occupational cancer risk.[12]

Under-reporting of conditions including chrome ulcers—a warning sign of exposures that could lead to chromium-related lung cancers—indicate that HSE's intelligence on many occupational carcinogen exposures is lacking. The proliferation of small firms means more workers are likely now to be working in firms with inadequate systems to recognize and deal with risks, and will remain almost entirely off the HSE's radar. Workplaces enforced by HSE can expect an inspection only once every thirteen years, or three times in a person's working lifetime. This is about half the inspection frequency of seven years ago.[13] At the same time, as the HSE claims great progress on occupational health,[14] the occupational health staff employed by HSE have shrunk to such small numbers that former employees seriously doubt if the group can function properly at all[15] and their capacity to address the challenges of occupational cancer appears very restricted.

HSE initiatives to address occupational cancers are a small component of an HSE disease reduction program, which is in turn a small part of the HSE illness reduction program, which is itself only a small part of the HSE Fit3 program. This is not enough. The HSE plan to inspect only where there are cancer "exposures." This assumes knowledge of where carcinogens are, yet there is no basis for that assumption within the HSE, and their inspections will not normally be sufficient to identify all carcinogens, especially if deficient Material Safety Data Sheets are used.

In an HSE presentation posted in 2007 on an online silica forum, the HSE said findings from its surveys conducted in 2006 and 2007 in the stonemasonry, brickmaking, construction, and quarrying sectors showed it had grossly underestimated the size of the over-exposed population and the levels of crystalline silica encountered in the workplace. In stonemasonry, for example, both the HSE and the industry had estimated no workers were exposed to above 0.1mg/ m^3. In fact, the survey findings suggest 3,150 workers could be exposed above that level, and 1,425 were potentially exposed to 0.3mg/ m^3 or more of respirable crystalline silica.

The HSE's estimates of those at risk of, and developing, occupational cancers fail to take adequate account of the rapid increase in the numbers and volumes of substances used in the workplace. About one hundred thousand chemicals are in industrial use, an estimated thirty thousand used in the European Union in high volumes (manufactured or imported in volumes over 1 tonne).

The UK Chemical Industries Association in 2006 reported that over the last decade the chemical industry had grown more than five times faster than the average for all industries. It noted "the chemical industry accounts for 2 percent of UK GDP and 11 percent of manufacturing industry's gross value added. Turnover, which includes the sales of merchandised goods (e.g., chemicals imported and then resold), was estimated at £50 billion in 2003. Over the same period sales of domestically produced chemicals were £34 billion."

The industry's own figures show that in 2004, while almost 50 percent of chemical industry sites had implemented environmental management systems, fewer than 15 percent had equivalent health and safety management systems.[16] The UK industry employs directly about 230,000 workers.

Chemical usage is not just an issue for those in primary manufacturing or processing. Vulnerable workers, for example hairdressers and cleaners, use highly toxic chemicals routinely and work largely unseen by statutory safety authorities and without occupational health guidance or access to health and safety expertise.

When assessing the impact of work cancers on the working population, it is also important to note that almost all the risk is concentrated in a relatively small segment of the workforce. Work-related cancer is far more common in blue-collar workers—there is an undeniable correlation between employment in lower status jobs and an increased risk.[17] Studies have found, for example, that 40 percent of the lung and bladder cancer cases in certain industrial groups are caused by occupational exposures.[18] French records published in 2005 found one in eight workers was exposed to carcinogens at work, but that the figure was 25 percent for manual workers and just 3 percent for managers.[19]

The 1998 CAREX report for Great Britain[20] concluded workplace exposures to carcinogens were restricted to about one-fifth of the working population. If the occupational cancer risk was equal across the population, based on HSE's figure of six thousand deaths a year, this would equate to 1 percent of all deaths being caused by occupational cancers in any given year. However, the responsible exposures are limited to a much smaller group who bear most of the risk, suggesting that 5 percent or more of deaths in this group could be caused by occupational cancers.

Nor are all the exposed workers in big firms with occupational health facilities, health and safety professionals, and sophisticated control systems. Each year members of the UK Chemical Business Association (CBA) distribute more than 2.5 million tons of chemicals. CBA estimates that 95 percent of Europe's chemical industry is composed of small- and medium-sized enterprises.

Cancers in workers in small firms are unlikely to be attributed to work unless they are otherwise rare cancers, and the workers are unlikely to have access to informed occupational safety or medical advice. Research on small firms has shown that they have very limited understanding of the risks of hazardous substances and relevant legislation, and that HSE guidance often does not reach them.[21] A 2006 UK Federation of Small Businesses report, "Health matters: A small business perspective," reported barely one in twenty survey respondents (6.5 percent) provided access to occupational health services. The FSB report concluded small businesses "need incentives to enable them to promote healthy workplaces and provide occupational health support to their staff."[22] So, there is still ineffective health and safety management in small- and medium-sized enterprises, insufficient staff in local authorities and HSE to check such workplaces and no possibility that effective cancer prevention policies and practices can be introduced under the current system.

The UK strategy fails to take adequate account of complex workplace exposures—multiple exposures at one time and multiple changing exposures through a working lifetime. The use of more substances in higher volumes in a greatly increased number of products and processes creates the potential for highly complex working environments with complex, combined exposures to workplace carcinogens or substances that could increase vulnerability to carcinogens. A general dusty environment, for example, can overwhelm the body's mucociliary clearance system, allowing easier passage of airborne substances into the body. Existing exposure standards and control policies do not reflect this total carcinogen dose nor the complexity of some mixed workplace exposures, which could create a gross exposure greatly in excess of the exposure limit for any single substance.

The number of jobs per working lifetime has increased markedly in the last thirty years, with most workers now having ten or more jobs in the period between joining the workforce and retirement. New technologies and processes mean workplace exposures will in many instances change markedly throughout a working lifetime.

As Great Britain has no occupational cancer registry or systematic measures to ascertain or register exposures, HSE does not know who has been exposed, to what, where, or when. This means only a minority of cancers—generally otherwise rare and work-specific—stand any chance of being recognized. This has implications for both prevention and for workers' welfare. Potentially hazardous conditions will not be recognized or addressed and victims of occupational cancer are unlikely to be compensated or receive a timely diagnosis and treatment.

INACTION ON KNOWN RISKS

Even where the Health and Safety Executive recognizes a workplace exposure may cause cancer, this is frequently overlooked in its practical guidance. HSE's metalworking fluid web pages[23] omit any mention of the occupational cancer risk from the general health risks section and guidance for occupational health advisers, and treat exposure as a general hazard "to be prevented where reasonably practicable" rather than a cancer hazard where far more stringent stipulations should apply. Recent evidence suggests there is even more reason for HSE to issue an explicit cancer warning. A Harvard University report noted that existing studies substantially underestimate the metalworking fluids cancer risk.[24]

When medium-density fiberboard (MDF)—a composite creating potential for exposure to two recognized carcinogens during manufacture or machining— became the subject of a recent safety controversy, HSE entirely backed the industry line on potential health problems, failing to acknowledge the cancer risk.[25] It did not modify this position when formaldehyde was upgraded in 2004[26] to the International Agency for Research on Cancer's top cancer risk category, Group 1.[27] Wood dust was already rated as an IARC Group 1 carcinogen.

On other substances, HSE has trailed behind other national regulatory agencies in recognizing a workplace cancer risk in at least one instance actively promoting the use of a cancer-causing substance. In February 2000, chemical manufacturer Dow failed in a bid to stop Australia's chemical standards body, NICNAS, labeling the common industrial solvent trichloroethylene as a carcinogen and mutagen. It was two years before HSE issued an equivalent warning.

HSE's 2002 alert said employers should consider using an alternative solvent or cleaning process or, if this was not possible, enclosing the degreasing process as far as possible. Prior to this, HSE had for a decade—including the two years in which Australian workers had been warned of the cancer risks—been explicitly recommending trichloroethylene use as an "ozone friendly" alternative to the more worker-friendly trichloroethane. UK unions in the 1970s had run successful campaigns to get rid of trichloroethylene, in some cases negotiating trichloroethane as a safer alternative. Alternative processes, friendly both to the environment and the workforce, had been available when HSE was recommending trichloroethylene use.

In 1988, NIOSH recommended that perchloroethylene be labeled a potential occupational carcinogen,[28] yet as late as 2000, the HSE was producing leaflets that did not mention any cancer link with exposure to this substance in dry cleaning.[29]

Many important workplace cancers are entirely overlooked by HSE. Breast cancers are not treated as a serious work-related risk to be addressed in HSE's strategy, despite evidence that large numbers could be at risk.[30, 31]

HSE also misses entire categories of workers known to have an elevated cancer risk. Its list of targeted work cancer risks does not include "painting." However, painters comprise a large occupational group classified as facing a Group 1 cancer risk by the International Agency for Research on Cancer, the top risk rating.[32]

On wood dust, another Group 1 IARC carcinogen, HSE says this on the cancer risk: "Established for cancer of the nasal cavity or sinuses in cabinet makers and machinists exposed to wood dust." In fact, wood dust is a nasopharyngeal cancer and possibly lung cancer risk,[33] and has been identified in almost *all* woodworking occupations, not just for cabinet makers and machinists.

Other occupational groups recognized elsewhere and in the literature as facing an elevated risk for a range of cancers are also ignored. This includes the increased risk for non-Hodgkin's lymphoma and other cancers in farm workers and a range of cancers in firefighters, including primary site brain cancer, primary site bladder cancer, primary site kidney cancer, primary non-Hodgkin's lymphoma, primary site ureter cancer, primary site colorectal cancer, and primary leukemia.[34] Firefighters in Canadian provinces such as Manitoba, Alberta, Saskatchewan, British Columbia, and Nova Scotia are already entitled to compensation for work-related cancers (TUC Risks May 2007; Ontario Ministry of Labour news release May 4, 2007). No such measures are on the horizon in the United Kingdom and there is little or no evidence that HSE is actively working to address the risks of this occupational group and recognize such cancers.

Even for substances like asbestos, HSE limits its analysis primarily to the risk of lung cancer and mesothelioma, despite known associations with many other cancers. Cancers including gliomas, head and neck cancers,[35] breast and hematopoietic cancers, all linked to work exposures, are among those largely or entirely ignored.

HSE is overly reliant on data from the EU and IARC. For example, its briefings on benzene, cadmium, and diesel exhaust are dangerously outdated, and greatly underestimate the potential cancer risk. Nor has HSE practical systems to review and act upon new information in a timely manner or to revise assessments.[36,37] For instance, Germany and Denmark recognize bladder cancer in the metal industries, where exposures to cadmium and epoxy resins may occur. Denmark officially notes the use of azo dyes by painters: a link not made in the United Kingdom despite recognizing the hazards to printers. The Sheffield Occupational Health Project (now SOHAS) identified a series of bladder cancer cases where exposure to cadmium had occurred, ranging from smelting to TV repairs and cutlery work.

On a rare occasion when HSE revisited the occupational cancer estimates, they were revised down. The ratio of asbestos-related lung cancers to mesotheliomas are now lower than 1 to 1—a 2005 HSE paper[38] puts the ratio of asbestos lung cancers to mesotheliomas at between 2/3 and 1 to 1—much lower than many other estimates. The authors acknowledge their figure will miss some cancers because it underestimates the effects of chrysotile (white asbestos), which has been the dominant exposure since 1970. And their analysis only includes cancer deaths up to the age of seventy-four, whereas many asbestos-related lung cancer deaths occur in older ex-workers. While many observers believe the ratio of asbestos-related lung cancers to mesothelioma may be closing, as fewer workers are experiencing the very high exposures that were linked to much higher numbers of lung cancers, and a drop in smoking will reduce those caused by the synergy between smoking and asbestos exposure, HSE's new estimate is significantly lower than generally cited figures.

The HSE data sources are also inadequate. Its chemical-by-chemical approach relies on the limited work already done. Yet, relatively few chemicals in use in the workplace have been thoroughly assessed for chronic health risks, fewer still providing sufficient satisfactory data to be listed as a human cancer risk by either IARC or the EU. Many substances used in the workplace and likely to present a substantial cancer risk are assumed safe as a result of HSE's approach, whereas lack of data means no adequate assessment of the cancer risk has been undertaken. This is not a basis for a protective approach, and leaves workers facing relatively uncontrolled exposures to substances that may, as data accumulate, be proven to be cancer-causing.

Further, HSE's exposure standards for known carcinogens fall below the levels expected elsewhere. For example, HSE's assessment that at an exposure level for chromium of 10 μg/m³ "no further risk reduction measures are needed" would be completely unacceptable in Germany, where this no requirement to act stipulation would only be accepted if the exposure level was a tenth of this, at 1 μg/m³, and then only in the short-term. Long-term, no further action would only be required if the airborne chromium levels were 0.1 μg/m³, one-hundredth the UK level.

The HSE's approach is entirely about limited controls on a limited number of carcinogens in a limited number of circumstances. It does nothing to reduce the overall number or volumes of carcinogens at use in workplaces.

A more responsible approach would be to set targets for "sunsetting" the most potent carcinogens, and to introduce a Toxics Use Reduction approach to ensure safer methods and processes are used where they are effective.[39] Toxics Use Reduction is an approach that has not only been used effectively, but has also received strong support from industry.[40] Such forward-thinking strategies are supported elsewhere. The Canadian Strategy for Cancer Control (CSCC), a coalition of cancer prevention, health service and other bodies, has made a public stand in favor of this "primary prevention" of occupational cancer.[41]

Many researchers have warned that failure to act promptly on early warnings has in the past led to entirely avoidable epidemics of occupational disease, including workplace asbestos, benzene and radiation cancers.[42]

Large groups running a small risk from exposure to workplace carcinogens still amount to a large number of affected workers, a public health burden entirely missed by HSE. For example, a report this year identified a five-fold increase in breast cancer in developed industrial regions was in part due to exposure to industrial chemicals.[43]

Equally unlikely to be classified as occupational are the many lung cancers caused by exposure to "nuisance" dusts, for example general building or foundry dusts. Lung cancer is the standout cancer killer, but is overwhelmingly attributed to smoking. Latest evidence suggests that not all these "smoking" lung cancer deaths are caused by smoking. As smoking levels decline in developed nations, a much larger than expected number of "never smoked" lung cancers are being seen. Occupation is a clear contributory factor to these cancers.

A *Journal of Oncology* paper in 2007, for example, concluded one-in-five lung cancers in females and almost one-in-ten in men occur in people who have never smoked.[44] That would equate to approaching three thousand non-smoking lung cancer deaths in UK women each year, and two thousand deaths in men.

Obviously, workplace exposures would be a cofactor in the lung cancers experienced by the smoking group too—smoking does not make you immune to occupational lung carcinogens. The evidence suggests it does in fact greatly increase the likelihood of getting a work-related cancer.

In the great majority of cases, HSE is failing to provide workers and former workers information about the cancer risk posed by their past and current exposures to workplace carcinogens. This has three main detrimental effects.

Firstly, these workers are not in a position to make informed decisions about their working environment and seek improvements. Secondly, they are not in a position to seek the health surveillance necessary to improve the chances of an early cancer diagnosis and therefore treatment. Survival rates in the United Kingdom for some of the major cancer killers, for example lung cancer, are low compared to other developed nations. This is in a large part due to late diagnosis.

Finally, lack of awareness and support means most workers developing occupational cancers receive no compensation or related benefits, even for extremely well-known causes of work cancer like asbestos. For example, in 2002, 1,862 people died from the asbestos cancer mesothelioma, but only 54 percent of those people received Industrial Injuries Disablement Benefit. However, far fewer still receive this benefit for asbestos-related lung cancer. Despite it being accepted that there is at least one lung cancer death for each mesothelioma death—and this is a conservative estimate—only sixty lung cancer payments were made in 2001 in the United Kingdom. Contrast this with Germany, where 767 benefit payments were made for asbestos-related lung cancer and 665 benefits for mesothelioma in 2001.[45] Only some twenty people per year received Industrial Disablement Benefit for occupational bladder cancer despite this being a condition which, even by HSE's conservative estimates, affects several hundred workers every year.

Most occupational cancers occur in older workers, so there is also a compelling case for health agencies other than HSE to greatly increase the resources available to provide advice, screening, and support for retired workers at risk of developing work-related cancers.

MISTAKES ON SHORT LATENCIES

The HSE makes an assumption that occupational cancers have a long latency period, with today's cancers the result of exposures occurring a working generation ago. This has two damaging effects. It allows HSE to assume today's cancers are the result of historic working conditions, much worse than those in workplaces today, while also allowing it to downplay the risk facing the current working generation.

For example, on wood dust, the HSE says: "There is a latency of twenty years between exposure and tumor development." However, many cancers including those caused by wood dust can have much shorter latency periods. For wood dust, latency can be under ten years. The HSE also says the mode of action is "uncertain." In fact the occupational cancer risk from wood dust is as a result of inhalation, and is therefore easily preventable.

In Germany and at the Sheffield Occupational Health Advisory Service in the UK, there is a recognition that minimum latency and exposure times for occupational cancers may sometimes be much shorter than the UK system recognizes (see below).[46]

MINIMAL LATENCIES FOR OCCUPATIONAL CANCERS IN THE GERMAN COMPENSATION SYSTEM.[47]

Agent	Site	Minimum exposure time (yrs)	Minimum latency (yrs)
Chromium	Lung, nasal, URT	2	4
Arsenic	Lung, nasal, URT	0.5	3
Aromatic amines	Bladder, UT	0.25	1
Halogenated hydrocarbons (VCM etc.)	Liver, Bladder, UT	5	11
Benzene, Benzene homologs, Styrene	Leukemia	0.5	2
Halogenated alkyl, aryl or alkyl aryl oxides	Lung, UT, skin, nasal, larynx, stomach, etc.	2	8
Ionizing radiation	Lung, leukemia, skin, Mesothelioma	<1	10
Asbestos	Lung	<0.25	8
Asbestos	Mesothelioma	1 day	15
Nickel	Lung, nasal, URT	1	6
Wood dust	Nasal adenocarcinoma	5	8
Soot, crude paraffin, tar anthracene, pitch and related compounds	Skin cancer	3	4

HSE makes unprovable assumptions about improved occupational hygiene standards and risks, and about the willingness and capability of firms to recognize and control risks. HSE's own studies have shown many chemical companies had, at least until the mid- to late-1990s, little or no knowledge of their duties under the chemical control regulations and most were unaware of relevant occupational exposure limits. At the time, research suggested many products, including potentially carcinogenic dyes, were being imported without adequate warnings.[48]

Assumptions about exposure levels and risk based solely on exposures in the workplace underestimate the total toxic load many workers experience. Workers can be exposed at work and in the general environment. Women exposed to cancer-causing endocrine-disrupting chemicals at work, for example, will frequently have additional exposures to substances acting in the same way outside of work. Again, there is little evidence that such exposures are yet built into the HSE assessments.

Similarly, farm workers exposed to pesticides may face household, environmental and dietary exposures to the same or related chemicals. A 2007 study found agricultural workers exposed to high levels of pesticides have a raised risk of brain tumors. All agricultural workers exposed to pesticides had a slightly elevated brain tumor risk, but the paper reported the risk was more than doubled for those exposed to the highest levels. The study, published online in the journal *Occupational and Environmental Medicine* in May 2007, also found a significant risk among people who used pesticides on houseplants.[49]

CHANGING INDUSTRY

HSE's chemical-by-chemical approach fails to take account of the rapid evolution of industry and industrial processes. Evidence of an emerging cancer problem in the microelectronics industry[50] has not elicited prompt, precautionary action from HSE, a failing that has attracted international criticism.[51] Similarly, while HSE, at least theoretically, advocates a precautionary approach in the fast emerging nanotechnology industry, in practice there is little understanding of the hazards posed or how they might be controlled. The industry, meanwhile, largely free from the attention of the resource-depleted enforcement agency, is growing at a startling pace.[52]

The problem is not limited to those employed in new industries, but also has an impact on the much greater number affected by the changing nature of existing jobs or job functions. More workers performing routine tasks are exposed to chemicals as a result of the tendency to opt for quick chemical fixes applied by poorly skilled workers as an alternative to labor- and resource-intensive skilled labor. For example, many municipal authorities are opting to use pesticides for routine weed control as an alternative to employing skilled parks and garden staff.

Over three million workers in the United Kingdom work in excess of forty--eight hours per week, with the potential for work-time exposures considerably in excess of those assumed under existing occupational exposure limits, based on the standard working week. In addition, new age discrimination regulations and government moves to raise the retirement age mean many workers are likely to have more years of exposure to potential risk. The United Kingdom already has one of Europe's highest proportions of older workers in work.[53] The changing nature of employment—long hours, frequent changes of job, frequent changes of job task, irregular hours, and shift work all impact occupational cancer risks. Breast and other cancers have been linked to shift work, something that HSE staff is aware of, but, to date, no significant policies or practice recommendations have emerged from the organization.

Women are now better represented in the workforce and consequently are likely to spend longer in the workforce and do a much wider range of jobs. Since 1975, men's employment has declined from around nine out of ten to eight out of ten (79 percent) for men of working age (sixteen to sixty-four). At the same time, women's employment has increased from around six out of ten to seven out of ten (70 percent) for women of working age (sixteen to fifty-nine).

The HSE's approach fails to take adequate account of the increasing participation of women in the labor market or of the risks to women, or of risks in women-dominated employment areas. For example, HSE's estimates of risks in the health sector include far fewer jobs, cancers and exposures than the equivalent guidance from the US National Institute for Occupational Safety and Health.

The HSE fails to present any credible assessment of the occupational cancer risks faced by women or the number of cancers in women related to workplace exposures. For example, breast cancer is the most common cancer in the United Kingdom and one of the top cancer killers. However, it does not appear on HSE's priority action list nor in its estimates of the numbers affected by occupational cancer, despite clear evidence associating industrial exposures with elevated cancer risk. An October 2005 report, "Breast cancer—an environmental disease: the case for primary prevention," concluded there was "incontrovertible evidence" that many industrial chemicals and radiation are major contributors to overall breast cancer rates.[54]

The concentration by the HSE on occupational cancers fails to take account of the interaction of occupational and supposedly "lifestyle" cancers. For example, work stress is associated with poor behavior patterns, including smoking and other substance abuse behaviors outside work.[55–59]

Workplace exposures can also "potentiate" the effect of tobacco smoke. For example, the synergy between asbestos exposure and tobacco smoke is well reported, the combination creating a massively increased risk compared to exposure to either carcinogen alone. A 2005 paper concluded exposure to wood dust increased the chances of developing not only nasal cancer but also lung cancer, finding the risk of lung cancer was increased by 57 percent with wood dust exposure in those who did not smoke, by 71 percent in those who smoked but were not exposed to wood dust but by 187 percent for individuals who were exposed to both smoking and wood dust.[60]

The impact of work exposures can also be intergenerational with the impact on workers' children wholly ignored in HSE's analysis. For example, a 2003 University of Massachusetts Lowell report noted "evidence increasingly indicates that parental and childhood exposures to certain toxic chemicals including solvents, pesticides, petrochemicals, and certain industrial by-products (dioxins and polycyclic aromatic hydrocarbons) can result in childhood cancer."[61] Recent research has reinforced this evidence.[62]

And para-occupational cancers—cancers in those incidentally exposed to carcinogens via exposure to asbestos on the clothing of a parent or spouse, for example—are being seen with increasing frequency.[63]

The increase in overall life expectancy and declining death rates from other causes mean that for the current working generation cancer will have longer to develop and less competition as a cause of death. And while mortality from cancer might be falling in certain cases, as a result of improved diagnosis and treatment, the incidence of cancer is not, supporting the case for greater preventive efforts.

The policies and practices of the HSE are clearly affected by many of the influencing factors discussed in other chapters of this book and, while changes are needed in relation to many of these underlying causes, a whole series of measures could be put in place, especially in relation to all those employed in risk industries.

Occupational cancer prevention should be recognized by the UK government as a major public health priority and should be allocated resources accordingly. A national occupational cancer and carcinogens awareness campaign should be launched as a matter of urgency. Current independent sources about occupational cancer can be found at a www.cancerhazards.org.

The Health and Safety Executive should convene a tripartite working party, including representatives of unions, health and safety campaign organizations and occupational disease victims" and advocacy organizations, to review its occupational cancer strategy.

Wherever possible, IARC Group 1 and Group 2A carcinogens should be targeted for "sunsetting"—a phase-out within a designated time-frame—to be replaced by safer alternatives. Toxics Use Reduction legislation, already used successfully in some US jurisdictions, should be introduced to encourage the use of the safest suitable substances and processes. The precautionary principle should be applied to substances suspected of causing cancer in humans.

A national system of occupational health records should be developed to ensure adequate recording of workplace exposures and other occupational cancer risk factors. Employers must have a duty to inform any workers of their exposures to known or suspected workplace cancer risks and carcinogens. A National Exposure Database should be created and should not rely on inadequate Material Safety Data Sheets to identify carcinogens.

The Health and Safety Executive should provide resources for training of union safety representatives. This training should cover "lay epidemiology" techniques for the early recognition of work-related diseases, including cancer, and training in lay exposure-reporting systems, because trade union reps, lawyers and individual workers will be critical to finding carcinogens and, through REACH-type mechanisms, feeding back information to other users, suppliers and HSE on their location. The value of such an approach in revealing "hidden cancers" and other occupational diseases is considerable.[64]

The United Kingdom should implement properly the European Union law requiring workers to have access to occupational health services. The government Industrial Injuries Benefit Scheme should be revised and extended to include a wider range of occupational cancers in its scope. There should be a consideration of the introduction of a "rebuttal presumption" of work-causation for cancers with an established association with work. Those exposed to carcinogens should be adequately covered for compensation. Exposures, not specific and narrow occupational categories, should determine compensation.

Chapter 16

SPIN IN THE ANTIPODES— A HISTORY OF INDUSTRY INVOLVEMENT IN TELECOMMUNICATIONS HEALTH RESEARCH IN AUSTRALIA

Don Maisch, PhD

The potential for conflict of interest can exist whether or not an individual believes that the relationship affects his or her scientific judgment. Financial relationships (such as employment, consultancies, stock ownership, honoraria, paid expert testimony) are the most easily identifiable conflicts of interest and the most likely to undermine the credibility of the journal, the authors, and of science itself.[1]

The International Committee of Medical Journal Editors, 2007

As universities turn their scientific laboratories into commercial enterprise zones, and select facility to realize these goals, fewer opportunities will exist in academia for public-interest science—an inestimable loss to society. . .The roles of those who produce knowledge in academia and those stakeholders who have a financial interest in that knowledge should be kept separate and distinct.[2]

Sheldon Krimsky, 2003

INTRODUCTION

In March 2009, three Australian neurosurgeons, Drs. Vini Khurana,[3] Charles Teo,[4] and Richard Bittar,[5] wrote a Letter to the Editor to the medical journal *Surgical Neurology*. Titled "Health risks of cell phone technology," the letter expressed the neurosurgeons' concerns over what they considered was a serious emerging public health risk from the ubiquitous use of the cell phone and the increasing evidence for harm, including brain and salivary gland tumors, male infertility, behavioral disturbances, and electrosensitivity. The authors concluded by strongly recommending that children's cell phone use should be restricted.[6]

Khurana and Teo, with coauthors Michael Kundi, Lennart Hardell, and Michael Carlberg, have also written a peer-reviewed paper published in *Surgical Neurology* titled "Cell phones and brain tumors: a review including the long-term epidemiologic data." This paper concluded that "there is adequate epidemiologic evidence to suggest a link between prolonged cell phone usage and the development of an ipsilateral brain tumor" and "it is likely that neurosurgeons will see increasing numbers of primary brain tumors, both benign and malignant."[7]

On previous occasions, Khurana, Teo, and Bittar have publicly expressed their concerns over what they were seeing in their surgeries. For example, Dr. Teo stated in a *60 Minutes* interview (April 3, 2009) that he was seeing a rise in the incidence of brain cancer and as a result the public should be informed as to all the potential causes of the disease. Teo said that he was "incredibly worried, depressed at the number of kids I'm seeing coming in with brain tumors. . . . Just in the last three or four weeks, I've seen nearly half a dozen kids with tumors which should have been benign and they've all been nasty, malignant brain tumors. We are doing something terribly wrong."[8] Khurana shared Teo's concerns as he, too, was "seeing too many young people with such tumors."[9]

Teo's concerns were backed up by statistics that found brain tumors were now apparently the leading cause of childhood cancer mortality in the United Kingdom. While childhood leukemia mortality had decreased 39 percent between the years 2001 to 2007, childhood brain tumor deaths had increased by 33 percent over the same period. In addition, according to a UK charity, Brain Tumour Research, in 2009 more children and adults under the age of forty were dying from brain tumors in the United Kingdom than from any other form of cancer and that the incidence was increasing with some experts seeing a recent doubling of brain tumor cases.[10]

Concerns over an apparent increase in brain tumor incidence in young people also were raised in US congressional hearings in September 2008. Ronald Herberman, Director of the University of Pittsburgh Cancer Institute, testified that in his examination of government statistics the incidence of brain cancer has been increasing over the last ten years, particularly among twenty- to twenty-nine-year-olds. Herberman pointed out that as the latency for brain tumors is more than ten years and if cell phones were responsible for the increase, brain tumor rates might not peak for at least another five years. At the congressional hearings, both Herberman and David Carpenter, Director of the Institute for Health and Environment in Albany, New York, cited research findings by Lennart Hardell from Sweden that indicated people who started using cell phones before the age of twenty were five times more likely to develop a glioma, frequently a type of malignant brain tumor. According to Carpenter, "this observation is consistent with a large body of scientific studies that demonstrate that children are more vulnerable than adults to carcinogens." Carpenter stated at the hearing that "the evidence is certainly strong enough for warnings that children should not use cell phones." He warned that, "the failure to take [strong preventive action] will lead to an epidemic of brain cancer."[11]

Concerns also were raised in France with the Environment Minister, Jean-Louis Borloo, announcing legislation in January 2009 that would ban advertising of the mobile phones to children under twelve years of age—and he would legislate a ban on the sale of any phone designed to be used by those under six.[12]

In March 2, 2009, the Russian National Committee on Non-Ionising Radiation Protection (RNCNIRP) issued official advice that the "health of the present generation of children and future generations is under danger" from cell phone use and therefore the committee has recommended that cell phone use be restricted for people under eighteen years of age. The RNCNIRP called for the dissemination of information specifically for parents, teenagers, and children on the dangers of cell phone use and called for the banning of cell phone advertising targeting children.[13]

In addition to the above concerns, in April 2009, Professor Bruce Armstrong, the head of the Australian section of the international thirteen nation Interphone Project, studying the possible long-term hazards from cell phone use (below), saw that for long-term users a suggestion of an increased risk of gliomas on the same side of the head that a cell phone was usually used and as a result recommended that cell phone exposures should be limited, especially for children.[14]

Earlier, in June 2000, Australian calls for concern over the unrestricted use of cell phones by children were expressed by the Commonwealth Science and Industrial Research Organisation (CSIRO) in 2000 and the Australasian College of Nutritional and Environmental Medicine (ACNEM) in 2003. Dr.

Gerry Haddad, head of the CSIRO's Telecommunications and Industrial Physics Department, stated in Senate hearings that there was a need to "restrict use of mobile phones for children for essential purposes. . .a precautionary principle would seem to be a good idea."[15]

In 2003, the Australasian College of Nutritional and Environmental Medicine (ACNEM) published a paper by this author that detailed reasons why extra precautions needed to be taken for children and cell phone use. The paper included a number of statements of concern specific to this issue from scientific and medical organizations internationally. These included the UK's Independent Expert group on Mobile Phones (IEGMP), the International Institute of Biophysics, Germany, the German Interdisiplinary Association for Environmental Medicine, and the World Health Organization's Director General Dr. Gro Harlem Brundtland, to name a few. The ACNEM paper concluded with the question: "Is it worth the risk" to continue to allow unrestricted cell phone use by children?[16]

In stark contrast to the above concerns, however, Australian Centre for Radiofrequency Bioeffects Research (ACRBR), until it closed in June 2011, was apparently of the opinion that it was worth the risk. On the ABC Lateline program (April 4, 2009) Dr. Rodney Croft, then Director of ACRBR, stated: "There really has been a lot of research done to date and the research has very clearly shown that there aren't any effects. With children, I really don't think there is any evidence suggesting that this might be a problem. There isn't anything to suggest that we may have to be a little bit more cautious."[17] To visually back up ACRBR's dismissive viewpoint on children and cell phone use on the ACRBR web site was an animated GIF image that included images of children happily using cell phones.[18]

THE INTERPHONE STUDY

Differing expert interpretations of scientific findings on cell phone use are seen in statements over the findings of the thirteen-nation Interphone study, which examined brain tumor (glioma and meningioma) risk in relation to mobile phone use in the participating countries.[19]

As for the overall findings, Dr. Elizabeth Cardis, Director of the Interphone study, stated the following:

> The study is very complex and the interpretation is not clear. And we have not demonstrated consistently that there's a risk, but I think it's really important to note that that does not mean that there's no risk. We have a number of elements in the study which suggest that there might actually be a risk, and particularly we have seen an increased risk of glioma, which is one type of malignant

brain tumor, in the heaviest users in the study—in particular on the side of the head where the tumor developed and in particular in the temporal lobe which is the part of the brain closest to the ear so closest to where the phone is held, so that's the part of the brain that has most of the exposure from the phone.[20]

Dr. Christopher Wild, Director of IARC, said in the IARC press release of the study findings, the following:

> An increased risk of brain cancer is not established from the data from Interphone. However, observations at the highest level of cumulative call time and the changing patterns of mobile phone use since the period studied by Interphone, particularly in young people, mean that further investigation of mobile phone use and brain cancer risk is merited.

Professor Elisabeth Cardis added in the press release the following statement:

> The Interphone study will continue with additional analyses of mobile phone use and tumors of the acoustic nerve and parotid gland. Because of concerns about the rapid increase in mobile phone use in young people—who were not covered by Interphone—CREAL is co-ordinating a new project, MobiKids, funded by the European Union, to investigate the risk of brain tumors from mobile phone use in childhood and adolescence.[21]

In stark contrast, however, Rodney Croft, Director of ACRBR, simply summed up that the "The Interphone results provide a clear indication that there is no association between mobile phone use and brain tumor rates—or at most, that if there was ... it would be too small to be detectable by even a study of Interphone's magnitude."[22]

Despite Croft's dismissive statements, on May 31, 2011, due to the Interphone findings, the IARC classified radiofrequency radiation from wireless (mobile) phone use possibly carcinogenic to humans (Group 2B).[23]

Readers at this point would be forgiven if they found somewhat confusing the huge disparity between ACRBR's stance on the safety of cell phone use and those of Khurana, Teo, Bittar, and the rest. In order to seek to clarify why such a disparity exists this paper looks at the development of the Australian research effort into the possible hazards of cell phone use and the commercial and political influences that have been brought to bear on the scope, interpretation, and use of that research. Also examined are the organizations that have taken over the research after ACRBR's closure in June 2011.

The starting point for this inquiry is to examine the important role previously played by the Commonwealth Scientific and Industrial Research Organization (CSIRO), which was the prime mover in creating the first Australian telecommunications frequencies[24] standard setting committee under the auspices of the Standards Association of Australia (SAA) in 1979. During this time, and later under Standards Australia, CSIRO's Division of Radiophysics took the position that technology should be applied with public safety as a prime consideration.

THE CSIRO AND RADIATION POLITICS

The history of the CSIRO, Australia's premier scientific research organization, begins in 1916 when the federal government established an Advisory Council of Science and Industry (ACSI). The goal for ACSI was to gather information on Australian scientific work, undertake research, review existing research, and collect and disseminate scientific information to the public. In 1920, the Commonwealth Institute of Science and Industry (CISI) was established under the directorship of physicist and statistician Sir George Knibbs.

In 1926, the British government's Balfour Declaration established the British Commonwealth of Nations and the Empire Marketing Board was created to foster closer economic, scientific, and technical cooperation between Commonwealth countries. As a result, the Australian Prime Minister Stanley Melbourne Bruce arranged for Sir Frank Heath of the British Department of Scientific and Industrial Research to report on reorganizing CISI. His report resulted in legislation being passed in 1926 that established a successor agency, the Council for Scientific and Industrial Research (CSIR), charged with carrying out scientific research for the benefit of primary and secondary Australian industries. Scientific advice to the government on the setting up of CSIR argued strongly that creative scientific research required a type of working environment not usually found in government departments. As a result, CSIR was set up as a statutory authority with a governing council to oversee appointments and staff management run by an Executive Committee of three. In 1936, the government extended the role of CSIR to provide scientific assistance to secondary industry. With the creation of the National Standards Laboratory, the Aeronautical Laboratory and the Division of Industrial Chemistry in the years 1937 to 1940, CSIR played an important part in the rapid wartime development of Australian industry. As part of the wartime effort, CSIR established the Radiophysics Advisory Board and the Division of Radiophysics in 1939. After the war, research expanded to include areas such as building materials, wool textiles, coal, atmospheric physics, physical metallurgy, and assessment of land resources.

Because of conflicts between the need to maintain its scientific freedom during the early years of the cold war with the Soviet Union, CSIR ceased all secret or classified work of a military nature under the Science and Industry Research Act of 1949 and was reconstituted as CSIRO, the Commonwealth Scientific and Industrial Research Organization. Over the next thirty years, CSIRO research covered almost every area of primary, secondary, and tertiary industry. In addition, it expanded into areas affecting the community, such as environment, human nutrition, conservation, urban and rural planning, and water supplies. In 1978, the approximately thirty existing research divisions were grouped into areas of compatibility called Institutes, with Directors appointed to oversee an integration of planning, research, and resources within their area, such as agriculture, industrial technologies, or minerals. In 1986, a Board of external members plus a Chief Executive to lead CSIRO was formed. Among other changes was a decentralization where much of the central administrative work was devolved to the Institutes.

The current corporate structure of CSIRO is a result of the Board Review's recommendations from 1996. The Chief Executive is supported by four Deputy Chief Executives who oversee part of the research activities and one or more corporate functions. The Institute structure was abolished with fewer but larger divisions established. These divisions operate as semi-autonomous business units reporting to the Deputy Chief Executives. Sector Advisory Committees have been established to provide advice on strategic research directions and to improve "the interface with industry and society."[25]

As mentioned previously, the CSIRO was the driving force in creating Australia's first national telecommunications radiofrequency and microwave (RF/MW) standard setting committee in 1979, as well as assisting in drafting the first Australian RF/MW exposure standard (AS 2772-1985). CSIRO took an active interest in non-ionising radiation health effects, from cell phones to ultrasound, and played a leading role for many years on the radiofrequency standards committee, having high regard for public health and safety.

In early 1994, Spectrum Management Agency (SMA)[26] commissioned the CSIRO's Division of Radiophysics to undertake a comprehensive review of the available worldwide research on the biological effects of RF/MW exposure on the human body.[27] Funding for the study came from the national carrier Telecom (later Telstra), and the carriers Optus and Vodafone, and the review report was authored by Dr. Stan Barnett from CSIRO's Ultrasonics Laboratory, Division of Radiophysics.

Barnett's report listed many well-documented adverse bio-effects from exposure to RF/MW at power levels well below the threshold for thermal effects,[28] which the Australian and International exposure standards were based on. It also listed many laboratory studies that reported bio-effects at power levels well below the maximum standard limit of 1mW/cm^2, with implications for possible adverse effects on the human immune system. The importance of non-thermal interaction[29] with the human body was a central feature of the CSIRO report. For example, in the Section 9.0, "Mechanisms of Interaction" it is stated (in part):

> The reported effects are unexpected from the existing knowledge on physical interactions since they do not appear to be described by classical intensity or dose-response relationships. It seems to be unlikely that a single bio-physicial interaction mechanism will be adequate to explain all of the reported non-thermal effects of RF and microwave radiation.

In his report, Barnett pointed out that the research database to date was inconclusive, and called for the establishment of an effective research program to determine threshold levels for the onset of RF/MW bio-effects. This research was to span from the level of molecular biology to whole-body physiological reactions and included consideration of possible non-thermal low-level bio-effects. CSIRO considered that the creation of an independently verified database was necessary to be able to develop meaningful safety standards and achieve the trust of the public. The report went on to recommend specific areas of research that it felt was needed and called for the formation of an expert committee to oversee such a program.[30]

The CSIRO report, however, was very controversial as it contradicted the opinion of the telecommunications industry that there were no known non-thermal effects from RF/MW. The report also brought into question the credibility of government policy to promote telecommunications and as a result, the report was classified "Confidential" and withheld from publication. This was the case until its existence was leaked to the magazine Communications Day and the office of Australian Democrats Senator Robert Bell in March 1995.[31]

The CSIRO report, after its distribution by the Australian Democrats, became an alternative source of expert knowledge for the public who were concerned about possible unintended hazards from the rapid proliferation of wireless technology. This development would have been of concern to the federal government as it was a majority shareholder in Telstra and therefore had a vested interest in protecting its investment and promoting telecommunications technology and its safety. Sociologist Sheila Jasanoff has written of similar situations where "the credibility of governmental actions in contemporary knowledge societies depends crucially on the public evaluation of competing knowledge claims and the consequent production of reliable public knowledge."[32] Considering Jasanoff's words, the CSIRO report could be seen as a threat to the government's credibility in relation to government statements on the safety of telecommunications technology.

After pointing out research priorities in the report, CSIRO's Department of Radiophysics[33] applied several times to the National Health & Medical Research Council (NH&MRC) for funding to research the potential effects of mobile phone radiation on DNA and cancer. However, despite the fact that the Division of Radiophysics was arguably well qualified to conduct the research, it was in both instances rejected. This rejection was possibly due, not only because the government considered CSIRO to be in conflict with government policy, but because various people from government, Telcom (Telstra), Optus and Vodafone had claimed that the CSIRO report was merely a blatant attempt to gain research funding.[34] If CSIRO had been successful in gaining funding for research, it would have been conducted by their own researchers who did not necessarily share government and industry views on the safety of telecommunications technology. The history of CSIRO's telecommunications policy on standard setting illustrates that they consistently weighed up conflicting viewpoints on safety. The knowledge thus generated by a CSIRO research program would have been considered as an unknown quantity (a "loose cannon," so to speak) with the potential to conflict with both government and industry policy and generating what Jasanoff called "competing knowledge claims."

The government subsequently removed the CSIRO from any involvement with the mobile phone research program later established by NH&MRC, and was also removed from any future involvement with non-ionising research altogether in 2003.[35] It was at a time when the federal government was instigating changes to the CSIRO management, appointing an executive with experience in venture capital expertise to build partnerships with industry and re-model CSIRO as a profit-centred corporate business. In January 2001, the federal government appointed Dr. Geoff Garrett as CEO of CSIRO and he was re-appointed in April of 2005. One of Garrett's pledges to the government when he first took up his post was to increase external funding to CSIRO by encouraging industry partnerships and commercialising patents for CSIRO discoveries. One initiative was to replace key CSIRO executives with people with "venture capitalist expertise."[36] In an October 2005 interview on CEO Insight, Australia's leading web site for corporate CEOs, Dr. Garrett talked about "traditions that need to be preserved and those that were simply historical responses to conditions that may no longer apply." A major part of Garrett's changes was in the area of communication, which he considered to be 60 percent of the overall necessary changes to the organization. Garrett saw as essential that with communication, key stake-holders—by which he meant industry—needed to hear the same messages.[37]

In order to "improve" CSIRO communication, in May 2002 Garrett removed Julian Cribb as Director of National Awareness (public communication) at CSIRO. Cribb, the principal of Julian Cribb & Associates, specialists in science communi-cation, was eminently qualified for his former communications appointment at CSIRO. He was Adjunct Professor of Science Communication at the University of Technology Sydney and had authored a book with Tjempaka Hartomo titled *Sharing Knowledge: A Manual for Effective Science Communication.*[38]

In early 2004, Dr. Garrett with the approval of Science Minister Peter McGauran took an unusual step by announcing the creation of a new CSIRO senior staff posi-tion of "Director of Communications" as one of his initiatives to make CSIRO into more of a money making "corporate business" instead of an agency doing research predominantly in the public interest.[39] A number of CSIRO staff objected, since the position had been created and imposed on the organization from above, and not by any normal procedures involving the scientific committees of the organization.[40] In spite of these objections, Donna Staunton was selected and took up the new staff position at CSIRO, on March 1, 2004, on a three-year contract staff position with salary of around $330,000 a year, placing Staunton in the top four earners in CSIRO at roughly three times the salary of a senior research scientist. When CSIRO management made a brief announcement to their staff of her hiring, it did not mention her background qualifications but said she "is highly regarded in political and corporate spheres."[41] According to science journalist, Dr. Peter Pockley, writ-ing in Australasian Science, it was widely considered that Staunton was selected on Garrett's personal recommendation.[42] The job specification did not require the appointee to have any experience in science or its communication. Staunton stated that her expertise is in "risk management and reputation management."[43] According to her consultancy's website at the time, Staunton "brings a very deep knowledge of the corporate sector to this business. She understands the way the corporate sector needs to successfully interact with its many stakeholders—the media, government, shareholders, the investment community, staff, customers and the general public."[44] As CSIRO Director of Communications, one of Staunton's tasks was liaising between the media and agency scientists, essentially working as a censor through which agency scientific findings would be put before releasing to the media and public.[45]

Donna Staunton's previous experience illustrated that conflict of interest was a non-issue in the new corporate CSIRO. She had previously been a lawyer with the legal firm Clayton Utz where her job was to handle work for tobacco cases on behalf of the industry. She later became Chief Executive Officer of the

Tobacco Institute of Australia and Vice President for Corporate Affairs of the Philip Morris Group.[46] Guy Nolch, Editor of *Australasian Science* raised concerns over Staunton's tobacco past on March 30, 2004, when he wrote that: "It's unlikely that trust in science can improve in Australia when public comment from its premier scientific research organization is filtered by a manager who has used science to put corporate interests ahead of community health."[47] Nolch put it more strongly in a May 28, 2004, email to CSIRO CEO Dr. Garrett: "Staunton's appointment is an endorsement by CSIRO of the tobacco industry, and signals CSIRO's desire to employ the methods Staunton used to put the interests of the tobacco industry ahead of the interests of public health."[48]

Stanton also held a position on the board of the Institute of Public Affairs (IPA), an organization that proclaimed that it was "Australia's Leading Free Market Think Tank." As for its position on climate change, IPA considered global warming a natural cyclic event and all climate scientists who thought otherwise were suffering from the disease of "Mother Earthism" with a "touching belief in the Garden of Eden, the halcyon state of the Earth in times before the wicked Industrial revolution."[49] Such strong statements were in sharp contrast to the CSIRO's climate change division where they have stated: "Over the past two hundred years, human activities have significantly altered the world's atmosphere."[50] As a reflection of how the CSIRO had changed under the guidance of Garrett and Staunton, in 2005, the Media, Entertainment and Arts Alliance (MEAA) gave CSIRO management a special commendation in its George Orwell Awards for those who have done the most to suppress press freedom.

According to investigative journalist Stewart Fist a close link is seen between the Liberal Party, the tobacco industry and Staunton in that the then Deputy Leader of the Liberal Party, Julie Bishop, was previously a lawyer at Clayton Utz from 1983 to 1998. While working at the firm, Bishop as managing partner worked on behalf of the Tobacco Institute fighting a high-profile passive smoking case (Burswood Casino) and opposing an active anti-smoking lobby in Western Australia. In their intersecting roles, Bishop and Staunton would have been close working associates. After resigning from Clayton Utz Bishop became a Liberal candidate for the federal seat of Curtin and won the seat in the election held in October 1998.[51]

THE NH&MRC AND RADIATION POLITICS

Even though the Liberal government had eliminated CSIRO from the non-ionising radiation issue altogether by 2003, the 1994 CSIRO recommendations for a research program were later largely adopted by the NH&MRC, the national peak body offering grants for health and medical research. The CSIRO report had called for an expert committee to be established to oversee an Australian research effort that would critically evaluate the dosimetry and bio-effects of published studies, and create direct lines of communication between research, regulatory, and political sectors. It would also design research protocols for critical areas of research and collaborate with international organizations to verify research.[52]

In 1996, NH&MRC did establish an expert committee along the lines of the CSIRO recommendations. Concerned about the potential involvement of the telecommunications industry in this process, Sarah Benson, a researcher for Senator Lyn Allison, wrote to the NH&MRC in early December 1996 asking about industry representation. On December 30, Richard Morris, Assistant Secretary of the Health Research Branch, replied, stating that members of the telecommunications industry would not be involved:

> In regard to your concern about the involvement of industry in the NH&MRC process, let me assure you that members of the NH&MRC Expert Committee will be active researchers without links to the telecommunications industry. This independence from industry is seen as being of great importance to NH&MRC.[53]

Despite this assurance from the NH&MRC, when it came to appointing a key expert radiation adviser to its EME Expert committee, they chose Dr. Ken Joyner, Motorola's Director of "Global EME Strategy and Regulatory Affairs."[54] Dr. Joyner has also represented the Australian Mobile Telecommunications Association, an industry group, on the telecommunications standards committee[55] and had also represented the Mobile Manufacturers Forum.[56]

Such a complete reversal of their former stance that "independence from industry is seen as being of great importance" was most likely a result of direct political interference by the federal government. Joyner has been closely associated with the formulation of government policy on RF exposure. This is seen in the Bioelectromagnetics Newsletter of July/August 1998. In his article titled "Australian Government Action on Electromagnetic Energy Public Health Issues," Joyner's affiliation was given as representing the Australian Federal Department of Communications and the Arts.[57]

When asked by Senator Lyn Allison about the advisability of Dr. Joyner being appointed to the NH&MRC Expert Committee to advise on submitted proposals for mobile phone research, Minister Senator Richard Allston saw no conflict of interest because (in part):

> Dr. Joyner's involvement in the EME Expert Committee in relation to communications technology is as an individual and not as a representative of the telecommunications industry or his employer, Motorola.[58]

Despite Allston's assurance of Dr. Joyner's advice being independent from Motorola's corporate objectives, it must be noted that Motorola has been active in attempting to influence mobile phone research internationally. For example, Motorola has played a central role in the European Union's cell phone research effort. This was not without complaints. As reported in Microwave News (1999), there was a fair amount of discontent on part of European scientists with Motorola's involvement with the EC research and telling European scientists how to spend research funds.[59]

The NH&MRC has long established conflict of interest guidelines for a wide range of possible situations with a requirement for "Disclosure of interests," which applied to membership of the EME Committee. To quote:

> In the case of direct pecuniary interest, members may not take part in any deci-
> sion to which the potential conflict of interest pecuniary interest applies, and
> must physically absent themselves from all or any part of a formal meeting or
> other discussion at which the matter in question is being discussed.[60]

If this requirement was vigorously applied, then it is difficult to see how Dr. Joyner could have been involved at all when the matter in question was mobile phone research. However this requirement could conveniently be waived because of an opt-out clause that states: "the Chair of the Expert Committee, in consultation with the other uninvolved members of the Expert Committee, will determine the extent to which a member may be involved in the discussion or decision concerning the matter involving the potential conflict of interest."[61]

In January 2009, Dr. Joyner announced that he was leaving his Director position at Motorola after twelve years and was "looking for new opportunities to work in the telecommunications industry."[62] In that same year, Dr. Joyner was listed on the NH&MRC's Peer Review Honour Roll which acknowledged its many peer reviewers and external assessors who had exhibited "excellent track records and wide-ranging expertise in Australian and international health and medical research fields." However, under the section "Administering Institution/ Employer" he was listed as simply "consultant"[63] even though during his time on the NH&MRC committee as an expert reviewer, his employer was Motorola.

Joyner was later appointed as expert advisor on the thirteen member Victorian Radiation Advisory Committee. This committee advises the Minister or the Secretary on any matters relating to the administration of the radiation legislation referred to it by the Minister or the Secretary. In other words, when radiation issues arise for the government the committee's advice would very much influence the state government's position. Dr. Joyner's inclusion on the committee coincided with the Victorian government's decision to mandate the statewide rollout of new wireless electrical meters (called advanced or smart meters) in all homes and other buildings. This caused a significant level of public opposition and even spawned a new political party specifically opposing the roll-out of the new meters. This opposition was primarily a result of health complaints reported by some people after the meters were installed. These complaints would obviously be sent to the Radiation Advisory Committee for its expert advice. Dr. Joyner was the only person on the committee to give such advice as he was the sole member with expertise in "non-ionizing radiation."[64] In this respect it is essentially a committee of one.

THE ACRBR AND RADIATION POLITICS

In 2003, the NH&MRC awarded $2.5 million in funding to establish a so-called "Centre of Excellence," the Australian Centre for Radiofrequency Bio-effects Research (ACRBR), based at the Royal Melbourne Institute of Technology (RMIT) University in Melbourne, Victoria. ACRBR was to investigate and advise on possible biological effects arising from exposure to radiofrequency radiation (RFR) from telecommunications technology. The person selected by the NH&MRC's EME Committee to take up a position as the first Director of ACRBR was Associate Professor Vitas Anderson,[65] a close associate of Dr. Joyner, and a former Telstra employee who represented Telstra's interests on the former Standards Australia TE/7 standards committee. On that committee, Anderson opposed CSIRO's scientific position regarding the existence of nonthermal bio-effects from telecommunications RFR, which he saw as purely hypothetical. He saw the real task as being the need to "comfort the community" about the safety of wireless communications.[66]

In 2001, Anderson appeared on the Australian SBS TV Insight program *The Mobile Phone Debate*. Anderson appeared at the behest of the transnational public-relations agency Burson Marsteller, one of the world's biggest PR firms, well known for its work on behalf of the tobacco industry,[67] and the industry group the Australian Mobile Telecommunications Association (AMTA) of which Burson Marsteller is listed as one of AMTA's "Support Industries."[68] Anderson was introduced on the program as a "Mobile Phone Industry Consultant."[69]

As taken from the transcript of that program, Anderson's views on the mobile phone health issue were as follows:

> The issue of mobile health effects is something that's been looked at for a long time and it's something that's been under review almost continuously, at least

for the last 20 years quite intensively, and the evidence that we have to date, clearly indicates that there is no real reason for concern from the evidence that we have so far.[70]

The presenter, Gael Jennings, later asked Anderson: "Are you saying that as a scientist, you don't accept that there may be a mechanism whereby cells can be harmed in the laboratory, you don't accept that research? Are you saying that?" To this Anderson replied:

Well, actually it's not just a matter of myself not accepting it. Actually, it's merely the consensus of the general scientific community. There has been review, after review, after review on this topic. You'll find that some agencies may recommend one [a precautionary approach] in terms of dealing with the social issues of mobile phones but in terms of a health effect, there really is no substantive reason to recommend a precautionary approach.[71]

Anderson further elaborated his doubts about a precautionary policy for mobile phones in a paper titled, "Mobile Telephony and the Precautionary Principle—A Phoney Debate?" published in *Radiation Protection in Australasia* in 2001. Anderson considered that the precautionary approach itself generated risks. Anderson wrote that:

In its worst form the PP [precautionary principle] can create arbitrary and onerous regulatory measures without regard to new community risks and costs that may be generated (e.g., denying or delaying public access to the social, economic, and public safety benefits of mobile telephony; redirection of limited community resources away from more important public safety issues; protracted legal argument (and costs) over the vague definitions inherent in the PP; undermining of the integrity of the scientific method in determining the true level of any health risk from direct exposure to low-level EME). Inappropriate occupational and public risk behaviors based on an exaggerated concern of EME as implied by the PP.[72]

Anderson then introduced the concept of a precautionary approach to the precautionary approach, when he concluded that:

There is little published data to quantify these risks, though a strong prima facie case exists for a cautious approach to the PP. A considered decision on the PP that protects the public interest will require quantitative analysis of the risks generated by the PP described above.[73]

Considering the above it was surprising that the issue of a conflict of interest was not apparently raised at the time about Anderson's appointment as the first Director at ACRBR.

With research into the effects on public health from non-ionizing radiation exposures being taken from the CSIRO by the government, RMIT University became a base for ACRBR.

RMIT University is "renowned for collaborating with industry, providing solutions, new ideas and processes that deliver real outcomes for business."[74] A cooperative relationship with Telstra was ensured by the already close working relationship between the two organizations. RMIT University was also home to the "Telstra Home Team: a different way of thinking," a team consisting of five postgraduate researchers funded by Telstra. The Team "undertakes research projects for Telstra while studying full time at RMIT."[75] RMIT University was also a partner in the Australian Telecommunications Cooperative Research Centre (ATCRC), whose focus was on "developing and commercializing the technologies that will drive a new generation of telecommunications."[76] RMIT University, therefore, was charged with conflicting duties of both commercialising communications technology and researching for possible health effects from that technology. This should have raised the question of a possible conflict of interest within the university.

In order to answer the conflict of interest question it is necessary to consider RMIT University's Conflict of Interest policy, "Business risks to the University," where it is stated that a conflict of interest may exist when:

- The potential for employees to act in a way that is not, or is perceived not to be, in the best interests of the University.
- The potential for financial loss by the University because of the employee's actions.
- The potential for the boundaries between the University and its interests, and the external company and its interests to be blurred.
- The potential for the University to be joined in legal proceedings because of the employee's position on the board.[77]

Although these points seem straightforward for addressing individual (employee) conflicts of interest, this chapter will examine how these can be interpreted in various ways, especially when it comes to the larger issue of institutional conflicts of interest.

With such a close working relationship between RMIT University and Telstra, there is little risk of a conflict of interest arising between the two as both have a shared interest in developing and commercializing the technology. Such shared goals between university and business interests were first termed the "university-industrial complex" by Martin Kenney in the title of his 1986 book *Biotechnology: The University-Industrial Complex.* Kenney, an assistant professor of agricultural economics at Ohio State University, raised concerns over the development of close business ties between many universities and large biotechnology corporations, and how this "university-industrial complex" would affect educational institutions, agriculture, and society in general.[78]

Sheldon Krimsky in *Science in the Private Interest* (2003) examined the ethical quandary whereby university research has generally become deeply entangled with entrepreneurship and commercial interests—to become what Krimsky called an "inevitable tide of corporate and academic partnerships and the commercialism of knowledge." Krimsky concluded: "As universities turn their scientific laboratories into commercial enterprise zones, and select faculties to realize these goals, fewer opportunities will exist in academia for public interest science—an inestimable loss to society."[79]

In relation to the first three points in RMIT University's conflict of interest business policy (above), a conflict of interest could arise, for example, if ACRBR researchers at the university found evidence that telecommunications technology had adverse health effects. This was a concern mentioned by Telstra in bold type in its 2004 Telstra Annual Report where it was stated, under the heading "Risk factors" that "[t]he establishment of a link between adverse health effects and electromagnetic energy (EME) could expose us to liability or negatively affect our operations."[80] Consequently, any research effort into this possible link would be of vital importance to Telstra, not because of the truth it may uncover but its potential to adversely impact on litigation, regulation, and the corporation's bottom line. It is interesting to note that in the same year Telstra was informing its investors that a risk existed, it was also telling the Australian public that there was no health risk from their use of mobile communications.[81] As for the focus of Telstra's corporate research interests, according to Krimsky (2003), "corporations view science not as a generator of truth but as one among many inputs into production."[82] Thus, depending upon what ACRBR research finds, the following could apply in relation to RMIT University's Conflict of Interest policy:

If a link between telecommunications technology and adverse health effects were found by ACRBR researchers at the university, this would pose a risk to both Telstra's and the university's operations—and also the university's shared ventures with Telstra. Thus, if this were to be the case, it could conceivably be said that the researchers who had found the risk had inadvertently acted "in a way which is not, or is perceived not to be, in the best interests of the University" and the interests of its partner Telstra. This situation would create a "potential for financial loss by the University because of the employee's actions." Such a situation would be likely to create conflict between Telstra's corporate interests and the university's interest in maintaining an unblemished image as an esteemed research organization.

In relation to RMIT University's conflict of interest policy on the "potential for the University to be joined in legal proceedings," it is worth noting the case of Dr. James Kahn and his employer, the University of California at San Francisco. Kahn had conducted a study on the effectiveness of an AIDS vaccine. When he found that the vaccine was ineffective, the drug company that provided the funding refused to supply more data and took action to block publishing of the study. Much to the credit of the university, rather than admonishing Dr. Kahn for creating a conflict with their corporate sponsor, they supported Dr. Kahn with the publishing of the study in the *Journal of the American Medical Association* in 2001. The company then proceeded to file a $7 to 10 million legal case against both Dr. Kahn and the university.[83] Besides a conflict of interest, this case clearly demonstrates the pitfalls that can occur in university-industry partnerships when research uncovers scientific findings not to the liking of the industry partner.[84]

However, while ACRBR became the center stage for Australia's research on the health impacts of telecommunications equipment, the situation was quite the opposite at CSIRO. In September 2003, Dr. Stan Barnett, author of the CSIRO report, circulated a letter to announce that he had been forced to accept "involuntary redundancy" from CSIRO and that his division had been told by senior management to cease all further research into the bio-effects and safety of ultrasound and non-ionising radiation. This was despite the fact that CSIRO ultrasound research had found that pulsed Doppler ultrasound, widely used in Australia on pregnant women, could cause significant heating of up to five degrees in the fetus, particularly near the bones. Barnett's research also indicated that fetal tissue was vulnerable to physical change from the heating, including cell differentiation, which could have significant consequences for the developing fetus. Barnett had stated that the clinical implications of possible non-thermal effects from the use of ultrasound had not been fully evaluated, and that the ultrasound scientific database was incomplete and could not keep pace with technological development of modern equipment.[85] Barnett's preliminary ultrasound work raised serious questions about a widely used technology that was being increasingly promoted as a safe procedure for the unborn child. For that reason a priority was evident to continue the research in the public interest. However, if further research confirmed Barnett's findings, there was the potential for a substantial risk for both the ultrasound industry and medical facilities using the equipment.

Barnett stated in his 2003 letter the following:

> CSIRO has chosen to stop all research into bio-effects and safety of diagnostic ultrasound and cease any involvement in safety of non-ionising radiation in general. It seems that research for the good of the community is not considered a priority area unless it is politically attractive or able to attract funding from industry. Clearly, that is not the case for safety related research in a taxpayer-funded research organization.[86]

Henceforth, any research into possible health impacts of mobile phones or other health issues related to telecommunications would be solely through the NH&MRC's EME committee, ACRBR, and its partner Telstra.

It has been argued on many occasions that the best people to involve in research are people with expertise in the field, and most of these people obviously work for industry. This was the argument put forward by Senator Richard Alston, Minister for Communications, Information Technology and the Arts in 1998. As a justification for selecting Dr. Joyner as the radiation advisor to NH&MRC's Expert EME Committee he stated: "If experts who have had any involvement with industry in the past were excluded from participation, it would be almost impossible to establish an Expert Committee."[87] What Alston didn't mention, however, was why CSIRO and its proven expertise on the issue were not represented on the committee. Senator Alston would have been aware that an expert radiation advisor, or several for that matter, could most likely have been drawn from the CSIRO's Division of Telecommunications and Industrial Physics (TIP). If this had been the case then NH&MRC's EME Committee would have not needed any industry representation in order to do their task. After all, this was of great importance to NH&MRC in 1996 when, as mentioned previously, an NH&MRC senior spokesperson stated: "independence from industry is seen as being of great importance to NH&MRC."[88] Obviously, from the government's perspective, the advice of Motorola on telecommunications health research issues was preferable to that of independent scientists from CSIRO.

Although RMIT University has a conflict of interest policy in relation to individuals, there is no provision for addressing possible institutional conflicts of interest. Therefore, no questions were apparently raised about possible conflicts when Telstra became a major part of the ACRBR research team. Ray McKenzie, from Telstra's EME Research & Standards section, was appointed Research Director at ACRBR.[89] Under the heading of Distinguished Directors of ACRBR

Dr. John Stocker, a Telstra Director, was also listed.[90] At an October 2004 joint ACRBR/Telstra Workshop, held at the Telstra Research Laboratories in Clayton, Victoria, Professor Mays Swicord was an invited participant. Swicord was referred to as a representative from the Mobile Manufacturers Forum, Geneva and an "internationally renowned RF Bio-effects researcher." Swicord was also a senior scientist for Motorola and has been editor of the Bioelectromagnetics Newsletter. According to the ACRBR web site, this workshop "provided the ACRBR with an update on international industry and academic perspectives on the Bio-effects Research area."[91] This is a clear indication of the close partnership between industry and academia where conflicts of interest can morph to becoming a shared interest.

Earlier that year, Swicord reported in the Bioelectromagnetics Newsletter on the heat shock protein (HSP) workshop held in Helsinki, Finland, in April 2004, which was hosted by Dariusz Leszczynski of the Finnish Radiation and Nuclear Safety Authority (STUK). However, Swicord omitted from his report much of Leszczynski's data that supported a HSP effect even though the findings had been one of the major reasons for organizing the workshop. As a result of this significant omission, a group of Bioelectromagnetics Society members called for an editorial board to ensure that this would not occur again.[92] Swicord's omission of inconvenient data confirms Krimsky's observations that corporations on numerous occasions have suppressed study findings that they funded when those findings were in conflict with their commercial interests.[93]

INSTITUTIONAL CONFLICTS OF INTEREST

Most institutional conflict of interest policies deal with individual trust and responsibility; however, of greater concern is the lack of safeguards in organizational partnerships, such as those between RMIT University/ACRBR and Telstra. Such safeguards are obviously needed in order to prevent institutional conflicts influencing the representation and interpretation of research results. This problem has been explored by Harold Barnes in his book *Social Institutions—In an Era of World Upheaval*, (1942) According to Barnes, institutional conflicts of interest can have a far greater impact on an organization than individual conflicts of interest as they set an expected level of behavior (establish an institutional culture) for all members of the organization. Barnes found that this can affect the actions of dozens or even thousands of individuals, both within and outside an organization). In relation to universities, he found that:

Faculty members depend heavily on the institution's administration for their salaries, promotions, tenure, space, teaching assignments, annual increases, and committee assignments. This power relationship makes it extremely hard for faculty members to be truly independent and objective toward the demands or perceived demands of the institution. This imbalance of influence provides an avalanche of pressure for expediency, conformity [and] intellectual lethargy.[94]

Thus, the institutional conflict of interest issue in relation to Motorola and Telstra employees influencing and directing the research effort at ACRBR would most likely result in an overall research program that conforms to the objectives of these corporations. This situation is clearly reflected by the statement published on conflict of interest in 2006 by the International Committee of Medical Journal Editors (quoted in part):

> Conflict of interest exists when an author (or the author's institution), reviewer, or editor has financial or personal relationships that inappropriately influence (bias) his or her actions (such relationships are also known as dual commitments, competing interests, or competing loyalties). These relationships vary from those with negligible potential to those with great potential to influence judgment, and not all relationships represent true conflict of interest. The potential for conflict of interest can exist whether or not an individual believes that the relationship affects his or her scientific judgment. Financial relationships (such as employment, consultancies, stock ownership, honoraria, paid expert testimony) are the most easily identifiable conflicts of interest and the most likely to undermine the credibility of the journal, the authors, and of science itself.[95]

The potential for conflict of interest was also addressed in a national conference titled "Conflicted Science" in July 2003, and sponsored by the Center for Science in Public Interest (CPSI) in the United States. The conference examined how the increasing commercialization of science is undermining science itself. At this conference, journalists, researchers, and university professors from a wide range of fields (from environmental planning to pediatrics to criminal justice) recounted how the commercializing of science was stifling or corrupting their disciplines. The conference concluded that there was a significant societal loss of trust in "science," even when it came from what appeared to be independent sources. Nonprofit organizations, public universities, and health charities, all too often dependent on corporate money, have become the messengers for corporate interests. Investigations by the CSPI have shown that "[t]here is strong evidence that researchers' financial ties to chemical, pharmaceutical, or tobacco manufacturers directly influence their published positions in supporting the benefit or downplaying the harm of the manufacturer's product."[96]

REJECTING "COUNTERINTUITIVE" RESEARCH[97]

One of the research studies considered by the NH&MRC's EME Expert Committee was a study by Dr. Pamela Sykes from Flinders University in Adelaide, South Australia. Syke's study, funded by the government's EMR Program, involved exposing mice to GSM cell phone radiation at a power level of 4 Watts per kilogram (4W/Kg). The aim was to test for changes in DNA, one of the issues CSIRO wanted to research had funding been approved. Her preliminary study findings, published in Radiation Research, November 2001, found that the exposed mice had fewer DNA changes than expected. Although this might suggest a beneficial or protective effect from the microwave exposure, Sykes pointed out in her paper that some proven genotoxic agents can also express this same effect, suggesting that cell phone microwave exposure may be genotoxic.[98] Sykes then applied to the EME Expert Committee for further funding to continue the investigation with a larger number of mice to see if her finding could be replicated. The review committee turned this request down because they claimed that her preliminary results were "inconclusive" due to the small number of mice used in the initial study and that the findings did not support her original test hypothesis that exposure to RF promotes more DNA breakages than normal in transgenic mice. The expert committee concluded that, as the study found less DNA breakages than what would normally be expected in non-exposed mice, there was no point in conducting further research in this area.[99] This conclusion, however, failed to address the issue of possible genotoxicity that was raised by Sykes. Microwave News (2001) notes that the EME committee stated, "[a]lthough it may be interesting, from a perspective of scientific curiosity, to further explore the phenomena . . . is, however, unfortunately outside [our] scope." The committee then suggested that Sykes re-apply to NH&MRC for a grant that was not specifically tied to RF bio-effects. This application was, however, also rejected. The committee wrote back, stating that while it "recognized the great potential significance of her results," it considered them "somewhat counterintuitive."[100]

The use of the word counterintuitive as a reason to reject research findings is of concern as it indicates that an assumption had been made that as Sykes' findings did not fit with what would have been expected they did not need to be further investigated. It is expert decision making at a level of "intuition" or "common sense" and therefore outside the norms of scientific objectivity. It indicates that a dismissal of the importance of Sykes' preliminary findings was made because it conflicted with the official stand of the Australian government (and industry) as stated in a government fact sheet: "Although there have been studies reporting a range of biological effects at low levels, there has been no indication that such effects might constitute a human health hazard, even with regard to long-term exposure." And: "The weight of national and international scientific opinion is that there is no substantiated evidence that exposure to low-level RF EME causes adverse health effects."[101] Therefore, research findings that ran counter to this frame of reference could be rejected as "un-useful" knowledge.

A comparison can be made here with research conducted by Dr. Ross Adey, et al., and published in Cancer Research in April 2000. This research exposed Fisher laboratory rats to an RF signal simulating exposures that would be expected in the head of a digital mobile phone user. Overall, the two-year study showed a trend toward a reduced incidence of central nervous system (CNS) tumors in the exposed rats in comparison to unexposed controls, thus indicating a protective DNA repair effect from exposure. Although this could be considered as evidence of danger of mobile phone use causing brain tumors, Adey, et al. pointed out that the findings needed to be followed up because they indicated a possible non-thermal (low-intensity) effect. To quote: "[T]here is considerable evidence in the literature to support the suggestion that low frequency modulated radiofrequency fields are capable of interacting with biological systems when applied at athermal (non-thermal) levels, involving interactions with key messenger and growth regulating enzyme systems." Adey, et al. went on to explain that the findings of the study were consistent with an action of the RF fields in lowering tumor incidence and suggested further research into non-thermal exposures.[102, 103] These suggestions cast doubt on the mobile phone industry's assertion that athermal (low intensity) RF exposures were of no consequence, as there could be no interaction with biological tissue at levels that did not cause heating. Adey's request to Motorola for further funding to do a replication was refused. Motorola then confiscated all the essential equipment, including field generators and exposure chambers. Adey stated in a sworn affidavit this was done "to ensure that we could not pursue any further studies."[104]

Considering that a standard practice in science is to replicate a study in order to establish a biological effect, it could be surmised that further research to explore possible biological effects from low intensity RF exposure did not suit Motorola's interests. With both Sykes' and Adey's (et al.) research, the unwillingness to attempt a replication of scientific findings of an effect (protective) between RF exposure and DNA suggests the findings were "counterintuitive" to strongly held beliefs that there can be no biological effects from RF exposures below the heating threshold.

As Jasanoff (2005) pointed out, political controls over science are pervasive in restricting scientists' "ability to pursue certain lines of inquiry, the conditions under which their advice is sought, and the extent to which research trajectories are subordinated to political imperatives...."[105] It can be argued that this was certainly the case with the government's removing CSIRO from the issue and establishing a research effort under the firm guidance of the telecommunications industry.

SWINBURNE UNIVERSITY TAKES UP THE BANNER

In June 2011, Rodney Croft as Executive Director of ACRBR announced, that as of June 10, 2011, the organization would cease operations because it had been unable to secure further funding to continue its research activities. Croft did announce, however, that many of the Directors would be able to continue their radiofrequency research but no longer under the banner of the ACRBR.[106] A number of the former ACRBR directors then continued their work under the banner of the Bioelectromagnetics Research Group, part of the Brain and Psychological Sciences Research Centre (BPsyC) at the Swinburne University of Technology. The Swinburne group had long been associated with ACRBR.

To quote from the university website:

> The Bioelectromagnetics Research Group explores biological and health effects of exposure to electromagnetic fields (EMF) such as produced by mobile phones, broadcast towers and power lines, particularly how this may affect the brain. It incorporates measurement and analytical tools for assessing EMF exposures in the environment and inside living systems, and an in-vitro laboratory (the Cellular Neuroscience laboratory) for conducting biological experiments. The centrepiece of the Group is the Radiofrequency Dosimetry Laboratory. Specific research interests include EMF safety exposure assessments, complex modeling of EMF and thermal patterns inside living systems, bioelectromagnetic cellular studies and biophysical aspects of neurophysiological equipment (led by Professor Andrew Wood).[107]

The Radiofrequency Dosimetry Laboratory is jointly funded by Telstra Corporation and the University and consists of equipment formerly used by the Telstra EME Safety group. As well as being available for research projects, it is used by Telstra for checking compliance of Telstra's assets with several Team Telstra employees assigned to the Lab.[108]

Such a close working relationship between the University and Telstra is not new. In fact, the Chancellor of Swinburne University, Mr. Bill Scales (2005 to 2014) was previously Telstra's Group Managing Director, Regulatory, Corporate and Human Relations, and Chief of Staff at Telstra. He was also Telstra's Director of IBM Global Services Australia Ltd. and a Director of the Telstra Foundation.[109]

INDUSTRY-BASED LEARNING

Rather than maintaining an arms-length from industry, Swinburne has a long history of working alongside industry with a program of Industry-Based Learning that was introduced into Swinburne engineering programs in the 1960s. To quote:

> Swinburne's industry connections extend well beyond the classroom. We collaborate with industry from the earliest stages of research through to commercialization, drawing on partnerships for resources, financial support and industry-based expertise. We also deliver customized training and short courses to businesses and organizations. Swinburne is a leader in the delivery of workplace training, with more than fifteen thousand students studying in their workplace. Our students also benefit from relevant and effective industry engaged learning, such as taking an Industry-Based Learning placement as part of their course, working for host organizations. Industry representatives sit on our course advisory boards, ensuring curriculum anticipates the future needs of industry so we can help develop work-ready graduates.[110]

Swinburne University may well be a suitable academic institution for meeting the needs of industry by conducting product development research and training graduates for a future career in industry. However, as with RMIT examined previously, an academic institution that is focused on what industry needs is arguably a highly unsuitable place for conducting research that may pose a risk to an industry partner. This should be especially the case when that partner (Telstra) has previously stated in writing its concerns over research which could established a link between its activities and adverse health effects thereby exposing it to possible liability or negatively affect its operations.[111]

SWINBURNE AND THE INTERNET OF THINGS (IOT)

In 2011, Swinburne partnered with Greenwave Systems, a home energy management company to open an Energy Management Research Centre (EMRC). Greenwave is a software and services company whose singular focus is to drive the mass adoption of Internet of Things, a concept where every device we use will one day all be connected wirelessly via the Internet.[112] EMRC's activities include "training and technology transfer of new intelligent solutions for energy management in smart grid to business and community in Australia and internationally."[113] Essential to the concept of the Internet of Things is the introduction of smart metering technology,[114] also called Advanced Metering Infrastructure (AMI), which sends building electrical consumption data back to the utility via a 900 Mhz radio frequency signal. This raises a conflict of interest if Swinburne's Brain and Psychological Sciences Research Centre is called upon to research possible health issues that directly conflict with EMRC's goals.

The problem of university/corporate partnerships was examined in a 2012 report by the Union of Concerned Scientists. Their analysis examined the effect on scientific inquiry when powerful corporate interests are involved in research. The report found that corporations "exert influence at every step of the scientific and policy-making processes, often to shape decisions in their favor or avoid regulation and monitoring of their products and by-products at the public's expense." The report highlighted five ways how corporations are able to influence scientific inquiry:

- Terminating and suppressing unfavorable research
- Intimidating or coercing scientists and academic institutions into silence with threats of litigation and loss of jobs/contracts
- Manipulating study designs and research protocols
- Ghostwriting scientific journal articles that actually promote their products
- Publication bias (selectively publishing positive results and burying or underreporting negative results)[115]

THE AUSTRALIAN CENTRE FOR ELECTROMAGNETIC BIOEFFECTS RESEARCH (ACEBR)

In August 2012, Federal Minister for Health Tanya Plibersek announced the establishment of a new $2.5 million NH&MRC Centre of Excellence, the Australian Centre for Electromagnetic Bioeffects Research (ACEBR) to be based at the University of Wollongong and led by Professor Rodney Croft, now head of the School of Psychology at Wollongong.[116] One of the central university partners of the ACEBR research effort is the previously mentioned PBsyC research group at Swinburne University. As stated on the Swinburne University's website: "ACEBR has embarked on a multidisciplinary five-year research program to address the most pressing radiofrequency (RF) radiation exposure questions to better protect the health of the Australian community." Among other things, Swinburne's research focus will be on accessing characteristic RF EMF emissions, exposure scenarios and corresponding exposure levels for new and emerging RF technologies.[117] Besides Wollongong and Swinburne universities, RMIT University, IMVS Pathology and the Victor Chang Cardiac Research Institute are involved in the research effort.[118]

FUTURE TRENDS: ACEBR SCIENCE & WIRELESS 2013

Overall, the proposed future ACEBR research program is very impressive, but what role will industry and other vested interests play in possibly influencing this research to protect their own interests? To possibly answer this question a brief examination of ACEBR's Science & Wireless 2013 seminar "Health & Future RF Technologies" is an indication. In the seminar acknowledgments, the following was stated: "The ACEBR gratefully acknowledges the financial support of the National Health & Medical Research Council of Australia and Telstra Corporation, which has enabled SW2013 to run."

The focus of the 2013 seminar was on new and emerging wireless technologies with presentations by industry representatives on 4G and especially RF transmitting smart meter technologies. It stands to reason that a discussion of smart meters featured prominently at the seminar. In Victoria there was, and is, an active and vocal level of public opposition to the rollout of smart meters and a number of concerned citizens were in attendance at the seminar. Much of this opposition was based on a growing number of Victorians reporting health problems after a smart meter was installed on their homes, often located externally on a bedroom wall.[119] What was especially concerning these people was that even though these health complaints were being reported worldwide,[120] after smart meters were introduced, absolutely no research had been conducted into these complaints.[121]

In Rodney Croft's introduction to the presentation by Mr. Mike Wood from the Australian Mobile Telecommunications Association (AMTA) on "4G telecommunications technologies," he said the following, in part:

> "Clearly what we see here is a whole lot of new technologies which are going to come about. How do we know what's going to be most relevant to us? Well, in the short-term I think that our industry representatives are going to give the best indicator of this."[122]

The presentation by Mr. Richard Hoy from the industry trade group Energy Networks Association was titled "Smart-meter technologies." In his talk he focused on the public's concerns that smart meters may affect health due to their RF transmission. As for the WHO's International Agency for Research on Cancer (IARC) 2013 ruling classifying radiofrequency (RF) radiation *from wireless phones* as a class 2B possible human carcinogen, he pointed out that typical smart meter exposures were far less than from a mobile phone, suggesting that this therefore was not a concern. He mentioned than there is some twenty-years research on the frequencies used by mobile phones and that the results of this research "apply even more so to the signals that are coming out of smart meters." He said that these transmissions only occur in short bursts, which might be quite a few but typically are less than 1 percent to 3 percent of the time (very short transmission period). Hoy said that by drawing some conclusions from the mobile phone work " we can pretty much decide where we are going" (with smart meter health issues). He claimed that "it can be said that there is no substantive evidence for health effects from exposure to AMI (smart meter) RF fields." In regard to electrosensitivity (EHS) in people claiming to be affected, Hoy quoted a WHO document that stated that EHS had no clear diagnosis criteria and there "is no scientific basis to link EHS symptoms to EMF exposure." He then added, "this gives the industry some relief" and that "no health effect from smart meters has been proven scientifically." Hoy concluded by saying that "some further research into people's concerns about smart meter health effects could be worthwhile." Note that he referred to research into "people's concerns," and not the reported health effects,[123] perhaps suggesting a psychosomatic disorder was at play.

Hoy's claim that mobile phone research data can be directly applied to smart meter exposures is open to argument as there are significant differences in exposure. Consider: The claim that smart meters transmit only 1 to 3 percent of the time paints a deceptive picture. Hoy mentions that the meters are transmitting very short bursts but not that they are doing this constantly. These bursts can happen up to 190,000 times over a twenty-four-hour period. This is well illustrated with diagrams in the published survey conducted by Richard Tell Associates in 2013. Smart meter emissions generally happen all through the day[124] and most smart meters remain relatively active in terms of brief signals being transmitted.[125]

THE FREQUENCY USED MAY ALSO BE AN ISSUE

Besides the constant pulsing of smart meter emissions, there is the issue of the frequency range used. In 1976, Lin concluded that 918 MHz energy constitutes a greater health hazard to the human brain than does 2450 MHz energy for a similar incident power density. In addition, studies of diathermy applications consistently show that electromagnetic energy at frequencies near and below 900 MHz is best suited for deep penetration into brain tissue.[126] So a possibility exists that in situations where people are sleeping in close proximity to an active smart meter, the combination of the frequent transmission bursts at around 900 Mhz constitutes a new and unique human exposure situation, quite unlike using a mobile phone, that may have unintended biological effects, especially on sleep.

A PANDORA'S BOX

As many of the health complaints (mainly an inability to sleep) are coming from people who have had a smart meter installed on a bedroom wall, close to their bed, this should be a high priority research area for ACEBR. Such a research program would necessarily include sleep studies to determine if smart meter transmissions interfere with sleep patterns. This is straightforward research but the implications for a positive finding (an effect on sleep) are enormous for the development and rollout of new technology, the so-called Internet of Things. Obviously this research would have to be done with a firm "firewall" between the researchers and industry affected by the possible findings of that research.

ACEBR's Science & Wireless 2013 seminar "Health & Future RF Technologies" dovetailed quite nicely with Swinburne's and Greenwave System's joint Energy Management Research Centre (EMRC). As EMRC is focused solely on developing and promoting future RF technologies, this is a clear conflict of interest when it comes to objectively investigating claims of possible ill health from these technologies.

CONCLUDING DISCUSSION

This examination of the history of telecommunications research in Australia indicates that the telecommunications industry sector, aided by a government policy to encourage economic development, had conducted a very successful campaign strategy. This was firstly, to eliminate CSIRO's independent involvement, and secondly, to become actively involved in the research effort themselves with a goal to ensure that industry goals would never be endangered by research that could possibly find that their technologies were a possible hazard to health. All this was orchestrated under the Howard Liberal government (March 1996 to December 2007), which had been a major shareholder in Telstra and obviously was acting to protect its investment.

However, the Howard government's actions were not limited to telecommunications. Hamilton and Maddison's book *Silencing Dissent* (2007) exposed how from 1996 to 2007, the Howard government systematically undermined dissenting and independent expert opinion in many areas of scientific debate. Those attacked were charities, academics, researchers, journalists, judges, public sector organizations, even parliament itself.[127]

The uncomfortable truth is that it was this caldron of suppression of alternative scientific viewpoints that gave birth to the current research effort on possible bio-effects from telecommunications technology in Australia.

It must be said here that there are obviously benefits for university/industry partnerships in the area of technological development. The problem arises, however, when the same university is also involved in medical health research that may conflict with its technological development partnerships with obvious financial implications. The challenge, at this late date for Australian universities, is how to maintain an effective "firewall" between the two. As David Korn wrote in JAMA in 2000:

> Conflicts of interest are ubiquitous and inevitable in academic life, indeed, in all professional life. The challenge for academic medicine is not to eradicate them, which is fanciful and would be inimical to public policy goals, but to recognize and manage them sensibly and effectively.[128]

Will Australian universities as well as the NH&MRC and ACEBR address this problem? If so, how would they make the necessary changes? And do they even want to consider it? These are questions that urgently need to be answered.

Chapter 17

WESTLAKES RESEARCH
INSTITUTE

Janine Allis-Smith

Did you ever expect a corporation to have a conscience, when it has no soul to be
damned, and no body to be kicked?
                    Lord Edward Thurlow, English jurist and statesman (1731–1806)

The Sellafield site on the Cumbrian coast in northwest England, originally
called Windscale, and chosen for its remoteness and because of its operational safety fears, was acquired by the Government as a munitions factory during World War II, transferred to the Ministry of Supply in 1945 for use in the
United Kingdom's weapons, and handed over to the newly formed United Kingdom Atomic Energy Authority (UKAEA) in 1954.

The United Kingdom's politically driven weapons program of the 1950s, via the
two Windscale Pile reactors, saw the rural West Cumbrian coastal site transformed
from a small wartime facility into a burgeoning nuclear complex. Benefiting from the
demise of the area's traditional industries of coal, steel, and shipbuilding, Sellafield
grew to become West Cumbria's foremost employer, and its operations came to
dominate not only the local landscape but also the local economy.

Ownership was again transferred in 1971 to British Nuclear Fuels plc
(BNFL), a company wholly owned by the government. The consequence of the
expansion was the creation of mounting stocks of wastes and materials which,
in the early development of the site, were produced with no thought about their
eventual disposal. Similarly, with scant understanding of their long-term behavior, radioactive discharges were made into the environment at levels that today
are acknowledged as being dangerously unacceptable.

Following a restructuring in 2004, site operations were delegated to one of the company's four main business groups, British Nuclear Group (BNG). In April 2005, ownership of the site was again transferred—to its current owners, the Nuclear Decommissioning Authority (NDA).

The full extent of the environmental legacy of this early military work and later commercial reprocessing operations has, over the last few decades, become clear, both in scale, damage to health, and cost.[1]

The 1957 Windscale Fire was Britain's worst ever nuclear accident.[2] On October 10, No. 1 Pile caught fire and, with the population kept in the dark, eleven tons of uranium ablaze and the reactor in danger of collapsing, a plume of radioactive material spread over the area. Those living next door to the plant were not evacuated, nor were they advised to stay indoors or close their windows.

Life went on as normal and as workers were told to keep quiet, babies were wheeled out in prams, and children played in the gardens. Not until three days later, and not until dangerously high levels of radioactive "Iodine 131" had been measured on grass in the area, did the Ministry tell local people not to drink local milk and stop farmers from distributing it. For nearly a month, over two million liters of milk, collected from about two hundred square miles surrounding the plant, were poured into the Irish Sea.

In 1983, the National Radiological Protection Board finally admitted that the radiation released from the Windscale Fire could have caused as many as thirty-three deaths. It has been estimated that the incident caused 240 additional cancer cases.[3]

During the 1960s, accidents at Windscale continued on a regular basis. Together with radioactive leaks, spillages and fires, many workers suffered plutonium exposure. According to the government's health and safety executive, by the early 1970s the Windscale plants had deteriorated to such unsatisfactory levels that safety standards were said to be compromised. BNFL promised improvements, but the accidents continued.[4]

Nothing changed during the 1970s. In 1973, a radioactive "Blow Back" accident seriously contaminated thirty-five workers and closed the B204 reprocessing plant forever. With excavation works in 1975, high levels of radiation were found in the soil and it was finally realized that radioactive water had been leaking from a fuel storage pond, probably since 1972. In 1978, another spillage was discovered.

All this came at a sensitive time for BNFL. There was public opposition to an application by BNFL for outline planning permission to build a new Thermal Oxide Reprocessing plant (THORP), to reprocess irradiated oxide nuclear fuel from both UK and foreign reactors. At the one hundred–day Windscale Public Inquiry,[5] environmentalists drew attention to the increases in radiosensitive cancers they had found along the Cumbrian coastal strip and warned of the possible health effects resulting from remobilization of plutonium and other radionuclide discharges by Windscale into the Irish Sea, and their subsequent return to land.[6] Even so, the Hon. Justice Parker found in favor of THORP.

As Windscale's national and international notoriety grew, so did opposition to the plant's operations. Its re-christening as Sellafield in 1981 by its British Nuclear Fuels operators was seen merely as a desperate public relations exercise.

Local opposition came from CORE (Cumbrians Opposed to a Radioactive Environment), founded in January 1980, after Greenpeace called a public meeting in the port of Barrow in Furness to highlight the import of highly radioactive spent fuel from overseas. Over two hundred people attended, including teachers, lawyers, nurses, bus drivers, office workers, sailors, workers from the local nuclear submarine shipbuilding yard, as well as some Sellafield staff. Many expressed their concerns over the safely of the foreign waste shipments, their transport by rail to Sellafield, and the high number of cancers in the area, which many thought were linked to both accidental and routine releases from the plant.

Initially as the "Barrow & District Action Group Against the Import of Nuclear Waste," CORE began to draw on a bigger membership across the county, playing a leading role in exposing accidents at Sellafield, the extent of radioactive environmental contamination from its discharges, the problems with managing radioactive wastes on-site, and the levels of childhood leukemias around the plant.

I was not involved with CORE during those first few years. Born in the Netherlands, I had come, in the early 1960s, to the United Kingdom to improve my English. I took a job at a boys' boarding school near Ambleside in the center of the English Lake District. I fell in love with Cumbria, its lakes, mountains, and its laid-back culture. Instead of going home, I got married, had two sons, and moved to a small hill farm, where I tended my small flock of Herdwick sheep and spent long sunny days on the nearby beaches, blissfully unaware that we lived less than twenty kilometers downwind from a place called Sellafield which was destined to dominate the rest of my life.

I wondered how safe those beaches had been when, on November 1, 1983, Yorkshire TV's *Windscale, the Nuclear Laundry* documentary showed the extent to which Windscale's radioactive discharges had contaminated the local coastal environment. Producer James Cutler and his team had found a dramatically high incidence, nearly ten times the national average, of childhood leukemia in

Seascale, the village next to the plant, and also an excess in other childhood cancers along the coastal strip. The film suggested that radiation from Sellafield was to blame.[7]

The program caused a national public outcry and confirmed many people's fears that emissions from Sellafield were linked to local cancer deaths. BNFL denied responsibility. Official and public complacency was further shattered a few weeks later by Sellafield's worse nightmare, a highly radioactive discharge accident. When taking silt samples from the end of the discharge pipe, Greenpeace divers had suffered serious contamination. Initially the public was warned against using a 200 meter stretch of beach but, when five days later heavily contaminated items were found, both north and south of the pipeline, the Department of the Environment (DOE) extended the closed area to forty kilometers. The warnings stayed in place for six months. It is ironic that BNFL was later fined £10,000 for causing the leak and Greenpeace was fined £80,000 for trying to stop it.[8]

After YTV's *Nuclear Laundry,* an immediate government inquiry, led by Sir Douglas Black, was launched.[9] "The Black Report," published in July 1984, was an exercise in public reassurance and concluded that it was impossible to prove or disprove the theory that Sellafield was responsible for the high rates of childhood leukemia in the local area. No evidence had been found of any general risk to health for those living near the plant when compared to the rest of Cumbria. Sellafield and the nuclear industry considered themselves innocent once again.

Somewhat miffed by Douglas Black's appreciation of James Cutler's award-winning documentary, a BNFL memo written at the time and produced in the High Court of Justice in 1992/3, said the following:

> It is somewhat galling that Black acknowledges that YTV may have performed something of a public service, and I find it even more galling to have to accept that YTV has so easily identified what Black calls unusual mortality rates of leukemia among young people, when the local health experts have failed to do so.

Nine months later, my twelve-year-old son was diagnosed with leukemia. With the *Nuclear Laundry* documentary still haunting me, I wondered if Sellafield was to blame. After three long years of hospital stays and visits, harsh and painful chemotherapy, and life-threatening infections, my son won the battle to beat his leukemia, but my war against Sellafield had started with his diagnosis.

With the Sellafield leukemias still hitting the media headlines, I was taken aback by health professionals' hostility and their unwillingness to discuss my questions about the possible link between Sellafield, the beaches, and my son's cancer. Was there a cover-up?

As CORE had a high profile in the local papers, I turned to them for advice. They gave me a crash course on Sellafield and, while staying in hospital with my son, I learned about BNFL's discharges and the effects of radiation. Being given the opportunity to talk to world experts, including Alice Stewart and Rosalie Bertell, I became convinced that the radioactivity from Sellafield was linked to my son's leukemia. I started to volunteer for the group, initially as one of the first parents prepared to tell the media that I believed in the Sellafield connection. We visited local graveyards, examined their church burial records, and found that at least nine cancer cases had not been recorded in the original Black Report. In 1990, I joined CORE as a full-time health campaigner.

One recommendation of the Black Report had been the establishment of a new government advisory body called the Committee on Medical Aspects of Radiation in the Environment known as COMARE. Its first report, published in 1986,[10] concluded that there had been a huge release of radioactivity from Sellafield that had not been disclosed to the authors of the Black Report. COMARE therefore considered that the level of uncertainty about the information available and the risk to the population from the Sellafield discharges was now greater than at the time of the publication of the Black Report.

With the Seascale excess confirmed in a study by Professor Martin Gardner and West Cumbria District medical officer Dr. John Terrel,[11] in 1988, COMARE agreed with the 1987 findings of a Scottish office study that there was an excess incidence of childhood leukemia around Dounreay in Scotland.[12] The Scottish researchers concluded that the similarities between the cases at Dounreay and Sellafield, as well as a third suspected cluster near the Aldermaston nuclear weapons facility in Berkshire "appeared to be a cause for concern." In 1987, Sir Douglas Black himself confirmed the likelihood of a genuine link.

"This is the evidence we have been waiting for," said solicitor Martyn Day in a press release, announcing his advertisement that appeared in the *Whitehaven News* on July 21, 1988. He invited parents interested in pursuing a claim against BNFL to contact him. Martyn Day believed that there might now be sufficient scientific evidence to persuade the courts in this country that some leukemia cases were caused by the action of BNFL, which would enable the victims to be compensated.

By October, Leigh, Day & Co. had been formally instructed by some twenty-five families, including my son, and their application for legal aid had been referred to the Law Society. In a civil action of this kind, the plaintiffs would have to prove, on the balance of probabilities, the leukemias had been caused by the emissions of radiation from Sellafield. Without having to prove negligence against BNFL, it would be crucial to prove the link between the plant and the leukemias.

Just before Christmas, BNFL solicitors blocked the families' legal aid, and therefore their claims, by telling the Law Society that these were based on incorrect assertions.[13] In March 1989, after an appeal and accusing BNFL of using the Law Society as "Judge and Jury," the legal aid offer was reinstated. The first writ was issued in August that year and would be followed by a Statement of Claim, requests for information and discovery, where solicitors would exchange documents relevant to the case. As the cases would probably take three years to come to trial, it was going to be an extremely long and arduous time for the families. It was very important they were provided with as much support as possible. CORE would keep the families up-to-date on developments and offer moral support.

With the plaintiffs having to show that, on balance of probabilities, radiation from Sellafield was the cause or part of the cause of each leukemia case, a general review of environmental radioactivity in Cumbria, Sellafield's historic discharges, the behavior of artificial beta emitters introduced into the environment, and conventional dose models, would have to be carried out.

Soon after the Leigh Day advertisement, the *Lancet* published Dr. Leo Kinlen's suggestion that a virus, brought in by people from outside moving into the area, rather than radiation, could be causing leukemia,[14] but initially many dismissed this theory as BNFL-funded wishful thinking. Six months later, however, the *Daily Telegraph* carried the story that, according to Professor Sir Richard Doll, then Britain's most famous epidemiologist, radiation was looking increasingly unlikely as the cause of excess childhood leukemia around nuclear power installations, but that there could be a link between leukemia and an unlabeled virus.

I wrote to Sir Richard Doll and asked him whether my son would now be pointed out and shunned for carrying this dangerous virus. When other concerned parents contacted the office, CORE campaign coordinator Jean McSorley asked Sir Richard Doll the same question.

Richard Doll reassured me that the children would not be infectious. "I am personally far from convinced that a virus plays any part in the production of childhood leukemia but that the idea is scientifically attractive" and "Only one factor is firmly established as a cause of childhood leukemia: namely, ionizing radiation."[15]

In his reply to Jean McSorley, one day later, he copied his response to me. The "Only one" factor had overnight become "two" firmly established factors: namely, "ionizing radiation and some of the drugs used in the treatment of or to facilitate organ transplantation."[16]

So why did Sir Richard Doll become such an advocate for the virus theory? In 1989, the United Kingdom Coordinating Committee on Cancer Research (UKCCR) had initiated a five-year program of research into the possible role of ionizing radiation in cancer, in particular childhood leukemia. The program was funded by donations from the UK Atomic Energy Authority, Nuclear Electric, British Nuclear Fuels, Westlakes, and Scottish Nuclear, of £3 million over five years. Industry representatives would have no hand in deciding what projects would be funded, nor would they have any role in deciding what information would be published.[17] Both Sir Richard Doll and Dr. Leo Kinlen were members of the committee.

In July 2003, having been invited to a CERRIE (Committee Examining Radiation Risk of Internal Emitters) workshop meeting, I looked on while Sir Richard Doll took the homage paid to him—by others of distinction—for granted.[18] During questions following his presentation, I reminded him of his letter to me. He remembered, but just shrugged his shoulders and said he'd changed his mind.

These days, the nuclear industry claims there is no risk to children living around Sellafield, that historic discharges were always too low to account for the leukemias, and that the Kinlen hypothesis remains the favored cause of the Seascale excess.[19] Blaming levels of unusual population mixing, a virus, infectious agents, or antibodies to them have yet to be identified. Their enthusiasm for population mixing is not shared by the wider international scientific community, and recently a German radiation scientist dismissed population mixing as "a hypothesis, primarily arisen to explain away the risks from radiation."[20]

Professor Sir Richard Doll's name hit the headlines again when, in October 1989, he testified as BNFL's chief witness in the Merlin case.[21] Leigh Day & Co. represented the Merlin family's claim against BNFL for the blight caused to their seaside property by the Company's radioactive discharges.

Measurements of their house dust samples showed manmade radionuclide levels of plutonium-239 that were 905 times—and Americium-241, 17,000 times—background level. Professor Doll conceded that even using conventional dosimetry, if every house was contaminated to the extent of the Merlins', there would be a hundred more cases of cancer. Nevertheless, he dismissed the risk to the Merlins' young sons as trivial and no more than that caused by smoking two cigarettes per year. The judge ruled that, as there had been no actual physical damage to the property, the Merlins had no right to compensation.

While preparing for the leukemia litigation, and with the dramatic findings of the 1990 Gardner Report in 1990, the Leigh Day team changed focus. Professor Martin Gardner's research had found that men who had worked at

Sellafield and had received a cumulative radiation dose of at least 100 mSv before a child was conceived, or a dose of 10 mSv in the six months prior to its conception, were at an eight times higher than normal risk of having a child with leukemia or non-Hodgkin lymphoma.[22]

BNFL panicked when, at a meeting with workers, their own director of health and safety, Roger Berry, said that the company was considering advising its Sellafield employees not to have families, in order to avoid the risk of fathering a child with leukemia.

With the "Gardner Theory" and Paternal Preconceptual Irradiation (PPI) in mind, Martyn Day decided that two test cases would be taken forward, those of Elizabeth Reay, whose ten-month-old baby daughter Dorothy had died of leukemia, and Vivien Hope who had been diagnosed with non-Hodgkin lymphoma. Both fathers had received a high radiation dose while working at Sellafield.

WESTLAKES SCIENCE AND TECHNOLOGY PARK

The Westlakes Science and Technology Park has its origins in the West Cumbria Initiative, established in 1988 as a partnership of the private and public sectors—British Nuclear Fuels, Cumbria County Council, and the district councils of Copeland and Allerdale. The West Cumbria Initiative consisted of three integral parts—the West Cumbria Development Fund (WCDF), the West Cumbria Development Agency (WCDA), and Westlakes Properties Limited.

During the early 1980s, communications with the local community had become even more difficult, particularly after the 1983 Windscale documentary and the beach incident. People believed that cover-ups were taking place, with BNFL being misleading and evasive.

In their report *Public Perception and the Nuclear Industry in West Cumbria*,[23] Lancaster University researchers confirmed that, despite significant investment in public relations, BNFL had suffered a generally poor public image in terms of openness and honesty over the years. With people feeling dependent on BNFL, and with little or no choice, it had robbed them of any sense of power they had. Many felt stigmatized by their servile dependency on the plant and the perception that West Cumbria had been the only place in the country compliant and dependent enough to accept it.

One of the main messages to come from group discussions was that people felt that further development was inevitable, even though they were worried about the risks. Acceptance of Sellafield was fatalistic rather than positive, a typical remark was: "We're stuck with the place so we must make the best of it."

In his book *Inside Sellafield,* BNFL Director Harold Bolter describes how BNFL, accused of being evasive and misleading, had come under renewed pressure to help the community and eventually agreed to do so in the form of grants to local authorities, tourist organizations, and individuals. Between 1984 and 1988 this had amounted to over £3 million. "We simply gave in when the pressure seemed too great to resist," he says. It is not clear whether Bolter suggested that BNFL had felt blackmailed by responding only in the aftermath of an incident at Sellafield or when a sensitive planning application had been held up by Copeland Borough Council, but he considered this "the main mechanism Copeland had for squeezing the last drop of financial support out of BNFL."[24]

In recognizing West Cumbria's need for developing a wider, more diverse industrial base, Bolter commissioned a study in 1987, led by business and marketing consultant Professor John Fyfe. The study was constrained by BNFL Chief Executive Neville Chamberlain's insistence that any money put into a new initiative should be kept under BNFL's effective control. This annoyed the Cumbrian local authorities who were afraid that the poor image of the nuclear industry could act as a deterrent to inward investment, especially in the tourism and food processing industries.

Eventually, in late 1987, two organizations were formed. Operating separately, the West Cumbria Development Fund (WCDF), with Harold Bolter as chairman, was responsible for the overall allocation of finances and the West Cumbria Development Agency (WCDA) had as its main role helping to create and develop small businesses and promote industrial developments in West Cumbria. As might have been expected, with duplication of functions and the funding of "lost causes" by both organizations, there was a great deal of internal rivalry between those running the WCDA and the WCDF staff, who were mainly provided by BNFL. John Fyfe was commissioned to take another look at the structure and relationship between the two organizations. He recommended the amalgamation of the two bodies, to be known as the West Cumbria Partnership.[25]

In 1989, Westlakes Properties Ltd. was formed to acquire the forty-acre Ingwell Estate and develop the Westlakes Science & Technology Park, which would provide facilities for clients and access to BNFL specialist and technical services.[26]

That more than just rivalry had been going on was suggested by the editor of the *Whitehaven News* on October 22, 1992. The West Cumbria Partnership, the West Cumbria Development Agency, and departure of its boss, Tony Winterbottom, had been the subject of many whispers for twelve months and more.

The editor thought it was probably because word got around that the agency's track record was being examined. Tony Winterbottom had been highly regarded for his enormous efforts on West Cumbria's behalf. "So why did some-one, who worked so many long hours, who traveled the length and breadth of the country trying to get companies and jobs into West Cumbria, take the ulti-mate decision to leave?" the editorial asked. Writing about the West Cumbria Partnership, the editor said the following:

> The question now has to be whether BNFL will want more responsibility for matters outside their operations at Sellafield and demand, as fair reward for their time and cash, control of the reconstituted and combined WCDA and the WCDF. If they do, will others vitally concerned through making a cash contri-bution of £50.000 a year, accept being dominated by BNFL? Neither Copeland, Allerdale, nor Cumbria councils have so far raised their voices in protest and the way seems clear for the new Agency to get under way.
>
> Only the naïve would underestimate the financial and political power of BNFL, who carry an enormous commitment from a government determined to see them operate successfully and well into the foreseeable future. It is therefore feasible to say what BNFL wants it will usually get.[27]

Even though some saw the nuclear industry as an invaluable resource, the impor-tance not to be too reliant upon one industry was recognized. With the prospect of large job losses after the completion of BNFL's Thermal Oxide Reprocessing Plant (THORP) project, the aim was to encourage outside investment and new businesses to locate, especially at Westlakes, but with BNFL boardroom influ-ence at Westlakes, evidence of independence from BNFL remained as conspicu-ous by its absence as was the employment it should have created for the man in the street.

WESTLAKES RESEARCH INSTITUTE

In 1991, BNFL Company Director Harold Bolter, in his dual capacity as chair-man of the West Cumbria Development Fund, announced a £2.5 million high-tech development in the shape of an independent research institute to be sited on the Westlakes Science and Technology Park. Bolter promised that the Westlakes Research Institute, on land purchased by BNFL and constructed with BNFL money, would bring in new investment and create local jobs.

In support of the institute, BNFL's own in-house and on-site genetics group laboratory, together with its BNFL scientists and staff, had already been relo-cated to the Westlakes Science Park site. BNFL's Geoffrey Schofield Laboratory (named after the late BNFL Medical Officer), once charitable status had been obtained, would become part of the independent Westlakes Research Institute.

Together with Sellafield workers' radiation dose records, and blood and tissue samples, tested for chromosome abnormalities, the laboratory held information on the incidence of leukemia in local children. BNFL had, for many years, provided a free amniocentesis testing service, analyzing for abnormalities for both the Whitehaven and Carlisle hospitals.

The institute's corporate structure comprised two companies—Westlakes Research (Trading) Ltd. and Westlakes Research Ltd. As the name implied, the former, as a private company limited by shares, "traded" for the latter and became registered as a charitable company.

Scrutiny of the companies' structures showed that they shared the same secretary and members, all of whom came from BNFL. The trading company had nine directors, eight of whom were highly ranked BNFL personnel. The charitable company had four council members, three from BNFL. All four members were also directors of the trading company.

So how independent was the Westlakes Research Institute? Given that such staff under contract to Westlakes were still paid by their original employer, and given the BNFL-dominated management structure of the companies which constituted and ran the research institute, it was difficult to see how any measure of independence from British Nuclear Fuels could be claimed.

Indeed, the Westlakes Research Institute's own glossy brochure,[28] published by BNFL's corporate publishing in Risley, pointed to its dependence upon BNFL, at that time and in the short-time future, clearly identifying the BNFL interest in the form of director and management appointments.

The institute's chairman, Dr. Gregg Butler, had joined the BNFL board, while director of the institute, Professor Roger Berry, was also BNFL's director of health and safety. Westlakes Research director of occupational health, Dr. Andy Slovak, had risen to BNFL's chief medical officer in 1990. Tim Knowles was the institute's business director as well as head of BNFL's UK Group Corporate Affairs, general manager of the West Cumbria Development Fund, Westlakes Properties Ltd., director of the Northern Development Company, and CBI councilor, all of which gave him "an extensive network of political and individual contacts which would be essential for the development of the research institute." Graham Smith, chairman of Westlakes Properties, was head of Sellafield. research institute spokesman Dr. Duncan Jackson had been BNFL information manager.

As director of environmental science, Professor Steve Jones's additional role as BNFL's corporate environmental adviser was not mentioned in the brochure. Through links with mainly northern-based universities, the research institute would aim to bring added value to West Cumbria by developing into an institution of higher education and would both carry out and manage a balanced program of applied research on contract to local industries.

The brochure said: "Although the institute will initially have its primary fund of expertise and probably its primary market for research services at Sellafield, its long-term success will depend upon how rapidly the institute develops into a truly viable stand-alone academic institution."

On this basis it was difficult to understand how such an institute could be deemed in any way to be independent from BNFL. Indeed, try as one might, it was hard to find a body more dependent on the nuclear industry than the Westlakes Research Institute, not only in terms of personnel but also in funding. The general opinion was that the institute was still the BNFL laboratory but had moved offsite.

On October 26, 1992, Elizabeth Reay and Vivien Hope took their claim against BNFL to the High Court of Justice in London to be heard before the Hon. Mr. Justice French. Although it was never disputed during the ninety-day trial that exposure to radiation and in particular to plutonium, increased the risks of cancers, including leukemia, the issue in the plaintiffs' case would be specific. The dispute centered on Professor Martin Gardner's hypothesis and whether someone not exposed to radiation could contract leukemia because, before their conception their father had been exposed to it.

According to the Westlakes Research Institute newsletter *View from the Park,* the institute from February to June 1993 "had seen considerable involvement in the leukemia litigation." Jan Tawn in London, had been joined by other members of her staff, and they were providing technical expertise to the defense.[29]

Resulting from collaborative work between the Epidemiology Group at the Westlakes Research Institute and the Child Health Department of Newcastle University, the draft Parker/Wakeford report was presented as evidence by Richard Wakeford, a principal BNFL scientist. Wakeford argued that the Gardner theory of Paternal Preconceptual Irradiation was not a plausible cause of the leukemias.[30]

On January 13, 1993, the thirty-first day of the trial, Professor Martin Gardner died. Many were, therefore, shocked when BNFL expert, Sir Richard Doll, considered the world's leading epidemiologist, accused Gardner and the whole prosecution team of fixing their report results and suggested that Gardner had only decided on the parameters of his study once he knew the results. This had been totally denied by Gardner before his death, but Sir Richard Doll, with virtually nothing to support it, persisted with the allegation in the witness box.[31]

The Kinlen hypothesis regarding population mixing was a cloud that had hung over the case, with BNFL failing to produce Kinlen, despite the fact that he was advising them behind the scenes. It was interesting that Kinlen, having produced only four studies in the four years prior to the beginning of the trial, produced three studies in the period between the closing of the plaintiffs' epidemiological evidence and the closing of the trial and Martyn Day's experts were unable to give their full views on Kinlen and his theory.

Professor Steve Jones, in his dual role as the Westlakes Institute Director of Environmental Sciences and Corporate Adviser to BNFL, gave evidence on historic environmental discharges from Sellafield, based on figures produced by his new SEAM model, which had taken him and two of his team two years to develop. Although plaintiffs' QC, Ben Hytner, expressed deep suspicions on the accuracy of Professor Jones' figures, he did not contest them, as an attempt to prove their inaccuracy would have been extremely costly to the Legal Aid Fund and, at the time, would not have advanced their case. He reserved the right to argue the point in other cases which might be pending.[32]

Elizabeth Reay and Vivien Hope lost their high court case against BNFL. On October 8, 1993, Mr. Justice French ruled that the Gardner theory was not to blame.[33]

"CLEARED!!" wrote Dr. Andy Slovak in the *BNFL News*. In his dual role as independent Director of Westlakes' Occupational Health Department BNFL and BNFL Chief Medical Officer, Slovak accused our statements in defense of our case as "rushing to find dafter and dafter reasons for why they aren't wrong." Those daft reasons were that Mr. Justice French had not in fact "cleared" BNFL of the allegations that radiation from Sellafield had caused leukemia in children. And neither had the plaintiff's deep suspicions of the accuracy of BNFL's historic discharges been tested in court.

"Had it proved necessary to explore this issue to the full," Mr. Justice French later commented in his judgment, "this would have involved calling about ten expert witnesses to give technical evidence regarding the quantities of radionuclides emitted by the various stacks on the Sellafield site, the nature of those radionuclides, the deposition rates within circles round the site drawn at varying distances from the site; the extent to which individual inhabitants were likely to inhale or ingest the various radionuclides directly from the atmosphere or when re-suspended, for example by passing traffic or ingested because taken up by farm produce or seafood."[34]

What French failed to say was that this was exactly what a good epidemiologist should do and he was using an argument that Doll and others had frequently used in relation to such things as chemicals and exhaust particulates—that the matter was too complex for scientific inquiry.

Pending the outcome of further research, Martyn Day had asked the court permission to keep some of the legal aid certificates of the follow-on cases open for a year, but they were discharged after a few months. Because of the thirty-year statutory limitation period, Mr. Justice French said the families could again bring proceedings if future scientific evidence became available.

According to the Westlakes Institute's newsletter, the uncertainty of deposition and re-suspension of relatively large particles around Sellafield had been investigated since October 1992 by Ellis Evans, who had joined Westlakes as one of their first research students. The institute considered that his project was progressing well.[35]

In common with most companies that award research contracts, BNFL does insist on the right to change or veto publications, a consideration that sometimes appears to stretch beyond the academic rubrics governing PhDs. While Evans received his PhD in 1998, he was said to be unhappy that before its assessment he had been asked to change some of his conclusions to his thesis.[36]

Professor Jones, who is director of environmental research at Westlakes, said that Westlakes would attempt to dispel such doubts raised during the trial by publishing in scientific journals and by establishing a reputation for being proved right. On the sensitive question of whether BNFL would try to veto publication of important findings, he said:

> If BNFL got the reputation within the scientific community in which it works for taking that sort of line, then things could get pretty sticky. But in the past where BNFL has funded research in these areas, the results always have been published.[37]

Newcastle University's Department of Child Health received £685,000 from the Westlakes Research Institute in 1994 for projects on stillbirths, birth certification, and the Collaboration 2000 project—researching transgenerational effects of radiation exposure. CORE was told that a Westlakes/Newcastle research paper on stillbirths and birth defects "was being sat on." Neither department was willing to comment on whether a report existed or whether publication was due. The report, published months later in the *Lancet* in October 1999, shows a "Statistical Association between Radiation and Stillbirths in Sellafield Workers."[38]

In 1994, the press announced that publication of Newcastle's research into the Kinlen viral hypothesis, a theory that a virus rather than radiation is the cause of the childhood leukemias around the Sellafield plant—a theory much favored by the nuclear industry—was imminent. It never came. In 1995, Dr. Louise Parker of Newcastle told CORE that publication had been delayed until 1996. In August 1999, the report was confirmed as having been abandoned.

THE NORTH CUMBRIA COMMUNITY GENETICS PROJECT ABOVE BOARD OR UNDERHAND

Suspicion of the BNFL/Westlakes/Newcastle partnership increased in 1994, when on May 16 Newcastle University announced they had been given permission, in principle, to take blood and tissue samples from babies born in West Cumbria.[39] The North Cumbria Community Genetics Project (NCCGP) samples would be stored at BNFL's Geoffrey Schofield Laboratory at Westlakes, and their genetic make-up studied by BNFL scientist Dr. Jan Tawn, who had been with the Sellafield's own genetics unit since 1978 and would be playing an important role in the development of the project.

Generally speaking, academics at Newcastle tended to see their cooperation with BNFL altruistically. I spoke to people who welcomed the BNFL money and saw their contribution to such things as a genetic data bank as a contribution to the community.

With BNFL funding for the project via a Westlakes Research (Trading) contract, a store of DNA, plasma, and viable cells from around eight thousand babies—born at the West Cumberland Hospital in Whitehaven—would, with maternal consent, be collected over a five-year period. Newcastle University Professor John Burn (Department of Human Genetics) and Dr. Louise Parker (Department of Child Health) would be leading research, hoping to find out the frequency of common and less common genetic defects which might affect the health of children and adults.

They would focus on two genetic disorders known as M-CAD and DiGeorge Syndrome. The former was thought to be responsible for some cases of cot death (SIDS) and the latter for heart problems in children. The aim of the study was to determine the frequency of genes for the two diseases in the general population, since it was felt that these might be underestimated at present.

To ensure confidentiality, samples would be stored at BNFL's Geoffrey Schofield Laboratory at Westlakes for sixteen years until the donors became of age, with personal information from parents' lifestyle questionnaires stored separately at Newcastle. Since collection started, placental tissue from mothers has also been included.

Many people thought this research was going too far. "It's like the fox knocking on the farmer's door offering to look after his chickens," someone commented on local radio.

Among the questions that CORE was asked, perhaps the most pertinent was: "If BNFL had applied in its own right to the West Cumbria Health Authority to research West Cumbrian babies, would they have been given permission? If not, why were they allowed access through the back door?"

As early as 1984, West Cumbria District Medical Officer, Dr. John Terrell, had questioned the ethics of a planned BNFL study of placental material and had written to the DHSS: "We debated the wisdom of going on with this in view of the possible criticism of the BNFL connection."[40] Nevertheless, they had approved the study.

With the researchers claiming that the project had the approval, in principle, of the West Cumbrian Ethics Committee, they soon realized that they would require not only the full backing of the health authority and local health professionals but, more importantly, the support of the local community. In spite of their strong promotion in the local media for the need to perceive the Westlakes Research Institute as being "independent," many Cumbrians considered the influential BNFL link as being insensitive and undesirable, particularly in the case of health studies. The clarification in the *Whitehaven News* by Head of Genetics Dr. Jan Tawn that, in May 1994, her BNFL genetics unit and all its staff had become independent, was not convincing.

There was also a strong feeling that before any agreement to the project, even in principle, had been reached by the West Cumbria Health Ethics Committee, full public and open consultation should have taken place in the area. Additional concerns were that members of the ethics committee had been chosen rather than elected and that discussions on confidentiality, coding, and publication of results had already taken place behind closed doors, without any input from local parents and with the confidential minutes unavailable for public scrutiny.

Knowing that ethical debate both with professionals and with the local community would be required to gain goodwill and support and that without their full backing the project would not be able to go ahead, the team promised a full and extensive public consultation in the Whitehaven area with information about the project publicly available.

When I put the questions, "Why West Cumbrian babies?" and "Would Sellafield be studying radiation effects?" to Dr. Louise Parker, she replied that, although her work to "explain" the Seascale leukemia excess had so far failed, it would continue. She denied that the North Cumbria Community Genetics Project was specifically concerned with either Seascale or Sellafield, although it would of course include children from Seascale families and some of those whose parents worked at Sellafield. She did not consider that the two groups of children in West Cumbria were different.[41]

BNFL did suggest that there could be a second agenda of radiation research. The *Sellafield Newsletter*, their weekly in-house publication, hailed the study as a "Pioneering Health Project," and "Europe's first DNA bank" and said: "Whilst it could also help research into the effects of radiation, BNFL believes the study will prove there is no difference between the genetic make-up of children born around Sellafield and those from the rest of the region."[42]

A local GP said it was obvious that the area had been chosen because of Sellafield; a Canadian scientist warned that we might be part of a bigger study within international nuclear circles and a Welsh MEP asked questions about the project in the House of Commons. One of the scientists on the Project's Ethics Advisory Group took the concerns of CORE "extremely seriously," while a second member thought that the large number of BNFL employees at the Westlakes Research Institute needed to be kept in mind in any discussions on the ethics of the project.[43]

However, even with publicly accessible information about the DNA project a prerequisite, and the pledge that extensive consultation with both professionals and members of the public in the Whitehaven area would take place, nothing happened: the silence was, said the *Whitehaven News*, proving "embarrassing." Initially the West Cumbria Community Health Council wanted to hold a public consultation meeting on the issue. Then the North Cumbria Health Authority asked to see the proposed study's protocols, so that all the contractual details, such as who controls access to data or the publication of research findings, were known before public opinion was tested. They took over the matter and started to arrange meetings.

A public meeting on June 13 was canceled. The Westlakes Research Institute rescheduled it to June 22, but this one was also canceled. Admitting that this was a great embarrassment and that the issue was a delicate one, Westlakes promised to arrange a meeting in July, but this never materialized.[44]

Eventually, on October 5, 1994, GPs and health authority employees only were consulted. Their major concern was that individual parents would not be entitled to specific information and feedback about their child.

It was total inefficiency, rather than foul play, when finally the announcement came that the general public was invited to give their views on the North Cumbria Community Genetics Project. Two meetings had been arranged, both on November 7, the first at Whitehaven in the afternoon and the second at Workington that evening, at the same time as a very well-publicized meeting on disposal of nuclear waste in West Cumbria was to take place. As advance advertising of the North Cumbria Community Genetics Project's consultation meetings had been extremely poor, few people were aware that the meetings were taking place. A check on local libraries showed that none had received the promised information handouts.

It was not surprising, therefore, that turnout was poor and, with some people going to both meetings, only around forty members of the public attended.

Two days later, we went out onto the streets to ask people's views about the meetings. We found that from the 441 people interviewed, only seven had been aware the meetings were taking place, 320 had never even heard of the project and the remainder had vague recollections of hearing something about it on television after the event. The "DNA bank is mystery to most." the *Whitehaven News* reported.[45]

At the meetings, with desperate efforts to allay people's fears, Professor John Burn told the audience that BNFL's backing for the project was a gamble and the DNA findings could shut Sellafield. As doctor in charge of the Northern Region Genetics Services, as well as the North Cumbria Community Genetics Project, he had long thought about storing a sample of blood from the whole population, so that they could match diseases to genes and learn how to prevent certain illnesses and treat others better.

Referring to the Westlakes Research Institute, he said that, for several years, the nuclear industry had been working with the Department of Child Health in Newcastle University to study the possible health effects of low-level radiation. He had known Dr. Janet Tawn since he took over the Genetics Clinic at West Cumberland Hospital in 1984, as her genetics laboratory at Sellafield was doing a free chromosome testing service for the West Cumberland Hospital. With the transfer of BNFL scientists to the Westlakes Research Institute, they had asked for joint research in the field of genetics. They would not, Professor Burn assured, have personal data and any medical studies would depend on work done in Newcastle University.

Although any powerful advance had dangers if misused, Burn said that he was convinced that well-developed professional controls, with a network of active Ethics Committees, were in place. There would be safeguards, he said. Taken with mothers' permission, samples would be discarded if they changed their minds; these would be kept for sixteen years only and, if the decision was taken to continue the study at a later stage, they would be asked again. Commercial and insurance companies would be denied access and, unless backed by a court order, so would the police. Admitting that BNFL would clearly have a legitimate interest in this kind of data, he said they would have no right to veto the outcome of research.

It had always been his intention that the North Cumbria Community Genetics Project's research would be extended to the whole of North Cumbria.

CORE organized a press conference. As well as those involved with the project, we invited genetics expert Dr. David King, editor of *GenEthics News*, an independent newsletter of ethical and environmental issues raised by genetic engineering. He warned "It is not desirable that such a bank be held in the hands of a private organization which is not directly accountable to the public or to those who have donated samples . . . particularly in the case of BNFL, which is a major local employer, and is certain to encourage fears about Big Brother."[47]

Speaking of the risks of "moving towards a genetic underclass of people who supposedly have 'bad' genes," Dr. King said: "The bank will contain both samples of DNA and blood and will therefore contain much sensitive personal information. In the next few years, with the avalanche of information from the Human Genome Project, it will become possible to do further tests, with even more personally sensitive implications."

He considered that the research should be conducted by entirely independent researchers. There was, unfortunately, a well-documented history, particularly in the United States, of nuclear installations suppressing information damaging to itself. He did not suggest this would occur here, but, with the precedent, there might be pressures on the researchers as the system of coding and confidentiality was not watertight, nor could it be made so. It was therefore essential to allow access to the raw data by outside scientists and any concerned local people. He proposed that a monitoring group was set up.

If samples were traced to individuals, how could this information be abused? One obvious possibility was that individuals with a high level of somatic mutations might be denied future employment at nuclear installations. The researchers should give a clear undertaking that they would not patent any material from the DNA bank, not attempt to commercialize nor allow anyone else to commercialize or patent the material.

David King was particularly critical that Sellafield would provide the money to fund a midwife attached to the study, rather than appoint an independent unbiased and non-directive trained counselor, not employed by the project. She would train hospital midwives and it was possible that parents would be pushed into allowing samples to be taken without properly understanding the implications.

Within a short time, a *second agenda* related to the research was confirmed. Director of Public Health, Dr. Joan Munro, confirmed the DNA bank's aim to screen babies of Sellafield workers. Although this had not been aired at the public meetings, the "professional body" had been aware of it, but she added that the study had not yet been applied for and nothing could go ahead without the ethics committee's consent.[48]

CORE commissioned Dr. David King to research this "second agenda," as for West Cumbrians this became the project's most controversial issue. His report, "Glycophorin: a somatic mutation assay," concluded that this research method was inadequate and predicted it would not be sensitive enough to pick up radiation damage in babies of Sellafield workers.[49]

On December 21, however, members of the North Cumbria Health Authority voted unanimously in support of the North Cumbria Community Genetics Project.[50]

As any claim of independence from Sellafield was a myth that could not go unchallenged, we were glad that both Dr. David King and Seascale GP Barry Walker had been asked to join the project's Supervisory Ethics Committee.

In 1995, with approval for the research, the frequency of somatic mutations of the glycophorin-A (GPA) gene were measured in red blood cells from a series of newborn babies and related to various epidemiological and lifestyle factors in order to identify those factors that might influence the mutation rate before birth.[51] As predicted by David King, no association with occupational radiation exposure was found.

The North Cumbria Community Genetics Project began sample collection in 1996 and, by the year 2000, specimens from over 4,200 babies had been received. In their report in 2000, they detailed the ten research studies that samples had been used in, both by the genetics project team and as part of collaborations with recognized experts in various medical research fields, including heart defects, breast cancer, neural tube defects, cancer susceptibility, and adverse response to radiotherapy and cystic fibrosis.[52]

The issue of informed consent was raised in a draft study by Erica Haimes and Michael Whong-Barr of the Newcastle University's Department of Sociology and Social Policy, which investigated women's perceptions of their reasons for donating to the NCCGP project and their reasons for refusing.[53]

Several of those who chose not to donate cited a lack of control over the samples, possible future abuse, and that it was not only their own consent but their child's as well they had been asked to give. The research acknowledged that the voices of the children who had also donated to the DNA bank would not be heard for quite some time. Until they reached the age of sixteen, they were essentially silent donors whose materials would contribute to medical research but without their consent.

Following the announcement by the government in 2001 of BNFL's technical bankruptcy, a 2002 strategic review on the future management of the United Kingdom's nuclear legacy led to the company's restructuring into a "holding company" working with government toward the creation of the proposed Liabilities Management Authority (subsequently renamed as the Nuclear Decommissioning Authority). Created under the Energy Act 2004, the NDA, as a statutory non-departmental public body, took ownership of Sellafield on April 1, 2005, together with BNFL's assets and liabilities.

During BNFL's restructuring 2002 to 2005 period, Sellafield's management was undertaken by in-house subsidiaries, including BNFL Alpha, British Nuclear Group, and Sellafield Ltd.

In 2007, Westlakes Research changed its name to Westlakes Scientific Consulting, but continued its extensive services to the nuclear industry and consultancy services in environmental and health science. British Nuclear Group's Project Services announced the opening of a "groundbreaking" new facility. Costing £200,000, the extension to the Geoffrey Schofield Laboratory was officially opened by ex-Sellafield PR man and Copeland's MP, Jamie Reed, who said the facility would "see West Cumbria become a future world leader in nuclear sciences" and went on to say that Sellafield's Project Services "understands the area's incredible potential and wants to be involved at the outset."

SELLAFIELD "BODY PARTS INQUIRY"

In April 2007, the then trade and industry secretary, Alistair Darling, made an emergency statement to the House of Commons in which he revealed tissue had been taken from sixty-five individuals, mainly workers at Sellafield, and analyzed for radionuclide content.[54] The government asked Michael Redfern QC to try to establish when, where, by whom, and by what means the taking of organs/tissues was requested and authorized. He would also be asked to report on whether informed consent was obtained from families and find out the reasons why the tests were conducted. The inquiry began with the Westlakes Research Institute.

Dr. David Macgregor had been appointed BNFL's Company Chief Medical Officer in 2003. His responsibilities included oversight of all BNFL's medical and epidemiological research projects. In May 2005, he had been notified by Westlakes Research Institute of a proposal to reexamine data obtained from radiochemical analysis of organs removed from former nuclear employees at post-mortem examination, which had led to his obtaining more information about the extent of the earlier work by one of his predecessors, Dr. Geoffrey Schofield.

He discovered that, in many cases, the cause of death could not have been related to radiation and that there was no evidence to suggest consent to the removal and radiochemical analysis of organs; he noted also that the coroner appeared frequently to have notified the medical department at Sellafield of employees' deaths, and considered this to be odd.

Dr. Macgregor discussed his concerns with BNFL management and the Sellafield trade unions, but before further investigations were carried out, the press became aware of the issue, which in turn attracted the attention of the government.

Government ministers chose a "good, bad news day" to publish the Redfern Inquiry Report's findings, picking November 16, 2010, the day when the announcement of the engagement of Prince William to Kate Middleton dominated all the media headlines.

The "Report of the inquiry into human tissue analysis in UK nuclear facilities" said that nuclear workers and their families had been let down. It had seen no evidence that the legal and ethical issues raised by the nuclear industry's retention of organs at post-mortem had been adequately considered, nor had the requirement for the consent of the relatives of the deceased been adequately addressed.

At Sellafield, an informal arrangement had existed between the late BNFL Chief Medical Officer, Dr. Geoffrey Schofield, the driving force behind the analytical work, and the pathologists at West Cumberland Hospital, which meant that he was told when a post-mortem was to take place on the body of a former Sellafield worker.

In cases of particular interest to him, Dr. Schofield appeared to have taken somewhat dubious steps to obtain organs; the attempts which he sometimes had made to ensure that deaths were reported to coroners could have been regarded as a manipulation of the coronial process. The range of body parts removed for analyses, including liver, ribs, kidney, as well as testes, brain, heart, and tongue, had been extraordinary.

The report concluded that although Dr. Schofield and his colleagues had made no attempts to conceal their research, there was no suggestion that they considered their actions to be untoward and neither did they appear to have given any consideration to the ethical implications of their work.

Newcastle and the National Radiological Protection Board had also been involved in the analyses of body parts, mostly vertebrae and liver, removed at sixteen hospital post-mortem examinations on children, for which consent had been obtained. The study was organized by Professor (now Sir) Alan Craft, Professor of Child Health in Newcastle, and most of the children had been under his care. It had received formal approval from ethics committees in West Cumbria, Newcastle, and North Tyneside. The results were published only in two internal NRPB papers in 1985 and 1986.

The House of Commons expressed "heartfelt regret" and apologized to the relatives of those involved. For the families, one of the hardest parts of the process had been that each person affected had felt as if they had re-experienced bereavements at different stages of the inquiry as and when the true facts had come to light.

At the start of the inquiry many boxes of CORE's archived papers had been offered to the Redfern team. These dated back to the early 1980s, when the group had raised funds and had enabled Sellafield workers or their families to access legal advice and secure compensation for work-related cancers. Our papers, including notes of interviews with Sellafield workers, widows, coroners' reports, death certificates, and correspondence with the unions and lawyers had given an inquiry solicitor "a valuable lead into everything at an early stage" and for that he had been most grateful.

With BNFL funding for the North Community Genetics Project becoming more difficult, on July 16, 2010, blaming the downturn in sales and the scale of the company's "significant" pension scheme deficit, the Westlakes Research Institute was put into administration, putting sixty-five jobs at risk. It was trading as Westlakes Scientific Consulting and was now a subsidiary of the University of Central Lancashire. PricewaterhouseCoopers LLP had been appointed joint administrators, working closely with key stakeholders to identify a positive outcome for the administration.[55]

Although most West Cumbrians had only vague memories of the publicity surrounding the controversial North Cumbria Community Genetics Project, several mothers who had donated wanted to know what would now be done to their samples. There had been rumors that the administrators would turn off the fridges. Parents had a right to know.

Communications with the Newcastle project team proved difficult. We therefore raised our questions at the Sellafield Stakeholder Group's Environmental Health Sub-Committee (EHSC), a watchdog body providing public scrutiny of the nuclear industry in West Cumbria, and taking account of the health of the community.

Professor (now Sir) John Burn replied to the committee that, when Westlakes closed, all DNA and tissue samples collected as part of the North Cumbria Community Genetics Project were to be transferred to the Newcastle University Biobank. As the study had not been set up to allow routine contact with the donors, the project's Research Ethics Committee had agreed that this move had not represented a substantive enough reason to attempt to contact the donor community. He added that, had the Newcastle Biobank been established when NCCGP started collecting samples, his team would probably have considered using them from the outset, though a factor in the discussions had been to involve Westlakes Research Institute wherever possible, in order to help them develop a research presence and support local employment.[56]

Their consent clearly stated that they were not permitted to retain identifiable samples on any child beyond the age of sixteen years without renewed consent. This would become an issue in 2012 and an extensive dialogue with the ethics committee was taking place. If the current efforts to raise funds were successful, they would design a new project to re-consent the participants and extend the remit and scope of the project to take account of the rapidly developing field of genomics.

"So what about the Human Tissue Act 2004 which, if applicable, would require appropriate consent for storage of human tissue samples?" CORE had asked. Professor Burn replied that the Human Tissue Act 2004 did not apply to stored DNA.

Professor Burn had "made it clear," according to Professor John Haywood, EHSC's chairman, "that the North Cumbria Genetics Project was not aimed at or used for the study of environmental health factors. The EHSC's remit was limited to environmental health issues. If, at some future time the samples taken were used to investigate environmental health factors, then that activity would fall within EHSC's remit and EHSC could follow it up." We, the involved public, did not have the right to know.[57] In 2012, there was a short statement that, without further funding the project samples were being retained and, as these reached the age of sixteen, the identifier for each sample would be deleted, ensuring their anonymity in future, and would not be used as part of a national database. A 2014 update request is still awaited.

With yet another rechristening, Sellafield Ltd. announced on March 11, 2014, a "New era, new name" for their former BNFL Westlakes Laboratory. It had been named after the late BNFL Chief Medical Officer, Geoffrey Schofield, who was instrumental in, and heavily criticized by the Redfern "body parts scandal" inquiry. Renamed Greeson Court, the laboratory is now owned by Cavendish Nuclear and offers nuclear, civil, and industrial sectors a wide range of leading-edge analytical techniques.

The Energy Coast's "Masterplan," mainly promoting all things nuclear, predicts that "by 2027 West Cumbria will be globally recognized as a leading nuclear, energy, environment, and related technology business cluster, building on its nuclear assets and its technology and research strengths."

The fate of the North Cumbria Community Genetics Project's samples remains unclear. The basic human right of NCCGP parents to know what happened should be respected. Since the publication of the Redfern Report into the shocking removal of tissue samples from the bodies of nuclear workers without informing their families, they need to know that their samples are not being viewed as just another piece of laboratory equipment.

We don't suggest that the NCCGP samples are, or ever have been, misused in any way, nor has CORE denied that they could help research into major diseases. We have never wished to impugn the integrity of any individual participating in the research program either directly or indirectly, but we remain convinced it was unnecessarily dangerous to have placed the sensitive NCCGP samples in the hands of a body so clearly and inexorably linked to an industry which has a vested interest in the outcome of any research.

Over a twenty-year period of my involvement with CORE, it has been clear to me that industry and government involvement in the nuclear industry has deprived the public of a real say in the environmental conditions of their own health. In the path already traveled, one is able to see the signposts to the future—if there were a major nuclear disaster in Britain, it would be covered up with the same aggressive propaganda that defends all major corporate mistakes.

The formation and the work of the Westlakes Research Institute was a classic corporate maneuver seen in other industries, to give a promotional gloss to the industry; in this case, however, the close involvement in the nuclear industry of the British government added even more power and greater secrecy to industry lack of accountability, while adding authority to the work of academics and scientists who carried out their jobs in almost asocial confinement.

CORE's current campaign is for the precautionary principle to be adopted in the form of publicly displayed signs or notices being provided on or adjacent to West Cumbrian beaches to alert the general public to the presence of radioactive "hot" particles. The right to know is a basic human right enabling individual choices to be made. I only wish I'd been given that choice all those years ago.[58]

Chapter 18

WILHELM HUEPER AND ROBERT KEHOE— EPIDEMIOLOGICAL WAR CRIMES

Devra Davis

The right to search for truth also implies a duty; one must not conceal any part of what one has recognized to be true.

Albert Einstein

Active and aggressive work in this field is like participating in a strange type of war, which, like any other type of war, had its cruelties and its casualties.

Wilhelm Hueper

War crimes," as Robert McNamara pithily noted in the Academy Award-winning film, *The Fog of War*, "Are what the losers get charged with." But sometimes conquerors behave so badly and their actions fall so far from accepted conduct that they are, if not criminal, then immoral.

What if a major figure in American business had gone to Germany right after World War II, and come back with evidence that the chemicals his firm was then producing caused cancer in German workers and would soon do so in their American counterparts? What if he then failed to pass that information on to those workers, or to government agencies then trying to set standards for those who worked with these materials? What if this, and other, evidence that workers were being harmed by the materials they were working with was systematically ignored, or hidden in plain view in the United States and elsewhere in the 1950s? What if a scientist who showed that these same chemicals induced cancer in animals and workers was hounded out of his job, vilified both as a communist sympathizer and former Nazi, and marginalized beyond recognition?[1]

At the start of the 1940s, the world was at war. Those economies that were still standing when World War II ended in 1945 recovered from the global depression by remaining highly militarized and industrialized. To understand the real-world constraints placed on research on environmental causes of cancer in the 1940s, we can do no better than to consider the stories of two major figures—Wilhelm Hueper, a German émigré pathologist to the United States, and Robert Kehoe, a founder of industrial toxicology. With an encyclopedic grasp of workplace causes of cancer, and a command of four languages, Hueper founded the field of occupational and environmental carcinogenesis. A pivotal figure in several major chemical firms, Kehoe, along with other founders of industrial toxicology and workplace epidemiology, established the basic rules by which analyses of worker health and safety would be carried out for the first half of the twentieth century.

Two people could not have had more fundamentally different views of the role of science and scientists in the crafting of public policy. To understand Hueper, it is necessary to imagine the world in which he grew up. The son of an impoverished south German family that repeatedly moved from one rental property to another, as a young man he was drafted into the German Army prior to the First World War. He dodged residues of poison gas that would waft back onto German troops during that conflict. After being discharged, he became a pacifist, and a critic of religious and reactionary politics.

Hueper arrived in the United States in his twenties in 1921 as a married physician and became a citizen within two decades. In 1934, during the depths of the depression, he was broke and unemployed. He put his furniture in storage, cashed in his life insurance policy, and with his young wife and children traveled back to Germany to try to find a job, just after the Nazis seized power. His letter seeking work at the time was signed *Heil Hitler*. In looking at Hueper's motives to return to Germany, the science historian, Robert Proctor, notes, it is not always easy to distinguish between conviction and opportunism in such matters.[2]

Hueper was stunned by what he found after arriving in Germany. Once the world's leader in scientific research, the Germany that he toured in 1933 had rendered research on dogs illegal for humane reasons but deemed some people lower than animals.

During the war, the Germans actually halted testing of rabbits, but continued to carry out studies on humans. Keeping up a tradition of human observation that stemmed from the turn of the twentieth century, German researchers had found that men producing some synthetic dyes (Farbenindustrie) often developed blood in their urine and blockages in their bladders—early signs of tumors. In 1895, less than two decades after production of synthetic dyes had begun in Frankfurt, Germany, an astute surgeon, Rehn, reported that one of every ten industrial dye factory workers had bladder cancer.

By 1906, physicians from every nation where such production had begun two decades earlier reported dozens of additional cases. In the 1930s, Germany and Switzerland officially agreed to pay those dye workers who developed bladder cancer—making this one of the first formally compensable occupational illnesses.

Disheartened by what they found in Nazi Germany, Hueper and his wife returned to the States, where he found low-paying work in pathology. But in 1937, Hueper got one of those once in a lifetime chances. The DuPont family's personal physician referred Hueper to the growing company. Within a few weeks, he had become a part of the company's new Haskell Laboratory for Toxicology and Industrial Medicine.

With a spirited start, Hueper set up novel experimental systems to study how animals responded to some of the dyes and solvents being manufactured at DuPont at the time. He also tried to monitor the health of workers with these same agents. Things did not go well. After Hueper lost his job with DuPont in 1939, he went on to hold a number of other research posts, developing experimental studies of suspect materials and ending up at the US government a decade later. From 1948 until his retirement in 1968, Hueper held what appeared to be a dream post. At the US National Cancer Institute, Hueper led its first section on environmental cancer. He was the person Rachel Carson would credit in her book *Silent Spring* for exposing the connections between the environment and cancer.[3]

Kehoe took a quite different path. Trained in medicine at the University of Cincinnati at the same time as Hueper, he became comfortable in a world of relative privilege and noblesse oblige. Those who were wealthy were not only expected to help those less fortunate, they were assumed to be better able to do so than ordinary people. Recognized early on for his brilliance and innovation in grappling with industrial workplace conditions and for his knack for the business world, Kehoe made a career of advising corporations under fire. He also remained a central figure in public health circles for more than forty years, and at one point was President of the American Academy of Occupational Medicine, and Director and President of the American Industrial Hygiene Association— groups that took on the task of setting standards for exposure to workplace hazards.

Kehoe's views on the values and dangers of industrial hygiene research reflected the corporate crucible out of which they emerged. Consider the position he took on leaded gasoline. On February 2, 1923, the world's first leaded gasoline had been sold, touted as a salve for engine knocks and pings caused by incomplete combustion. That same year in a small General Motors (GM) plant in Dayton, Ohio, the only two workers who had been responsible for bottling liquid lead died. The line was shut down in April 1924. Charles Kettering, chief of GM's effort to develop leaded fuels, blamed the workers.[4]

"We could not get this across to the boys. . . ." he said. "We put watchmen in at the plant, and they used to snap the stuff [pure tetraethyl lead] at each other, and throw it at each other, and they were saying that they were sissies. They did not realize what they were working with."

Kehoe, then a young assistant professor of pathology at the University of Cincinnati, was brought in to advise on how to prevent future such events. He counseled then what was undoubtedly true and what he fervently believed in most such situations—workers needed to be trained to be more careful. Realizing the value of being able to tap such advice on a regular basis, the Ethyl Corporation, General Motors, DuPont, and others provided the grand sum of one hundred thousand dollars in 1929 to build the industrial toxicology laboratory on the University of Cincinnati campus, which was named in honor of Kettering who headed GM's research operations at the time.

Kehoe became the lab's first director and provided toxicological advice to these firms over the next two decades on various products. He also served as medical director of the Ethyl Corporation and a corporate officer of GM. These overlapping positions speak volumes about the close relationships of business, government, and the university that continued throughout Kehoe's leadership at Kettering, until a stroke in 1963 ended his active involvement with the laboratory. Kettering Labs conducted studies of rodents and of "human organisms," according to contracts signed with Monsanto, DuPont, General Motors, Stauffer Chemical Company, the Tennessee Valley Authority, US Steel, Mobil Oil, and the Ethyl Corporation, among others. Each contract included a proviso that "the investigative work shall be planned and carried out by the university, and the university shall have the right to disseminate for the public good, any information obtained. However, before issuance of public reports or scientific publications, the manuscripts thereof will be submitted to the donor for criticism and suggestion."

This was not at all unusual at the time. Businesses routinely funded research at universities and even within the federal government, where support for basic research was negligible. The same businesses that produced materials that

Kettering tested also regularly decided what findings could and could not be made public. As we will learn, one consequence of these practices was that limited results from the confidential studies that Kettering undertook were ever published. But, private reports were made available to the producers of suspect materials, many of which never were released to the public.

As late as March 25, 1965, when Kehoe had retired from active management of Kettering, he sent a memo to the staff regarding papers prepared for publication that reminded people of the need not to refer to private reports. "It is undesirable, as a rule," the memo indicated, "to refer to reports of the laboratory made to sponsors in papers prepared for publication, since such references bring requests for these reports. As these reports often contain confidential information, they cannot be supplied, except confidentially, to other interested persons, and unless one knows that they are suitable for issuance to others . . . they should not be mentioned in public."

At the labs, Kehoe proved a mentor to many of those who would go on to lead distinguished careers in industrial hygiene, including Eula Bingham, who later became director of the Occupational Safety and Health Administration in 1976, and Paul Kotin, who would become the first director of the National Institutes of Environmental Health Sciences, in 1968.

Still, when it came to dealing with heads of corporations on matters regarding the safety of their products, Kehoe took an old-fashioned view. He believed that businessmen would listen to doctors and that workplace hazards could best be handled if they were kept confidential. These were not the only points on which he would be proved wrong.

Within two months after the war in Germany had ended, intelligence agencies from Britain and the United States began collating useful German information. One member of the US team sent to gather this intelligence was Dr. Kehoe. Shortly after the surrender of Germany in June of 1945, Kehoe went to Germany, interviewed key scientists, and brought back critical studies on topics ranging from chemical warfare to pesticides, pharmaceuticals, and industrial materials. He had lots to draw upon, as Germany had been the world's leader in science and engineering prior to the war and had pioneered experimental and human studies on toxic materials.[5]

A June, 1945, headquarters report by an Allied Service Forces intelligence bulletin reported on the testing of dyestuffs, textile finishes, and other chemicals for toxicological effects, when applied to that light pink delicate underside of a rabbit's ears and then tested on human skin. Eager to learn what had fueled the German war effort, and well aware of the eminent reputation of German science earlier in the century, teams of US and British field investigators combed through Germany right after the war, looking for scientific studies on poison gas warfare and other matters.

What Kehoe found made it clear: the Germans had understood much about the ways in which various toxic agents could kill people quickly and could also cause permanent damage that would lead to death more slowly. The average age of death from bladder cancer for men who had worked with 2-naphthylamine and benzidine was twenty years younger than for men without such exposures, according to information provided by Professor, Doctor of Medicine, H. Oettel, of Ludwigshafen am Rhein, Germany, in 1939.

Based on these findings, Germany had officially devised workplace rules that allowed only older workers to work with certain cancer-causing materials during World War II. Presumably, these older men would have gone off and died shortly after their employment with these lethal materials had ended.

The introduction to one report prepared for the British Intelligence Objectives Subcommittee on I G Farbenindustrie A G, Leverkusen, in January 1947, was straightforward: "the objective was to study incidence of and methods of prevention of bladder tumor among workers in the benzidine plant." I G Farben, as the firm was better known, stood for *Interessengemeinschaft* "Association of Common Interests" of fabric dyes. Among the numerous common interests of this group was the election of Adolph Hitler, for which I G Farben was the single largest funder. Members of I G Farben included BASF, Bayer, Hoechst, and other German chemical and pharmaceutical companies.

The I G Farben researchers had developed precise methods for calculating the amount of chemical residues found in urine of their workers, the percent of all those working who had developed bladder cancer, and how many years they had been employed at the plant. The bladder is a kind of natural storage system through which all sorts of poisons regularly flow out of the body. But things that move through the bladder, and especially through the long narrow ureter that empties at the end of a man's penis, can leave residues with long tracks.

To carry out their studies, German researchers regularly ran crude rubber tubing into the penises of workers up to their bladders, checking for residues of blood or early signs of tumors. Researchers complained that some workers were not especially cooperative and needed days off after they had been tested.

Still, the findings were quite simple: The longer a man had worked at Leverkusen, the greater his chance of developing tumors of the bladder. Every single one of those who had survived working for twenty years or more had cancer of the bladder. Half those working fifteen to twenty years had such tumors, while only one fourth of those working fifteen years or less had such tumors. This was an early and clear illustration of a basic concept in public health, called dose-response. The higher the dose, the stronger the response. This was yet another instance where stronger and longer was not better.[6]

Remarkable things were learned from the analyses conducted of these workers. It shows clear evidence that the longer workers were employed in the plant, the more of them got cancer. Within two decades every single one of the workers still alive had come down with bladder cancer.

So what happened to the evidence of workplace and other chemical sources of cancer produced by this German research? Where did it go? While the general public never heard much about it, right after World War II ended, a rich array of scientific information on industrial cancer hazards developed by the Nazis was translated into English by various field investigation offices, such as the one that Kehoe manned for the Allies. These detailed summaries of Nazi research on workplace and tobacco hazards made their way to many of the US corporations then engaged in producing these materials. That's where it apparently stopped.

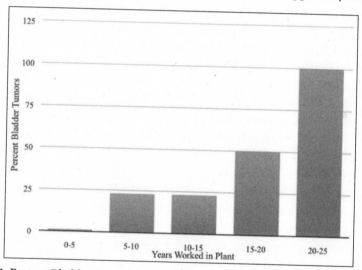

Figure 1. Percent Bladder Tumors in Benzidine Plant Workers, Leverkusen, Germany, 1946

We do not know all of what this unpublished material contained. But we do know that Dr. Kehoe would go on to pursue a highly profitable and distinguished career, working under contract with some major firms that were then, and are now, among the top producers of these and related materials. One of the principal funders of the Kettering Laboratories, DuPont, would in due course become one of the largest successful chemical companies in the world.

Like Kehoe and like physicians throughout the world at the time, Hueper wanted to believe that medical doctors would be held in higher esteem by the governments and corporations and that their advice would be heeded. Hueper's first contacts with DuPont were encouraging. They came about initially through the recommendation of the family physician of the DuPont family who had been impressed with Hueper's work in pathology. In 1937, Hueper had written directly to the chief of the firm, Mr. Irénée DuPont, warning that, based on his own experiences in Germany and elsewhere, Chambers Works dye-making employees were likely to contract bladder cancer. Shortly afterwards, Hueper was brought on board by DuPont to help shape the newly formed Haskell Laboratory for Toxicology and Industrial Medicine. This was pretty heady stuff for a German immigrant, granted a scientific platform in one of the world's leading firms in order to study the hazards about which he had warned. But, coming up with methods for studying hazards is one thing. Trying to do something to keep those hazards from affecting people is quite another.

In his unpublished autobiography, Hueper explained that his honeymoon with Haskell Laboratory proved short-lived. Hueper recorded how the bladders of dogs first became reddened, then scarred over, and finally produced tumors, after repeated exposures to some of the same chemicals then being produced at the Chambers Works. Eager to see at firsthand what went on in the manufacture of aromatic amines, one day Hueper set out to look inside the factories. Here is how he described his first and last visit to the beta-naphthylamine manufacturing plant just across the Wilmington River at Deepwater:

> The manager and some of his associates brought us first to the building housing this operation, which was located in a part of a much larger building. It was separated from other operations in the building by a large sliding-door allowing the ready spread of vapors, fumes and dust from the beta-naphthylamine operation into the adjacent work rooms. Being impressed during the visit by the surprising cleanliness of the naphthylamine operation, which at that occasion was not actively working, I dropped back in the process of visitors, until I caught up with the foreman at its end. When I told him "Your place is surprisingly clean," he looked at me and commented, "Doctor, you should have seen it last night; we worked all night to clean it up for you."[7]

When the inspecting group moved up the road to check out the actual benzidine operation, they entered a small building slaked with white powdery residues from the road, to the loading platform, to the window sills. The entire facility was covered in white dusts. Hueper never set foot in the place again.

The response of his directors at Haskell to Hueper's foray into the factory world was swift. He was ordered to stop studying humans. He was told to restrict his research to studies in experimental animals. By 1939, he had been fired and threatened with legal action if he tried to talk about or publish any of his findings. Another apparent consequence of the tumult over Hueper's work was that for the next twenty years the Chambers Works did not report on any new cases of bladder cancer in their workers. No national or state registries existed for reporting these cases at that time. Nobody was looking for them. Their existence was neither noted nor recorded. But, cases did keep accumulating, as reports that finally surfaced in 1981 revealed.

Unbeknownst to Hueper and other federal researchers at the time, Kettering Laboratories held private contracts with many major corporations from the 1950s through the 1960s, including Ethyl Corporation, Frigidaire, General Motors, DuPont, Lehman Brothers, US Steel, Minnesota Mining and Manufacturing, Tennessee Valley Authority, and Monsanto. The latter four firms all asked the labs to study "fluorine compounds in the human organism." How such studies were to be constructed, what those being exposed experimentally were required to be told, all of that remained at the discretion of the investigators at this time.

The lessons of Nuremberg did not yet extend to the practice of toxicology. The need to be sure that all those participating in such studies were fully apprised of the risks they might incur had not yet been put into American law or practice. It is one of those ironies of science history that though they never actually worked as collaborators, the efforts of Kehoe and Hueper crossed in ways that neither fully appreciated at the time.

In 1939, Hueper had been ordered to stop studying or talking about the cancers he had found increased in those men who labored with synthetic dyes and solvents. Eventually, he was also instructed not to disclose any evidence that animals exposed to these same compounds, or to coal tar derivatives, also developed tumors. In fact, research on these matters did not end with Hueper's suspension from Haskell. Under private contract with DuPont, Kehoe continued the work that Hueper had been ordered to stop, looking into the cancer-causing properties of synthetic dyes and coal tar contaminants of paraffin in workers and studying lab rats' responses to these same agents at the Kettering labs. One confidential agreement for research identified thirteen different formulations of paraffin oils that the labs would study in animals, ranging from naphthenic oil, solvent refined, to chlorinated sperm oil in sulfurized fat base. Keeping any findings on cancer-causing hazards of these and other workplace exposures secret was perfectly legal at the time. Many companies had their own laboratories. Others contracted with universities, like Cincinnati and elsewhere, under the stipulation that no results were to be reported without approval of the sponsors. This clandestine work at Kettering on coal tars and dyes never saw the light of day.

Kehoe took the position when it came to the hazards of lead, synthetic dyes, or other materials, that experimental work was of quite limited value. He insisted that those who would make more of lab findings on the dangers of these agents were merely engaging in speculation and offering opinions. What counted most, he claimed, were plain, hard facts, the sort of information that only comes from studying "human organisms"—looking at the health of real live, or sick, or dead workers.

In Germany, Hueper had charted the ruined lives of workers exposed to lead and aromatic amines. He knew that in America, Germany, Switzerland, England, France, Italy, Austria, Czechoslovakia, and Poland—basically every country where aromatic amines were used—within two decades outbreaks of bladder cancer would hit. While the Chambers Works stopped reporting their cases of bladder cancer in 1936, cases kept coming. By 1980, more than 364 cases at this single facility had been amassed.

In his autobiography, Hueper notes that there are three basic ways that industry can avoid attention to cases of occupational cancer. First of all, they can feign blindness, by not seeing or recording cases, as DuPont did with bladder cancers at the Chambers Works after 1936. Second, they can create negative evidence, by only counting diseases in workers who have been employed a short period of time and not including those with long-term experiences who are neither working nor alive. Or, they can pack the population that is studied with many with no exposures to the agent being examined, thereby diluting any evidence of an effect. Finally, they can engage in outright suppression or prolonged delays in publishing results.[8]

Sometimes legal proceedings end up revealing that all of these practices have gone on. At a deposition in the 1960s, as a witness for the US government, Hueper offered the expert opinion that three men whose cases he had reviewed had developed skin cancers because of their daily work with oil residues. Hueper's mimeographed autobiography reveals that it was during this case, twenty years after his research had been stopped at DuPont, that he finally found out that Kehoe had secretly carried out these studies. As part of what was discovered during a lawsuit on behalf of workers who sought compensation for their bladder cancers, the fact of this secret experimental and human research program was disclosed. Research on aromatic amines at Haskell Laboratories remained so secret that few others ever heard of them.

There is in the history of industrial hygiene a curious practice of seeking to soften the blows of what a chemical portends for human health by changing the wording that is used to describe what it can do, as though softening the language, in and of itself, can minimize the impact. Some of those who pushed for taking American coal tar off the list of cancer-causing agents paid a very heavy personal price. While the cancer-causing label was stripped from American coal tar, that did not wipe away the capacity of coal tars to cause cancer. One industry representative learned this firsthand.

> The irony of this decision [to remove coal tar as a carcinogen] was that the vice president of this tar company was suffering at the time of his visit with me from two small tar cancers on the skin of his neck from previous occupational contact with coal tar.

When it came to looking into patterns of scrotal tumors in petrochemicals workers, Hueper reported in his autobiography that a similar effort had gone on to make this problem appear to go away. For a while, it had appeared that what was once a big problem had been eliminated. Prior to 1920, a number of groups of workers were found to have increased rates of tumors in their scrotums. After the industry had reported cleaning things up, not a single case was recorded.[9]

This was ballyhooed as a triumph of improved industrial hygiene. It turned out to be no such thing. In fact, whenever a scrotal tumor appeared after 1920, it was simply called a venereal tumor—allegedly linked with sexually transmitted diseases. When these alleged venereal tumors were examined more carefully, it was clear that the epidemic of scrotal cancer had not ended, but had been literally defined away. Each one of these venereal tumors turned out to have been a scrotal tumor nonetheless.

In life, timing can be everything. In a remarkable bout of inauspicious happenstance, just weeks after the Japanese attack of Pearl Harbor, Hueper published what would prove to be a public health call to arms—a massive tome that covered laboratory and public health studies of workplace hazards in several countries, entitled *Occupational Tumors and Allied Diseases*. With the war finally under way, the only arms of concern to most people at the time were those that could provide for national defense. Hueper's amalgamation of studies from four continents over more than a century in this massive volume pulled together threads from experimental and epidemiologic research. He carefully explained that, despite the limits of available statistics on cancer in humans, there was much evidence that workplace factors were important and controllable causes of cancer and other illness. Richer people tended to have different tumors from poorer ones. Those who worked in dirtier, dustier trades developed distinct ailments.[10]

Despite his run-ins with DuPont, Hueper did find some receptive colleagues in parts of mainstream medicine after he left Haskell Laboratories. Up to 1950, he was tapped to write occasional editorials for the *Journal of the American Medical Association* on environmental cancer hazards, including those of solar radiation, aromatic amines, estrogens, coal tar products, arsenic, asbestos, and other environmental carcinogens.

In 1948, he acquired what appeared an ideal post, with the fledgling National Cancer Institute (NCI). In the early days of this work, he led the first environmental cancer section ever created, which was officially part of the Federal Security Agency, under the US Public Health Service. At first, this must have appeared kismet. In 1950, under Hueper's leadership, the NCI issued a pamphlet on Environmental Cancer that named a number of industrial, nutritional, and other causes of cancer.[11]

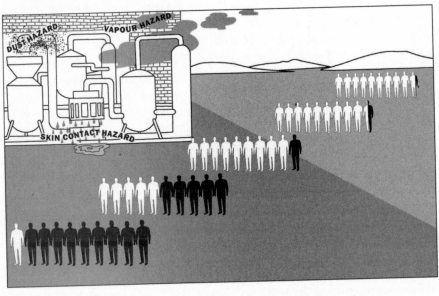

The twenty-page pamphlet began by pointing out that cancer has been a recognized medical problem since eight centuries before Christ. With the modern era patterns of cancer had shifted radically. Medical X-rays, dietary deficiencies, tobacco and drinking habits, sunlight, and toxic chemicals all played a role. When it came to the role of tobacco smoking in cancer, Hueper took the view that while smoking could be important, its role was easily exaggerated by those who wanted to downplay the impact of toxic chemicals. Not everyone who smoked got cancer, but every man who worked for more than two decades with certain synthetic dyes did develop bladder cancer.[12]

This NCI report reviewed major workplace causes of cancer, extending from radiation to specific toxic chemicals, including asbestos, aniline dyes, aromatic amines, paraffin oil, shale oil, crude oils, benzene, chromates, nickel carbonyl, and other residues. Above a small figure from this report is reproduced (Fig.2), as it concisely displayed the types of evidence then in existence regarding the cancer-causing properties of aromatic amines. The diagram shows that workers could be exposed through inhaling dusts or fumes, or through direct skin contact with residues.[13]

The risk of bladder cancer can be seen to vary relative to the amount of exposure that could take place. Workers in the immediate vicinity of manufacture would have the greatest risk. This is depicted below as nine out of ten highly exposed workers developing bladder cancer. Those in the general community surrounding the plant would not escape risk either, though it would be considerably smaller. This small diagram turned out to be more prophetic than Hueper could have realized at the time. Twenty years later, in 1975, the citizens of Salem County, home to the Chambers Works, had the highest rate of bladder cancer in the nation.

A memo written by Hueper in 1961 provides a sobering account of official corruption, obstruction of science, and suppression of information at the NCI during the 1950s. In some sense Hueper was one of many victims of the Cold War mentality that kept evidence of industrial hazards under wraps. Even his ability to speak to medical students as an official of NCI was restricted, "under the pretext that 'my time as a scientist at the agency is too valuable for engaging in such educational activities.'" Just as happened at DuPont, Hueper was soon ordered not to publish these findings and not to talk about what he also could not write about.

By 1961, Hueper found that he could no longer work at NCI freely, but had to submit all his papers for what seemed to be interminable reviews. He stopped trying to revise his major compendium on occupational causes of cancer, while at NCI, because he became convinced that the never-ending editorial reviews constituted a kind of censorship.

When is paranoia not paranoia? In Hueper's case, the feeling of persecution turned out not to be delusional but accurate. He eventually learned that the industries his work at NCI was criticizing had been given extraordinary access to his papers prior to their being submitted for publication. When he set out to show the cancer-causing properties of chromate ore, he ran straight into a fan blade of scientific criticism from which he could never recover. A medical consultant to the chromate-producing industry charged that the research activities of Hueper's NCI section on environmental cancer were injurious to this industry. Note, the consultant did not charge that the work was wrong, merely that it damaged business. As a result of these charges, Hueper was forbidden to continue research in this area or even to contact industrial or state health departments with information about the increased risk of lung cancer of chromate workers.

When he had landed at NCI, Hueper had hoped that DuPont would ignore him. But, that proved not to be the case. "I soon found out that I had underestimated its unrelenting spirit of personal persecution." Several weeks after meeting with a plant physician in Denver regarding aromatic amines and bladder cancer cases, Hueper received a letter from the Federal Loyalty Commission "informing me that I was under investigation for disloyalty." A colleague informed Hueper that he had been asked whether Hueper was a Nazi. A few weeks later, a letter from Dr. Gehrmann [Hueper's boss at DuPont] alleged that, "I had shown communistic tendencies." After these attacks, Hueper was summarily removed officially from conducting any studies of humans regarding the risks of bladder cancer due to aromatic amines, under his NCI mantle, and he was also barred from completing work he had begun with other researchers on chromates, beryllium, and other cancer-causing agents in the workplace.

What had happened to Hueper at Haskell played out again at NCI. Hueper was pulled off of any studies of workers and told to focus solely on experimental animals. The argument continued to be—we do not have proof of human harm from these exposures. So long as Hueper, and the state health departments with whom he was then working, were prevented from amassing proof of the damaging effects of chemical exposures on workers, of course, no evidence of harm could be said to exist. So long as studies of sick or dead workers remained secret, or were not tallied at all, then no evidence of hazard could be said to exist. Where Hueper had begun to amass evidence that validated his little sketch from 1950, showing how environmental exposures well outside the workplace affected cancer patterns, or the dangers to nuclear plant workers, he was forced to withdraw publications under threat of legal actions.

There is one matter on which it is important to fault Dr. Hueper. With his single-minded focus on chemical hazards, he tended to minimize evidence on the dangers of cigarettes. After all, smoking is nowadays understood as the best-established and greatest contributor to lung and many other cancers. But, Hueper had a fear. "It became clear that the acceptance of the cigarette theory would require the extermination of a great deal of factual medical knowledge . . . which was painfully and tediously acquired over many decades of medical science, and to replace it with an ill-documented, simple, Unitarian theory [of smoking] which appears to offer no plausible solution . . ." Hueper understood that smoking caused many forms of cancer. But, he feared that other workplace chemical causes of cancer would be ignored in the rush to finger a single villain. He also noted a number of paradoxes regarding cancer and smoking. Why did scientists fail to acknowledge that women with lung cancer were not always smokers and that lung and other cancers could occur in folks with no smoking history whatsoever? What vexed Hueper was the fact that while about one in ten smokers would come down with lung cancer, ten out of ten workers exposed to synthetic dyes would develop bladder cancer.

With the exception of his recalcitrant views on tobacco, the brief NCI pamphlet that Hueper produced in 1950 ended with a surprisingly clear set of proposals for a program of cancer control that remains pertinent today. These include goals to eliminate carcinogenic agents from industrial, civilian, or military use whenever practical and possible, institute safety procedures for the handling of any suspect materials, and provide careful medical monitoring of exposed workers for early signs of cancerous and pre-cancerous conditions that could be treated.

The conclusion of this pamphlet from half a century ago also bears repeating more than half a century later:

> Environmental carcinogenesis is the newest and one of the most ominous of the end-products of our industrial environment. Though its full scope and extent are still unknown, because it is so new and because the facts are so extremely difficult to obtain, enough is known to make it obvious that extrinsic carcinogens present a very immediate and pressing problem in public and individual health. It should become one of the most urgent tasks of all medical men, public health officials, labor and management leaders, and members of legislatures, to become familiar with the problems of environmental cancer. They must all work together to combat its causes at the source, before the dread disease spreads to more and more of our people.

The political pendulum had swung in a rather different direction a mere decade after Hueper's pamphlet had been issued. By 1959, when Hueper submitted an update of this popular pamphlet for publication, the editorial board of the NCI dallied so long that it never appeared. Later, he failed to get an update of his 1942 tome through official approval. In his final months of life, after his wife of more than fifty years had died, Hueper typed out his memoirs, with some resignation:

It is not surprising that the promotion and development and the factual evidence supporting the concept of environmental carcinogenesis as the dominant cause of human cancers has aroused more disbelief as well as objections and condemnations than any other concept advanced regarding the causes of cancer in man.

By 1950, knowledge of the ways that sundry physical and chemical agents affected cancer had been around for about 175 years.

While Hueper and Kehoe shared a naïve confidence that careful, methodical assembly of the right facts would lead directly to a better world, they held fundamentally different views of what that world might consist of and who would be in charge of making it right. What that world would look like, how we would know we had arrived there, and what it would take to keep it—all these matters were not at all agreed on. Neither of them quite appreciated that what passes for facts depends on to whom those facts are presented and other circumstances that can create receptivity or hostility to their existence. The world is not only stranger than it seems, it can be stranger than we are permitted to know. Science remains a quintessentially human enterprise, where giants of the field sometimes have feet of clay right up to their heads.

The failure of modern cancer policy to address occupational and environmental causes is no reflection of the absence of scientific research. Hueper believed that when fully informed of the dangers of occupational cancer causes industry would do the right thing and the government would facilitate that. The old conflict between Kehoe and Hueper epitomizes a very contemporary reality: scientific findings may be a necessary driver to reform policy but they are not sufficient in and of themselves. Whether the hazards of tobacco, vinyl chloride, butadiene, or other more modern workplace hazards, actions to reduce these have only been implemented after definitive evidence of their harm to humans has been obtained. Michael Gilbertson's Halifax Project has recently affirmed the importance of taking a systematic and precautionary approach to modern chemical or physical technology.[14] The failure to use experimental studies in animals to predict human harm effectively means that we are continuing to treat workers as experimental subjects in studies that have no controls.

Chapter 19

THE PRECAUTIONARY PRINCIPLE

Pierre Mallia

The emergence of increasingly unpredictable, uncertain, and unquantifiable but possible catastrophic risks such as those associated with genetically modified organisms, climate change, etc., has confronted societies with the need to develop a third, anticipatory model to protect humans and the environment against uncertain risks of human action: the Precautionary Principle (PP).

UNESCO: The Precautionary Principle. World Commission on the
Ethics of Scientific Knowledge and Technology (COMEST)

The precautionary principle enables rapid response in the face of a possible danger to human, animal or plant health, or to protect the environment. In particular, where scientific data do not permit a complete evaluation of the risk, recourse to this principle may, for example, be used to stop distribution or order withdrawal from the market of products likely to be hazardous.

The European Union

THE PRINCIPLE OF PRECAUTION

Imagine waking up one morning to find a very large satellite mast less than a few meters from your child's window on the roof of a neighbor's house. You are at first concerned about the size and the view it has destroyed. Over your morning coffee, you reflect that such a mast is too large for a television. Later during the day you meet the neighbor, who does not normally use the house but who happened to be there, and jokingly ask whether he is trying to get channels direct from Down Under. He replies that he was awarded a couple of thousand euros for having the mast on his rooftop. Since he does not use the place often it did not bother him. He tells you that it is a "relay station" belonging to a mobile phone company. You suddenly have goose skin. You remember you had heard stories about these masts and that the electromagnetic radiation they emit are harmful to children and that countries had reported many cases of leukemia in children at these sites.

You obviously take up the issue and try to calm down and gather as much information as possible. You confirm that the studies are recorded and make printouts. You write to the company and do your own research. You find that the company has breached the local planning authority rules, and indeed that MEPA granted an exception. You go to your local minister and have no luck. You end up going to the minister concerned, to the planning authority, to the MEP. All give you sympathy but say that no law, but only guidelines, exist. The local parliamentarian, however, contacts MEPA and asks for the nullification of the application and for the dish to be removed. The dish remains.

This is a true story. I have omitted identities and details that can reveal those involved. If I were the parent of two young girls, I would be concerned—who wouldn't be? The facts above are only a mere summary of what went on and, to be sure, I am not certain whether the parents knew about the application before the dish was installed. The neighbor, of course, either could not be bothered to find out, or did not know the facts. Would he have accepted the money knowing that young couples with children were in the vicinity? To date, the couple has contacted the minister of health who asked them to check whether there is an EU law to the effect in order for him to take action. The context of this chapter is not merely to convince the authorities but to show that if we mean business on bioethics, and if we are truly a caring society, we need not wait for children to get cancer before starting to move in the right direction.

It is true that politicians walk a tightrope between the business world, the economy, and the environment. It is not easy not to grant permits in such small countries such as Malta. But neither do we conscientiously have to wait for someone in Brussels to make a law. This is not about breaking laws; it is about common sense and following clear evidence. We should be the forerunners, making use of evidence before the need for law.

The only way that a small country can have an impact in the EU is to show that they mean business in areas that count. God forbid that this issue is politicized, and certainly walking in the shoes of a politician with such an issue in hand is not an easy task when you are faced with the duties of everyday life which, in turn, affect all of our lives. It is true that the days when a politician grabs the phone and shouts a command down the hierarchical ladder are gone.

People can and do use the force of the law, where it is known that a court case can take years to resolve. Parents, however, do not have years where the welfare of their children is concerned. By the time courts decide the damage is done.

The study of bioethics all started with such environmental issues. The person who actually coined the word "bioethics" was an oncologist who realized that we have to do something about the environment we live in, as it was the same environment that was causing much of the cancer he was recording. From passive smoking to power stations and radiation stations, he realized that if we had to wait for epidemiological evidence, we would be sacrificing the lives of too many people. It is true that the business world must move forward, but there should be social ethics that take on the biological impact of the environment we live in to prevent disease; hence bio-ethics.

It is also the case that the word bio-ethics has been corrupted. What the oncologist meant was to take into consideration the biological effects; what it has become is a term meaning an ethics of life, seeing that "bio" often is interpreted as "life." Be that as it may, the final effect is the same. UNESCO has, however, taken this environmental stand in its manifesto,[1] and it is spreading throughout the world.

In its studies and publications on the *Precautionary Principle*, it gives examples of how in the past, when precaution was taken, considerable damage was avoided. Today, since the use of litigation is commonplace, it is often years before things change. The UNESCO document cites the case of Dr. John Snow, a GP working in London during the time of the cholera epidemic, who noticed that the areas of London where cholera was mostly endemic were related to a particular water pump (in those days there were private companies, and different companies provided water for different areas). His recommendation to close down the station led to a decrease in cholera and to further studies that revealed how it was actually transmitted in water.

On the other hand, however, we have all heard about the long drawn out asbestos tragedy; the UNESCO publication describes it well. Times have changed since John Snow. Over time, no precaution was taken even though evidence accumulated about the effects of asbestos on the lungs, giving rise to cancer and cancer-like conditions, just as lethal. But asbestos was so much in use that it was difficult for countries to take action. When countries finally took a stand, many had died, and there are still many people suffering from the effects of asbestos— where it is mined—still used in industry, or exposed in public places, or removed from these places. Even in Malta, many ex-dockyard workers have this condition and the unions have only managed a collective agreement with insurers gaining these workers a pittance in compensation. The point is, however, that had action been taken earlier, many deaths and illnesses could have been avoided. We tend to think of asbestos and other environmental carcinogens historically, the product of other times in Malta, employment, and work came before theories of public health medicine.

Would it have been different today? In discussing this question, we must in all conscience admit that we have the problem on our plates again today—with radiation. Now the EU has adopted the Precautionary Principle. And the European Union has considered these relay masts and dishes and given guidelines that are clear. The European Environment Agency (EEA) calls for immediate action to reduce exposure to mobile phone masts. The EU says they should be distanced from schools and hospitals. But if they should be distanced from schools and hospitals, then why not homes? I have spoken to MEPs and they say that once one considers schools and hospitals, it is taken for granted that homes are included. There is no need for an actual law or directive, and governments are expected to follow up on these recommendations.

So we have the EU, the EEA (a European institution), and UNESCO all telling us the same thing. Of course we can err. But correcting that error takes courage and energy. Sometimes being in government means that you have the force of the Law and even where specific laws do not exist, you are in the position to do something about it.

The Precautionary Principle is clear. It has been adopted by the EU.[2] It tells governments that they do not need to wait for laws or for EU institutions to give directives. Actually, *neither do they need to wait for epidemiological evidence*, if the indications are clear. One uses the precautionary principle because lives are important and we know that producing evidence and passing laws takes time. In the meantime, we are told (as if we needed to "be told") that we *can* and *should* do something about it.

In the case I cited at the beginning of this chapter, we *also* have enough evidence that shows that such radiation emanating from such masts cause the growth of brain cancer cells, and especially the incidence of childhood leukemia, apart from headaches, memory loss, attention deficit (in children), increased blood pressure in healthy men, damage to eye cells, etc. There have been considerable resolutions by scientific bodies, including the Vienna Resolution,[3] The Salzburg Resolution on Mobile Telecommunication Base Stations,[4] reports to the EU by EC-sponsored studies (REFLEX),[5] etc. The WHO, FDA, International Agency for Cancer, National Cancer Institute, the European Commission, etc. have all spoken.

However, the Maltese Communications Authority acts in accordance with the ICNIPR—the International Commission on Non-Ionizing Radiation

Protection—which falls short of health issues—especially long-term ones like leukemia in children. The UK commissioned a report in this regard (the Stewart Report),[6] which concluding, states clearly that there is now scientific evidence that there may be biological effects from such masts; they also say that they cannot guarantee that even radiation below national and ICNIPR guidelines are totally without adverse effects. The report states that the gaps in knowledge *are sufficient to justify a precautionary approach.*

Taking a precautionary approach, using this principle of precaution reverses the way we should do things. It tells us to "stop" until we have the evidence, and not to stop *when* we have the evidence. It does not even speak about laws and it is pre-law—could it be otherwise? And to whom does it speak if not to our politicians? Taking a precautionary approach means picking up the phone right now and asking politely to remove that antenna. We all want the luxuries of our mobile phones. But I for one would not wish that that luxury comes at the cost of the lives of our children. It is not the onus of this particular family to bring to the minister any law that exists. I am sure the minister has people who can do this for him. But in the absence of such law, and even in the absence of evidence, there is a principle that we have been speaking about, which involves a moral law and a natural right. A feeble minster will dilly-dally. A courageous and morally sound one would use this invaluable tool that has been given to him. He is, at the end, the true bio-ethicist, given that as a matter of fact, there *is* the evidence. The Precautionary Principle recognizes that absence of evidence is not evidence of absence.

ON PRUDENCE AND PREVENTION

The precautionary principle (PP) should not be confused either with "Prudence" or with "Prevention." The first term is used often in philosophy, and the second used in medicine. Both have distinct meaning, which to the layperson may sound as if they overlap. In this section I will try to distinguish—so as not to *degrade*—the PP to these two terms which have found different places in technical applications.

Let me start with prudence. Prudence is considered a *virtue* in philosophy. Even in medicine, Virtue Ethics, mentions prudence as a character trait that the good health-care professional should have. By being prudent, I can be seen to be taking a precaution. But that is not the case. Acting prudently means acting in a way whereby I am cautious of not causing harm; it is about considering the *possibility* that there may be a consequence of my action that is unwanted. The PP would not go this far. An example often used in the Catholic tradition, invoking prudence, is for the use of emergency contraception. Emergency contraception works in three main ways. The first is by altering the lining of the uterus and the fallopian tubes in such a way that any sperm will find it difficult to reach the ovum which it usually will fertilize in the outer third of the fallopian tube. In the same way any fertilized egg will find it difficult to implant itself in the uterus, which is the second effect of the medication. The third effect is to delay ovulation if this has not occurred. Now the possibility of affecting an already fertilized egg has created a lot of controversy, for emergency contraception is thus seen as possibly abortifacient.

It is not within the scope of this chapter to argue in favor or against emergency contraception, but only to see how the application of prudence differs from the precautionary principle. Following a trial between the Society for the Protection of the Unborn Child (SPUC) and a major drug company that produces the "morning after pill," the British Episcopal Conference issued a document to explain to the Catholic population its opinion on the use of emergency contraception in instances of rape.[7] The trial, which was started by the SPUC against the company, was justified. In the United Kingdom, abortions are only legal for health reasons. Therefore, taking a pill to induce a miscarriage at such an early stage when one still cannot as yet establish whether there is a health reason, was thought to be considered breaking the law. It should be mentioned that women in the United Kingdom can buy the "morning-after" pill over-the-counter (OTC) and that, therefore, no visit to a GP is necessary. Moreover, since it is a GP (in fact, at the time, the signatures of two practitioners were needed) who identifies and confirms that the abortion will take place for health reasons, OTC delivery of drugs will definitely not satisfy the criteria required by law for the cause of an abortion or miscarriage. The drug company won the case on the technical definition of "miscarriage." One can only, in this interpretation, miscarry a pregnancy and the definition of pregnancy is when a fertilized egg has actually *impregnated* and thus implanted itself in the uterus. Therefore, the question was raised whether you can actually "miscarry" when you are not actually (by definition) "carrying."[8] The judges accepted this argument and threw out the case.

For the Catholic, however, life begins at conception and, therefore, any drug that will cause the elimination and/or prevent implantation of a fertilized egg, is in itself an abortion. This actually abounds by the fact that to abort means to eliminate from the woman's body and not simply "to kill." In fact, the Catholic Church has never agreed that pregnancy starts with implantation and identifies the start with conception—when life actually begins. Now, one can look at "carrying" in two ways. One can use the scientific definition meaning that implantation has had to occur. But one can also argue philosophically, and not less correctly, that if the woman has a fertilized egg in her tube, which has not yet implanted itself into the uterus, and she travels from the United Kingdom to the United States, she still actually "carries" the fertilized egg with her. The question is not so much as to when the pregnancy has actually started—whether in the United Kingdom (when conception occurred) or in the United Stated or on the way (when the impregnation occurred). This is answered according to the belief of the definition of when pregnancy starts. The question is whether technically and in actual fact the woman *did* carry with her the fertilized egg—and that she was, indeed, "carrying," which would, therefore, lead us to conclude that the morning-after pill does indeed cause a miscarriage. Is it not also the case that medically, if one carries a virus that is still lying on the mucus of the pharynx from one country to another makes no difference to the medical man who has to take a travel history? This is how malaria and influenza and all other microbes can get transmitted. Whether the virus had already "implanted" itself in the cell or not does not make a difference. The reality is that it was carried from one country to another. One cannot really blame the courts, for these rely on expert evidence and laws that are already written. One should blame the experts who decide on the definitions. The courts can only be blamed if they get to choose between differing expert opinions.

But at this stage we have to return to the main line of argument—that of prudence. The British Episcopal conference[9] issued a statement on whether a woman who is raped does not have the right to protect herself from pregnancy. Of course, the Catholic Church can only issue a statement on contraception within the context of rape, for any kind of consensual sex outside the scope of marriage is seen as illicit. But one can extrapolate the reasoning of the document even within the scope of consensual sex for the argument on prudence. The bishops pointed out that, indeed, a girl or woman who is raped has the right to protect herself from becoming pregnant, more specifically, to prevent fertilization from occurring. She can, therefore, use emergency contraception if this does not cause an abortion. In other words, if ovulation has not occurred, the morning-after pill can be used with the intent of prolonging ovulation and thus prolonging the time that an egg is released. Therefore, before ovulation there is minimal chance of conception. If ovulation has occurred, the document goes on, the chances of conception are higher, and even though the intention may not be to kill a fertilized egg, and even though the chances of having a fertilized egg may still be low, one has to be *prudent* and not use the drug blindly.

One might use a simpler example. Supposing I am a hunter used to shooting birds in the sky. If a large bird escapes my shot and goes down behind a bush, can I shoot blindly into the bush, given the extreme possibility that someone might be in those bushes (a child may be playing or someone may be resting in its shade). It is probably unlikely that someone is in the bush. So the argument of *probability* cannot hold as we shall see. The legal fact is that if I do shoot and kill someone, I should be legally held liable. There is a clear argument that I have acted negligently as I should assume that, even if the probability is extremely low of there being someone in the bush, it is always a possibility. Therefore, out of prudence, I should not shoot. In fact, there is a general duty within tort law that if breached, and harm is caused by that breach (the nexus), then there is a claim for negligence. For this reason, hunters should never fire into bushes.

With the same reasoning, if we are concerned about a fertilized egg and there is a possibility of there being one in the tubes, according to Catholic moral philosophy, we should not use emergency contraception. To be sure, although being a Catholic myself, I agree with the fact that abortion is caused even if you intentionally cause the elimination of an egg that has not yet implanted, I found issue with the argument of the Episcopal Conference[10] as it is quantitative and not qualitative. It argues that the *chances* of pregnancy increase, thereby admitting the scientific fact that pregnancy can actually happen almost throughout the menstrual cycle except during menstruation. Since immediately after intercourse the chances of a sperm fertilizing an egg are just about as much as before ovulation, then one should perhaps consider the principle of double effect whereby a foreseen but unintended harm is permitted, as in the case of an ectopic pregnancy where one has to destroy the embryo within, in order to save the life of the mother.

Precaution is therefore a personal virtue; one that is required by law under certain circumstances. In this case, it can become an obligation—the hunter is required to be prudent and failing to do so makes him or her incompetent to hold a gun license. How this does not make it precaution is due to the clear explanation and definitions given by the UNESCO document on the PP, which will be described in the next section. It should be made clear, however, that when one makes a *principle*, and hence the word precaution changes into a *principle of precaution*, this as will be seen appeals to law, insofar as law is based upon principles, but also appeals to prudence in the face of uncertainty.

We now turn to consider "Prevention." When in front of the Parliamentary Committee on Social Affairs discussing this issue,[11] a parliamentarian giving his comments and reaction to my presentation said he agreed with "prevention" and went on to laud what had been said. This was not a coincidence for the parliamentarian was himself a doctor and, therefore, was used to the concept of preventive medicine. But preventive medicine is different. Preventive medicine is about preventing harm *when there is evidence*, something that is quite different from precaution, which is contemplated when there is enough *reason to believe*. In the latter there may not be direct (or enough) evidence. Therefore, we may not have evidence that mobile masts set up close to the bedrooms of children have actually shown an increase in the number of brain tumors and leukemias in this group of children as compared to children who do not have such masts close to their bedrooms. But there are other studies that clearly show crops of these diseases in areas of high concentration of electromagnetic radiation that have caused authorities to take action—for example of not allowing such masts on schools.[12]

It is clearly not only being prudent because we do have clear reasons and other studies. Neither is it prevention however—which it will be only when you have actual evidence. It lies somewhere in between, which is why there is the necessity in health care for precaution. By the time we have enough evidence for a preventive approach, we will have lost lives unnecessarily, which is why the principle of precaution is introduced.

Preventive medicine finds itself dealing with evidence-based medicine. Thus, we know that smoking causes lung cancer. There are direct studies that link one to the other. Yet smoking continues not to be illegal, and indeed we do not punish (other than with taxes) smokers—they will still receive health care. Advising not to smoke is preventive medicine. Similarly, advising women to have a PAP smear is preventive medicine because studies *have* shown that this reduces the incidence of cervical cancer. Preventive medicine also leads to health promotion. We promote not drinking if you are going to drive; we promote not smoking, not because it will certainly harm your health but because it actually *does* so to the majority of people although you may be the exception. We promote eating healthy because we know that certain foods increase cholesterol and that obesity is associated with more morbidity and mortality. We have the evidence and having this evidence leads us to have an obligation to *prevent* harm and to *promote good*, which Beauchamp and Childress have classified under the Principle of Nonmaleficence.[13]

So, I can learn from preventive medicine and health promotion campaigns and I would then be prudent to follow the advice. Yet, we cannot take a drastic decision not to allow people to smoke or to eat hamburgers as a precaution, even though smoking may cause harm to others. Neither can we say that, as a precaution, we may make it law not to smoke in public places as passive smoking *has been shown* to cause harm. If we accept this definition of precaution, then we would not have the necessary strength to tackle such issues as mobile masts, as we would be attacking so many personal choices as to be seen by some as infringing the liberties of individuals.

Unfortunately, people have used the precautionary principle injudiciously, even though with good intentions. For example, a bishop invoked the precautionary principle when speaking about censoring the media.[14] This bishop rightly quoted that according to the European Commission, based upon this principle of precaution, when one suspects that something can cause harm to the public, then the authorities can remove this harm. He goes on to say, following a solid morality, that the authorities should censor the media.

While it is not within the scope of this chapter to argue this point, I do believe that there is a wrong interpretation of the PP in this argument used by the bishop, as the criteria of UNESCO—which he refers to as well—are clearly not fulfilled. If this were the case, we would probably resort to being a confessional state, and moreover remove all kinds of things that are suspected of causing harm in light of particular belief systems. We would only eat salads, and follow only a conservative fashion of clothes—good things in and of themselves, and morally laudable, but that in a free society will not hold. The criteria speak of invoking the PP in a free society and gives clear guidelines to which we must now turn.

UNESCO'S DECLARATION AND ITS MEANING

The concept of the precautionary principle was first adopted in the Earth Summit's Declaration of Rio. It was then adopted by the European Union, first in the Maastricht Treaty and later in the Lisbon Treaty.

> [In 2005, UNESCO] given its mandate in ethics of science and technology . . . has a role to play here in fashioning the precautionary principle into a form that Member States can properly use in making assessments of the choices science and technology present.[15] . . . In conformity with the mandate received from the Member States (31 C/5), UNESCO, together with its advisory body, the World Commission on the Ethics of Scientific Knowledge and Technology (COMEST), has brought together a group of experts to propose a clear definition of the precautionary principle and provide clarification of the possible uses of this principle, aiming at offering an ethical platform to ensure proper risk of management and correct information to the public and to policy makers, in view of the impact of new technologies.[16]

The scene is set by stating that human existence cannot continue if its effect on the biosphere, that provides the basis for all life, is destroyed. Clearly the fact that sailors sail on boats with lifeboats is not because they expect to be wrecked but because they know it would be irrational not to be prepared for such a danger.

This action is indeed a prudent action. The introduction goes on to say how countries, in order to prevent pollution, came out with a principle of "polluter pays," requiring that the polluter pays for any damage caused. It was clear that such a law could only work if accompanied by a preventive policy—that prevention is better than cure. Yet "the emergence of increasingly unpredictable, uncertain, and unqualified but possible catastrophic risks, such as that associated with genetically modified organisms, climate change, etc., has confronted societies with the need to develop a third, anticipatory model to protect humans and the environment against uncertain risks of human action,"[17] hence the PP. The PP has marked that change in paradigm from a post-damage control to a pre-damage control of events.

UNESCO noticed that within the previous years, many countries and international bodies adopted the PP, and yet there was disagreement and different views as to what precaution is. Clearly the PP was being interpreted in different ways. While everyone agreed on a principle that invoked a "look before you leap," and a "better safe than sorry" attitude, it was clear that these different interpretations necessitated UNESCO to help member states with rules on its application.

The evidence that John Snow provided for the causal link between cholera and the water pumps was relatively weak and there was no proof "beyond a reasonable doubt." It was probably his position as physician to the Royal Family (having personally administered chloroform to Queen Victoria when she was in labor), which helped him in his quest to close down the culprits. Nowadays things are quite different, and clearly governments depend on economies which in turn make the economy a significant force in policy.

Where arguments and conflicts can still occur are around the definition of "possible" risk as well as a definition of precaution. Clearly, even "possible" risk has to be established by scientific debate free of vested interest and it is here, for want of a level playing field, that the areas fit for the precautionary principle can sometimes remain undecided. Clearly one attitude for change is to have clear evidence. This gives the politician clout over the business world and the business world cannot but accept this proof, especially if it is repeatable, and change its attitude. But clearly such proof comes at a cost.

To be sure, even scientists are admonished not to continue with any research that is showing significant harm or benefit before the end of the stipulate period of time for the research activity. Why should a research subject continue to receive a placebo when the first results of the research clearly show that the drug or treatment under trial is of significant benefit? In the same way a multicentered trial on HRT was stopped when early in the research it was shown that the risk for cancer was greater than was expected and that the risk-benefit ratio was shifted. Doctors were told not to prescribe HRT for its benefits to heart, skin, and bone, as the risk outweighed these benefits. This problem was described clearly in the Nuremberg Code and later adopted by the Declaration of Helsinki.

Such was not the case with the asbestos saga where it took countries over a century to ban all forms of asbestos—the early signs being in 1898 when an inspector in a UK factory spoke about its harmful effects. There were already "reasonable grounds" from experiments on rats in 1911 that asbestos dust is harmful. Yet, the era of industry was strong, and clearly times had changed not only since John Snow but from other eras from a different political age. The Romans had stopped the use of lead pipes for the distribution of water when they realized the signs of lead poisoning. Proof was unnecessary other than a reasonable connection. Clearly the PP is then about political change—in democracies one cannot convince one responsible person, but has to convince parliamentarians, who at the end of the day are driven by two factors: morality and votes. Clearly, both are important and it is not the first politician to compromise morality for votes. UNESCO's guidelines can clearly be seen in the light of providing the politician with strong moral grounds on which to base his choice and convince voters of a strong moral position.

Despite all these quandaries about the precautionary principle, the document starts by mentioning key elements that the various definitions share:[18]

- The PP applies when there exist considerable scientific uncertainties about causality, magnitude, probability, and nature of harm;
- Some form of *scientific analysis* is mandatory; a mere fantasy or crude speculation is not enough to trigger the PP. Grounds for concern that can trigger the PP are limited to those concerns that are *plausible* or scientifically tenable (that is, not easily refuted);
- Because the PP deals with risks with poorly known outcomes and poorly known probability, the unquantified *possibility* is sufficient to trigger the consideration of the PP. This distinguishes the PP from the prevention principle: if one does have credible ground for quantifying probabilities, the prevention principle applies instead. In that case, risks can be managed by, for instance, agreeing on an acceptable risk level for the activity and putting enough measures in place to keep the risk below that level;
- Application of the PP is limited to those hazards that are *unacceptable*, although several definitions are more specific: Possible effects that threaten the lives of future generations or other groups of people (for example inhabitants of other countries) should be explicitly considered. Some

formulations refer to "damage or harmful effects," some to "serious" harm, other to "serious and irreversible damage," and still others to "global, irreversible and trans-generational damage." What these different clauses have in common is that they contain value-laden language and thus express a moral judgment about acceptability of the harm;

• Intervention should be proportional to the chosen level of protection and the magnitude of possible harm. Some definitions call for "cost-effective measure" or make some other reference to costs, while others speak only of prevention of environmental damage. Costs are only one consideration in assessing proportionality. Risk can rarely be reduced to zero. A total ban may not be a proportional response to a potential risk in all cases. However, in certain cases, it is the sole possible response to a given risk;

• There is a *repertoire of interventions* available:

1. measures that *constrain the possibility of the harm;*
2. measures that *contain the harm,* that is limit the scope of the harm and increase the controllability of the harm, should it occur;

• There is a need for ongoing systematic empirical search for more evidence and better understanding (long-term monitoring and learning) in order to realize any potential for moving a situation beyond the PP towards more traditional risk management.

The grounds for concern that can trigger the PP have therefore to be plausible or tenable. One needs to produce background knowledge and the concern must be consistent with this knowledge. "If the hypothesis requires one to reject widely accepted scientific theories and facts, then it is not plausible."[19] One should show that there is a causal mechanism and not simply a fear of it. The document, thus, postulates that the invocation of the precautionary principle must be based on a threat to human life or health, or a serious and effectively irreversible effect, or inequitable to present or future generations, or imposed without adequate consideration of human rights of those affected.

Here are generally three situations or classes where the precautionary principle is *not* applicable.[20] "The first class is when the scientific uncertainties can be overcome in the short-term through more research, or when the uncertainties are simply understood as low probability of harm (in that case it is only a question of the chosen level of protection). However, in some cases the potential consequences can be of a nature and magnitude that make them morally unacceptable even if the probability is very low: for instance, extinction of mankind. The second class is when the potential harm is not morally unacceptable, for example, when the harm is restricted to individuals who voluntarily engage in the activity and are informed about the possible consequences. The third class of cases is when the harm is reversible, and it is likely that effective counteraction is not becoming more difficult or costly, even when one waits until the first manifestations of the harm eventually occur. In this case a "wait and see" strategy might be used. "The PP (therefore) provides a rational framework for managing uncertain risks. However, the PP in itself is not a decision algorithm and thus cannot guarantee consistency between cases."

HOW CAN IT WORK: THE APPEAL TO LAW AND POLITICAL REASON

It is clear that ethical and legal principles are the foundation of laws. Moreover, principles assist in the interpretation of the law. Thus, when one appeals to principles in medicine such as beneficence and respect for autonomy, it may be unclear as to which principle trumps the other, for example whether one should respect a request for euthanasia or whether this breaks the medical principle of doing good and the principle of doing no harm. Yet, these clearly are debated internationally. However, in the face of laws of individual countries, decisions have been taken according to previously laid principles and ethical norms, and to date no country has found in favor of any case that appealed to euthanasia unless there was an already existing law. Principles thus become guidelines, but to what extent they become binding depends on the recognition of a *value*, and secondly on how much existing law can uphold the value.[21]

Therefore, although not legally binding, principles of law are important tools to conceptualize new values and concepts as is the principle to take precaution. Article 38 of the Statute of the International Court of Justice states that, "The Court, whose function is to decide in accordance with international law such disputes as are submitted to it, shall apply:

1. International conventions, whether general or particular, establishing rules expressly recognized by the contesting states;
2. International custom, as evidence of a general practice accepted as law;
3. The general principles of law recognized by civilized nations;
4. Subject to the provisions of Article 59, judicial decisions and the teachings of the most highly qualified publicists of the various nations, as subsidiary means for the determination of rules of law.

To this effect, according to UNESCO's document, the PP seems to be legally relevant among the principles emanating from international law. "From the moment that the PP is recognized as an element of international law, it also becomes part of the general principles of environmental law, with undisputed legitimacy in guiding the interpretation and the application of all legal norms in force."[22]

Insofar as the politician is concerned, there are clear roads to follow. Certainly for such drastic measures as the removal of mobile phone masts, the decision of one minister alone in many countries may not be sufficient and adverse lobbying can indeed be harmful to that minister without the support of his or her colleagues. It is more of a matter of claiming a high moral ground that is supported by sufficient scientific evidence and showing that in the face of uncertainty the appropriate action be taken given the above guiding rules. The implications that this has for policy and governance is that one cannot make a decision based merely on speculation. A parliament has to be faced with clear reports, insights, and experts' advice. Expert advice in turn has to come from diverse fields that may have competing interests, such as science and the humanities. Clearly advancing science and its profitability cannot be seen solely as the enemy as it is the scientific evidence of the harm or potential harm that is the only real evidence available. Listening to alternative and competing views—with declared interests—is mandatory as otherwise the final decision will not be based on a fair hearing.

Nevertheless, governments have to be held accountable, and because of this, they have to have highly dependable mechanisms of when and where to invoke such a principle that can be upheld in local and international courts and presented to the people, who are ultimately final arbiters as well in the judgment of decisions and policies. A flaw in the mechanism of invoking the PP may lead to an about-turn of a decision following an election. Therefore, governments must feel the tort responsibility of the consequences of neglecting to consider such a principle, without the need to impede the forward movement of progress.

In the particular case of mobile antennae, cited at the start of this chapter, the local government took the necessary action of creating a parliamentary committee for social affairs on the particular issue. It clearly would need to find solutions that are not seen as retrogressive steps (one does not want to be accused of taking the country back to smoke signals for communication). But it is not merely a utilitarian balance of the need of a commodity versus rare diseases that is in question. For while everybody uses mobile phones, only a few get leukemia or brain cancer, and the overall balance in public opinion may be in favor of the mobile phone. Clearly, this would be the result of inhumane consideration, for even if the diseases are rare, if a causal link is probable, one cannot merely treat it as a form of pollution that is tolerated, as is the case with cars. Even the latter requires due consideration to reduce emissions, but the uncertainty of something not seen will create a fear of the unknown that has to be balanced against the serious consequence on children, for example, when it will simply be too late to use a "wait and see" policy. No country should tolerate an increase in cancer because of the free marketing of a commodity. While power stations are not "deliberate" agents of pollution, communication means are more so. Mobile phones are a commodity, as are cars, and clearly one can tolerate them up to a certain extent, dependent upon an education to safeguards and constant review of the seriousness of the conditions caused.

Policies, however, need not include a total banning of the means. As for cars, precaution may be making better public transport systems that allow consumers to use their cars less. It is certainly imprudent to allow *all* mobile phone companies to have their own masts, and locate them where they will, when mast-sharing and allocated locations could be a means of reducing both the risk to human health and the number of masts. The three Rs for environment (Reduce, Reuse, Recycle), and for animal research (Replace, Reduce, and Refine), are clear example of application of rules to satisfy principles—that of protecting the environment and of not harming animals in research unnecessarily. Clearly *reduction* of masts is possible; *refining* regulations, such as regulating the distance from home, is possible, and sometime one should consider *replacing* policies. If one accepts the principle of safeguarding public health by not allowing such masts on or adjacent to school premises, where children spend fewer hours than they spend at home, then it makes sense to remove masts from crowded urban areas where they are close to and continuously affecting the "private" environment of children—such as domestic bedrooms.

In conclusion, the precautionary principle should be introduced when one is strongly suspecting a causal factor, and not merely an associated factor. It is there to save lives and time. Whether it works is another matter. The masts are still there. Governments change, and those who previously were in power and considered the oppressors suddenly become the advocates, and vice versa.

Chapter 20

THE PRECAUTIONARY PRINCIPLE IN THE PROTECTION OF WILDLIFE— THE TASMANIAN DEVILS AND THE BELUGA WHALES

Jody Warren

[W]hen human activities may lead to morally unacceptable harm that is scientifically plausible but uncertain, actions shall be taken to avoid or diminish that harm.
COMEST

[W]e feel that abnormal hormonal environments during early postnatal (and antenatal) life should not be underestimated as to their possible contribution to abnormal changes of neoplastic [cancerous] significance later in life.
N. Takasugi and H. Bern

Since the 1970s it is estimated that 30 percent of vertebrate species have become extinct and many more are threatened.[1] In 2002, the parties to the Convention on Biological Diversity set a target to significantly reduce the rate of biodiversity loss by 2010. This date has come and still many species, including mammals, continue to be threatened.

Following the Earth Summit, in order to protect biodiversity, progressive governments adopted the precepts of sustainable development. Fundamental to this approach was the precautionary principle, a crucial tool for decision makers,

380 CORPORATE TIES THAT BIND

to act to mitigate environmental harm caused by human activities when scientific knowledge is uncertain.

This chapter will investigate the role of the precautionary principle in mitigating environmental harm to protect biodiversity. It will also briefly investigate its relevance to the regulation of atrazine,[2] an endocrine-disrupting chemical, and the secret ties that prevent decision makers from regulating it. Endocrine disrupters are particularly challenging for decision makers because the scientific knowledge of their harmful effects is uncertain. By analyzing two case studies, the first, the Tasmanian devil cancer on the east coast of Tasmania and the second, the beluga whale cancer in the St. Lawrence River estuary, Canada, a clearer picture should emerge as to how these ties operate to prevent the protection of biodiversity. In both cases, these populations are endangered and facing extinction from rare and deadly cancers. Both cancers are recent and are two of only four documented accounts of cancers in wildlife, apart from fish.[3]

The Tasmanian devil cancer has been classified as a neuroendocrine tumor and named Devil Facial Tumour Disease (DFTD). While the beluga whale cancer is predominantly an intestinal cancer, a number of reproductive organ cancers have been recorded in females. These wildlife cancers in top-level predators, with greater exposure than humans to environmental contaminants, act as sentinels or bioindicators of human health, similar to the canary in the mine.

There are many similarities in the incidence of these wildlife cancers. Both wildlife species are mammals. Both are top predators, endemic to their regions and isolated from other sub-populations. These sub-populations, in less-contaminated regions, do not have the cancers.[4] Moreover, in both regions, there is an increased incidence of cancers in the human populations.[5] The causes of these cancers remains uncertain. However, within the geographical regions that these populations inhabit, the water is frequently heavily contaminated with industrial and/or agricultural chemicals.

While both geographic regions are frequently contaminated with many pollutants, water monitoring has revealed atrazine to be the most frequently detected hazardous chemical and at the highest concentrations. Atrazine is one of the most widely used herbicides in the world. However, because of its dangers as an endocrine disrupter and its potential to contaminate groundwater, its use has been banned in the European Union (EU). The EU, by implementing the precautionary principle under the Registration, Evaluation, and Authorization, and Restrictions of Chemicals (REACH) Program has banned or restricted many dangerous chemicals. Meanwhile, the regulatory bodies in the United States, Australia, and Canada have failed to follow the EU's use of the precautionary principle to ban atrazine.

There have been some minor restrictions of atrazine in the United States and Australia, while Canada has restricted its use to corn because of Canada's recognition of atrazine's persistence, bioaccumulation, and toxicity. The failure of regulatory bodies to act more decisively is due to the close ties and undue influence exerted by vested interests—such as Syngenta, the manufacturer of atrazine, the corn growers in Canada, and the forestry industry in Tasmania—on decision makers and those who inform them.

THE PRECAUTIONARY PRINCIPLE

The precautionary principle is a commonsense approach to decision making based on timely action taken by policy makers to avert unnecessary, unethical, or irreversible harm. It goes beyond risk assessment and management being implemented when environmental factors cannot be quantified because of scientific uncertainty or ignorance. Quantifying within an environmental context how much chemical is used, when, where, and by whom, is often not possible; even when monitoring is conducted it is often by the user, not by an independent assessor. In response to this commonsense precautionary approach, the chemical industry has insisted on risk assessment based on "sound science," when assessing the harm caused by chemicals in the environment. "Sound" and "Science" placed together are code words for "do nothing until harm has been scientifically proven." This "sound science" approach has created a great deal of controversy over the harm caused by chemicals and the need for them to be regulated, restricted, or banned. The chemical industry has achieved relative success in preventing the implementation of the precautionary principle to limit or restrict the use of hazardous chemicals, even though this principle is the mainstay of sustainable development.

The precautionary principle is both a legal and legislative instrument adopted by progressive authorities across the world in an effort to live in a sustainable manner. It is a reasonable and rational way of dealing with uncertainty; taking a precautionary approach to evidence of harm that human activities may be causing in the environment. When the risks faced by human society cannot be quantified, when scientific evidence is lacking or missing, then it is the precautionary principle that must be applied. It is clearly important that we continue to acknowledge that the resources of the planet are finite and we owe to future generations the ability to live in a stable environment with a reasonable standard of living.

According to the World Commission on the Ethics of Scientific Knowledge and Technology (COMEST), a definition of the precautionary principle is "[W]hen human activities may lead to morally unacceptable harm that is scientifically plausible but uncertain, actions shall be taken to avoid or diminish that harm."[6]

This is particularly pertinent to life-supporting ecosystems. It is the responsibility of those charged with protecting human life and the environment to make decisions to alleviate harmful human activities.

SCIENTIFIC UNCERTAINTY AND ECOSYSTEMS

The precautionary principle has become increasingly necessary as a strategy for assessing and managing risks within the context of scientific uncertainty.[7] It applies to specific environmental problems that are of a complex nature, especially with regard to their causal relationships, and which exhibit unquantifiable scientific uncertainty limiting the applicability of traditional risk assessment.[8] This apparent move away from scientific certainty has caused critics to view the precautionary principle as unscientific. However, as stated in the introduction to the COMEST paper "[t]he Precautionary Principle is not unscientific; it acknowledges uncertainty in scientific practice."[9] As Professor Sharon Beder writes, in respect of chemical use in the environment, "Scientists are usually unable to tell policy makers exactly where and how far a pollutant will spread, how it will interact with other pollutants, and how it will affect the health of people and the functioning of ecosystems."[10]

This view was supported by the late Danish Professor Poul Harremoes and his colleagues who state that "[N]o matter how sophisticated knowledge is, it will always be subject to some degree of ignorance."[11] David Kriebel, professor at the Lowell Center for Sustainable Production, and his colleagues state the "cumulative and interactive effects of multiple insults on an organism or ecosystem are very difficult to study"[12] and they refer to the recent problems with endocrine disruption as an example:

> So shocking was this revelation [about the widespread observation of endocrine disruption in wildlife] that no scientist could have expressed the idea using only the data from his or her discipline alone without losing the respect of his or her peers.[13]

The precautionary principle is dependent on scientific methods to inform precautionary policy. Kriebel and colleagues acknowledge that in environmental sciences observational studies are the rule because often experiments are not feasible or are unethical; hence they explore other types of evidence such as the accumulation of plausible conclusions from various independent lines of study.[14] They suggest some of these study lines into environmental causes of cancer may be provided by "the geographic distributions of cancers; time trends in cancer frequency; . . . and experimental knowledge of chemical pathways of cancer induction."[15] While any one line may prove inadequate, "[I]t is the preponderance of evidence that finally prevails."[16] However, Magnus Breitholtz of the Stockholm University and his colleagues call for more decisive rules which "stipulate that when relevant ecotoxicological information (i.e., sufficient test data is lacking), this automatically calls for precautionary actions."[17]

Meanwhile, Nicholas De Sadeleer, Professor of Environmental Law at the University of Oslo, argues that "[T]his type of complexity is the rule, rather than the exception, in ecosystems." However, scientists still have an obligation to carry out science that protects both human health and the environment. In this situation, the precautionary principle provides a "standard that is to be observed, not because it will advance or secure an economic, political or social situation deemed desirable, but because it is a requirement of justice or fairness or some other dimension of morality."[18] It is, therefore, a tool to support both scientists and decision makers in carrying out their obligations to protect both humans and the environment.

ADOPTION OF THE PRECAUTIONARY PRINCIPLE TO MANAGE DANGEROUS CHEMICALS

The precautionary principle has been widely adopted in the management of dangerous chemicals at the international level, within the EU and in the United States. In the international arena, the 1985 Vienna Ozone Convention is considered the first treaty referring to precaution.[19] It was followed up in 1987 by the Montreal Protocol which required, in the absence of scientific certainty and consensus, relatively strict measures to mitigate depletion of the ozone layer. Then later in 1987, an explicit reference to the precautionary principle was given at the second North Sea Conference. In 2004, the principle was included in the Stockholm Convention on Persistent Organic Pollutants (POPs),[20] which states in Article 1 the following objective:

> Mindful of the precautionary approach as set forth in Principle 15 of the Rio Declaration on Environment and Development, the objective is to protect human health and the environment from persistent organic pollutants.[21]

In both the EU and the United States, the need to manage chemicals grew out of struggles by communities and individuals who realized the impact industrial chemicals were having on their health and the environment. However, the precautionary principle, in order to manage this impact, acquired a different status in the United States as opposed to EU. In the United States, environmental health advocates, policymakers, and scientists held the Wingspread Conference in 1998, from which they produced the Wingspread Statement on the precautionary principle.[22] This Statement, however, was not an official US government policy statement.

The United States had once been a leader in precautionary legislation; the Clean Air Act and the Clean Water Act, both enacted in the 1970s with bipartisan support, explicitly allow regulators to act in the face of scientific uncertainty.[23] However, the US government does not presently accept the precautionary principle as a basis for policy.[24] Regardless of the advances made to incorporate the precautionary principle into decision making, industry maintained that the chemicals should be considered safe based on findings of company risk assessments.[25] Consequently, the precautionary principle has only been adopted piecemeal within the United States and was rejected by the Bush administration as an unjustified constraint on business.[26]

In contrast, the history of precautionary measures in the EU has a long and vital history, particularly in Sweden, where the concept was first implemented in 1786. A royal prohibition restricted the sale rights of any kind of toxic substances to pharmacists, and made them obliged to "take all necessary and legally required precautionary measures."[27] It was also implemented in Germany during the 1970s and 1980s in an effort to save the Black Forest from acid rain and was subsequently transformed into the German principle of law as the Vorsorgeprinzip, literally, the "forecaring principle."

The precautionary principle's adoption as the basis of the REACH Program by the EU has the potential to normalize precaution in the management of dangerous chemicals. The EU enacted to prevent the continued degradation of the Black Forest from acid rain.[28] This is REACH policy in 2007. Registration requires companies to provide data on their products including toxicity and information about how humans or the environment might be exposed to them. This reverses the burden of proof and places the responsibility and cost of information about the industry's products on the industry.[29] The precautionary approach also calls for substituting non-toxic or less-toxic alternatives in place of dangerous chemicals.[30] The EU adoption of the REACH program could have far-reaching regulatory implications for the chemical industry worldwide, a fact not missed by those affected by it.

THE CHEMICAL INDUSTRY AND THE PRECAUTIONARY PRINCIPLE

The fact that the precautionary principle attempts to manage risks posed by human activities, such as the use of dangerous chemicals, inevitably meant it faced considerable opposition from vested interests. This opposition to the precautionary principle began when it was used to control CFCs in the depletion of the ozone layer. Early in the 1980s, the American Chemistry Society complained that any restriction on CFCs production would represent "the first regulation to be based entirely on an unverified scientific prediction." This statement was supported by a DuPont spokesperson who protested, "We are going a very long way into the regulatory process before scientists know what's really going on."[31]

Likewise, the recent negotiations on the establishment of the REACH policy witnessed further struggles between the proponents of the inclusion of the precautionary principle into the REACH policy and the chemical industries of both the United States and the EU. The EU chemical industry was concerned that the EU governments may misuse the precautionary principle to ban or restrict chemicals;[32] the US opponents were more concerned with what they saw as protectionism and the possibility that the EU would use the precautionary principle to prohibit imports of US chemicals.[33] US opponents also feared that similar legislation would be adopted in the United States.

The United States had already engaged in a dispute with the EU over a ban on the import of hormone-treated beef. The United States, the main exporter of hormone-treated beef, challenged the ban before the WTO and the trade body ruled that the ban was not based on "sound science" and was therefore an illegal trade barrier.[34] The European chemical industry's fears of over-regulation seemed to be confirmed when the EU launched an emergency precautionary ban on PVC teething toys that contain phthalates.[35] This application of the precautionary principle had been made against the advice of the Scientific Committee on Toxicity, Ecotoxicity and the Environment (SCTEE), which found phthalates posed no risk. The European Commission went further in deciding to ban another four phthalates as a precautionary approach to prevent the chemical industry using them as substitutes for the initially banned substance.

The US chemical industry's opposition had the support of the Bush administration. Although the United States has incorporated the concept of a precautionary approach into its legislation, the precautionary principle was not embraced as an official government policy. In fact, the Bush administration was totally opposed to both the precautionary principle and the REACH policy.[36] The American Chemistry Council, the industry's main trade group, contends that the EU wants to "eliminate all risks from daily life" and "replace science with speculation." Documents obtained from anonymous sources and through the Freedom of Information Act lay out elements of a full-fledged, closely coordinated lobby campaign to weaken REACH. The campaign was being waged by narrow chemical industry interests and the Bush administration's Environmental

Protection Agency (EPA), State Department, Commerce Department, and United States Trade Representative (USTR).[37] As part of this campaign the US chemical industry pushed for greater US involvement in EU policy making, for US-style risk assessment, and for no regulation of existing chemicals.[38]

In 2004, the aggressive campaign to undermine REACH caught the attention of the Congress. A US Senate report described the effort as "a case study of how a well-connected special interest can reverse US policy and enlist the support of numerous federal officials, including a cabinet secretary, to intervene in the environmental policies of other countries."[39] However, the US chemical industry was not only engaged in a struggle to curb the influence of the REACH policy in Europe, it also had a local struggle against the adoption of the precautionary principle by the city and county of San Francisco. A leaked memo written by the American Chemistry Council (ACC) stated: "For too long, the 'commonsense' appeal of the PP has gone unopposed," and "[m]oreover, California is a bellwether state, and any success enjoyed here could readily spill over to other parts of the country."[40] The chemical industry was beginning to fear the normalization of the precautionary principle in the regulation of dangerous chemicals.

AN ENDOCRINE-DISRUPTING CHEMICAL—ATRAZINE

There is a great deal of scientific evidence that endocrine-disrupting chemicals are dangerous, but their mode of action is extremely complex. Not only is there a diversity of hormones and receptors but there are also countless ways in which toxic chemicals can disrupt the endocrine system.[41] This situation is further complicated by the uncertainty surrounding the use and dispersion of chemical substances within the environment.[42] However, there are precedents for toxic chemicals used in the environment being recognised as causing harm, even if their mode of action is unknown. One such example is Rachel Carson's book *Silent Spring*, in which exposure to DDT was linked to harm in birds such as raptors before the science was certain.[43]

There are many endocrine-disrupting chemicals in the environment but the high volume use and persistence of atrazine in the environment marks it as a chemical of great concern. Atrazine was banned under the new EU REACH program soon after that Program's implementation, although the United Kingdom delayed its ban until the end of 2008. Atrazine is a member of the triazine group of chemicals and, together with its metabolites and related chemicals, is classified as an endocrine disrupter.

The danger of these chemicals was first brought to the attention of the public in Theo Colburn's book *Our Stolen Future*, which quotes Takasugi and Bern as stating "[W]e feel that abnormal hormonal environments during early postnatal (and antenatal) life should not be underestimated as to their possible contribution to abnormal changes of neoplastic [cancerous] significance later in life."[44] Since the publication of *Our Stolen Future*, there has been both a steady increase in evidence that atrazine poses a harmful threat to the environment and human health and an equally steady increase in the refutations of this evidence of harm by the chemical industry.

Atrazine was first synthesized in Switzerland in 1955 by scientists at JR Geigy, SA, and early tests suggested it would have a similar level of effectiveness on weeds as DDT had on insects.[45] Syngenta was formed in 1999 from the merger of agrochemical and seed division of Novartis (formed by the merger of two Swiss giant chemical/pharmaceutical companies Ciba-Geigy and Sandoz) and the agrochemical and biotechnology research division of AstraZeneca (part of which was formerly the British company Industrial Chemical Industries, or ICI). Syngenta has evolved into a giant in the crop protection business and has become the largest agribusiness company in the world, and the largest manufacturer of agrochemicals.[46] Syngenta produces and sells atrazine under a number of retail names. Syngenta's total sales for 2005 reached $8.1 billion,[47] while in 2006 selective herbicides, which include atrazine, accounted for the highest share of sales at $1.8 billion.[48]

Atrazine has been identified as an endocrine-disrupting chemical in more than two dozen human and animal disorders, including reproductive and developmental abnormalities, immune dysfunction, cognitive and behavioral pathologies, and cancer.[49] As an immune suppressor, laboratory experiments have corroborated the association between atrazine exposure and increased infection and limb deformities in frogs.[50] It is also known to act in synergy with other chemicals.[51]

Endocrine-disrupting contaminants interfere with the normal chemical signaling between cells and can adversely alter reproduction, growth, and immunity in living organisms.[52] As described by Louis Guillette and D. Andrew Crain, "[These] chemicals have been observed to mimic hormones, act as antihormones, or alter the synthesis and/or degradation of hormones."[53] Research into the effects of atrazine as an endocrine disrupter on aquatic organisms, prompted in part by the worldwide decline in frogs, has produced further new evidence.[54] Collaborative research by a team of scientists in both Japan and the United States published in 2007, states, "Current findings are consistent with atrazine's endocrine-disrupting effects in fish, amphibians, and reptiles; the induction of mammary and prostate cancer in laboratory rodents; and correlations between atrazine and similar reproductive cancers in humans."[55] This study confirms the importance of atrazine as a risk factor in endocrine disruption in wildlife and reproductive cancers in laboratory rodents and humans.

Many countries have been sufficiently convinced of the dangers of atrazine contamination to take regulatory action. The EU, invoking the precautionary principle, banned the use of atrazine in 2003.[56] Other precautions have been taken worldwide that set limits for atrazine contamination in drinking water. The World Health Organization (WHO) has set a limit of 2 parts per billion (ppb), the United States has set a limit of 3 ppb, and the EU has set a limit of only 1 ppb of any pesticide residue in either drinking or groundwater.[57] However, contrary to this trend, the Australian Drinking Water Guidelines[58] for atrazine has set a health value[59] limit at 40 ppb. The Canadian Environmental Water Quality Guides for the Protection of Aquatic Life (CCME) for atrazine in freshwater is 1.8 ppb, but there is no recommended guideline for marine aquatic life.[60]

ATRAZINE—A SITE OF CONTROVERSY

Scientific research into the hazards of atrazine to frogs has become a more recent site of controversy. Professor Tyrone Hayes from the Department of Integrative Biology, University of California, Berkeley and his fellow researchers showed in 2001 conclusively, in both laboratory studies and in field study sites across the United States, that atrazine exposure at extremely low levels equal to 0.1 ppb resulted in retarded gonadal development and hermaphroditism in leopard frogs (*Rana pipiens*).[61] Hayes had earlier conducted similar studies on frog populations with funds provided by the manufacturer of atrazine, Syngenta, through Ecorisk Inc. But when his studies showed negative effects, Syngenta tried to suppress his findings and launched an aggressive campaign to discredit Hayes.[62] Ecorisk Inc.'s previous clients include the Chlorine Chemistry Council, Dow Chemical, and the Ciba-Geigy Corp.[63]

The Mayo Clinic's Dr. Alan Hoffman said Hayes's research was courageous because "[H]e's fighting this company, this big agriculture business, about an important thing—and he's playing fair. He's doing good science. And we know in this world when business runs up against things, they produce not such good science."[64]

Meanwhile, Hayes and his work on frogs, the results of which have appeared in *Nature* and other peer-reviewed journals, continues to be the focus of attack by Syngenta and a chorus of supporters, including the Kansas Corn Growers Association, a Fox News commentator, the industry-sponsored Center for Regulatory Effectiveness, and the Hudson Institute,[65, 66] a conservative think tank whose goals are to combat limits to technological advances.[67, 68] The Center for Regulatory Effectiveness invoked the US Data Quality Act to marginalize published research about atrazine toxicology. The Data Quality Act was an attempt by the Bush administration to require scientific data to be more certain before it can trigger regulatory action, thereby defeating the precautionary principle trigger of plausible but uncertain scientific evidence.[69]

The biologist James A. Carr of Texas Tech University in Lubbock, Texas, a member of the industry-financed scientific team, which also included Keith Solomon, Professor, Department of Environmental Biology, University of Guelph, Ontario, Canada, criticized Hayes stating "[T]here are not a lot of details published in "Hayes work"[70] but EcoRisk/Syngenta had no such criticisms of Hayes's original work, only his adverse findings. The Hudson Institute in their publication, *Centre for Global Food Issues*, also published a scathing attack on Hayes discrediting his research.[71] However, a subsequent US EPA science panel was to level harsh criticisms at the industry-sponsored studies for their poor design and careless implementation.[72] As a result of the conflicting studies, the knowledge surrounding the endocrine-disrupting hazards of atrazine remains in a state of uncertainty.[73]

ATRAZINE AS A CARCINOGEN

Atrazine's role as a carcinogen has also been the site of scientific uncertainty. In 1991 and 1999, scientific findings by the International Agency for Research on Cancer (IARC) concluded that although the human and animal epidemiological studies on the carcinogenicity of atrazine were not definitive, the animal studies provided sufficient evidence that atrazine causes cancer.[74] Similarly, a study by McMullin et al. of Sprague-Dawley rats showed that high doses of atrazine not only disrupt normal neuroendocrine function but have carcinogenic effects.[75] Similarly, research by Wetzel et al. into the effects of high doses of atrazine on female Sprague-Dawley rats found not only an increase in endocrine changes but also earlier and/or increased incidence of mammary tumors.[76] A further study by Stevens, et al. pointed out that the results were strain-specific to Sprague-Dawley rats, and therefore the results are not applicable to human biology.[77] However, both Wetzel and Stevens were employed by Novartis Crop Protection Inc. (now Syngenta) while conducting their research.

In 2003, the Natural Resources Defense Council (NRDC) filed a legal motion charging that the US EPA had failed to evaluate the link between cancer and atrazine. The NRDC charged that the EPA had "ignored a court order mandating independent scientific review of its unfounded conclusion that atrazine does not cause cancer."[78] The matter was not resolved because, as the NRDC later found, the EPA had cut a deal with Syngenta.[79] Syngenta would not have to test 96 percent of the streams at risk and only report on contamination if it reached a "level of concern." Nevertheless, the Californian EPA set their public health goal for atrazine in drinking water based on mammary tumors (adenocarcinoma and fibroadenoma) observed in females in a carcinogenicity study in Sprague-Dawley rats fed atrazine.[80]

THE REGULATION OF ATRAZINE

The mounting evidence against the use of atrazine and its known contamination of surface and groundwater has produced various responses in the regulation of atrazine from authorities in different countries. The EU has discontinued the registration and use of atrazine. In Canada, the use of atrazine continues primarily on corn with restrictions on application rates, and with no aerial application allowed.[81] In the 1990s, the US EPA, in the face of growing evidence, listed endocrine disrupters as a research priority and devised a strategic plan to implement new policies.[82] However, this action stalled and the EPA finally released a draft list of compounds to screen for endocrine disruption in June 2007. This list should have been completed in 1999.[83]

Under industry pressure, the EPA has since reclassified atrazine from "possibly carcinogenic to humans" to "not classifiable as to its carcinogenicity to humans" in alignment with the IARC, which has also made the reclassification.[84] This reduced caution in classification prompted one former IARC director to warn, "[I]f tests show those hypotheses to be incorrect, or if they do not account adequately for the wider range of susceptibility in humans, serious consequences for public health may follow."[85] Australia has followed the US regulatory policy on atrazine, which allows for the aerial spraying of atrazine on forestry plantations.

However, the US EPA has come under intense criticism as it further delays action on atrazine.[86] In 2003, in the lead-up to the re-registration of atrazine, the EPA and atrazine manufacturer Syngenta held approximately fifty private meetings, the outcome of which was the establishment of two advisory committees, with members from both the EPA and Syngenta, to determine how atrazine should be regulated and where it should be monitored.[87] Subsequently, the data used to regulate atrazine has primarily come from industry-sponsored research.[88] In addition, the review did not include data on the hormone-disruption activity of atrazine.[89]

In the EPA's April 2007 update, it has now sought additional data to reduce uncertainty with regard to the study conducted for the manufacturer, Syngenta Crop Protection Inc., of the incidence of prostate cancer in workers at an atrazine manufacturing plant in Louisiana.[90] In relation to the effects of atrazine on amphibians, the EPA is waiting for Syngenta "to conduct a study that will enable the Agency to determine if exposure to atrazine can affect amphibian gonadal development."[91]

In Australia, the Australian Pesticides and Veterinary Medicines Authority (APVMA) is the body responsible for the approval of the active constituent of atrazine, the registration of the products containing atrazine and their associated labels. The APVMA has taken its regulatory lead from the United States in continuing the registration of atrazine rather than following the European ban. It states that its assessment is based on scientific data and takes a weight of evidence approach.[92] Meanwhile, the regulation of the actual use of atrazine rests with state and local government bodies.

In a recent review of atrazine the APVMA, following the US EPA's findings, concluded that "[I]t appears unlikely that atrazine, when used in accordance with the label recommendations will contaminate waterways to any extent likely to present a hazard to the environment or to human beings through the consumption of contaminated drinking water."[93] The APVMA also cited the EPA's recent findings of an inconsistency and lack of reproducibility across studies, and an absence of a dose-response relationship in support of its conclusions. It has also stated that the issue of atrazine and amphibians may be revisited if additional data demonstrates that atrazine is likely to impact on frog populations at realistic levels of exposure. But it considers such outcomes to be unlikely.[94]

In Canada, a re-evaluation of atrazine as a risk to human health was conducted by the Pest Management Regulatory Agency (PMRA) in November 2003.[95] It concluded that the use of atrazine and its end-use products did not entail an unacceptable risk to human health. However, according to Environment Canada's website published in 2007 CEPA Environmental Registry, atrazine meets the criteria for persistence and/or bioaccumulation and is inherently toxic to aquatic organisms and humans.[96] Studies found the acute aquatic toxicity experimental value was 0.011 mg/L.[97]

The Canadian Government accepts that there is evidence of adverse effects due to endocrine disruption exposure seen in fish and wildlife in Canada.[98] Environment Canada has published a brochure on *Endocrine Disrupting Substances in the Environment*, which lists atrazine as an endocrine disrupter.[99] It also states that Environment Canada has made endocrine disruption a research priority to produce the knowledge necessary for informed policy and regulatory decisions. In partnership, Environment Canada and Health Canada manage the Toxic Substances Research Initiative, which includes support for research on endocrine disruption. There has also been research on endocrine disruption in the major Regional Ecosystem Initiatives. However it states this research "will produce sound scientific assessments of the potential impacts of endocrine disruption on the Canadian environment."[100]

Further, the Canadian government funds research on endocrine disruptors through the Canadian Institute of Health Research, the National Sciences and Engineering Research Council (NSERC), Toxic Substances Research Initiative, and Northern Contaminants Program. It states that Canadian scientists are involved in international efforts to harmonize ways of assessing the risks posed by endocrine disruptors through the Organization for Economic Cooperation and Development (OECD).[101] Another Canadian group conducting research into the effects of low levels of endocrine disruptors on development and reproduction is the Canadian Chemical Producers' Association (CCPA). CCPA states on its website that "the jury is still out on endocrine disrupters."[102] CCPA is also sponsoring several research initiatives, primarily through the Canadian Network of Toxicology Centres (CNTC).[103] During the years 1999 to 2002, the CCPA supported CNTC studies into the environmental risks posed by endocrine disruptors, which were carried out in part by Dr. Keith R. Solomon and GJ Van der Kraak, both from the University of Guelph.[104]

Solomon is on the CNTC Board of Directors, as well as on the Network Management Committee and a Director of the Centre for Toxicology at the University of Guelph. He was a collaborator with James A. Carr, John P. Giesy, and Glen Van Der Kraak, a Syngenta-funded research team that attempted to discredit Professor Tyrone Hayes's studies on the effects of atrazine on frogs.[105, 106] In Solomon's opinion, there exists a common misconception, based on anecdotal evidence, that pesticides cause disease such as cancer.[107]

The University of Guelph receives funding from Syngenta Crop Protection (Canada) Inc., as does the Natural Sciences and Engineering Research Council of Canada (NSERC), which receives cash and in-kind funding.[108] Research funds received by the departments in the College of Biological Science for the period May 1, 2005, to April 30, 2006, from both Syngenta (US) and Syngenta Crop Protection Canada Inc. totalled $403,436.[109] The NSERC fosters partnerships with universities, industry, government, and other organizations. The NSERC is a Canadian federal agency that came into existence in 1978 and now has a budget of $1 billion. The collaboration between the Canadian governments, Syngenta, and the University of Guelph also extends to the Canadian Corn Pest Coalition (CCPC). A conflict of interest threatens to arise when the university (Guelph) is carrying out research into the cost-effectiveness of atrazine as well as its potential harm.[110] Further conflicts of interest, undue influence and close ties between governments, industry, and scientific research can be seen in the following two case studies.

CASE STUDY ONE—TASMANIAN DEVIL CANCER

In Australia, the precautionary principle was adopted in February 1992 through the Intergovernmental Agreement on the Environment (non-binding), whereby the Commonwealth, states, territories, and local governments agreed to follow the precautionary principle as part of a commitment to ecologically sustainable development.[111] The Australian government has since implemented the Convention on Biological Diversity under the Environment Protection and Biodiversity Conservation Act 1999 (EPCB). The object of the Act, through the promotion of ecologically sustainable development, is the protection of biodiversity. The Act commits Australia to the precautionary principle with the direction that "[T]he Minister must consider the precautionary principle in making decisions"[112] and its objective of ecologically sustainable development[113] that includes the precautionary principle."[114]

In Tasmania, the precautionary principle has not been implemented to protect the Tasmanian devil. An incident in the northeast of the state in 2004 involving a helicopter crash, while spraying chemicals on plantations, followed by a flood event, resulted in the mass deaths of oysters and other organisms in the Georges Bay. An inquiry into the incident by the Tasmanian Department of Primary Industries, Water and Environment (DPIWE) concluded that the deaths were due to an influx of fresh water.[115] This incident was the culmination of many years of oyster abnormalities which had also been investigated by DPIWE.[116] Frustrated by the finding, oyster growers commissioned an independent study by Dr. Marcus Scammell, a marine ecologist, and Dr. Alison Bleaney, the local area medical officer.

Although Scammell and Bleaney were unable to make a causal link between the use of chemicals and the oyster deaths at the time, they could correlate, in time and space, the increase in forestry plantations, the use of chemicals, the oyster abnormalities, and the Tasmanian devil cancer. Faced with scientific uncertainty, they recommended the implementation of the precautionary principle until further scientific studies could be carried out. The government ignored their call for the implementation of the precautionary principal and has taken no action to either halt aerial spraying of chemicals or further restrict the use of chemicals used in plantations. Although there has been considerable scientific research into the Tasmanian devil cancer, focusing on the hypothesis that it is a transmissible tumor— the allograft theory—there has been no research into a chemical aetiology for the tumor.

The Tasmanian devil cancer has been named Devil Facial Tumour Disease (DFTD) and scientific consensus has termed it a neuro-endocrine tumour (NET). The disease was first detected in 1996 when a wildlife photographer captured an image of a diseased animal in the northeast of the state. Since then the devil population has plummeted to below 50 percent of its 1996 numbers on the eastern side of the state while those on the western side remain disease free. The DFTD scientific research is controlled by the Department of Primary Industries, Parks, Water and Environment (DPIPWE) (formerly DPIWE) in close association with the University of Tasmania (UTAS). This scientific research has endeavored to provide support for the allograft theory—that the cancer is a contagious disease spread from devil to devil via biting.

The allograft theory was published as a Brief Communication,[117] which are relatively informal articles of preliminary results, in the prestigious scientific journal *Nature* in 2006 by Anne Marie Pearse and her technician, Kate Swift.[118] It is based on the observation that the chromosomal rearrangement in the cancer cells of one devil was different from that devil's normal cells. From this observation, and a precedent of a canine transmissible venereal tumor, the hypothesis that the cancer was contagious was adopted. Although Pearse and Swift concluded their article with the remarks that the cancer could have a chemical aetiology and that further DNA tests would be needed to confirm their hypothesis, little scientific research has been conducted along these lines. There has been no published data on studies carried out on toxin levels in Tasmanian devils. The scientific research that has been pursued by the government-sponsored project has been to confirm the allograft theory. This has led to a further hypothesis that the cancer is transmissible due to a lack of diversity in the devils' major histocompatibility complex (MHC).[119]

Investigations into a chemical aetiology of the disease were not totally abandoned. Following public pressure through the media, DPIPWE finally carried out limited toxicology studies of diseased devils. However, the data from these studies was only released after a Freedom of Information request from *The Australian* newspaper. Two letters of opinion by independent scientists based on statistical analysis of the data by Professor Hamish McCallum, head of the DPIPWE Tasmanian devil disease project, were published. The toxicology studies found high levels of PCBEs or flame retardants in the fat tissues along with traces of other chemicals. These studies were carried out at the National Measurement Institute in Sydney.

The triazine chemicals, atrazine and simazine, both widely used in plantation forestry as herbicides, were undetected in the devils' tissues. These studies were carried out in house by the Analytical Services Laboratory, funded by DPIPWE and located within the University of Tasmania and accredited by the National Association of Technical Authorities (NATA) to analyze water and sediment samples, only not biological samples, such as devil tissue.

Notwithstanding, scientific studies into the effects on Tasmanian devils of any one chemical or a combination of the chemicals used in forestry have not been carried out.

Atrazine and simazine have continued to be detected in surface water in Tasmania since the early 1990s with a recent contamination of the city of Hobart's drinking water. So serious has been the contamination of drinking water that the public/private enterprise, Forestry Tasmania, has banned the use of atrazine on its plantations. Given the weight of evidence against chemicals such as atrazine, relevant toxicological experiments would constitute normal scientific practice. A recent study by Holly Ingraham and colleagues found atrazine altered hormonal signaling in human cells and in zebrafish. Ingraham, a UCSF Professor of Cellular and Molecular Pharmacology, stated in an interview, "[T]hese fish are very sensitive to endocrine-disrupting chemicals, so one might think of them as 'sentinels' to potential developmental dangers in humans."[120]

There are close ties and the potential for conflict of interest in Tasmania between the DPIPWE, charged with monitoring chemical use and protecting endangered species, and UTAS. The university receives scholarships and funding for research and education from the forestry industry. For example, plant development at UTAS is funded by the Southern Tree Breeding Association (STBA), whose members include Forestry Tasmania and timber giant Gunns Limited. Meanwhile, scientists at UTAS working on the devil project receive their funding through DPIPWE. Sheldon Krimsky, Professor of Urban & Environmental Policy & Planning, Tufts University, writes that universities that rely on industry funding for their research in any area are sensitive to adverse results emanating from other research schools within that university.[121] He suggests a "firewall" should be erected within the universities to isolate different schools from undue influence.

Further evidence of conflict of interest is demonstrated in the lead-up to the environmental assessment of the proposed Gunns Limited pulp mill. There has been an aggressive push by the state government, supported by the previous Premier Paul Lennon, to establish the proposed Gunns pulp mill at Bell Bay. However, a lack of transparency in the process has given rise to considerable opposition prompted by environmental concerns. The resulting controversy culminated in an appeal to the federal government to resolve the issue. The outcome was the establishment of a panel of scientists to review the environmental impacts of the proposed pulp mill.

The federal government appointed the Australian Chief Scientist to chair an expert scientific panel to investigate the environmental impact of the proposed pulp mill. However, the Australian Chief Scientist, Dr. Jim Peacock, has close financial ties to the manufacturer of atrazine, Syngenta. Peacock, along with Peter Gerner, CEO Oceania, Syngenta International AG, is a Non-Executive Director of Graingene, whose business is the commercialization of Graingene technology. Graingene is an alliance between the Australian Wheat Board, CSIRO, Grain Research & Development Corporation (GRDC), and Syngenta, each with a 25 percent share-hold.[122] The commercialization is carried out by LongReach Plant Breeders, which is 50 percent owned by Syngenta. Peacock is a plant molecular biologist who headed the CSIRO Division of Plant Industry and a leading promoter of genetic engineering in Australia. He is quoted as saying, "We are looking forward to working with Syngenta researchers."[123] He instituted the Graingene Initiative and is a Director of Gene Shears, a biotechnology company, and the HRZ Wheat Company.[124]

Also on the panel was the Senior Scientist, Professor Hamish McCallum from the DPIPWE Tasmanian devil disease project.[125] In all the environmental impact assessments of the proposed pulp mill, the use of pesticides, such as atrazine, in plantation forestry management has not been raised as a potential problem. The expert scientific panel terms of reference were confined to the pulp mill site.

CASE STUDY TWO: THE ST. LAWRENCE RIVER ESTUARY BELUGA WHALE CANCERS

In Canada, the precautionary principle underpins both the Canadian Endangered Species Act 1998[126] and the Canadian Environmental Protection Act 1999.[127] The management of chemical substances is a major part of the *CEPA 1999*. Sustainable development and the incorporation of the precautionary principle underpins the *CEPA 1999* and is incorporated into the Preamble, which states:

> Whereas the Government of Canada is committed to implementing the precautionary principle that, where there are threats of serious or irreversible damage, lack of full scientific certainty shall not be used as a reason for postponing cost-effective measures to prevent environmental degradation.[128]

Contrary to this statement, *CEPA 1999* decisions regarding chemicals are made on a "risk-based" method. It states that "[R]isk is determined by looking at the harmful properties of the chemical substance and how much exposure there is for people or the surrounding environment." The precautionary principle goes beyond normal risk assessment, which relies on quantification, giving decision makers a tool to act to mitigate harm when scientific evidence is unquantifiable because it is uncertain.

This reliance by Canada on the US model of chemical risk assessment for regulation is also apparent under Environment Canada's Chemical Substances ecoACTION; ecoACTION is a challenge to assess two hundred substances of the highest priority.[129] This initiative moves away from the precautionary principle toward a risk management approach and a "strong science" approach. Further impediment to controlling dangerous chemicals is the need for them to be added to the List of Toxic Substances before they can be restricted. Although atrazine has been added to the Domestic Substances List as of December 27, 2006, it has not been added to the List of Toxic Substances for assessment.

Consequently, in Canada there has been no official implementation of the precautionary principle to mitigate the harm to the St. Lawrence River Beluga Whales. Liz Armstrong, Guy Dauncey, and Anne Wordsworth in their book *Cancer: 101 Solutions to a Preventable Epidemic*,[130] call for the implementation of the precautionary principle to halt an epidemic of cancers including the beluga whale cancers. However, a look at the close ties that exist between the manufacturer of atrazine, Syngenta, the scientific research into the beluga whale cancer, and those charged with protecting endangered species in Canada will shed some light on the situation.

In 1982, the first dead beluga whale was discovered. Over a period of seventy years, the population had been reduced from 5,000 to approximately 650 individuals.[131] In 2002, Dr. Daniel Martineau, a veterinary pathologist at the University of Montreal, and his colleagues carried out a study of beluga whale carcasses reported stranded between 1983 and 1999.[132] They found the main cause of death was cancer (27 percent incidence).[133] It is higher than the rate of any other wild mammal species. Cancers detected included intestinal and mammary gland cancer—a first for marine mammals. The human population in the same region also has a particularly high incidence of stomach, digestive system, and breast cancer compared to other regions of Quebec and Canada.

Martineau et al. proposed that polycyclic aromatic hydrocarbons (PAHs) from local aluminium smelters "present in benthic invertebrates . . . may contribute to the elevated rate of digestive tract cancers . . ." in the St. Lawrence River estuary beluga whales.[134] Beluga whales feed by diving deep down to the bottom of the river to feed on fish that have consumed plankton.[135] The study states that "causal relationship between intestinal adenocarcinoma and PAHs is further supported by the observation that in mice, chronic ingestion of coal tar mixtures (which contain benzo[a]pyrene) causes small intestinal adenocarcinoma."[136] Scientific proof that PAHs play a role in the beluga whale cancers has not been established. Research into immune system functions, which also play a role in cancer, is incomplete and its role is unknown.[137] As a consequence, the research into St. Lawrence beluga whale cancers is confounded by scientific uncertainty and ignorance.

However, while chemical monitoring of the St. Lawrence river has revealed concentrations of PAHs, it is atrazine (used extensively on corn) that is most frequently detected, and at the highest concentrations. Environment Canada, through the St. Lawrence Centre, monitors water quality in Quebec. The degraded state of the St. Lawrence River prompted the St. Lawrence Centre in 1990 to established a research program in order to quantify contaminants in the drainage basin. Because of its prevalence, its persistence, and its potential toxicity, atrazine was chosen as a contaminant of concern.[138] Based on its ability to inhibit photosynthesis, it has the potential to affect the growth of phytoplanton and hence the dynamics of the aquatic food chain.[139]

PAHs and benzo[a]pyrene are ubiquitous atmospheric contaminants, which usually result from wood burning, although they can subsequently be deposited in water. Monitoring by Environment Canada had found that PAH concentrations in the river were comparable to 1990 with only a slight increase in suspended particles since 1995.[140] The highest concentrations occur during winter and are probably due to the increase in the combustion of wood and other fossil fuels. In contrast, atrazine concentrations, measured between 1995 and 2002, were higher in summer due to the application of pesticides on farmland and lower in winter due to snowmelt.[141] In 2002, atrazine concentration recorded at Quebec City was the highest it had been since 1995.

While it is unusual in an environmental context to be able to identify a particular chemical as the cause of cancer, the Martineau finding blaming PAHs and benzo[a] pyrene is supported by the Binational Toxic Strategy, a US and Canadian Great Lakes strategy. The strategy reports that benzo[a]pyrene is moderately persistent, a probably human carcinogen (Category 2B) according to the EPA, and an animal carcinogen according to the IARC. However, it lists the main sources of PAHs as residential wood combustion and petroleum refining but does not include aluminium smelting. The Martineau study was partly funded by the aluminium company Alcan. Alcan now claims new technology reduces PAH emissions from aluminium plants by 82 percent. At this time, Alcan had been a major contributor to the St. Lawrence National Institute of Ecotoxicology (SLNIE), which in its short history gained notoriety for its work on the beluga whales and its "Let's adopt a Beluga" program. It was founded in 1987 and published its last newsletter entitled "Beluga" in 2002, which gave an overview of its research programs.[142] Dr. Pierre Beland, who was chairman in 2001 and 2002, published a book called Beluga: A Farewell to Whales in 2002.

There were many studies into the beluga whale cancer between 2002 and 2006 in which Martineau was involved—none of which included the effects of atrazine. However, these studies were funded by bodies that received funding from Syngenta. In 2003, a study, partly funded by the Canadian Cooperative Wildlife Health Centre (CCWHC), was carried out into the possible cause of hyperplastic lesions of the thyroid gland in Beluga whales.[143] Although the lesions are linked to PCBs (found in the beluga whale tissues), they recommended that these not be considered the only possible carcinogens, and their findings remained inconclusive. Syngenta is a part founder and funder of the CCWHC, which was established in 1992 with leadership from Environment Canada and funds from the Max Bell Foundation. The Max Bell Foundation received $170,150 in funding in 2004 from the Donner Canadian Foundation, which funds conservative think tanks and organizations.[144] Daniel Martineau is listed as staff and an associate of the CCWHC in the 2006 Annual Report. The University of Guelph is also a partner.

Although studies were carried out into the beluga whales from 2004 to 2006, they were funded by NSERC. Syngenta, the manufacturer of atrazine, is a research partner in the NSERC and sponsors an NSERC Industrial Research Chair in Groundwater Contamination in Fractured Media.[145] Atrazine is a known groundwater contaminant that has the potential to leach out into the environment. In these studies, Martinueau and colleagues studied the role of Canadian Arctic beluga as models for St. Lawrence beluga[146] and conducted studies into the effects of pollutants such as PBDEs,[147] but none of the research looked at the role of atrazine.

The scientific research into the beluga whale cancers was initiated in 2002, and because of the highly contaminated environment in which they live, linking the cancers to a cause has been problematic. The research, rather than supporting the supposition that PAHs are responsible for the cancers, has confounded the problem—the science has increased in uncertainty. However, the studies carried out since 1990 into the contaminants has shown a slight reduction in PAHs, which could be attributed to a reduction in emissions from aluminium smelters. In contrast, there has been a steady increase in atrazine contamination. Beluga whales are still threatened with extinction and the Canadian government has failed to implement the precautionary principle to mitigate the harm.

A NEW APPROACH TO THE PRECAUTIONARY PRINCIPLE

The proponents of atrazine call for a "strong science" approach when there is a lack of local evidence of harm and considerable scientific uncertainty. They insist on the application of traditional risk assessment and the need to quantify the level of harm. They argue that no regulatory measures should be taken until a direct causal link has been established between the use of atrazine and harm. The Australian APVMA and the Canadian authorities, following the EPA lead, have re-registered atrazine based on this appeal to "sound science." The EPA has sought to limit regulation through the Data Quality Act while the APVMA has stated that it has not seen any direct evidence that atrazine is a health risk. Therefore, those who defend the use of atrazine claim that the lack of scientific evidence of atrazine-caused harm precludes the adoption of the precautionary principle.

It is unclear whether the precautionary principle should be applied in a situation where there is strong international evidence that atrazine causes harm but weak evidence that atrazine is causing harm in the local environment (see Table 1 below). Nor is this sort of situation discussed in the precautionary principle literature. It is therefore proposed that two further elements be introduced to help clarify when the precautionary principle should be applied.

TABLE 1. INTERNATIONAL *VERSUS* LOCAL EVIDENCE (PP = PRECAUTIONARY PRINCIPLE)

	Strong international evidence chemical causes harm	Weak international evidence chemical causes harm
Strong local evidence chemical causes harm	pp triggered	pp triggered
Weak local evidence chemical causes harm	pp trigger debatable	pp not triggered

The first element is the extent of the harm already caused. Where the local evidence that a certain chemical causes harm is weak, but international evidence that the same chemical has the capacity to cause harm is strong—in other words the evidence is mixed—the precautionary principle may be debatable. However, if there is also strong evidence that there is local harm of the type thought to be caused by the chemical elsewhere, then this should be enough to trigger the precautionary principle. This appears to be the case in Tasmania and the St. Lawrence River Estuary.

The second element is the issue of necessity, which can also be introduced to further aid in deciding when to invoke the precautionary principle (see Table 2 below).

TABLE 2. EVIDENCE *VERSUS* NECESSITY (PP = PRECAUTIONARY PRINCIPLE)

	Strong evidence chemical causes harm	Mixed evidence chemical causes harm
Low necessity for chemical	pp triggered	pp triggered
High necessity for chemical	pp triggered	pp trigger debatable

If there are alternatives for the chemical in question that can be used and are being used by others, then the level of evidence needed to trigger the precautionary principle should be much lower.

It would appear that the banning of atrazine under REACH in the EU, its restriction in Canada to use only on corn, and the banning of atrazine by Forestry Tasmania in Tasmania means that alternatives to atrazine are available and should be used. Currently atrazine is only used in privately owned Tasmanian plantation forests and on corn in Canada. It is argued that this lack of necessity should lower the threshold for the implementation of the precautionary principle. Therefore, the case for adopting the precautionary principle in both Canada and Tasmania to prevent the use of atrazine is strong. It would be prudent therefore to implement the precautionary principle to ban atrazine, as has been done in the EU, as a measure to protect not only wildlife and the environment, but more importantly human health.

CONCLUSION

Both case studies provide evidence of chemical contamination in the environments of the Tasmanian devils and beluga whales. In fact, it is fair to say that they inhabit a toxic soup of agricultural and/or industrial chemicals, all of which are potentially dangerous individually and as combinations. There is also strong and credible evidence of serious and possibly irreversible harm being caused in both the wildlife and the human populations in Tasmania and Canada. However, the evidence that atrazine is the cause of harm in both Tasmania and Canada is weak due, in part, to a lack of studies. If there are further delays, while the regulators seek "sound science," many more cancers will eventuate that could have been avoided. The successful implementation of the precautionary principle, through restricting, banning, or seeking to introduce the use of safer alternatives to dangerous chemicals, reflects a determined and sophisticated effort to protect the health of the environment and the public.

The precautionary principle, a common sense approach to mitigating harm, has generated completely different responses in the EU as opposed to the United States, Canada, and Australia. There is strong evidence of contamination of both the Tasmanian devil and beluga whale environments by harmful carcinogenic and endocrine-disrupting chemicals, such as atrazine, but there has been no scientific research that has linked the harmful chemicals to the cancers. Political will or undue corporate influence plays a part in this lack of evidence, due to lack of research funding compounded by uncertain scientific knowledge or ignorance. Policymakers therefore are morally bound by the precautionary principle to prevent harm by restricting or banning harmful chemicals. These wildlife species cancers are bioindicators of human health, and there is evidence that humans in both geographic regions are suffering a higher than normal incidence of cancer. It is therefore time to act, not delay further restrictions of known endocrine disrupters and carcinogens such as the widely used chemical atrazine.

Chapter 21

DUST, LABOR, AND CAPITAL— SILICOSIS AMONG SOUTH AFRICA'S GOLD MINERS

Jock McCulloch

South Africa's gold mines were the first in the world to compensate silicosis and tuberculosis as occupational diseases. They were also the first industry subject to a state regulated system of medical surveillance. Despite that degree of state control, official disease rates showed that by 1920 the mines had all but eradicated silicosis. The industry is currently facing a massive class action by former miners for uncompensated lung disease. The historical evidence suggests that the mines were never safe and that the more data the mines and the state collected the less the disease burden was visible.

The gold mines of South Africa are the largest and deepest in the world and historically they have been among the most dangerous. One of the hazards facing miners has been silicosis, which is a life-threatening disease caused by the inhalation of free silica dust. The disease, in which scarring or fibrosis reduce lung function, usually results from moderate exposure over a prolonged period. At first, shortness of breath may occur during exercise, but eventually it will appear even during rest.[1] The disease is insidious and it will progress after a man or woman has ceased to work in a dusty atmosphere.

Since it is not possible to ban silica in the way that has been done with asbestos, silicosis can be said to be embedded in industrialism. States can ban certain uses of silica such as sandblasting, but the material itself is ubiquitous. China records in excess of five hundred thousand cases of silicosis annually with more than twenty-four thousand deaths. In the United States, it is estimated that more than a million workers have occupational exposure to free silica dust. The ILO/WHO International Program on the Global Elimination of Silicosis, launched in 1995, aims at the reduction and eventual elimination of what is an incurable disease. Exposure to silica also greatly increases an individual's chances of contracting pulmonary tuberculosis. That is particularly true in the developing world, where most cases of silicosis nowadays occur. In terms of morbidity, mortality, and the cost of litigation, silicosis has arguably been the most important of the modern industrial diseases.

Silicosis also has claims to being the quintessential occupational disease. The first occupational health crises in South Africa, the United Kingdom, Australia, and the United States involved silicosis, which was formally recognized as a disease of the workplace in Anglo American jurisdictions after 1880. The elevated dust levels created by power tools proved particularly lethal to hard rock miners and foundry workers. Those crises, which were provoked in large part by trade union militancy, led to numerous public inquiries and in the United States to a flood of litigation. Silicosis also provoked a questioning of the new systems of production.[2]

Outside of the industrial heartlands, silicosis was linked to imperialism, which drew labor between centers and peripheries. Thus, many of the Cornish miners who worked in South Africa, the United States, and Australia contracted silicosis and returned home to die. It was their plight which precipitated the first commissions into silicosis in the United Kingdom and South Africa. Researchers and legislatures on the imperial rim also played an important role in the global response to the disease: in 1909 an Australian physician, John H. L. Cumpston, invented the classificatory system for silicosis, while South Africa became the first state to compensate silicosis (1912) and tuberculosis (1916) as diseases of the workplace. Silicosis is of particular interest to historians because it exposes the complex and highly contested relationships between labor, the state, and capital.

In August 2004, the case of *Mankayi Mbini v. American* was filed in the Pretoria Supreme Court. Mbini had worked as a gold miner for sixteen years at Welkom and is now suffering from silicosis and tuberculosis, for which he sought compensation.[3] Mbini claims that Anglo American knew or should have known that silica dust causes silicosis and that it failed to protect him from the risk of injury. Mbini's was the first case of its kind to be brought before a South African court: it has long been assumed the various Mines Acts stretching back to 1911 preclude such litigation.[4] If successful, Mbini's claim may be the initial step in a class action involving hundreds of thousands of miners from South Africa, Lesotho, Malawi, Swaziland, Mozambique, and Botswana, all of which supplied labor to Anglo American mines. Such a class action could cost employers as much as R50 billion (approximately $5 billion in USD).

· The gold mines of South Africa, which are concentrated within a single geological deposit around Johannesburg and the Free State, are distinguished by their depth, their scale, and the size of their labor force. Those features have encouraged the dominance of a few mining houses, such as Anglo American, which, because of their centrality to employment, foreign exchange, and state revenue, have enjoyed considerable political influence. For much of the twentieth century, the gold mines were by far the largest single employer in South Africa.[5] At their peak in the 1980s, those mines employed well over half a million men, most of whom were migrant workers drawn from neighboring countries. While migrancy has been common to industrial states, in South Africa, it has been unique in the depth of its political foundations and in its negative impact upon labor-sending communities.[6] Under minority rule, racist legislation determined job specializations, rates of pay, and compensation for disease or traumatic injury. White labor, which was represented by powerful trade unions, was well compensated for silicosis: black labor, which had no unions, was not.

At the beginning of the twentieth century, South Africa's mines faced a crisis over silicosis among white miners who represented less than 10 percent of the workforce.[7,8] Rock drilling was skilled and highly paid work reserved for whites: it was also a particularly hazardous job. As a result, in the first decade of mining hundreds of drillers died from acute silicosis. A series of commissions into miners' phthisis (silicosis) in 1903, 1910, and 1912 saw the introduction of new blasting regulations, watering down, and dust extraction technologies. Instruments, such as the konometer, to measure dust levels were also used for the first time. The South African mines were also the first to use routine X-ray screening of workers, which helped make Johannesburg the world center for research into dust disease.

By 1916, these innovations had greatly reduced the palpable dust, thereby transforming silicosis from an acute disease, which would kill miners within a few years, to a chronic disease. In spite of the reduced risk, continuing demands by militant white trade unions resulted in more public inquiries and commissions into silicosis in South Africa than in the United States, Australia, and Western Europe combined. For each commission there was at least one Act to further regulate the industry and often to increase the levels of compensation. By 1930, the compensation for white miners and their dependents was the most generous in the world.

The compensation schemes assuaged to some extent the white Mine Workers' Union (MWU), created the image of hygienic work environments and foreclosed on litigation. Even so, to compensate only 10 percent of the work-force proved expensive. The legal adviser to the Chamber of Mines, G. E. Barry, remarked at the 1930 Silicosis Conference in Johannesburg that the compensation scheme imposed such a heavy cost on employers that some mines had been forced to close.[9] H. W. Sampson, minister of posts and telegraphs, told the delegates that compensation had cost the gold mines almost one million pounds per year or 15 million pounds in the period from 1911 to 1929.[10] Under the Miners' Phthisis Legislation, blacks had a right to compensation but few were aware of that privilege and very few applied. Even fewer were successful. If blacks, who accounted for 90 percent of underground workers, had received adequate compensation, many mines would have been rendered unprofitable.

After 1916, the Chamber of Mines and employers like Anglo American maintained that there was little silicosis among gold miners. That claim was repeated at numerous commissions and it was supported by the official data on the disease rates. Those data were based on the number of successful claims for compensation decided by the Miners' Phthisis Bureau and later the Silicosis Bureau. In 1937 the Miners' Phthisis Prevention Committee, which included representatives from the white MWU, and the Chamber, produced what in effect is an official history of silicosis. The report maps out the lowering of the silicosis rate from 1902 by reference to four variables: changes to blasting regimes, the application of water, rock drill designs, and dust measurements.[11] The Committee found that every discovery regarding prevention had found its way into the legislation.[12] According to the official data in the period from 1918 to 1935, there was a constant fall in the disease rate.[13] In the absence of figures, the committee could only guess that prior to 1917 the silicosis rate was probably between 23 percent and 30 percent.[14] In the period from 1917 to 1920, the rate among white miners was 2.195 percent.[15] By 1935, it had fallen to .885 percent. The rate for black miners was even lower. In 1926 to 1927 it was .129 percent and in 1934 to 1935 it had fallen to .122 percent.[16] The picture, which survived until the end of apartheid, was one of ceaseless improvement in which South Africa led the world in prevention and compensation.

Despite the reassuring data, there is evidence from the 1920s that at least one South African scientist was concerned about the continuing problem of silicosis. Dr. Anthony Mavrogordato, who had worked with J. S. Haldane in the United Kingdom, was appointed Fellow in Industrial Hygiene to the South African Institute of Medical Research in 1919. He worked closely with the Department of Mines and the Chamber on dust counting and ventilation. From his appointment until his retirement in 1939, Mavrogordato published only twelve papers.[17] That modest output is curious, given the significance of his work.

In 1926, Dr. A. Mavrogordato wrote a 120-page review of the medical literature reflecting upon the issues of risk and its management.[18] Mavrogordato identified three key problems on the Rand: the difficulties of diagnosis, the synergy between silicosis and tuberculosis, and the intractability of the dust burden. He noted that more cases of silicosis were picked up at autopsy than during routine X-rays. For example, a man killed in an accident after only three years underground would at autopsy show definite signs of fibrosis even though he was at the time of death in apparent good health.[19] That suggested the disease rates might be higher than was officially recognized. Mavrogordato also believed that the minor changes to lung tissue, found at autopsy but invisible in X-rays, greatly increased the risk of tuberculosis.[20] That in turn suggested that tuberculosis was being exported from the mines into the labor-sending areas, a problem the industry has always denied.[21, 22]

The most important aspect of Mavrogordato's paper deals with dust. He distinguishes between income dust, which is the dust generated by each day's work, and capital dust, which is the dust always in circulation underground.[23] Income dust had been greatly reduced by the use of water sprays but sprays had no effect on capital dust, which Mavrogordato believed was sufficient in itself to produce silicosis. Capital dust also made it unsafe to use mine air for ventilation. Mavrogordato acknowledged that improved air quality would greatly increase production costs.[24] In summary, Mavrogordato concludes that silicosis and tuberculosis remained a serious hazard and he suggests that it was impossible to reduce dust to a level at which those diseases would not occur. His findings, which have been borne out by subsequent research, were not cited in the literature and Mavrogordato did not raise any of his concerns about capital dust and lung disease at the 1930 Silicosis Conference in Johannesburg.

Since majority rule in 1994, research conducted by the National Institute of Occupational Health (NIOH) in Johannesburg and the University of Cape Town has identified a pandemic of hitherto undiagnosed and uncompensated silicosis.[25] A published survey of Basotho miners who had worked at Welkom shows that over 23 percent have the disease.[26] That study of men employed at the President Steyn Mine, the mine at which Mbini worked in the Free State, was commissioned by Anglo American and took ten years to be released. It confirms the data from other major surveys showing a silicosis rate of between 22 and 24 percent. The rates of silicosis in South Africa's gold mines are among the highest in the world.

The under-reporting of silicosis raises the specter of a backlog of compensation claims. In his work on Botswana miners Steen found that the Medical Bureau for Occupational Diseases (MBOD) has underestimated the rate of

silicosis by a factor of between four- and tenfold. That is in line with Anna
Trapido, who suggests there are 196,000 former miners in South Africa and a
further 84,000 in neighboring states with compensable silicosis.[27] Extrapolating
from Churchyard, eight thousand men currently employed in the mines are eligible for compensation.[28] Given the rate at which the workforce has replaced
itself over the past twenty years, there could be a further two hundred thousand
compensable cases in the neighboring states of Southern Africa. Neil White costs
the immediate shortfall in compensation at around R2.8 billion.[29] Under common law, to those figures must be added the costs of pain and suffering, the areas
in which working class plaintiffs usually have the strongest claims for compensation. For that to happen, a number of legal barriers must first be negotiated.

INVISIBLE DISEASE

The current disease rate among black miners is as much as two hundred times
higher than was the official rate seventy years ago. South Africa's gold miners
have long been among the most heavily medicalized workforces in the world,
which makes the gap between the new and old data remarkable. How could such
a disease burden have gone unrecognized for so long? There are three possible
explanations: the labor process, and with it work conditions, may have deteriorated dramatically in the past thirty years or so; the means of diagnosis may have
improved; or the official data produced by the regulatory bodies may have been
false. I believe that the last of these explanations is correct and that for decades
the actual disease burden was carefully hidden from public scrutiny.

Silicosis is not easy to diagnose, especially in its early stages. As early as 1920
it was recognized that X-rays alone are an unreliable guide to diagnosis: they are
even less reliable for assessing disability. A proper diagnosis requires an X-ray and
a careful medical examination augmented by the taking of full medical and work
histories. All gold miners were required to undergo pre-employment and periodic
medicals. White miners were assessed by interns at the Silicosis Bureau. Black
miners were examined either at the Chamber's recruitment depot in Johannesburg
or at individual mines. The Bureau interns were obliged to conduct an X-ray
examination of each miner and complete a Form A, which entailed a detailed
medical and work history. Because of the volume of work, such details were rarely
recorded. In 1951, for example, the Bureau carried out 54,772 medicals or 5,472
examinations per intern.[30] Allowing for an hour-long daily meeting to adjudi-
cate on compensation claims and other duties required each intern to examine
on average five patients an hour. At most, the twelve minutes allowed for each
examination were never adequate to identify silicosis among white miners. That
tendency to under-diagnose and therefore under-compensate disease is borne

out by the repeated protests from the MWU. The process was even less rigorous with blacks, with as many as a hundred men being examined by a mine medical officer in a single hour. No details of work or medical histories were taken. It is not surprising that much of the disease burden was missed.

The Chamber of Mines, along with the Departments of Health and Mines in Pretoria, enjoyed a monopoly over the disease data. In the period from 1930 until the 1990s the Chamber made no attempt to monitor the health of black miners once they had left the industry nor did it commission independent research. Once migrant workers left the mines they disappeared.

Migrant workers were viewed as temporary employees who worked for short periods then returned home to rural areas to recuperate. According to employers their very low rates of silicosis were due to their periodic employment on short-term contracts. The lack of biomedical care in rural South Africa and in the labor-sending states of Lesotho, Swaziland, and Mozambique further obscured the incidence of silicosis. Underfunded and under-resourced health systems were at their worst in dealing with a chronic disease for which there is no easy diagnosis and no treatment.

A third contributing factor was the lack of independent medical research. In the first decades of the twentieth century, South African scientists, including I. G. Irving, A. Sutherland Strachan, F. W. Simson, W. Watkins Pitchford, A. Mavrogordato, Spencer Lister, and A. J. Orenstein, largely defined the research and regulatory agendas on silicosis. The research community in Johannesburg to which they belonged was close-knit and scientists were employed either by the state or the mining houses. That tended to blur the boundaries between employers and the state. The major research center, the South African Institute of Medical Research (SAIMR), founded in 1912, was jointly funded by the mining industry and government.[31] The leading research center in the United States, Saranac Laboratories, was also funded by industry. There was no employment for researchers outside of the Chamber or the state, and it was the Chamber that largely set the research agenda and decided upon the models of data collection. Under minority rule, the state was reluctant to give researchers access to labor-sending communities. When Marianne Felix from the National Institute of Occupational Health began pioneering work among asbestos miners at Mafefe in the late 1980s, she encountered resistance from the Departments of Health and Mines.[32] The same happened five years later when Anna Trapido began work on silicosis in the Eastern Cape

Perhaps the most important factor that hid the disease burden was the potential cost of compensation. The legislation of 1912 saw South Africa become the first state to recognize silicosis as a compensable disease. Initially, compensation was paid from a levy based on the number of men employed at each registered mine. Levies were set according to an estimate of dust levels. Sampling was done by the Chamber of Mines or the Government Mining Engineer each three years and an index was calculated using a complex formula. From that index a levy was imposed per ton of ore extracted. By 1925, more than one hundred thousand dust samples were being taken annually and it is likely that more dust samples were collected on the Rand than in the rest of the world.[33] Those samples were expensive to collect and yet the Chamber did not publish any studies from that data. Benefits were based on wage levels, and so white miners received more generous compensation than did blacks.[34, 35] In addition, black miners were migrant workers and few were aware of their rights.

In the three years to July 1916, the total compensation for whites was thirty times greater than that paid to black mine workers.[36] Over the period from 1912 to 1946, fifteen further silicosis acts were passed, most of which improved the benefits paid to white labor. The MWU, founded in 1913, was so effective in promoting the interests of its members that each commission increased the compensation levels.[37] No effort was made by the South African parliament or by the Chamber to reduce the barriers facing African claimants. And there were no parallel commissions into viral pneumonia or meningitis, which probably killed as many black miners as did silicosis. Since the 1930s, employers had argued that compensation for white miners was forcing marginal mines to close and compromised the profitability of the industry as a whole. It is certain that if all black miners with silicosis had been compensated it would have had a profound impact upon the industry's viability.

The challenges posed to employers by silicosis in South Africa have been very different from those found in the United States. Silicosis in the United States has been spread over a range of industries including glass, steel, and iron foundries, located in dozens of states and involving thousands of individual employers. By the late 1930s, all dusty industries that used sand faced the same problems of lung disease and litigation. In New York State, over $30 million in silicosis lawsuits were filed in 1933 against the foundry industry.[38] Employers quickly resolved the crisis to their advantage by having the issues of risk and compensation referred back to regional legislatures.[39] In South Africa, silicosis has been a disease of gold miners. So long as the price of gold was fixed, the only way employers could improve profitability was to reduce production overheads. The most important of those costs were wages. Francis Wilson has shown that the Chamber was so successful in controlling the price of labor in real terms that wages for black miners did not rise from 1910 to 1970.[40] In addition to wages, compensation was one of the few avenues where costs could be controlled.

The extent to which the issue of compensation was politicized can be seen by the number of factors which should have made the disease burden obvious. The Weldon (1902) and Haldane (1904) commissions into the fate of Cornish miners offered employers a model for monitoring the health of labor drawn from outside South Africa's borders. In addition, the unparalleled levels of medical surveillance and state regulation should have made the disease burden apparent. At their peak the Rand mines employed over five hundred thouand men. This meant silicosis may well have been a factor in the declining economies of the Reserves into which most of the black population was driven. That decline was well documented by the 1943 Commission into African Wages.[41] There was also the research community in Johannesburg, which until 1940 was one of the best in the world. There were plenty of skilled scientists to monitor the health of migrant labor if only the Chamber had been willing to commission such research. Perhaps the most important factor was the synergy between silicosis and tuberculosis. Pulmonary tuberculosis is easy to diagnose. It is also highly infectious, particularly when brought into communities with little previous exposure. The impact of imported tuberculosis was felt in Malawi and Swaziland from the 1920s.[42] That drew protests from colonial administrations that the Chamber was repatriating infected men without notifying regional health authorities. Those practices continue to the present day.[43]

CONCLUSION

The history of silicosis in South Africa is riven with paradoxes. The Rand mines were the first in the world to invest heavily in dust extraction technologies and instruments, such as the konometer, to measure risk. Yet, as the current data suggest, those mines have remained among the most dangerous in the world. South Africa was the first state to compensate silicosis (1912) and tuberculosis (1916), yet benefits went principally to white miners who represented less than 10 percent of the workforce. South Africa's mines were the first to use X-ray screening (1912), which soon became the basis for diagnosis and compensation in Australia, North America, and Western Europe. And yet it appears that South Africa was less successful than Australia or the United States in reducing risk or in providing adequate compensation. The major paradox is between the intense public debates about silicosis and the invisibility of the disease burden. In addition to the more than twenty commissions, there were a dozen select committees into silicosis. And yet the more the Department of Mines and the Chamber talked about silicosis and the more data they collected, the less the disease burden was visible.

The stories of asbestos and silicosis litigation in South Africa share much common ground. They are connected by the careers of the leading medical researchers such as Ian Webster and J. C. Wagner, who is generally credited with having discovered the link between asbestos and mesothelioma. From the 1930s, researchers in the United Kingdom, the United States, and South Africa tended to work on both silicosis and asbestosis. Silicosis and asbestos disease are also connected by US corporations, such as Johns Manville and Union Carbide, which over a period of decades have faced litigation from employees suffering from those diseases. Within South Africa, the connections are more intimate. The legal settlements against the asbestos companies Cape plc and Gencor in 2003 and the current Anglo American cases have involved the same lawyers: Richard Meeran and Richard Spoor. Meeran has remarked on the parallels: "The chronology of the hazard is also very similar. In this case, the mines and the government had specific knowledge of the dangers of dust and the fact that it caused silicosis. While the asbestos issue was subjected to litigation for years—since the 1960s— the gold mining industry has managed to escape justice."[44,45] The two cases have also involved the asbestos mining company Charter Consolidated. Charter was an Anglo American subsidiary, which gave the parent company an immediate stake in the claims for compensation being made by asbestos miners.

There are also parallels with the global scandals over asbestos disease and the pandemic of asthma and bronchitis among British coal miners. In both instances, recognition of occupational injury and the awarding of compensation took decades to achieve.[46–48] In South Africa the labor markets, the economic importance of gold mining, and the political environment have made recognition even more difficult.

Minority ruled South Africa was probably the ideal setting in which to hide a pandemic of occupational disease. The majority of the workforce was denied civil liberties, including the right to trade union representation. There was a racialized political culture, which after 1948 was ruthlessly enforced. A migrant labor system allowed the costs of injury in the workplace to be externalized and thereby in effect made invisible. Finally, before 1994 there was no politically independent research community to challenge the fictions about low disease rates promoted by employers.

Chapter 22

COMMUNITY EPIDEMIOLOGY[1]

Andrew Watterson

If you give a man a fish he is hungry again in an hour; if you teach him to catch a fish you do him a good turn.[2]

When an incident involving toxic chemicals, biohazards, or illness relating to other environmental factors occurs in any community, it is important at the outset for those who think they may have been exposed to record their experiences, what they have been exposed to, under what circumstances, at what levels, and with what adverse effects. Even though this should be publicly available information, it may be unavailable or difficult for victims to obtain. The problems of investigating chemical exposures and the nature of the current system for generating and evaluating information about toxins has led to a crisis of public confidence in a number of cases.[3]

The process whereby environmental pollution investigations have been communicated by professionals to communities has also often been flawed, as with the Camelford aluminium sulphate water pollution case in the United Kingdom and many others. Finding out about which pesticide or other toxins have affected you or may affect you in the future, how much, and in what form, is vital information that should be immediately available to the affected public.

Such information and such studies may provide essential evidence for a clinical diagnosis of your individual problem and also help with an understanding of any collective "poisoning." It may also be of use to check whether there are long-term and possibly chronic effects from any exposure. Studies of these long-term effects are called epidemiological studies. Illness (morbidity) and death (mortality) are investigated, where possible, for small or large populations.

Lay epidemiology has been defined as "the process by which laypersons gather statistics and other information and also direct and marshal the knowledge and resources of experts in order to understand the epidemiology of disease."[4]

The premise underlying this kind of epidemiology is that not only are the populations, be they occupational or residential, more in touch with the lives of the community than are outside professionals, only rarely are they attached to corporate interests.

Community, lay worker epidemiology may provide a better way forward for employees and those in communities, than that carried out by professional epidemiologists. Investigations of hazards and their spread might also be carried out in conjunction with sympathetic professionals.[5]

This approach is proving increasingly effective among employees in workplaces.[6] For example, in the United States, lay investigations of childhood leukemia clusters near a chemical plant at Woburn, Massachusetts, were carried out.[7] The plant produced pesticides and other chemicals. Professional epidemiologists and lay people involved in the investigations had different views on collecting, interpreting and using data.[8]

PROBLEMS WITH CONVENTIONAL EPIDEMIOLOGY FOR PESTICIDES

The professional epidemiologists tend to look only at data they think "scientific" while discarding other forms of data collected by communities; they use only traditional methods of analysis and discount less orthodox methods; they rely on "statistical significance" as the key guide to results while ignoring data that was clearly significant but not statistically so.

Epidemiology explores the occurrence and distribution of diseases and deaths in populations: the populations may be very large or small, and based on small areas. The larger the populations studied, the greater the weight often given to results because of their statistical significance. However, large studies may also dilute the effects of exposures on a small group and fail to show a serious adverse effect on a small group (or cluster) of workers or a small population. Epidemiology shows correlations between various factors. It does not show causes of disease for individuals. This is why in pesticide health and safety, toxicology, and occupational hygiene are the key preventative scientific disciplines. Epidemiology checks that the other disciplines are right and working.

There have been enormous problems with epidemiology. Perhaps the most alarming and detrimental to any scientific process is that many professional epidemiologists work in cooperation with corporations which are held by the community to be responsible for the problem. Some epidemiologists work with statistical information analyzed and bundled up by the companies and it is the companies rather than the "affected" or their representatives who chose the interviewees.

Particularly this is relating to the difficulty of getting good data to assess what exposures people may have had to toxic agents and good data on what specific illnesses they have contracted. Sometimes exposure data may not exist and sometimes the medical and scientific professions may not be able to diagnose certain effects of exposure to such things as pesticides or may disagree about the effective measures and indicators of exposure.

Sometimes there may be confounding factors in studies that will mean results are not useful: for instance tobacco smoking, gender, and age are obvious confounders, as might be occupation. Epidemiological studies will attempt to allow for such effects and where necessary adjust figures of diseases and deaths accordingly.

There may also be problems with identifying a control group with which to compare the exposed populations. This has happened frequently with epidemiological studies of people exposed to pesticides where finding a control group with no or limited exposure may be difficult. This is because most people almost anywhere in the world will have some exposure to pesticides through water, food, or atmosphere. Recent studies of sheep dipping also ran into problems when trying to identify non-exposed rural workers as a control group.

Other problems come from what have been termed "negative epidemiological studies." "Negative" epidemiology or rather "non-positive studies" in this context mean the presentation of results as evidence that no risks exist from a potential hazard when the studies are not large and not sensitive enough to be more than inconclusive and limited.[9] This relates to the problem of studies that are unable to show whether a correlation exists or not, because of methodological problems or small populations or whatever.

Negative epidemiological studies have sometimes been used to argue that pesticides and other environmental hazards are not hazards to the public at all. Yet, these studies cannot demonstrate either effects or non-effects and they demonstrate the truism that: the absence of evidence is not evidence of absence. The need to involve workforces in workplace health research has been widely acknowledged,[10] but good practice in the field is still lacking. Such an approach would ensure that epidemiology is located in the community and workplace in ways that have rarely happened in the recent past: to the detriment of both community and epidemiology.[11]

The approach would involve the public or specific communities in an important educational and information process and help them identify serious hazards and risks rather than spurious ones. The very process of involvement would ensure that there was greater public confidence in both studies and results than has hitherto been the case.

A related problem can sometimes occur later in the process when "the affected" make civil claims against companies in court cases. Such court cases rely in the main on the testimony of "expert" witnesses. There have been occasions in recent years where experts for claimants have been denigrated in the public media and where experts brought before the defense might not be who they appear. The courts need to be "opened" in such cases, so as to give "the affected" a much stronger voice.

COMMUNITY EPIDEMIOLOGY NECESSITIES AND PROBLEMS

Lay or community-based occupational and environmental epidemiology should be "participative, non-expert; subjective; and collective in nature."[12]

Epidemiologists should be prepared, in some instances, to work for, rather than on, communities. Effectively, epidemiologists should help communities do their own epidemiology.[13] This type of approach, sometimes called "participatory research," involves the public, the worker, input into the research questions to be asked, accessibility of the results and their implications to groups affected by exposures, the means whereby data may be more than statistical, and experiences and subjective symptoms all play a part in the analysis.[14]

The approach is not without its problems, including methodological ones—the political issues of the status of professionals; the resistance of professional scientists to share with the lay public both methods and results. While basic factors like lack of funds can end lay research before it even gets off the ground, the concerns of the State and large corporation to control or restrict access to their data can be a stumbling block.

Nevertheless, community or lay epidemiology is still worth pursuing and has been successful in Scandinavia, even in parts of the United Kingdom and in the United States. The WHO European Charter on Environment and Health lays down a baseline for community and workplace action, stating that: every individual is entitled to information and consultation on the current state of the environment and plans, decisions, and activities that will affect the environment and health; the strategic need to consult and involve individuals and communities in managing their environment through, for instance, environmental health impact assessments; and finally, the strategic need to encourage and strengthen national and international programs in health education and information for the public on health and the environment.[15]

WHAT YOU NEED TO KNOW FOR LAY OR COMMUNITY EPIDEMIOLOGY

The rights of citizens and workers to know about the hazards they have been or may be exposed to and the risks following from those hazards should be fundamental in any democratic society. The right may create problems relating to doubt and worry about future health risks, but workers should be informed about hazards affecting them.[16]

There is also the problem of the extent to which epidemiology has been interpreted negatively on the basis of restricted data. Workplace and environmental health problems have been neglected by some scientists and/or ignored by governments.

Lay people getting involved in community epidemiology need to start with a checklist of important facts upon which they can build. They need to note the names of pesticides being used and have the data sheets that apply to them. They need to know who manufactured or formulated them and what solvents and adjuvants the toxins were used with. Such research has to be combined with information about previous problems or history of health adverse effects for the specific chemicals.

The application of toxins like pesticides is important. How were the pesticides applied or released? If applied, with what sort of sprayers, foggers, granules, or applicators? What was the condition of the applicators? What amounts were used? If released accidentally, in what form were the pesticides when released? How much was released? Where did the released pesticides initially go (atmosphere, soil, or water)?

Clearly, companies and employers might well be obstructive to these inquiries but pressure might be brought on them by the court or simply by inquiries made by lawyers. Other information might be found from public bodies—what were the weather conditions at the time of exposure: windy, wet, warm, cold, etc. What was the prevailing direction of wind, if drift was likely, or the direction of the stream or current if in lake or sea?

Several years ago, the International Federation of Plantation and Agricultural Workers mooted the idea of a pesticide passport to be held by every agricultural worker listing the type, date, amount, and exposure of that worker to pesticides. This has finally been recognized by professional epidemiologists as a useful means to study exposures to pesticides and their effects. Communities should adopt a similar idea with either "a Community Pollution Passport" or passports for individuals in a community. The sort of information listed above should all be included on such a passport.

Some of the most important information will come from interviews by those affected by the toxins. With lay epidemiology—because it is not simply general statistical information that is needed, such as where and how the person works, sleep, or eats—long and quite detailed interviews might take place, with interviewers having the confidence of the interviewee. Simple things may be noted that might otherwise be missed by a statistical approach, for example the record of affected pets in relation to domestic toxins.

HOW TO START A LAY, WORKER, OR COMMUNITY EPIDEMIOLOGY STUDY

Those wanting to become involved in community epidemiology should collect as much data as possible about the incident they have been involved in. Discuss the case with sympathetic professionals who will support in principle the idea of a lay epidemiological study. In the beginning, cast the net as widely as possible; you never know when these professionals, scientists, or lawmakers might become useful in any campaign.

Speak to GPs, environmental health officers, local councilors, MPs and MEPs, and local lawyers. It is important that at the beginning of any study you do not draw the boundaries of the work too tightly around those affected. A visit to the local hospital casualty ward and a chat with doctors on duty could uncover cases. This might also be the case with all kinds of local professionals such as infant school teachers, practice nurses, health visitors, district nurses, and school nurses.

As the structure of a possible study begins to take shape, follow through with those people you think may have been exposed to pesticides. Try to get the people who have been exposed, or representatives that they wish to attend for them, involved in drawing up the design of the study (the protocol). Try to make sure that those exposed are involved in any steering group looking at the effects of the exposure over a period of time. Try to negotiate the involvement of independent experts of your choosing to look at the protocol and also to receive data not confidential as the study progresses. These steps will ensure public confidence in the outcome of any study and will automatically ensure good communications between public and experts throughout the study.

Try, at the earliest possible opportunity to get biological measurements of any toxins the group may have been exposed to. Ensure copies of records are available to individuals who have been so monitored.

POSITIVE CONCLUSIONS

This "community" approach has been adopted on several occasions by powerful national organizations—commercial, industrial, and governmental—in support of policies that may damage or at the least provide no indication of benefit to the public health.

The tobacco and the asbestos industries have been notable in the past for selecting, excluding, or suppressing epidemiological and toxicological data so that the health hazards attached to their industries or products have been neglected or distorted. "Any people exposed to a small risk may generate a large total of cases, albeit with no conspicuous risk to any one person or group."[17]

The tendency of some epidemiologists and medical practitioners in the past to ignore or minimize low-level environmental health risks to large populations from such things as pesticides may be corrected partly by the adoption of lay epidemiology. In the United States, lay epidemiology has shown greater concern about such low-level risks than some professional epidemiologists.[18]

The public is often unimpressed by epidemiological analyses that reduce the impact of hazards on individuals to very low statistical risks when perceptions of risk vary so much. Lay epidemiology could, therefore, have an important role to play in monitoring "non-positive epidemiological studies," flagging up concerns and worries about hazards, which could be investigated at an early stage, possibly to be discounted or put in context as insignificant risks at a later date. This will help to ensure firstly that the possibilities of low-level exposures leading to unforeseen ill health are not forgotten by professionals and secondly that public panics about health fears are reduced when public and professional groups together find them to be unfounded.[19]

Chapter 23

DOWNPLAYING
RADIATION RISK

Nicola Wright

On the 31st of May 2011, the WHO/the International Agency for Research on Cancer (IARC) classified radiofrequency electromagnetic fields as possibly carcinogenic to humans based on an increased risk for glioma, a malignant type of brain cancer, associated with wireless phone use.

(WHO press Release no 208, 31 May 2011)[1]

The United Nations' authority on public health categorized mobile phone frequencies as "possibly carcinogenic" and published that warning. So mobile phone and other wireless signals are now in the same category as lead and DDT.

For some people, it came as a shocking surprise that a technology so central to everyday life suddenly has a powerful official health warning attached to it. For others, those scientists, researchers, and victims who, for so long, had been fighting to warn the public about the health dangers implicit in this technology, this categorization came as a real breakthrough.

But for most people, this information passed by unnoticed. It wasn't something that many consumers of this technology wanted to hear anyway, or those in the mobile phone industry wanted heard.

The warnings however had been there for a long time. Dr. Gerald Hyland expressed it in 2000 as follows:

If mobile phones were a type of food, they simply would not be licensed because there is so much uncertainty surrounding their safety.[2]

The average mobile phone user would be surprised to hear this from a leading UK professor emeritus of biophysics. Surely there are structures and processes in place to ensure that new inventions are safe before they enter the market? And why have we heard so little in the media from eminent professors such as this one?

Barrie Trower, a physicist and ex-government advisor on microwave radiation said:

> The (UK) Government, the (mobile phone) Industry, and government scientists will be responsible for more deaths of civilians in peace time than all the terrorist organizations ever.[3]

The implied complicity between the government, mobile phone industry, and "soft" government scientists hiding the truth on the dangers of this technology might also be a surprise to the consumer. But how has this come about?

In this chapter we are going to look at how the telecommunications industry has taken control of the institutions that set exposure guidelines, those that research the health effects of exposure to microwaves, and those that disseminate information to the public.

THE SCIENCE OF MICROWAVE RADIATION

Firstly though, we need to be clear about what makes this technology unhealthy and what symptoms can occur when humans are exposed to it.

Importantly, electromagnetic microwave radiation used to transmit data is not only used in mobile phones. It's also used in Wi-Fi systems, DECT phones (cordless home phone systems), cordless baby monitors, Wii systems, and all mobile phones, laptops, and other handheld devices that can connect remotely such as PlayStation and XBox. Of course these signals are networked via mobile phone masts and digital TV and TETRA transmitters that span the country.

Microwaves are part of the electromagnetic spectrum. Lower down than microwaves on the spectrum are radio waves. Higher up on the spectrum at a higher frequency we have light, X-rays, and gamma rays. Their frequency is inversely proportional to the wavelength and they travel at the speed of light. Microwaves transmitted by mobile phones are often called "radio waves" by those attempting to downplay the danger that they pose. This is because they know that the public look upon radio waves as "safe" but are less certain about microwaves because of the microwave oven, which does use the same frequency as Wi-Fi.

The microwaves act as a "carrier wave" along which data (voice, text, pictures, etc.) is sent in bundles by modifying the amplitude, frequency, or phase, depending on the system. This results in an effective low-frequency "pulse" that is unfortunately close to the low frequency electrical signals used by our bodies' biological communication system, heart rhythm, and brain waves.

Taking some of the technologies in turn—firstly mobile phone masts. The antennae transmit a microwave radiation signal all the time. Eighty percent of the radiation is contained in the "main beam" and covers up to 500 meters for a 15 meter high mast.

Secondly, digital (DECT) cordless phones. These also emit all the time from the main base, even when not in use. The levels from a cordless phone system measured inside a house are of the same order of magnitude as those measured in the main beam of a mast coming in from outside. The more powerful mast is obviously further away and so the signal drops off as it enters the house; the cordless phone base station is transmitting from within the house.

Thirdly, Wi-Fi routers. These are also in the middle of the living space and generally never turned off. They emit levels similar to a cordless phone. If a neighboring house also has a "BT Home Hub" Wi-Fi router (and cordless phone), the effect is compounded. One only has to look at the available networks on a computer to see how many signals one is being exposed to from other networks in a city environment.

Then, in order for the signals to travel long distance between cities and into the countryside, there is also the more powerful system called WIMAX, which crisscrosses the land.

So, from various sources, a large number of microwave pulsed signals are continually passing through our bodies, all subtly different as they perform different "wireless" tasks. The result is that the everyday background radiation is now a trillion times what it was fifteen years ago. We are, however, told not to worry since these levels of exposure are way below the ICNIRP exposure guidelines to which the United Kingdom and much of the rest of the world subscribe.[4] The government uses the guidelines to assure the public that this technology is safe, irrespective of whether it has been tested or not.

The question is, are they safe and how did ICNIRP come up with those guidelines? The rather frightening answer is that the guidelines are set to prevent the heating-up of human tissue over a six-minute period. They are not intended to protect against long-term exposure and do not take cumulative effects into account. And so this is the nub of the industry and government arguments when presented with cancer clusters around phone masts or children with migraines in schools with Wi-Fi transmitters. "It's below the ICNIRP guidelines so there can't be any effect."

Some countries have their own health protection agencies and have slightly varied minimum guidelines. But on the whole, most take advice and collaborate with the World Health Organization (WHO), who has played a large part in setting standards with ICNIRP.

ICNIRP—THE RADIATION GUIDELINES

ICNIRP, or the International Commission on Non-Ionizing Radiation Protection, was formed in 1992 by a group of mainly self-appointed engineers.

It says it is a body of independent scientific experts and was constituted in Germany as a non-profit organization. It aims to disseminate information and advice on the potential health hazards of exposure to non-ionizing radiation. ICNIRP carries out scientific reviews and, in collaboration with the WHO, risk assessments resulting in exposure guidelines. It consults with many other organizations including the Institute of Electrical and Electronics Engineers, IEEE.

The ICNIRP guidelines allow for exposures of up to 61 V/m (or 10 W/m^2). However, in scientific studies, intensity levels of 0.01 V/m have been shown to cause adverse health effects. It is not known if there is such a thing as a "safe" level of exposure but current levels (that in reality only average 0.5 V/m) are still widely regarded as being unsafe by independent researchers.

It is also worth comparing the maximum exposure limits in some countries to those in Britain and the United States.[5]

Russia & China: max exposure up to 6 V/m (or 0.1 W/m^2)

Salzburg Region: max indoor exposure 0.02 V/m (or 0.0000011 W/m^2)

THE WHO

Recent actions taken by the WHO to categorize mobile phone signals as a possible carcinogen might suggest a move toward tougher guidelines in the future. However, the WHO, in its own words is merely a "coordinating authority on international public health," and in this capacity makes policy suggestions based on information offered to it. The result is that it is open to being influenced by the likes of the mobile telecommunications industry who make sure that only certain information crosses its desk.

However, the recent classification of microwave radiation as a class 2B carcinogen must have slipped under their radar, having come from a WHO linked agency called the International Agency for Research on Cancer (IARC). But no doubt it will have no effect on changing the guidelines set by ICNIRP. Too much industry influence resides there. And revealingly, in the WHO fact sheet no. 193 dated June 2011, a few paragraphs below the carcinogen warning, one can still read: "to date, no adverse health effects have been established as being caused by mobile phone use,"[6] Is this sloppy web-management, or does it show how little impact the new information is having on the "coordinating authority on public health?"

Looking back, the WHO has always stuck to the same line on electromagnetic frequencies (EMF's), declaring this in 1999:

> The main conclusion from the WHO reviews is that EMF exposures below the limits recommended in the ICNIRP international guidelines do not appear to have any known consequence on health.[7]

This was in contrast, for example to the German Federal Radiation Protection Agency who published the following in 1992 in the early days of the development of mobile technology. They clearly referred to non-thermal, biological effects of microwave radiation.[8]

> Effects which are not related to heating have been described in the scientific literature for approximately fifteen years. If a high frequency radiation is amplitude modulated with another frequency, field effects can occur, which do not exist under unmodulated radiation. These manifest mostly as changes in the permeability of the cell membranes. For example, it has been found that with high frequency radiation with a frequency of 147 MHz, which was modulated with frequencies between 6 and 20 Hz, the calcium efflux from cell cultures was significantly increased (by 10 to 20 percent) for certain frequencies. Generally, a complex dependency of these effects on intensity and frequency has been observed, showing that certain frequency windows are particularly active. These membrane effects have been replicated many times, so that their existence has become established scientific knowledge.
>
> It needs to be noted that the SAR values used in some studies were lower than 0.01 W/kg, and therefore significantly below the threshold of thermally relevant intensities.

WHO FUNDS THE WHO EMF RESEARCH PROJECT?

In 1996, The WHO set up the EMF Project to research the health effects of microwave radiation under the chairmanship of Dr. Michael Repacholi, an Australian physicist. Dr. Repacholi had performed research in 1995, when at the Royal Adelaide Hospital, that showed a doubling of lymphoma in transgenic mice exposed for one and a half years to the same microwave radiation used in the 2G phone network.[9]

The WHO EMF Project was what they term "softly funded," which meant that it was to raise funds. These were sent to the Royal Adelaide Hospital, (RAH) and then transferred on to the WHO. For many years the accounts of the RAH were not audited and Repacholi continued to deny receiving industry funding until his retirement in 2006.

In 1999, Norm Sandler, a Motorola spokesman, told the publication, *Microwave News*, "This [sending money to the RAH] is the process for all the supporters of the WHO program." At the time, Motorola was sending Repacholi $50,000 each year. That money was later bundled with other industry contributions and sent to Australia by the Mobile Manufacturers Forum (MMF), which gave the project $150,000 a year.[10]

After Repacholi left The WHO in 2006, this arrangement ceased and the WHO now state on their website; "The (WHO EMF) project is fully funded by participating countries and agencies."[11] and in the 2006 progress report they state: "Through an agreement set up in 1995 between the WHO and the Royal Adelaide Hospital (RAH) in Australia, RAH provided financial management of funds received from contributions of non-governmental entities [i.e., presumed to be Industry] on behalf of the Project. Dr. Repacholi was seconded from RAH to WHO from the time of the agreement until his retirement from WHO in June 2006. Following Dr. Repacholi's departure, the agreement was terminated in early 2007. New funding sources are now being sought."[12]

Dr. Repacholi finally admitted in 2007 that the project had been funded by industry, although he claimed that industry funding made up less than half of the total amount.[13]

Research obviously needs to be funded by those without vested interests if a clear position on guidelines and advice is to be given from an organization perceived to be acting in the public interest such as the WHO.

Interestingly as is the case with so many of these committee members, Repacholi was also on the UK government committees of the MTHR and the Stewart Committee. In 2000, he was the only member of the Stewart Committee to vote against warning UK children not to use mobile phones.[14]

THE TOBACCO INDUSTRY AND THE WHO

In 2000 in Geneva, the WHO heard the results of a report into the strategies employed by the tobacco industry into undermining the WHO's scientific assessment of the effects of secondhand smoke. Information had been gathered from tobacco industry documents made available on the Internet as a result of a lawsuit found against Philip Morris in 1998.[15]

Part of the WHO's fifty-eight recommendations were the following:

> The WHO should clarify, strengthen or expand the process and rules in place
> to guard against potential conflicts of interest involving the tobacco industry.

Additional safeguards should be put in place to protect against tobacco company attempts to distort scientific research sponsored by, or associated with, WHO and affiliated organizations.[16]

It seems that the WHO has not been able to apply these lessons to the phone industry. Moreover they are working in partnership with the industry. One can see how pleased the industry is with the WHO by looking at Vodafone's 2001 CSR report, which confidently points to all the WHO's findings and recommendations on EMF research! They state on p11[17] "Vodafone also provides funding to the WHO International EMF Project." This, despite the fact that the industry is not supposed to fund the project!

THE PRINCIPLE OF NO-PRECAUTION

Between 1992 and 2010, the industrialized world experienced an explosion of commercial microwave technology for wireless applications. It is possible to suggest that to acknowledge the adverse sub-thermal effects of this technology simply became politically and economically impossible as the industry grew in economic and political weight.

Even as far back as 1971, an American report compiled by the Electromagnetic Radiation Management Advisory Council, an expert panel of nine scientists ordered to look at electromagnetic radiation by the President's Office of Telecommunications Policy, was published. The report: "Program for Control of Electromagnetic Pollution of the Environment," stated as follows:

Unless adequate monitoring and control based on a fundamental understanding of biological effects are instituted in the near future, in the decades ahead, man may enter an era of energy pollution of the environment comparable to the chemical pollution of today. The consequences of undervaluing or misjudging the biological effects of long-term, low level exposure could become a critical problem for the public health, especially if genetic effects are involved.[18]

Many independent scientists criticize the ICNIRP guidelines. In Dr. Neil Cherry's ICNIRP critique of 1999, he stated that the guidelines should be set initially at 0.45 v/m (0.0005 W/m^2). (ICNIRP are at 61 V/m (or 10 W/m^2). Dr. Cherry produced a more detailed critique in early 2000, in which he said the following:

For ICNIRP to concentrate on a single biological mechanism, tissue heating, is inappropriate and wrong... WHO, ICNIRP and their international and national counterparts have developed a highly sophisticated system of approaches to dismiss all epidemiological evidence and animal and cellular evidence which conflicts with their RF-Thermal view of the world. As the epidemiological and laboratory evidence has grown stronger and stronger, the dismissive methodology has lost all sophistication and, as demonstrated by ICNIRP, it is blatantly selective, reductionist, biased and scientifically dishonest" (1998).[19]

A quote from the late Professor J. R. Goldsmith, Department of Epidemiology and Health Services Evaluation, Faculty of Health Sciences, Ben-Gurion University of the Negev, illustrates this, too:

> There are strong political and economic reasons for wanting there to be no health effect of RF/MW exposure, just as there are strong public health reasons for more accurately portraying the risks. Those of us who intend to speak for public health must be ready for opposition that is nominally, but not truly, scientific.[20]

THE WHO AND THE EASTERN BLOC

In 1997, the WHO grandly developed a research agenda with the stated intention of incorporating work from laboratories around the world.

But research going back eighty years on the effects of microwave radiation, and literally thousands of studies showing adverse health effects to non-thermal levels in the current telecommunication environment were not taken into account.

In the Eastern bloc, the a-thermal biological effects of microwaves have been extensively researched and acknowledged. Effects on the central nervous system, on the electrolyte balance in the body, on DNA structure, on the cardiovascular system, on metabolism, and on circadian rhythms are well understood.

To this day, Russia has refused to sign up to the ICNIRP guidelines for obvious reasons despite tremendous pressure by the WHO and other international bodies who want to "*harmonize* legislation."[21]

The current Russian guidelines are lower than ICNIRP's recommendations in power flux density terms by a factor of 100. They acknowledge the higher damage potential of pulsed radiation and therefore set stricter limits for exposure to pulsed radiation than for non-pulsed. They also acknowledge the cumulative effect (duration of exposure) and reflect the special sensitivity of children and pregnant women.[22]

Russia's precautionary approach extended beyond this, too. In the ex-USSR, every worker occupationally exposed to electromagnetic fields had to undergo yearly health examinations, specifically geared to detect the potential damage linked with this type of exposure. The diagnostics included all normal clinical symptoms, but also neurophysiological and neurological symptoms as well as depression. Based upon this very large pool of data, a large body of epidemiological and occupational long-term studies were conducted, some covering periods as long as twenty years.

There is no comparable body of knowledge anywhere in the West, where research focuses on short-term effects. Germany did review the Russian data though in 1996, led by Professor emeritus Dr. Med. Karl Hecht and Dr. Balzer at the behest of the German Federal Office for Telecommunication, (The German regulatory equivalent of OFCOM in the UK).

Hecht and Balzer reviewed the Russian literature that began in 1960, looking at the effects of electromagnetic frequencies on human health. Of the 1,500 studies pre-selected for the review, 878 met the criteria to be included. This has become the most extensive review of long-term epidemiological and occupational studies ever on the subject.[23]

The highest incidence of long-term effects found were as follows:

- Neurasthenia (a condition characterized long-term effects by chronic fatigue, dizziness, headaches, anxiety, depression)
- EEG changes (disruption of alpha rhythm in the brain)
- Sleep disturbance
- Blood pressure variations
- Heart arrhythmia
- Other cardio-vascular conditions
- Hyperthyroidism
- Impotence
- Digestive Problems
- Hair loss
- Tinnitus
- Higher susceptibility to infections

This list of conditions is identical to the more current list of symptoms published by various International Doctors' Appeals[24] and is also identical to the symptoms described by people who are suffering from electro-hypersensitivity. In their research contract, the German Federal Office for Telecommunication committed to publishing and publicizing the review, but unsurprisingly this never happened.

The WHO Research Agenda for Radiofrequency Fields in 2006 stated in its "mission statement" that research in this field should ideally cover:[25]

Large-scale studies of subjects with high occupational RF exposure, including cohort studies as well as the use of the RF occupational exposure data within large scale case-control studies. Rationale: Workers exposed to RF fields in some occupations receive high exposure levels (often to large areas of the body, and sometimes exceeding ICNIRP guidelines). Thus, these populations may be well suited to assess whether a health impact of RF exposure exists.

Oddly though, the WHO showed no interest in the Russian Hecht and Balzer Review, which offers access to precisely this type of material. To this day, no funding is available to translate the Hecht and Balzer Review into English and so it is not included in the WHO's database. The UK's Health Protection Agency, HPA, and Mobile Telecommunication and Health Research Program, MTHR have been approached, but all seem disinterested in paying for a translation.

Instead, in the United Kingdom, the Stewart Report undertaken in 2000 is relied upon when referring to health and EMFs.[26]

This review of some of the scientific literature was undertaken by the specially formed Independent Expert Group on Mobile Phones, IEGMP, chaired by Sir William Stewart, who later became head of the HPA.

Dr. Repacholi was also a member of this group as was Professor Anthony Swerdlow, who was also a member of ICNIRP, chairman of the NRPB's (now the HPA) Advisory Group on non-ionizing radiation, AGNIR,[27] and head of epidemiology at the UK's Institute of Cancer Research He also led the Breakthough Breast Cancer study on the causes of breast cancer.

The Stewart Report concluded:

1.16 Despite public concern . . . rather little research specifically relevant to these emissions has been published in the peer-reviewed public literature.
1.17 The balance of evidence to date suggests that exposures to RF radiation below . . . do not cause adverse health effects to the general population.

However it did go on to concede the following:

1.18 . . . there is now scientific evidence . . . which suggests that there may be biological effects occurring at exposure below the(se) guidelines.
1.42 We recommend, in relation to macrocell base stations sited within school grounds that the beam of greatest intensity should not fall on any part of the school grounds or buildings without agreement from the school and parents. Similar considerations should apply to macrocell base stations sited near to school grounds.

What became known as the "precautionary approach" was recommended in the light of this, but there is no evidence of anything changing at all on the side of government policy or exposure guidelines.

CRITICISM OF THE STEWART REPORT

The results of the review could have shown a lot more; it was claimed by many critics. Although the report did concede to the existence of biological effects from microwaves, the *Observer* newspaper reported that vital research was kept from Stewart's committee by the National Radiological Protection Board, NRPB.[28]

The research, on one thousand school children in Latvia,[29] was significant because the subjects had been exposed to pulsed microwave signals, whereas nearly all the other research that IEGMP reviewed was of the effects of exposure from continuous waves. The children aged nine to eighteen suffered impaired memory and attention span among other effects. (The exposure strength was the same as received by mobile phone masts and school Wi-Fi networks.) There is no other research on effects on children, despite that they are all exposed daily to Wi-Fi in their schools!

Independent scientist, Roger Coghill, also a member of the Stewart Committee at the time, went further in criticizing the whole premise of the Stewart Report:[30]

> The entire NRPB Consultation document is presumptively based on a serious logical flaw. The present guidelines, standards and limits being adopted in the West are based on bad science, and influenced by commercial not biological considerations....

Another independent scientist who has been committed to this area of work, Professor Henshaw, Bristol University, pointed out further shortfalls in his subsequent critique HPA-RPD (formerly NRPB), called the Report of an Independent Advisory Group on Non-ionizing Radiation(AGNIR): Power Frequency Electromagnetic Fields, Melatonin and the Risk of Breast Cancer. June 2006:[31]

> Overall, the substantial evidence supporting the hypothesis that exposure to power frequency EMFs affects melatonin levels or the risk of breast cancer is not brought out (in the report) ...

Ex-government physicist Barrie Trower mentioned here earlier was commissioned by the Police Federation to write a report on TETRA[32] in 2001. He criticized the fact that virtually none of the NRPB's reports are peer reviewed and that evidence was supplied to them by what he felt was a dubious source—by a senior consultant to Orange, Dr. Camelia Gabriel.

Gabriel is a director of MCL Technology Ltd, MCL, and advises the Home Office and the Health & Safety Executive, while being chairman of the European Standardization Body. Dr. Gabriel has jointly authored the Orange Base Stations Health & Safety Manual and her son, Sami, also of MCL's sister company Sartest Limited, confirms the safety of transmitters for Orange plc in school playgrounds. Dr. Gabriel is also on the Biological Effects Policy Advisory Group (BEPAG) of the Institution of Engineering and Technology, IET (formerly IEE).[33]

THE ECOLOG REPORT FOR T-MOBIL

While the Stewart Report was being debated in the United Kingdom, T-Mobil in Germany in 1999 commissioned exhaustive research into the health effects of mobile technology by the highly respected independent research institute in Hannover, The Ecolog Institute.[34]

The resulting study reviewed more than 220 peer-reviewed and published research papers and "found clear evidence for" the following:

- "the cancer initiating and cancer promoting effects of high frequency electromagnetic fields used by mobile telephone technology."
- ". . . genotoxic effects of these fields, like single- and double-strand DNA breaks and damage to chromosomes."
- "carcinogenic effects" leading to "influence cell transformation, cell growth promotion and cell communication"
- "teratogenic effects and loss of fertility, in animal studies"
- "loss of memory and cognitive function. . ."
- "disruptions of the endocrine and the immune system"
- "increased production of stress hormones" leading to "a reduction of the concentration of the hormone melatonin in the blood."

It was plain to see that the Ecolog Report for T-Mobile came to dramatically different conclusions as compared with the Stewart Report. The extended list of evidence for health effects paints a very different picture. The Stewart Report said there "may" be biological health effects and recommended "caution." The Ecolog Report called for an "immediate downward regulation of the power flux density that should be allowed by the guidelines, by a factor of 1,000."

The results of the Ecolog Report were shocking and revealing, and obviously not what the commissioning body, T-Mobil, wanted to hear. Unfortunately, too, for T- Mobil, the details of the study became known prior to them being able to have any control over the information released. In an attempt to defuse the impact, T-Mobil commissioned three smaller studies. Dr. H. Peter Neitzke, one of the Ecolog scientists explained that T-Mobil broke the original agreement with regards to the procedure and commissioned further experts from whom no critical results or recommendations were to be expected.

After T-Mobile successfully deflected the initial impact of the study, the report was kept quiet for nearly five years until a whistle-blower leaked the document to the United Kingdom. With the authorization of the Ecolog Institute, the study was translated into English and a copy of the summary was sent to the then British Office of the Deputy Prime Minister, ODPM. The reply was dismissive of the findings, using the argument that:

> . . . in this very contentious field, too much weight shouldn't be put on a review led by one person. This subject has, as you know, been reviewed by other groups of scientists. . . . who came to somewhat different conclusions. (Referring to the Stewart Report findings).

Ecolog's Dr. H. Peter Neitzke said it certainly was not a review conducted by just one person:

> This study was produced by a team of scientists, consisting of Dr. Kerstin Hennes (veterinary medicine), Dr. Hartmut Voigt (biophysics), Dr. Gisa Kahle-Anders (biology), and myself.[35]

In April 2007, the story was published in the *Sunday Times* newspaper. However, only a few copies carried the full story. One can only presume that overnight someone thought better of it and made sure that further editions reduced the story to a few lines in the margin.[36]

DR. CARLO AND WTR

Trouble for the mobile telecommunications industry had begun early in the United States. In 1993, a very public lawsuit took place in Florida filed by a businessman called David Reynard whose wife had died of a brain tumor. Their surgeon claimed on *Larry King Live* that the tumor was right where the radiation from the phone would have impacted.[37]

The media researched the industry's claims of safety and found that all the research they had quoted was to do with microwave ovens and not applicable to mobile phones. The lawsuit nonetheless was dismissed for "lack of valid scientific evidence." But as with many such lawsuits that passed through the US courts, the effect was for congress to put pressure on the mobile telecommunications industry to set up the Wireless Technology Research (WTR) program at a cost of $28.5 million USD.

The program ran over five and a half years and was comprised of fifty-six studies, including in vivo and in vitro studies, provocation studies, and epidemiological studies. It was supervised independently by the Harvard School of Public Health, with several layers of peer review built in.

The program was chaired by Dr. George Carlo, a public health scientist, epidemiologist, and lawyer. He had successfully represented other industries in litigious situations. The eventual findings were so surprising to Dr. Carlo that he reported to have had certain experiments replicated before trusting the results. The main findings showed the following biological effects at non-thermal levels of exposure:

- Opening of the blood-brain barrier with subsequent leakage of large albumin molecules into the brain.
- Formation of micronuclei, an indication for the triggering of cancer
- Disruption of DNA function, including negative impact on DNA repair mechanisms (found at SAR values of 0.7 W/kg, i.e. less than half of what is allowed by the ICNIRP guidelines)
- Higher cancer mortality (although people had only been using phones for circa five years)
- Significant increase of acoustic neuroma (a benign tumor of the auditory nerve) after six years of use.
- Significant correlations between the side of the head where the phone was held and the location of tumors

Dr. Carlo reported these results to the CTIA and recommended an urgent further research program, yet no follow-up ever happened.[38]

Dr. Carlo wrote a letter to the chairman and CEO of the AT&T Corporation (1999) expressing his concerns and frustration at the industry's inertia in the face of such a significant growing public health problem. His later testimony before the Energy and Environment Subcommittee of the Committee on Science, US House of Representatives, of July 15, 1998, said the same.

Dr. Carlo has subsequently written a book[39] about this experience and is lobbying for more independent research and the implementation of the precautionary principle in the United States.

In a radio interview in December 2006, Dr. Carlo claims that after he published his findings, the US insurance industry refused to give product liability insurance to the mobile operators. He explains that they are now basically self-insured, meaning that in a litigation case, any liability would have to be paid out of the company's profits.

THE CONTEMPORARY WORLD

As evidence showing the negative health effects of mobile telecommunication equipment mounts up, the industry has had to be all the more active in trying to win back public perception on its safety.

As an example, in August 2007, a collaboration between fourteen international EMF and health scientists published "The Bioinitiative Report."[40] They were all independent of industry, three being past presidents of the Bioelectromagnetics Society, which specialized in health effects from RF signals. In their report they reviewed over 2,000 studies and concluded among other things that the ICNIRP guidelines were totally inadequate to protect public health.

Unfortunately, the *Sunday Independent* was the only one of the mainstream press to mention the report.[41]

Others dismissed the report on the basis that it hadn't been formally published in a medical journal and so should not be regarded as valid. Proponents of the report argued that it had been published as individual papers which appeared in a special issue devoted to EMFs in the *Journal of Pathophysiology* published that August.[42]

Industry supporters had thus deployed their primary tactic of discrediting and ignoring the validity of the study in order to defuse its impact. The second tactic was to publish a counter-study. Twelve days later in the United Kingdom, the MTHR unexpectedly released their report.[43] This organization, MTHR—Mobile Telecommunication and Health Research Programme, is co-funded by the telecommunications industry and UK government. The MTHR report refuted any negative health effects—having looked only at short-term exposure. It was deemed to be a "rushed job" as only twenty-three of the twenty-eight studies were actually completed, Many studies concerned processes (such as dosimetry—how to take measurements), rather than looking at the actual health effects.

The MTHR Report was launched at the Science Media Centre.[44] The Science Media Centre only invited selected national media reporters to attend the announcement of the study so that few challenging questions would be asked. No one was allowed to see a copy of the full report until after the press briefing. By this time the stories had been written based on the factually misleading press release.

It is worthwhile for a second to hear about the Science Media Centre's (SMC) role in influencing public perception on mobile technology and health. On their website's "About Us"[45] page, they say they are "an independent press office for science when science hits the headlines." They say they "will provide journalists with what they need in the form and timeframe they need it when science is in the news." Among its sponsors are Vodafone, the Wi-Fi Alliance, Monsanto, and other multinationals producing harmful toxins.[46] On controversial areas of science reporting the BBC and daily papers the *Guardian*, *Times* and *Independent* appear to follow the SMC line.

Steered by the SMC, the UK news was full of the outcome of the "major" MTHR counter-report. An analysis of the papers reveals: "Odds of mobile link to cancer very low" from the *Times* Health Editor, the *Guardian* report was similar.[47] The *Telegraph* did better and interviewed Alasdair Philips, someone not put forward for interview by the SMC and a long-time researcher running the group Powerwatch. He commented on Hardell's findings of a 2.4 times increase in brain tumors.[48]

In actual fact, in some parts of the MTHR report (those parts not fed in the press release to the media) health problems relating to microwave technology were found. Professor Swerdlow of Cancer Research UK and ICNIRP and Dr. P McKinney, IET, had found an increase in glioma after ten years mobile use.[49] The MTHR reported that their own study showed no effects on cells in vivo and failed to mention the major European REFLEX project where seven countries collaborated to research on cells in vivo. They found double-strand DNA breaks and chromosome damage occurred from the radiation, effects which are an accepted mechanism for cancer.[50]

A week later on September 16, 2007, Geoff Lean at the *Sunday Independent* reported "Europe's top environmental watchdog (the European Environment Agency) is calling for immediate action to reduce exposure to radiation from Wi-Fi, mobile phones and their masts. It suggests that delay could lead to a health crisis similar to those caused by asbestos, smoking and lead in petrol."[51]

Geoff Lean had a scoop previously that year with a report on German research on bees that showed that they vanished and did not return to their hives when exposed to radiation levels similar to those from phone masts.[52] The *Sunday Independent* received more than a million hits on its website, something not achieved by any other paper. The following year, a meta-analysis by an eminent German biophysicist, Dr. Warnke in 2008 was presented at the Royal Society to a team from the WHO and HPA showing how radiation from the phone masts has greatly exacerbated colony collapse disorder. It details exactly the mechanism by which this occurs by interfering with the bees' navigation and communication as well as causing immune system damage as it does to humans and all living matter.[53]

However, the WHO and the HPA seem not to be interested in this research.

THE CORPORATE TAKEOVER OF SCIENCE

By the end of the first decade of the new century it is becoming clearer that all is not as it seems in the field of science when there are corporate interests at play.

> Our academic institutions have given up all pretense of being citadels of higher learning and disinterested enquiry into the nature of things; least of all, of being guardians of the public good. The corporate take-over of science is the greatest threat to our survival and the survival of our planet. It must be resisted and fought at every level.[54]

Scientists studying the telecommunications industry are as affected as any. The process of undermining science starts with funding research. Most studies in the United Kindgom are funded by the Mobile Telecommunications and Health Research Programme (MTHR), which is cofunded by the mobile phone industry and the government.[55] There is virtually no other research in the UK on EMF health effects.

A second problem is that research can be skewed by setting the parameters of the study in such a way as to expect to see no effects. An easy example is to do a study using exposures of an hour only. This can tell us nothing about what would happen over twenty years. Another example is the Interphone research, which is discussed in more detail below.

Prof. Lai did an analysis of 252 studies. Where they were industry funded no adverse effects were found in 81 percent of the studies. Independently funded studies showed the opposite![56]

The third most serious problem presented by skewed research is the review bias. Public health decisions are taken based on evidence provided by "official" science reviews. This means a selected panel of scientists chooses certain peer-reviewed and published studies and draws conclusion from these. The process is so controlled and managed that the outcome always favors the telecommunications industry, as evidenced by the growing vocal criticisms of independent scientists.[57]

The fourth method, as pointed out by Michael Meacher, ex-environment minister and UK Member of Parliament, "companies have learned that small investments in endowing chairs, sponsoring research programs or hiring professors for out-of-hours projects can produce disproportionate payoffs in generating reports, articles, reviews and books, which may not be in the public interest, but certainly benefit corporate bottom lines."[58]

For example Li Ka-shing, GBM, KBE, through his corporation, Hutchison Whampoa (3G) funds various university scholarship places and in 2002 a new state-of-the-art cancer research center called the Hutchison/MRC Research Centre was opened in Cambridge. It was jointly funded by the Medical Research Council and Hutchison Whampoa, who donated £5.3 million. In 2007, the Li Ka-shing Centre was completed at a cost of £50 million funded equally by Hutchison, the MRC, and Cancer Research UK. It houses the Cancer Research UK Cambridge Research Institute.[59]

Cancer Research Institutes have also been partly funded by Hutchison in Oxford, Berkeley, Toronto, Stanford, Hong Kong, Singapore, and China.[60]

Meacher told a public conference in 2005 on science, medicine, and the law that we need independent science and scientists who take the precautionary principle seriously, and called for sweeping changes in science funding and scientific advice to the government that would have ensured the protection of independent science, and hence, the public.[61]

Of course none of this has happened! Instead it seems that the same group of "experts" is on the committees of virtually all institutions charged with looking at public health.

Take Dr. McKinlay. He heads the Physical Dosimetry Department in the Radiation Protection Division of the Health Protection Agency (HPA-RPD), and is also a member of AGNIR. He was chairman of the ICNIRP until 2004 and a member of the WHO International EMF Programme Advisory Committee and on the MTHR board. He is a founder member and president of the European Society for Skin Cancer Prevention (EUROSKIN).[62]

Dr. McKinlay was brought in as an expert witness during a court case in 1998. When he was asked about his qualifications and publications, Dr. McKinlay said he had obtained his PhD *after* he had started working for the NRPB, and that his *entire* working career had been with the NRPB. None of his papers had been subject to peer review and he had not authored any experimental studies. Dr. McKinlay admitted, too, that he had no biological expertise in relation to the case.[63]

The "experts" in this field belong to a number of self-serving committees and organizations such as the Biological Effects Policy Advisory Group, BEPAG, of the Institution of Engineering and Technology, IET;[64] the Radiation Risk and Society Advisory Group, RRSAG, formerly of the NRPB;[65] the Advisory Group on Non-Ionizing Radiation (AGNIR)[66] of the HPA; and the MTHR[67]

These expert groups are inevitably linked into industry and industry initiatives, such as the Guidelines on Science and Health Communication for

438 CORPORATE TIES THAT BIND

journalists,[68] National Grid Transco, the HPA, Institute of Cancer Research,[69] and Kings College School of Psychiatry under Professor Wesseley[70] who is also on the Science Media Centre (SMC)[71] board, and formerly the NRPB's RRSAG. Prof, Wesseley's team under Rubin (now on the AGNIR) have performed research into electrical hypersensitivity. They performed provocation studies but without even screening the room from external fields for which they did not control! Perhaps they were looking for a psychological response?[72]

As well as the HPA, the WHO is also looking at "risk perception and communication." As far back as 2002, the WHO published a book on Electromagnetic Fields entitled "Establishing a dialogue on risks from electromagnetic fields." It seems to be mainly concerned with managing "public perception of risk" than offering any concrete warnings.[73]

One could be forgiven for thinking that a presentation at a WHO EMF seminar in 2005 entitled "Regulating the risks of mobile phone base stations: a comparative study in five countries" was evaluating health risks. On inspection however, it was analyzing risk to the phone operators! It detailed that where there was consistency among a strong central government, the experts, and the courts, "[s]cientific, judicial, and social uncertainty" was low and hence the political risk and risk to the operators was low, too. The overall advice seemed to be that: States need to aim to strengthen the power of their central government, to speak with one voice with the operators, eliminate any power of decision at the local level, only give approved experts a public voice, and get the courts in line![74]

With the ability to decide who does the scientific research, the industry also dictates the research itself and how it is interpreted through press releases. Industry scientists create "counter-evidence" for every true finding so that it can be said that "the issue is controversial" and that "the scientists have disparate opinions" or that the effect is "not conclusively proven." Thereby doubt is created in the minds of the public and restrictive legislation is delayed. The tobacco industry employed this technique for many decades after it had been proven that smoking is harmful.[75]

A host of methods are employed, many of which seem to have been taken straight out of tobacco industry PR manuals. In his book "Heat," George Monbiot[76] details how after a major class action lawsuit in 1998, the tobacco companies were forced to publish their internal documents on the Internet. These documents reveal that after a report by America's Environmental Protection Agency was released in 1992 on the hazards of secondhand smoke, Philip Morris hired a PR agency called APCO to advise them how "to discredit the EPA Report" to prevent "passive-smoking bans."

APCO advised that they should create a "grassroots movement" to fight "overregulation." It should portray the danger of tobacco smoke as just one "unfounded fear" among others, such as concerns about pesticides and cell phones! APCO proposed to set up "a national coalition intended to educate the media, public officials and the public about the dangers of 'junk science.'" (Could this be where the UK term "Bad Science" came from?)

The grassroots movement was set up and called "The Advancement of Sound Science Coalition" TASSC. To industry epidemiologists, "sound science" meant industry-sponsored research demonstrating no adverse effects while junk science (bad science) meant studies that drew attention to adverse effects.

A memo from another tobacco company, Brown and Williamson, noted, "Doubt is our product since it is the best means of competing with the 'body of fact' that exists in the mind of the general public. It is also the means of establishing a controversy,"—which will result in delaying regulation for decades.[77]

Working with lawyers and PR agencies, the "Sound Science" movement was expanded to involve other industries. Philip Morris promoted a set of standards originally proposed by the Chemical Manufacturers Association called "Good Epidemiology Practices." By modifying the proposal and developing new opportunities to introduce it, Philip Morris sought to establish an arbitrary threshold for identifying health risk from secondhand smoke—a threshold higher than where adverse effects had already been found from exposure to secondhand smoke.[78]

The mobile phone industry seem to have taken a leaf out of the tobacco textbook when they had ICNIRP make the standards for non-ionizing radiation protection higher than the level at which adverse health effects had already been found!

Recently the wireless industry have gone even further than Tobacco. The European-wide REFLEX Report, 2004, is a thorn in their side as it replicates Lai and Singh's studies on double-strand DNA breaks. In 2008, at the Vienna Medical University involved in two studies, a research assistant was accused by the Rector Wolfgang Schütz of falsifying data. It is a complicated story but the Rector called for the two studies to be removed from the scientific literature. This shed doubt on the whole REFLEX Report. There was no convincing evidence against the research assistant. However, she had a breakdown and has lost her job. To date the research has not been withdrawn from the Journal. If it had been without proof of flaws, this would have been unprecedented. Hugo Rüdiger, the lead researcher, is suing the Rector Wolfgang Schütz for "promulgating false allegations."[79]

Because of this manufactured doubt, when the EU met at a later date to consider funding another project under the lead researcher Professor Adlkofer into human damage, funding was refused.

The World Health Organization's EMF Research Agenda states the following:

> Studies in tissues, living cells and cell-free systems play a supporting role in
> health risk assessment. Cellular model systems are excellent candidates for test-
> ing the plausibility of mechanistic hypothesis and investigating the ability of RF
> exposures to have synergistic effects with agents of known biological activity.

This approach would be eminently reasonable if it acknowledged the findings
of researchers actually describing cellular effects. Yet, the latest version of the
Research Agenda (2006) continues:

> There are several recently completed or ongoing studies (genotoxicity, apopto-
> sis, etc.) mostly reporting no effects.

This is a very strange statement (mirrored in the UK government's MTHR
report of 2007), considering the results of the REFLEX project. The REFLEX
Report doesn't appear on the WHO EMF database and so presumably has simply been ignored.

The REFLEX Project (Risk Evaluation of Potential Environmental Hazards
from Low Energy Electromagnetic Field Exposure Using Sensitive in vitro
Methods): was a recent four-year EU-backed study by twelve partners in seven
countries which reported in 2004. It cost 3 million euros.

Twelve research institutes in seven countries found genotoxic effects and
modified expressions on numerous genes and proteins after radio frequency and
extremely low-frequency EMF exposure at levels, below ICNIRP guidance, to
living cells in-vitro. These results confirm the likelihood of long-term genetic
damage in the blood and brains of users of mobile phones and other sources of
electromagnetic fields.

They concluded that in-vitro damage is real and that it is important to carry
out much more research, especially monitoring the long-term health of people.[80]

ROLE OF THE MTHR

As mentioned, the MTHR, or Mobile Telecommunications and Health Research
Programme, is cofunded by the Department of Health and the telecommunications industry. It is thus difficult to not be a little suspicious of the fact that its
primary purpose is probably nothing other than to conduct research that shows
that mobile devices are safe, and to disprove claims that they have negative health
effects.

Time and time again their research methods, what they choose to include, and how they analyze what they find, would tend to support this point of view. Epidemiology is ignored, short-term laboratory studies are set up designed to disprove health is an issue, and excessive time and money is spent discussing how to measure radiation and what sort of monitoring equipment should be used.

In the MTHR study in 2004, over half of the £3.5 million first-round research budget was wasted in this way, according to critics. More time and money is allocated to what they call "risk communication," and yet more toward the inclusion of studies from psychiatrists. Their job is to sow doubt on the validity of results that might show ill health effects by deeming symptoms as merely psychosomatic. And the money spent on "risk communication" makes sure that the results are "on message" for the industry.

The final report on the first round of the MTHR[81] study was interesting too because of the four studies it left out; they were not yet completed when the report was suddenly issued in 2007.

The largest singly funded project (at £960,000) was a study of leukemia and mobile phone use led by Professor Swerdlow.[82] Results were only published in late 2010. They found no link except possibly for fifteen years of use, which they dismiss. This is not surprising since leukemia is fairly rare. One would be unlikely to see an increase if any from mobile phone use after a short time. There may be an impact, but the more immediate link with phone use is to brain tumors and dementia. Leukemia is more likely to be caused by the impact of the longer term constant nighttime whole-body exposures in the vicinity of cordless landlines, Wi-Fi, and phone masts. Now a study looking at this would be far more likely to yield some results so this is precisely why we will not see one, at least not from the MTHR.

Another case-controlled study led by Professor Elliott (costing £247,000) was published in June 2010. It looked at cases of cancer in children living near base stations. It too found no correlations. However, this was a very poor study and it is surprising how it ever got published in the BMJ.[83] Instead of measuring actual radiation exposures in the houses of the cases, the exposure was merely estimated based on a model. The only accurate way to get the actual exposure is to take measurements. However the main flaw was that no other microwave sources were included. Thus someone may not live near a base station but have an even higher exposure from their own cordless landline or Wi-Fi network or that of their neighbor. The study did mention this in passing. However, it can be seen from the outset that this study was at best useless and at worst designed to get a media headline of "no link between childhood cancer and mobile phone masts," see also the *Guardian*.[84]

Dr. Sienkiewicz's animal study (costing £590,000) on RF effects on brain physiology was published on the MTHR website in December 2009. Dr. Repacholi oversaw the project. This complicated study concludes that there were no "lasting" effects from exposures in mice; however, some changes were seen in the brains of mice exposed to pulsed signals.[85]

Dr. Porter's work (costing £454,000) on interaction of RF with the human body was published on the MTHR website in January 2010. All it did was look at radiation absorption from various different transmitter types in a "phantom" body (i.e. a fluid-filled torso!)[86]

The studies that had been included in the early publication of the MTHR report, covered dosimetry (methods of measuring exposure), short-term exposure, and risk communication. And there were five studies on electrical-hypersensitivity (EHS) led by a psychiatrist who purported that EHS people could not tell when the signal was on or off—their symptoms were being made up.

If one looks carefully at the "experts" on the MTHR committee that allocate funding for studies, one can see that in the first round over £7 million[87] was awarded to the same small group on the committees of the IET, the HPA (NRPB), ICNIRP, MCL, Kings College School of Psychiatry, and the MTHR committee members themselves!

THE INTERPHONE STUDY

The MTHR cofunded the UK's participation in the worldwide Interphone study investigating the link between brain tumors and mobile phone use, coordinated by IARC, The International Agency for Research on Cancer. The University of Leeds, where one UK study was carried out, also received financial support from five UK-based mobile network operators.

Thirteen countries in all participated in the studies, those in Europe being funded by the EU, and the Mobile Manufacturer's Association, the GSM Association, and individual governments, and mobile phone companies.[88] With backers such as these, it was unsurprising that across the board in the different countries, press releases were issued on individual country results highlighting "no risk" for regular users.

In January 2006 the UK media reported on the UK team's research as follows: Mobile phones "don't raise brain cancer risk." *Daily Mail*[89]

The UK's Interphone study, led by Professor Anthony Swerdlow, was criticized as being fundamentally flawed for a number of reasons.[90]

The study does indeed find the "no increased risk" for the gliomas, but the sample used excluded a large majority of the high grade (fast growing) glioma cases because: "We interviewed [only] 51 percent of those patients with glioma who were eligible, mainly because rapid death prevented us from approaching all of them."

Amazingly, the data of the participants who died too quickly to be interviewed was not included in the study, confounding the result. Also, the press didn't inform the public that in the remainder of the group, significantly more glioma were found on the particular side of the head that participants usually held their mobile phones. To downplay this finding, the authors told the media that the participants probably couldn't remember which side they used for phone calls.

The researchers omitted also from telling the media that 1.8 times more acoustic neuroma after ten years mobile phone use was found in the study.

But the most fundamental flaw of all in the Interphone study was to do with their definitions of a regular user, a heavy user, and a non-user. The results of the study say that there is no increased risk for a "regular user"—which most people think applies to them. A regular user they define as a person who only uses a mobile phone at least once a week over a six-month period. A "heavy user" is defined as 1,600 hours of use over ten years (1/2 hour per day). A non-user would not have a mobile phone, but they were not questioned as to their use of home cordless landlines which emit just as much radiation to the head as any mobile phone. This would confound the control group, so the conclusions drawn are based on skewed categorization of phone use.

A first-draft analysis of all the Interphone brain tumor (gliomas and meningiomas) results were completed by 2005. However, the overall report was only published in 2010, much to the anger of the EU who had funded part of it. Even the *Economist* wrote an article called "Mobile Madness" in which they outlined how the researchers couldn't agree on the results.[91]

The delay might have been exacerbated by further Interphone groups undertaking work into what is called "recall bias."[92] Many of the results did show an obvious connection between phone use and brain tumors, and in order to scupper the release of these findings, researchers released reports saying that many of the participants "couldn't recall" aspects of their phone use habits, and so the results were inconclusive. This same tactic was frequently used by tobacco industry researchers in the 1990s to bring into question epidemiological evidence.[93]

Professor Hardell is an oncologist from the University Hospital in Orebro in Sweden and has been studying the use of mobile and cordless phones and the risk for brain tumors over the last decade. His team have consistently found increased risk of brain tumors from phone use, particularly for those who started using a phone before age twenty, who were found to have a five times increased risk after ten years' use.[94] Hardell and two Australian brain surgeons, Dr. Khurana and Dr. Teo, published a paper in 2009 in the *Journal of Surgical Neurology*[95] reviewing all the Interphone studies and all the independently funded work done by Dr. Hardell. They concluded that there is a doubling of risk of some brain tumors for people using mobile phones for over ten years. Dr. Khurana said that this was probably an underestimate due to the numerous flaws in the Interphone study.

In an investigative program on Australian TV in 2009, Dr. Teo stated the following:

> I'm incredibly worried, concerned, depressed at the number of kids I'm seeing coming in with brain tumors. Malignant brain tumors. Just in the last three or four weeks I've seen nearly half a dozen kids with tumors which really should have been benign and they've all been nasty, malignant brain tumors. We are doing something terribly wrong"[96]

THE WHO'S 2B BOMBSHELL

At the beginning of this chapter, we quoted the declaration by the WHO that classified "radiofrequency electromagnetic fields as possibly carcinogenic to humans based on an increased risk for glioma, a malignant type of brain cancer, associated with wireless phone use."[97] How indeed, was this point reached after all that we have heard? The following story reveals the degree to which various industry-biased individuals have been carefully placed in key organizations to influence all aspects of research, of information flow, and of regulation of the mobile telecommunication industry.

IARC set up a committee of thirty-two experts in 2011 to assess the Interphone studies to look for evidence of carcinogenicity from microwave radiation exposure. The chair of the committee was Professor Anders Ahlbom, Epidemiologist at the Karolinska Institute in Stockholm.

Professor Ahlbom has had a long history in this sector. As a member of ICNIRP from 1998 he participated in setting the guidelines for exposure. He led a review in the EU called SCENIHR that looked at effects of EMF's on human health. He also chaired every expert review for the Swedish radiation protection authority. He has repeatedly declared that there are no ill effects for exposures below the guidelines.[98]

In May 2011, Swedish journalist, Mona Nilsson discovered that Professor Ahlbom had set up a PR/lobby company with his brother Gunnar in 2010 to do consulting business in the EU, particularly in the telecommunications sector. Gunnar, who lives in Brussels, has worked in PR for the telecommunications industry since 1993. Anders Ahlbom had never declared his brother's work nor his directorship of his company to the IARC.[99]

Professor Ahlbom was removed from the IARC committee on May 22, 2011.[100] Two days later, the IARC met and began their review on the effects of microwave radiation on health, and on May 31, 2011, they declared it a class 2b carcinogen. It seemed more than coincidental that this was announced so soon after the removal of such a well-connected, influential individual such as Anders Ahlbom who seemed always to tow the line of the telecommunications industry.

WHO 2B CLASSIFICATION AND THE FUTURE

The WHO warning is now out in the public domain; it did appear in all the national newspapers in the United Kingdom, although predictably some publications such as the *Guardian*, the *Times*, the *Independent,* and the BBC did their utmost to downplay its significance.[101] They compared electromagnetic radiation to other carcinogens in the same category such as talcum powder, rather than mentioning that DDT and lead also reside in that group. (What they fail to recognize in their comparison with talcum powder is that it contains asbestos in its raw state.) The *Telegraph* and the *Sunday Times* did, however, seem to take the guidance more seriously and produced more balanced coverage.[102]

But what of the future? Since the announcement that mobile telecommunication is carcinogenic, ICNIRP have rereleased an old and flawed Danish study to downplay the IARC decision.[103] The WHO is left in a difficult position with two of their agencies, IARC and ICNIRP, now offering conflicting advice. This is reflected on their website, which still refers to no harmful health effects from microwave radiation although the IARC classification is now listed. The guidelines are exactly the same, being controlled by ICNIRP.

The next model of the Apple iPhone is on the shelves, everyone has a mobile gadget in their hand or against their heads without any warnings from the authorities about the dangers. 4G, digital TV, smart meters, wireless connectivity inside the home is also on the horizon, delivering more and more radiation across the globe.

Most importantly, our children are all becoming psychologically and sociologically dependent on this equipment that is so harmful to the health of growing young people.[104] We only have to look at the increases in brain tumors and cancers in adults and children to see that something dramatic has changed.[105] The Internet has modified itself to become the social catalyst for a generation, now completely mobile on equipment so powerful that our children are also exposed in what has been deemed the "largest epidemiological experiment ever."

To make matters worse, policy-makers blindly encourage the education system to introduce Wi-Fi into schools. On a BBC Panorama[106] documentary in 2007, it was demonstrated that the radiation intensity in a classroom with Wi-Fi was three times higher than in the main beam of a mobile phone mast, with two studies showing a tripling of cancer incidence after only five years' exposure in this strength of field.[107] The *Guardian* newspaper downplayed the issue attacking the engineer, Alistair Philips, who took the measurements.[108] This prompted the HPA to spend £300,000 on a two-year "study" to measure levels in a mock-up classroom. They came up with levels that were even higher than were shown in the documentary. However, they predictably announced that because they were still lower than the ICNIRP "guidelines," there wasn't a problem![109]

Many organizations have called for the removal of Wi-Fi in schools including regional governments in Germany, Austria, the ICEMS, the International Commission for Electromagnetic Safety, Paris libraries, and various individual schools.[110] In May 2011, the Parliamentary Assembly of the Council of Europe recommended that schools use wired Internet connections instead of Wi-Fi to reduce exposure to children.[111]

The UK Trades Union Congress states that: "caution should be used to prevent exposure to substances in group 2b. . . the regulations are clear that the first aim should be to remove the hazard."[112]

They go on to say that it is a legal requirement on employers to only use a carcinogen if there is no reasonable alternative. There are alternatives: the first is to cable up computers with Ethernet cabling, which provides a more secure connection and higher speeds.

There is a promising new development called "Visable Light Communications" whereby data can be sent using ordinary LED lighting.[113] It is believed to be much safer, as unlike microwaves, light cannot significantly penetrate the body. One possible effect may come from the flicker but of course this should first be safety tested.

Some people are looking for alternatives such as this. But the reality is that we are all responsible in some way for the growth of such a toxic industry since we buy these products that dominate our lives. We have all come to allow mobile gadgetry to mesmerize us to such a degree that we give no thought to its safety. The powerful institutions that control governments and health watchdogs, control university research, control portions of the media and supply, promote, and regulate this equipment have created a network of individuals and institutions all designed to keep rolling out more and more wireless technology at ever-higher frequencies and strengths, never mind the human cost.

Chapter 24

YOU HAVE CANCER: IT'S YOUR FAULT

Janette Sherman

You have breast cancer. You're told: "It's your fault." You did not eat the right foods, did not exercise enough, had your onset of menarche too young, menopause too old, didn't have children, or if you did, you didn't breastfeed, you grew too tall, became overweight, or worse yet had the wrong genetics. It's your fault.

Blaming the patient isn't confined to those who develop breast cancer; we blame those who develop cancer of prostate, lung, stomach, colon, and many others. You smoked, or lived with someone who did; you ate the wrong foods; you drank alcoholic beverages. The only ones we can't blame for their cancers are children, but even then, there is the unstated message that it is due to some failing of the child's parents.

Why is this so? There are many reasons, but top among them is the push for money and power, and the *secret, and not-so-secret ties* that link one to the other. If companies can sell us products, they make money. If they sell products we don't need or that are harmful, they still make money, and so do the corporations that supply their advertising. If companies can use ingredients or containers that contain harmful chemicals, they still make money. No better example than baby products contaminated with plastics or the pesticides chlordane, heptachlor and Dursban that were advertised to homeowners to control insects. And capping the efforts of these pushers of harmful products is their contributions to political candidates, where they buy access to writing legislation, inhibit enforcement by such agencies as EPA, FDA, OSHA, CPSC, DOE, NRC, and others, and control the airwaves and the press. Reaping the benefits too are the media and public relations (PR) companies who use every trick that Vance Packard warned of in his 1957 book, *Hidden Persuaders*.[1] Given that glitz and sex sells, and that critical thinking is not a hot topic in American education, the trifecta of corporations, the media, and public relation industries has taken over our thinking, and our government.

If we want to truly address the cancer epidemic, we have to address the base causes: *Carcinogens Cause Cancer*. These known carcinogens include a myriad of chemicals plus various forms of nuclear radiation. We don't know all of the chemicals and processes that cause cancer, but we know enough of them to do something about it. The contamination of our environment continues because we have not stopped the flow of money from these not-so-secret corporations, to the media, the purveyors of PR, and our elected officials.

Known chemical carcinogens are too numerous to name: pesticides, plastics, and pharmaceuticals, and a plethora of chemicals used in our workplaces, and purposely or inadvertently added to our food, housing, offices, carpets, personal care products, and general environment. The argument that cancer is due to lack of exercise doesn't make sense for those dancers, tennis players, athletes, and women who raise children and do their own housework but are diagnosed with cancer. As for the baseball and golf players who developed prostate cancer, lack of exercise pales as a reason beside the myriad of pesticides applied to playing areas. Does Lance Armstrong, the bicycle champion, have any idea what carcinogen(s) caused his cancer?

Many carcinogens make their way into our bodies through what we eat. Food suppliy sources and routes can be complicated in the United States. Our food supply comes from far-flung places and is transported thousands of miles from where it is produced. Who knows what was sprayed on food in the field, in the truck or train, in packaging, or in the store where we buy it? If you are a farmer you are pushed by corporate and agricultural extension agents to become dependent upon pesticides or bovine growth hormone (bGH). Worse yet, if you are a farmworker and have to keep your job, you have little to no say about what you are exposed to in the field. Fortunately, the European Union has lessened some of these problems for its citizens.

People with limited money, limited language skills, and limited access to information can't protect themselves and their families from food contaminated with toxic chemicals and radioactive substances. If adverse effects from exposure to toxic chemicals and nuclear radiation are withheld, the unaware public begins to accept the tragedy of cancer, birth defects, and other catastrophes as a "normal" course of existence.

Toxic chemicals alter our bodies. Grade-school girls are developing breasts and beginning their menses at younger and younger ages, while their mothers and grandmothers see their menses extended far beyond the usual age of fifty, either by use of hormonal drugs taken purposely or from inadvertent exposure to hormone-like chemicals hidden in foods, plastic products, or even cosmetics.

As an exercise in do-it-yourself epidemiology, go to any shopping mall and observe the next twenty or thirty teenaged boys as they pass by—many with fully developed breast tissue—a virtually unknown phenomenon fifty years ago in the United States, and rarely seen in other countries.

The issue of having or not having children and whether a woman breast-feeds her children is of consequence, because pregnancy and lactation are major hormonal events. Pregnancy is a detoxification route for the mother whereby chemicals stored in her body are transferred directly to the fetus, and to her infant in her breast milk.

Even if our milk is free from growth hormones, pesticides, and antibiotics, it can be a significant source of carcinogens if it comes from cows raised in the shadow of a nuclear power facility. Each reactor releases hundreds of radioactive isotopes including those of strontium, cesium, iodine, and hydrogen—the latter in the form of tritium.

The combined effects of nuclear radiation and chemicals interact with our basic genetic material or disrupt normal cellular or endocrine function resulting in cancer. We know the carcinogenic effects of many of these chemicals after decades of research and studies.

Perhaps the current biggest push by the trifecta of corporations, the media, and public relations upon our government is to support building more nuclear power plants, even as the nuclear power corporations themselves cannot raise the capital to do so. The plants are advertised as "no carbon" and "green" even though there is no truth to the claims.

Data from the recently released book about Chernobyl leaves no doubt that the isotopes released from nuclear power plants cause leukemia as well as thyroid and other cancers. Although over two decades have elapsed since the Chernobyl catastrophe, levels of radiation remain high across large areas.

Just living near a "normally" operating nuclear power plant has dangers. Work done by researchers with the Radiation and Public Health Project (RPHP) reveals that thyroid cancer incidence is rising rapidly and has more than doubled since 1980 in the United States. Of forty-four states studied from 1999 to 2002, Pennsylvania leads the country in the incidence of thyroid cancer for all ages, races, and genders. Of fourteen Pennsylvania counties with high thyroid cancer rates, thirteen are located east of local nuclear power plants. Radioactive iodine is a proven cause of thyroid cancer, and nuclear power plants are known sources of these isotopes that concentrate in the thyroid gland.

The half-life of any isotope can be misleading—to be completely decayed, ten half-lives must occur, thus for one form of iodine (I-131) that is released with a half-life of eight days, full decay requires eighty days (8 x 10 = 80 days.) For strontium (Sr-90) with a half-life of twenty-eight years, nearly three centuries are required (28 x 10 = 280 years.) Significantly, one of the iodine isotopes (I-129) released from reactors has a half-life of 15.7 million years.

Children born in proximity to nuclear reactors have higher levels of radioactive strontium (Sr-90) in their teeth, one of the main isotopes released during the generation of nuclear power. A study by RPHP scientists demonstrated an increase in infant mortality in children born within close proximity to nuclear power plants, and conversely a decline in childhood mortality after the nuclear power plants closed.

Dramatic increases in thyroid cancer occurred in those who consumed milk contaminated by fallout from nuclear bomb testing in the 1950s and early 1960s. During the Chernobyl catastrophe in 1986, an enormous amount of radioactive iodine was released and thyroid disease and thyroid cancer rose markedly. Many thyroid cancers could have been prevented had potassium iodine (KI) replacement been available to those in the fallout zones.

Following the Chernobyl meltdown, Dr. Vassili Nesterenko, then director of the Ukrainian Institute of Nuclear Physics, urged that iodine tablets immediately be dispensed. It was not done. Nor is it clear that potassium iodine is readily available for people living in proximity to the 439 plants currently operating worldwide.

According to the US Interagency Technical Evaluation Paper for Section 127(f) of the Bioterrorism Act of 2002,[2] if KI [potassium iodide] is given within two hours of an I-131 exposure the estimated level of protection is 80 percent, but if given twenty-four hours after an exposure it provides only 16 percent protection.[3] While prompt use of KI may be useful in preventing thyroid damage and thyroid cancer, a nuclear power plant "incident" will release many other nuclides such as the noble gases xenon and krypton, plus radioactive cesium and strontium and other isotopes.[4] To counteract or block these additional isotopes, KI will have no effect.

In January 2001, the US Nuclear Regulatory Commission revised a section of its emergency preparedness regulations. The revised rule requires that "states with a population within the ten-mile emergency planning zone (EPZ) of a commercial nuclear power plant consider including potassium iodide as a protective measure for the general public to supplement sheltering and evacuation in the unlikely event of a severe nuclear power plant accident."

It is important to note the language of the report: that states *consider* including KI, not that it would be mandatory. Notice too that KI would be used to *supplement sheltering* and *evacuation*.

From time to time, various US nuclear corporations indicate that iodine replacement will be dispensed at designated facilities, but we have no idea how many people will want or be able to travel within a fallout zone to obtain the KI tablets or the KI liquid preparation for their infants and young children. Conversely, if nuclear power plants, proactively distribute iodine replacement to all residents within a possible fallout zone, it could raise public awareness of living in a potentially dangerous place. Finally, potassium iodide administration will protect against radioactive iodine but provide no protection for the other isotopes.

Not only is there a high incidence of thyroid cancer, but published studies demonstrate a high incidence of breast cancer in women living in proximity to nuclear power plants, where isotopes precipitate onto the land and are taken up by dairy cattle, transferring radioactive isotopes such as strontium (Sr-90), cesium (Cs-137), and iodine (I-131) into the milk supply. This is why data collected from baby teeth in both the 1960s St. Louis, Missouri, study and the recent studies by the Radiation and Public Health Project are so useful. Sr-90 persists and can be measured—valid for scientific research, but dangerous for the contaminated person.

There is not a single dairy herd in all of Washington, DC, but the milk supply demonstrated elevated I-131 levels in 1986, along with a very high level of infant mortality. Did this contamination originate in the dairy industry in eastern Pennsylvania and Maryland, in proximity to the Peach Bottom, Three Mile Island, and Limerick Reactors? Did additional radioactivity come from the Chernobyl fallout that began in April 1986, as it was distributed across the entire northern hemisphere? The answer according to public documents is "yes," but as of this date, there is no evidence that the US Federal or DC government ever investigated the link between infant deaths and the elevated radioactivity in the milk supply.

Radiation-induced cancers come from multiple sources that include emissions from X-rays, CT-scans, medical radioisotope studies, and releases from nuclear power plants, nuclear production and research sites, and radiation-containing armaments, such as the depleted uranium (DU) munitions used in Iraq and Afghanistan.

Nowhere in the world is cancer randomly distributed—certainly not in the United States or Europe. Patterns of cancer distribution point to possible causes such as factory emissions, toxic dumps, and nuclear sites. By reducing these known sources of carcinogens the cancer epidemic could be lessened.

Shall we continue to believe that cancer is our own fault? Given the plethora of articles touting protective qualities of vegetables, exercise, certain food supplements, genetic modification, drugs, etc., the cancer rate continues to rise, and the pharmaceutical, chemical, radiation, and public relations industries flourish.

In the United States, we have been transformed from a country with a positive public health legacy that urged prevention of disease, to one that mostly promotes treatment, where incidentally, there is money to be made by the pharmaceutical and insurance corporations.

We once quarantined patients with communicable diseases, supported immunizations when they became available, and spent public moneys on public water and sewer systems, to the betterment of all citizens. Now we are on our own. In the past decade, the FDA, CDC, ATSDR, EPA, DOE, NRC, Department of Agriculture, and other agencies that were to promulgate laws and require that known carcinogens be kept from our food, water, air and consumer products have failed. Remember: *CARCINOGENS CAUSE CANCER.*

Primary among preventive health needs is to stop the development of new nuclear plants, close the existing ones, and develop a way to store the accumulated wastes as safely as possible.

By collective action, we the people of the United States outlawed slavery, obtained the vote for Blacks and women, and brought the Vietnam War to an end. Can we mobilize to stop the nuclear menace and contain the toxic mess that this technology has generated? It will be difficult and costly, but only then, can we say your cancer is not your fault.

> The natural world is deteriorating and human health is declining because those who make the important decisions aren't the ones who bear the brunt. Our purpose is to connect the dots between human health, the destruction of nature, the decline of community, the rise of economic insecurity and inequalities, growing stress among workers and families, and the crippling legacies of patriarchy, intolerance, and racial injustice that allow us to be divided and therefore ruled by the few.[5]

There are secret ties between the corporations that manufacture/import/sell harmful products, but many are obvious. The adage, "follow the money" must be done: from purveyors of products to the PR groups, the media, and to our politicians. Perhaps then we can stop the epidemic of cancer. A diagnosis of cancer is not your fault if you were given false information or no information at all by those entities, tied not-so-secretly.

REFERENCES

Dedication

1 J. Selikoff. J. McCulloch, G. Tweedale Int "Abstract from Shooting the Messenger: the vilification of Irving" *J Health Serv*, 37(4) (2007): 619–34.

2 Anthony Tucker. Obituary of Alice Stewart, Friday 28 June 2002. *The Guardian*.

Chapter 1: A Dark Culture, Martin Walker

1 George Orwell, *1984* (UK: Penguin Books Ltd, 2004).

2 A. Carey, *Taking the Risk out of Democracy: Corporate Propaganda versus Freedom and Liberty* (Champaign, IL: University of Illinois Press, 1995).

3 Noam Chomsky, *World Orders Old and New*.

4 T. O. McGarity, W. E. Wagner, *Bending Science: How Special Interests Corrupt Public Health Research* (Cambridge, MA: Harvard University Press, 2008).

5 K. Albrecht, "Microchip-Induced Tumors in Laboratory Rodents and Dogs: A Review of the Literature," http://www.antichips.com/cancer/index.html, (1990–2006).

6 "Union of Concerned Scientists. Heads They Win, Tails, We Lose: How Corporations Corrupt Science at the Public's Expense," (Cambridge, MA: UCS Publications, 2012), www.ucsusa.org/sites/default/files/legacy/assets/documents/scientific_integrity/how-corporations-corrupt-science.pdf.

7 G. Ruskin, "Spooky Business: Corporate Espionage Against Nonprofit Organizations," (Washington, 2013), www.corporatepolicy.org/spookybusiness.pdf.

8 D. Helvarg, *The War Against the Greens: The "Wise Use" Movement, the New Right, and Anti-Environmental Violence* (San Francisco: Sierra Club Books, 1994).

9 B. Ramazzini, *Diseases of workers. De morbis artificum diatriba. The Latin text of 1713*, revised with trans and notes by Wilmer Cave Wright (Birmingham, AL: Gryphon, Classics of Medicine Library, 1983).

10 Ole Daniel Enersen, http://www.whonamedit.com/search.php (2014).

11 June 1829 letter from Hahnemann to Dr. Rhul, cited in *Russell JR. The History and Heroes of the Art of Medicine* (London: John Murray, 1861).

12 Samuel Hahnemann.

13 Christoph Wilhelm Friedrich Hufeland, one of the most respected writers on medicine in the 18th century, was a close friend of Samuel Hahnemann and published many of his original writings in his journal.

14 J. R. Russell, *The History and Heroes of the Art of Medicine* (London: John Murray, 1861).

15 Young, S. Sue Young Histories, "*A Homeopathic History of Cholera*," http://web.archive.org/web/20140913091720/http://sueyounghistories.com/archives/2009/11/09/a-homeopathic-history-of-cholera/ (Nov. 2009).

16 Ibid.

17 Ibid.

18 The Committee for the Scientific Investigation of Claims of the Paranormal (CSICOP) was the first skeptics campaign organization set up in 1975, with which Maddox was linked. Led by Paul Kurtz, it grew from a US Marxist grouping into a major defender of corporate science. M. J. Walker, *Dirty Medicine: Science, Big Business and the Assault on Natural Health Care* (London: Slingshot Publications, 1993).

19 M. J. Walker, *Dirty Medicine: Science, Big Business and the Assault on Natural Health Care* (London: Slingshot Publications, 1993).

20 M. J. Walker, "Uncomfortable Science and Enemies of the People," *Medical Veritas* 6 (2009): 2061–66.

21 R. H. Sherard, *The White Slaves of England: Being true pictures of certain social conditions in the Kingdom of England in this year 1897* (London: James Bowden, 1897).

22 "The White Slaves of England," "The Cry of the Poor," "The Closed Door," and "The Child Slaves of Britain," Available as separate books. A series published in *Pearson's* and *The London Magazine*.

23 Sherard.

24 S. Salgado, *Workers: An Archeology of the Industrial Age* (London: Phaidon, 1993).

25 K. Bales, *Disposable People: New Slavery in the Global Economy* (Berkeley, CA: University of California Press, 1999).

26 Sherard.

27 Sherard.

28 *Leeds Times*, October 5, 1896.

29 R. H. Sherard, In response to the *Leeds Times* in an Appendix to the 1898 edition of White Slaves.

30 *The Textile Mercury*, September 5, 1989.

31 A. Besant, *An Autobiography* (London: T. Fischer Unwin, 1893).

32 O. Bennett, *Annie Besant* (London: Hamish Hamilton, 1988).

33 A. Besant, "White Slavery in London," *The Link*, June 23, 1888.

34 A. Stafford, *A Match to Fire the Thames* (London: Hodder and Stoughton, 1961).

35 "The Match Girls," The Matchcover Vault, http://matchpro.org/Archives/2009/Match percent20Girls percent20Strike.pdf (2009 Jul/Aug).

36 I. Tarbell, "The History of the Standard Oil Company," *McClure's Magazine*, (1902). I. Tarbell, *The History of the Standard Oil Company: Briefer Version*, Chalmers DM, ed. (New York: Dover Publications, 2003).

37   U. Sinclair, *The Jungle* (Chicago: Doubleday, Page and Co.,1906).

38   U. Sinclair, *The Autobiography of Upton Sinclair,* (London: W. H. Allen, 1963).

39   Ibid.

40   Ibid.

41   R. Carson, *Silent Spring* (Boston: Houghton Mifflin, 1962).

42   F. Graham, *Since Silent Spring* (London: Hamish Hamilton, 1970).

43   Ibid.

44   Ibid.

45   Carson.

46   Graham.

47   P. Brodeur, *Expendable Americans: The incredible story of how tens of thousands of American men and women die each year of preventable industrial disease* (New York: Viking Press, 1973).

48   P. Brodeur, *Currents of Death: Power Lines, Computer Terminals, and the Attempt to Cover Up Their Threat to Your Health* (New York: Simon & Schuster, 2000).

49   P. Brodeur, *The Zapping of America: Microwaves, Their Deadly Risk, and the Cover-Up* (New York: W W Norton & Co Inc., 1977).

50   B. Seaman, G. Seaman, *Women and the Crisis in Sex Hormones* (New York: BantamBooks, 1983).

51   M. J. Walker, *HRT Licensed to Kill and Maim* (London: Slingshot Publications, 2007).

52   Collaborative group on epidemiological studies of ovarian cancer. "Menopausal hormone use and ovarian cancer risk: Individual participant meta-analysis of 52 epidemiological studies," *Lancet*, (Pii: s0140-6736(14)61687-1), February 12, 2015.

53   G. Cannon, *The Politics of Food* (London: Century Hutchinson, 1987).

54   M. Norton, *The Borrowers* (London: Dent, 1952).

55   P. J. Quirk, *Industry Influence in Federal Regulatory Agencies* (Princeton, NJ: Princeton University Press, 1981).

56   J. Braithwaite, *Corporate Crime in the Pharmaceutical Industry* (London: Routledge & Kegan Paul, 1984).

57   M. Kenney, *Biotechnology: The University Industrial Complex* (New Haven, CT: Yale University Press, 1988).

58   S. Krimsky, *Science in the Private Interest: Has the Lure of Profits Corrupted Biomedical Research?* (Lanham, MD: Rowman & Littlefield, 2004).

59   Kenney, 1988.

60   R. W. Moss, *The Cancer Industry* (Brooklyn: Equinox Press, 1996).

61   S. S. Epstein, *The Politics of Cancer* (Rev. and expanded edition) (New York: Anchor/Doubleday Press, 1979); S. S. Epstein *The Politics of Cancer Revisited* (Fremont Center, NY: East Ridge Press, 1998).

62   Sutherland could not publish the original book, for fear of being sued. He died in 1950 and this revised version of his most comprehensive work was published in 1985. E. H. Sutherland, *White Collar Crime. The Uncut Version* (New Haven, CT: Yale University Press, 1985).

63   L. Doyal, S. Epstein, *Cancer in Britain: The Politics of Prevention* (London: Pluto Press, 1986).

64   R. W. Moss, *Doctored Results* (Brooklyn: Equinox Press, 2014).

65   S. S. Epstein, *Cancer-Gate: How to Win the Losing Cancer War. Policy, Politics, Health and Medicine Series* (Amityville, NY: Baywood Pub Co.,2005).

66   B. Lynes, *The Cancer Cure That Worked! Fifty Years of Suppression* (South Lake Tahoe, CA: BioMed Publishing Group, LCC, 1987). Lynes' website is at http://barry-lynes.com/.

67   B. Lynes, *Helping the Cancer Victim: Patient Rights, Medical Freedom & the Need for New Laws* (Marcus Books, 1989).

68   P. Tompkins, C. Bird, *The Secret Life of Plants: a Fascinating Account of the Physical, Emotional, and Spiritual Relations Between Plants and Man* (New York: Harper & Row, 1989).

69   C. Bird, *The Persecution and Trial of Gaston Naessens* (Tiburon, CA: H J Kramer, 1991).

70   M. A. Gerson, *Cancer Therapy: Results of Fifty Cases* (San Diego: The Gerson Institute, 1958).

71   B. Bishop, *A Time to Heal: Triumph over Cancer, the Therapy of the Future* (London: New English Library Ltd, 1989).

72   Walker, *Dirty Medicine: Science, Big business and the Assault on Natural Health Care.*

73   M. Gearin-Tosh, *Living Proof: A Medical Mutiny* (London: Scribner, 2002).

74   Dr. Hulda Clark. Hulda Clark died in 2009. She had been conscientiously defended throughout her last battles by Tim Bolen, who provides intelligence and legal advice for defendants and puts up-to-the-minute news about the increasingly failing court actions against alternative therapists on his website. Bolen is the best advocate for those who find themselves harried by quackbusters in the United States. http://bolenreport.com/

75   E. Richards, *Vitamin C and Cancer: Medicine or Politics?* (London: Palgrave Macmillan, 1991).

76   S. Goodman, *Vitamin C: The Master Nutrient* (New Canaan, CT: Keats Publishing, 1990).

77   S. Goodman, "Nutrition and Cancer: State-of-the-Art," *Green Library Publications* (1995).

78   G. Thomas, *Issels: The Biography of a Doctor* (London: Hodder & Stoughton Ltd, 1975).

79   G. Thomas, *Go Climb a Mountain* [film] BBC (1970).

80   P. Newton-Fenbow, *A Time to Heal* (London: Souvenir Press Ltd., 1971).

81   V. Brancatisano, *Di Bella, Un po' di verita sulla terapia. Un Po' di verita sulla terapia di Bella* [in Italian] (Rome: The Travel Factory, 1999).

82   V. Brancatisano, *Di Bella: The Nan, the Cure, a Hope for All* (London: Quartet Books, 1998).

83   Access to the therapy of Di Bella. The illustration and understanding of more than one hundred personal stories of successful treatment. V. Brancatisano, *Sentenze di Vita* [in Italian] (Rome: The Travel Factory, 2000).

84   M. Beljanski, C. Marcowith, H. Janecek, *Cancer: L'Approche Beljanski* [in French] (Paris: Guy Tredaniel, 2008).

85   M. Beljanski, *Mirko Beljanski ou La Chronique d'une "Fatwa" Scientifique* [in French] (New York: EVI Liberty Corp., 2001).

86   J. McCumiskey, *The Ultimate Conspiracy: The Biomedical Paradigm* (London: New Generation Publishing, 2012).

87   E. Hollister, Interview with Simoncini. http://www.curenaturalicancro.com/en/comments/interview-emma-hollister.

88   T. Simoncini, *The lies of orthodox oncology,* http://web.archive.org/web/20110123065344/; http://www.curenaturalicancro.com/en/dr-simoncini-writes/the-lies-of-orthodox-oncology/2010/10/02.

89   D. Davis, *The Secret History of the War on Cancer* (New York: Basic Books, 2007).

90   R. N. Proctor, *Cancer Wars: How Politics Shapes What We Know & Don't Know About Cancer* (New York: Basic Books, 1995).

91   K. Ausubel, *When Healing Becomes a Crime: The Amazing Story of the Hoxsey Cancer Clinics and the Return of Alternative Therapies* (Rochester, VT: Healing Arts Press, 2000).

92   This essay by Mark Lipsman is the most full and best-written description of the work, arrest, and imprisonment of Greg Caton. Mark Lipsman is a Boston-based writer, editor and holistic practitioner. M. Lipsman, *The FDA's Panacea* http://www.goodhealthinfo.net/cancer/fda_panacea.htm.

93   Ibid.

94   Ibid.

95   Ibid.

96   C. Caton, *Criminal FDA Gangsters Kidnap Greg Caton From Ecuador,* http://rense.com/general88/fedkidnap.htm (December 2009).

97   T. O. McGarity, W. E. Wagner, *Bending Science: How Special Interests Corrupt Public Health Research* (Cambridge, MA: Harvard University Press, 2008).

98   Ibid.

99   D. Michaels, *Doubt is Their Product: How Industry's Assault on Science Threatens Your Health* (New York: Oxford University Press, 2008).

100 E. Merlo, Memo to William Campbell [re: PM USA ETS actions]. Document no. 2021183916/3930. Available at: http://www.pmdocs.com. (February 17, 1993), Accessed September 24, 2001.

101 T. Lattanzio, *ETS Task Force update.* Document no. 2021178204. http://www.pmdocs.com. (May 20, 1993), Accessed September 24, 2001.

102 *The Advancement of Sound Science Coalition.* [Information sheet describing TASSC.] Document no. 2046989061, http://www.pmdocs.com. (1993), Accessed September 24, 2001.

103 M. Kraus, Letter to PM Director of Communications re: TASSC, Document no. 2024233677/3682, http://www.pmdocs.com. (September 23, 1993), Accessed September 4, 2001.

104 PM USA, *Corporate Affairs 1994 budget presentation,* Document no. 2046847121. http://www.pmdocs.com. (October 21, 1993), Accessed September 4, 2001.

105 E. K. Ong, S. A. Glantz, "Constructing 'sound science' and 'good epidemiology' tobacco, lawyers, and public relations firms," *Am J Public Health* 91 (2001) 1749–57.
106 D. Fagin, M. Lavelle, *Toxic Deception: How the Chemical Industry Manipulates Science, Bends the Law and Endangers Your Health* (New Jersey: Carol Publishing Group, 1996).
107 J. Strauber, S. Rampton, *Toxic Sludge is Good for You! Lies, Damn Lies and the Public Relations Industry* (Monroe, ME: Common Courage Press,1995).
108 P. R. Ehrlich, A. H. Ehrlich, *Betrayal of Science and Reason: How Anti-environmental Rhetoric Threatens our Future* (Washington, DC: Island Press, 1998).
109 L. Marsa, *Prescription for Profits: How the Pharmaceutical Industry Bankrolled the Unholy Marriage Between Science and Business* (New York: Scribner, 1997).
110 J. Crewdson, *Science Fictions: A Scientific Mystery, a Massive Cover-Up, and the Dark Legacy of Robert Gallo* (New York: Little, Brown & Company, 2002).
111 *What Doctors Don't Tell You*, http://www.wddty.com/.
112 L. McTaggart, *What Doctors Don't Tell You: The Truth About the Dangers of Modern Medicine* (London: Thorsons, 1996).
113 G. Tweedale, *Magic Mineral to Killer Dust: Turner and Newall and the Asbestos Hazard* (New York: Oxford University Press, 2000).
114 J. McCulloch, G. Tweedale, *Defending the Indefensible: The Global Asbestos Industry and its Fight for Survival* (New York: Oxford University Press, 2008).
115 G. Carlo, M. Schram, *Cell Phones: Invisible Hazards in the Wireless Age. An Insider's Alarming Discoveries About Cancer and Genetic Damage* (New York: Basic Books, 2002).
116 C. Medawar, *Power and Dependence: Social Audit on the Safety of Medicines* (London: Social Audit, 1992).
117 J. Harr, *A Civil Action* (New York: Vintage Books, 1996).
118 J. Harr, (book), S. Zaillan (screenplay). *A Civil Action* [film], (1998).
119 P. Brown, E. J. Mikkelsen, *No Safe Place: Toxic Waste, Leukemia, and Community Action*, Reprint Edition (Berkeley, CA: University of California Press, 1997).
120 Harr, *A Civil Action*, Vintage Books.
121 Ibid.
122 Harr, (book).
123 E. Brockovich, M. Elliot, *Take It From Me: Life's a Struggle But You Can Win* (New York: McGraw-Hill, 2002).
124 S. Soderbergh (director), S. Grant (writer), *Erin Brockovich* [film] (2000).
125 Wikipedia, *Erin Brockovich*, http://en.wikipedia.org/wiki/Erin_Brockovich.
126 W. Goolsby, *Erin Brockovich Talks Water Contamination in Midland*, 6 http://www.newswest9.com/story/10506941/erin-brockovich-talks-water-contamination-in-midland.
127 Walker, *Dirty Medicine: Science, Big Business and the Assault on Natural Health Care*.
128 Helvarg.
129 A. Rowell, *Green Backlash: Global Subversion of the Environmental Movement* (London: Routledge, 1996).

130 S. Beder, *Global Spin: The Corporate Assault on Environmentalism* (Devon, UK: Green Books, 1997).

131 Lobbywatch, *Complaint about Science Media Centre and the LM Group*, http://www.lobbywatch.org/archive2.asp?arcid=7761 (April 2007).

132 A. Rowell, "Seeds of Dissent: Monsanto's World Wide Web of deceit," *The Big Issue* 484 (April 2002).

133 E. Lubbers, ed., *Battling Big Business: Countering Greenwash, Front Groups and Other Forms of Corporate Deception* (Monroe, ME: Common Courage Press, 2002).

134 J. Grisham, *The Appeal* (New York: Dell, 2012).

135 J. Grisham, *The Runaway Jury* (New York: Dell, 1996).

136 G. Newman, Judge John Deed [television series]. BBC. The six series of JJD that stretched from 2001 to 2006 can found at: Judge John Deeds—DVD and Blu-ray. The two censured episodes, banned by the BBC, can sometimes be found on You Tube. A long and discursive article about the censorship of the two episodes can be found at: http://www.dvdtalk.com/reviews/54268/judge-john-deed-season-5/. Titled Judge John Deed - Season Five [Censored!]

137 A. Rusbridger (writer), R. Bennett (writer), B. Anderson (director), *Fields of Gold* [film]. BBC, (June 2002).

138 Ben Goldacre is the son of one of the "scientists" who had passed the damaging Urabe mumps strain MMR vaccination. His job, done in relation to the PR crisis in the pharmaceutical industry especially in relation to vaccines, has been rehabilitated—given an honest face and stashed in the cupboard to be brought out later in another crisis.

139 S. Rampton, J. Stauber, *Trust Us We're Experts! How Industry Manipulates Science and Gambles with Your Future* (New York: Tarcher, 2002).

140 Strauber, Rampton.

141 G. Palast, *The Best Democracy Money Can Buy* (New York: Plume Books, 2004).

142 L. A. Sobel, ed., *Cancer and the Environment* (London: Macmillan, 1979).

143 Ibid.

144 Ibid.

145 G. Green, *The Woman Who Knew Too Much. Alice Stewart and the Secrets of Radiation,* Reprint Edition (Ann Arbor, MI: University of Michigan Press, 2001).

146 D. Davis, *When Smoke Ran Like Water: Tales of Environmental Deception and the Battle Against Pollution* (New York: Basic Books, 2003).

147 Davis, *The Secret Histroy of the War on Cancer.*

148 S. Batt, *Patients No More: The Politics of Breast Cancer* (Charlottetown, Canada: Gynergy Books, 1994).

149 S. Steingraber, *Living Downstream: An Ecologist Looks at Cancer and the Environment* (Reading, MA: Addison-Wesley, 1997).

An interesting story is reported on the stopcancer.org site about Sandra Steingraber's book. Talking about the misuse of science, and phony science at every level of promotion, the site describes what happened when in 1997 the well-respected *New England Journal of Medicine* was taken to task following a review of Sandra Steingraber's book, Living Downstream. The review was written by an individual identified as Jerry H. Berke, MD, MPH, giving his home address. It turned out later when the review was researched that Dr. Berke, now retired, was Director of Medicine and Toxicology for W.R. Grace & Company, one of the largest chemical manufacturers in the United States. Among the company's offenses had been the payment of several million dollars in the mid-1980s to settle a civil court case for fouling drinking water in Woburn, Massachusetts, with a known chemical carcinogen, contributing to several cases of leukaemia. Even worse than not revealing Berke's secret ties, the *New England Journal of Medicine* knew about his affiliation, and—contrary to its own policy never to publish articles by authors who had a financial stake in the subjects they wrote about—permitted him to remain anonymous.

150 Gearin-Tosh.

151 L. Clorfene-Casten, *Breast Cancer: Poisons, Profits and Prevention* (Monroe, ME: Common Courage Press, 2002).

152 G. Monbiot, *Heat: How to Stop the Planet Burning*, (London: Penguin, 2007).

153 G. Monbiot, "The denial industry," *The Guardian*. (September 19, 2006) http://www.theguardian.com/environment/2006/sep/19/ethicalliving.g2.

154 Advisory Committee on Human Radiation Experiments, *Final Report of the Advisory Committee on Human Radiation Experiments* (New York: Oxford University Press, 1996).

155 A. J. Wakefield, *Waging War on the Autistic Child: The Arizona 5 and the Legacy of Baron von Munchausen* (New York: Skyhorse Publishing, 2012).

156 M. J. Walker, *Dirty Medicine: The Handbook* (London: Slingshot Publications, 2011).

157 B. Martin, "On the suppression of vaccination dissent," *Sci Eng Ethics* 21 (2015): 143–57.

158 Walker, *Dirty Medicine: Big Business*.

159 Walker, *Dirty Medicine: The Handbook*.

160 *Hazards Magazine*, http://www.hazards.org/.

161 In 2003 Egilman submitted an article for publication in the *Journal of Occupational and Environmental Medicine* (JOEM).

162 D. S. Egilman, "Suppression bias at the Journal of Occupational and Environmental Medicine," *Int J Occup Environ Health* 11 (2005): 202–4.

163 Marco Mamone Capria, an academic mathematician from the Italian Perugia University, set up the website and conference organization Science and Democracy. http://www.dmi.unipg.it/mamone/sci-dem/sci&dem.htm.

164 Capria M. Mamone, ed., *Science and the Citizen. Contemporary Issues and Controversies*,Lulu.com; 2013.

165 L. Suarez-Villa, *Technocapitalism: A Critical Perspective on Technological Innovation and Corporatism* (Philadelphia: Temple University Press, 2009).

166 R. Reich, *Supercapitalism: The Battle for Democracy in an Age of Big Business* (London: ICON Books Ltd., 2007).

167 J. Gledhill, ed., *Corporate Scandal: Global Corporatism against Society* (New York/Oxford, UK: Berghahn Books, 2004).

168 J. Bakan, *The Corporation: The Pathological Pursuit of Profit and Power* (London: Constable, 2004).

169 D. Rushkoff, *Life Inc: How Corporatism Conquered the World, and How We Can Take it Back* (New York: Random House, 2011).

170 R. Nader, *Getting Steamed to Overcome Corporatism: Build it Together to Win* (Monroe, ME: Common Courage Press, 2011).

171 D. C. Korten, *When Corporations Rule the World* (San Francisco: Berrett-Koehler Publishers, 1995).

172 T. Nace, *Gangs of America: The Rise of Corporate Power and the Disabling of Democracy* (San Francisco: Berrett-Koehler, 2005).

173 G. Moran, *Silencing Scientists and Scholars in Other Fields: Power, Paradigm Controls, Peer Review and Scholarly Communication* (Greenwich, CT: Ablex Publishing, 1998).

174 S. Lang, *Challenges* (New York: Springer, 1998).

175 Lubbers, *Battling Big Business*.

176 Moran, *Silencing Scientists and Scholars*.

177 Lang, *Challenges*.

178 Ibid.

179 European Environment Agency (EEA). "Late lessons from early warnings: the precautionary principle 1896-2000," *Environmental Issue Report No. 22*. Copenhagen: EEA; 2001.

Chapter 2: The Basis of Bad Science, David Egilman et al.

1 Parts of this chapter have been published before in: Bohme S. R., Zorabedian J., Egilman D. Maximizing profit and endangering health: corporate strategies to avoid litigation and regulation. Int J Occup Environ Health. 2005;11:338-48.

2 M. Friedman, "The social responsibility of business is to increase its profits, "*The New York Times Magazine*, September, 13, 1970, http://www.colorado.edu/studentgroups/libertarians/issues/ friedman-soc-resp-business.html., Accessed March 24, 2010.

3 L. E. Mitchell, *Corporate irresponsibility: America's newest export* (New Haven, CT: Yale University Press, 2001).

4 G. E. Markowitz, D. Rosner, *Deceit and denial: the deadly politics of industrial pollution* (Berkeley, CA: University of California Press, 2002).

5 T. S. Kuhn, *The structure of scientific revolutions* (Chicago, IL: University of Chicago Press, 1962).

6 P. Feyerabend, *Against method: outline of an anarchistic theory of knowledge* (Atlantic Highlands, NJ: Humanities Press, 1975).

7 P. Feyerabend, *For and against method: including Lakatos's lectures on scientific method and the Lakatos-Feyerabend correspondence,* (Chicago, IL: University of Chicago Press, 1999).

8 K. R. Popper, *1993. Realism and the aim of science* (London: Routledge, 1993).

9 D. Michaels, *Doubt is their product: how industry's assault on science threatens your health* (Oxford: Oxford University Press 2008).

10   OECD. *Research and development expenditure in industry/Les dépenses en recherche et développement dans l'industrie:1977/1998.* (2000).

11   L. Guterman, "Occupational hazards,"*Chronicle of Higher Education*, 51 (2005): A15.

12   L. Rosenstock, L. J. Lee, "Attacks on science: the risks to evidence-based policy," *Am J Pub Health* 92 (2002): 1.

13   L. L. Kjaergard, B. Als-Nielsen, "Association between competing interests and authors" conclusions: "epidemiological study of randomised clinical trials" published in the BMJ, *BMJ* (2002) 325:249.

14   D. Fagin, M. Lavelle, *Toxic deception: how the chemical industry manipulates science, bends the law, and endangers your health* (Monroe, ME: Common Courage Press, 1999).

15   Scout D. Egilman, "Corporate corruption of science: the case of chromium (VI)," *Int J Occup Environ Health* 12 (2006): 169–76.

16   Ibid.

17   D. Egilman, C. Fehnel, S. R. Bohme, "Exposing the 'myth' of ABC, 'anything but chrysotile': a critique of the Canadian asbestos mining industry and McGill University chrysotile studies," *Am J Ind Med* 44 (2003): 540–57.

18   H. M. Krumholz, J. S. Ross, A. H. Presler, D. S. Egilman, "What have we learnt from Vioxx?" *BMJ.* 334 (2007): 120–3.

19   Michaels, *Doubt is their product.*

20   Ibid.

21   Value of CIIT, Unpublished Corporate Document, 2005.

22   Unpublished CIIT document.

23   Exponent Annual Report, Form 10K SEC filing, (2003) Accessed June 26, 2005.

24   ChemRisk, http://www.chemrisk.com., Accessed June 27, 2005.

25   Minutes of the Chrome Coalition meeting with ChemRisk: Discussions and Recommendations. February 2, 1996. Chrome Coalition Ad Hoc PEL Committee. IHF archives.

26   T. F. Mancuso, Consideration of chromium as an industrial carcinogen. Proceedings of the International Conference on Heavy Metals in the Environment, (October 1975) Toronto, Ontario, p.343–56.

27   Ibid.

28   Ibid.

29   D. Paustenbach, Revised proposal to develop an alternative cancer potency factor for benzene, (American Petroleum Institute, 1990), Unpublished.

30   Ibid.

31   D. J. Paustenbach, R. D. Bass, P. Price, "Benzene toxicity and risk assessment, 1972-1992: implications for future regulation," *Environ Health Perspect* 101 Suppl 6 (1993): 177-200.

32   P. R. Williams, D. J. Paustenbach, "Reconstruction of benzene exposure for the Pliofilm cohort (1936–1976) using Monte Carlo techniques," *J Toxicol Environ Health* A 66 (2003) 677–781.

33   D. Capiello, "Oil industry funding study to contradict cancer claims. Houston Chronicle," April 29, 2005, AD; A1.

REFERENCES **463**

34 D. S. Egilman, "Public health and epistemology," *Am J Ind Med* 22 (1992): 457–9.
35 Ibid.
36 Ibid.
37 Ibid.
38 Ibid.
39 A. Rodgman, "The smoking and health problem—a critical and objective appraisal," Reynolds Tobacco Company, 1962.
40 Ibid.
41 Ibid.
42 Ibid.
43 D. S. Egilman, J. Kim, M. Biklen, "Proving causation: the use and abuse of scientific evidence inside the courtroom: an epidemiologist's critique of the judicial interpretation of the Daubert ruling," *Food Drug Law J.* 58 (2003): 223–50.
44 S. R. Johnson, "Solving problems with termiticides including Dursban," *Pest Control*, 1983, 6.
45 Unpublished CIIT document.
46 Int J Occup Envron Health narrative (see ref 1).
47 A. Hill, "The environment and disease: association or causation?" *Proc R Soc Med.* 58 (1965): 295–300.
48 Ibid.
49 K. P. Satin, W. J. Bailey, K. L. Newton, A. Y. Ross, O. Wong, "Updated epidemiological study of workers at two California petroleum refineries," *1950-95, Occup Environ Med* 59 (2002): 248–56.
50 S. Parodi, F. Montanaro, M. Ceppi, V. Gennaro, "Mortality of petroleum refinery workers," *Occup Environ Med* 60 (2003): 304-5, author's reply 305–6.
51 V. Gennaro, S. Parodi, M. Ceppi, F. Montanaro, "Cancer in oil refineries: absence of risk or misclassification?" *Epidemiol Prev* 27 (2003): 173.
52 V. Gennaro, L. Tomatis, "2005. Business bias: how epidemiologic studies may underestimate or fail to detect increased risks of cancer and other diseases," *Int J Occup Environ Health* 11 (2005): 356–9.
53 IARC (International Agency for Research on Cancer). "Monographs on the evaluation of the carcinogenic risk of chemicals to humans," Volume 45: *Occupational exposures in petroleum refining; crude oil and major petroleum fuels.* Lyon, France; IARC; 1989. http://monographs.iarc.fr/ ENG/Monographs/vol45/volume45.pdf. Accessed March 25, 2010.
54 Ibid.
55 Ibid.
56 Gennaro, Tomatis, "2005: Business bias . . ."
57 Ibid.
58 Lemen 1986.
59 Gennaro, Tomatis, "2005: Business bias . . ."
60 Ibid.
61 D. S. Egilman, M. A. Billings, "Abuse of epidemiology: automobile manufacturers manufacture a defense to asbestos liability," *Int J Occup Environ Health* 11 (2005): 360–71.

62 Gennaro, Tomatis, "2005: Business bias . . ."

63 Egilman, et al., "Exposing the 'myth' of ABC."

64 K. Crump, Crump's slides used during testimony for the Asbestos Information Association. Exhibit 237B OSHA H-033C docket. July 9, 1984.

65 D. Berman, K. Crump, "Final draft: Technical Support Document for a Protocol to Assess Asbestos-Related Risk," EPA # 9345.4-06. EPA, (2003).

66 Egilman, et al., "Exposing the 'myth' of ABC."

67 Egilman, Billings, "Abuse of epidemiology."

68 J. C. McDonald, "Asbestosis in chrysotile mines and mills," in: Bogovski P., ed. *Biological effects of asbestos; proceedings of a working conference,* (Lyon, France, October 1972) (Lyon; IARC Scientific Publications, 1973), p.8, 155–9.

69 Ibid.

70 A. Miller, Email re: Crump, to D. Egilman, June 20, 2005.

71 Cambridge Environmental Services, http://www.cambridgeenvironmental.com/services/litigation.htm., Accessed June 23, 2005.

72 Green L. Deposition. Cause No. 2004-03964. In Re: Asbestos Litigation. In the District Court of Harris County, Texas, 11th Judicial District, May 25, 2005.

73 D. Paustenbach, The roles of dose reconstruction and simulation studies in understanding historical exposure to asbestos. Montreal, Canada: Chrysotile Institute; 2006. http://www.chrysotile.com/en/conferences/speakers/dennis_paustenbach.aspx.

74 F. J. Solon, Interim position statement: Environmental health aspects of asbestos. May 31, 1996.

75 Cadwalader, Wickersham, & Taft, Letter to Dr. Selikoff, Oct 2,1964.

76 F. H. Edwards, Letter to L. Briley, Nov 29, 1965.

77 L. Grant, Letter to Brittingham R. President, Pittsburg Corning Corporation. Asbestos Textile Institute (ATI), Apr 22, 1966. Meeting minutes, Feb 4, 1971.

78 Ibid.

79 Ibid.

80 P. Bartrip, "Irving John Selikoff and the strange case of the missing medical degrees," *J Hist Med Allied Sci* 58 (2003): 3–33.

81 P. Bartrip, Deposition, *Kelly-Moore Paint Company vs. Dow Chemical*, No, 19785-BH02, District Court Brazoria County, 23rd Judicial District. Sep 22, 2003.

82 D. S. Egilman, G. Tweedale, J. McCulloch, W. Kovarik, B. Castleman, W. Longo et al., "P.W.J. Bartrip's attack on Irving J. Selikoff," *Am J Ind Med* 46 (2004): 151–5.

83 Jones, Day, Reavis & Pogue. *Corporate Activity Project. 2005*, http://tobaccodocuments.org/landman/37575.html.

84 I. Peterson, "Dow announces program to allay fear on dioxin," *New York Times*, June 2, 1983.

85 Hill & Knowlton (H&K), Program Recommendations, January 1, 1980.

86 Ibid.

87 Ibid.

88 Ibid.

89 Ibid.

90   "Third Party Technique. Center for Media and Democracy," *SourceWatch*, 2009, http://www.sourcewatch.org/index.php?title=Third_party_technique.   Accessed February 25, 2010.

91   Ibid.

92   Ibid.

93   Ibid.

94   Status Report of "Action Program" Activities. VCM-PVC Communications Committee, January 5, 1976, http://www.chemicalindustryarchives.org/search/pdfs/vinyl/19760115_004_ BA001939.PDF.

95   Hill & Knowlton (H&K), Public Relations Plan. Letter to James Gulick, Vice President of Planning and Administration. Brush Wellman Corporation, February 21, 1989.

96   Ibid.

97   H&K, Program Recommendations, January 1, 1980.

98   In Re: School Asbestos Litigation; *School District of Lancaster Manheim Township School District, Lampeter–Strasburg School District and Northeastern School District v. Lake Asbestos of Quebec, Ltd., et al.* March 17, 1988.

99   Hill & Knowlton (H&K), Preliminary capabilities presentation for the Alliance for Safe Buildings. June 11, 1984.

100 Ibid.

101 Americans for Nonsmokers' Rights Foundation (ANRF). The National Smokers Alliance exposed: a report on the activities of Philip Morris's #1 Front Group. http://www.no-smoke.org/document.php?id=257. Last updated June 1, 2005. Accessed February 25, 2010.

102 "Spinning out of control," *Ethical Consumer* 76 (Apr/May 2002).

103 Ibid.

104 Ibid.

105 Ibid.

106 PR Watch. Fourth Quarter Report, Center for Media and Democracy, 1997.

107 Ibid.

108 Ibid.

109 PR Watch. Third Quarter Report, Center for Media and Democracy, 2001.

110 Beder S. "Public relations' role in manufacturing grassroots coalitions," *Public Relations Quarterly* 43 (1998): 2.

111 PR Watch, Third Quarter, 2001.

112 PR Watch Fourth Quarter, 1997.

113 B. Burton, A. Rowell, "From patient activism to astroturf marketing," *First (95) Quarter Report.* Center for Media and Democracy, 10 (2003): 1.

114 Asbestos Textile Institute (ATI). Meeting minutes, 1973, http://www.ewg.org/reports/asbestos/documents/pdf/1973_ATI_Full. pdf. Accessed June 23, 2005.

115 Ibid.

116 B. Davis, "Rule breaker: In Washington, tiny think tank wields big stick on regulation," *Wall Street Journal*, July 16, 2004.

117 Ibid.

118 Ibid.

119 M. Dolny, "Right, center think tanks still most quoted," *Extra!* 18(3) (2005): 28–9.

120 *Daubert v Merrell Dow Pharmaceuticals, Inc.* WL: 9th Cir. 1995.

121 H&K Program Recommendations, 1980.

122 Ibid.

123 Ibid.

124 Ibid.

125 Jones, Day, Reavis & Pogue. Corporate Activity Project, 1998. http://tobaccod-ocuments.org/landman/37575.html.

126 W. M. Adler, "Will shill for nukes," *Austin Chronicle*, April 16, 2004.

127 Ibid.

128 D. Price, PR Watch. Second Quarter Report, Center for Media and Democracy. 2005.

129 Jones, Day, Reavis, & Pogue. Corporate Activity Project, 1998.

130 P. J. Hilts, *Smokescreen: the truth behind the tobacco industry cover-up* (Reading, MA: Addison-Wesley,1996).

131 Jones, Day, Reavis, & Pogue. Corporate Activity Project, 1998.

132 School Asbestos Litigation; *School District of Lancaster Manheim Township School District.*

133 VCM-PVC Communications Committee, 1976.

134 Leading Authorities, Inc. http://www.leadingauthorities.com., Accessed June 29, 2005.

135 J. Cohen, N. Solomon, "Tobacco wars: the first casualty is candor," *FAIR (Fairness & Accuracy in Reporting)*, July 20, 1994.

136 Ibid.

137 Stossel fabricated data on organics, researchers say. *FAIR*; August 1, 2000.

138 Agricultural Speakers Network (ASN),http://bureau.espeakers.com/agsn/.Accessed June 29, 2005.

139 FAIR, 2000.

140 Ibid.

141 "Code of Ethics and Professional Conduct," Radio-Television News Directors Association, September 14, 2000, http://www.rtdna.org/pages/media_items/code-of-ethics-and-professional-conduct48.php., Accessed February 26, 2010.

142 Ibid.

143 Ibid.

Chapter 3: A Battle Ground, Lennart Hardell

1 L. Hardell, "Soft-tissue sarcomas and exposure to phenoxy acids: a clinical observation,"*Läkartidningen* 74 (1977): 2753–4, (In Swedish).

2 R. Nilsson, "Chlorinated phenoxyacetic acids: evaluation of toxic effects on mammals including human beings,"*Produktkontrollbyrån. Statens Naturvårdsverk SNV PM* 527(Oktober 1974), (In Swedish).

3 "Polychlorinated-*para*-dioxins and polychlorinated dibenzofurans," *IARC Monographs on the Evaluation of Carcinogenic Risks to Humans*, Vol. 69, (1997) Lyon, France: IARC.

4   L. Hardell, "Pesticides, soft-tissue sarcoma and non-Hodgkin lymphoma: histori-
     cal aspects on the precautionary principle in cancer prevention," *Acta Oncol.* 47
     (2008): 347–54.

5   T. S. Carswell, H. K. Nason, "Properties and uses of pentachlorophenol," *Ind
     Engineer Chem* 30 (1938): 622.

6   Ibid.

7   R. Von Rumker, E. W. Lawless, A. F. Meiners, "Production, distribution, use
     and environmental impact potential of selected pesticides," EPA 540/1-74-001,
     Washington, DC. (1975), US Environmental Protection Agency.

8   E. W. Baader, H. J. Bauer, "Industrial intoxication due to pentachlorophenol," *Ind
     Med Surgery* 20 (1951): 286–90.

9   J. Kimmig, K. H. Schultz, "Occupational chloracne caused by aromatic cyclic
     ethers," *Dermatologica* 115 (1957): 540–6.

10   M. A. O'Malley, A. V. Carpenter, M. H. Sweeney, M. A. Fingerhut, D. A. Marlow, W.
     E. Halperin, C. G. Mathias, "Chloracne associated with employment in the pro-
     duction of pentachlorophenol," *Am J Ind Med* 17 (1990): 411–21.

11   K. Crow, "Chloracne: the chemical disease," *New Scientist* 78 (1978): 78–80.

12   R. Truhaut, G. Vitte, E. Boussemart, "Researches sur la toxicologie du pentachlo-
     rophénol. I. Propriétés. Caractérisation et dosage dans les milieux biologiques,"
     Arch Mal Prof 13 (1952): 561–7.

13   S. Nomura, "Studies on chlorophenol poisoning: report I. A clinical examination
     of workers exposed to pentachlorophenol," *J Sci Labor* (Tokyo) 29 (1953): 474.

14   D. Gordon, "How dangerous is pentachlorophenol?" *Med J Aust* 2 (1956): 485.

15   J. A. Menon, "Tropical hazards associated with the use of pentachlorophenol." *Br J
     Med* 11 (1958): 1156–8.

16   H. Bergner, P. Constantinidis, J. H. Martin, "Industrial pentachlorophenol poison-
     ing in Winnipeg," *Canad Med Assoc J* 92 (1965): 448–51.

17   R. W. Armstrong, E. R. Eichner, D. E. Klein, W. F. Barthel, J. W. Bennett, W. Jonsson,
     H. Bruce, L. E. Loveless, "Pentachlorophenol poisoning in a nursery for newborn
     infants. II. Epidemiologic and toxicologic studies," *J Pediatr* 75 (1969): 317–25.

18   G. E. Peterson, "The discovery and development of 2,4-D," *Agricultur Hist Rev* 41
     (1967): 243–53.

19   C. L. Hamner, H. B. Tukey, "The herbicidal action of 2,4-dichlorophenoxyacetic
     acid and 2,4,5-trichlorophenoxyacetic acid on bindweed," *Science* 100 (1944):
     154–5.

20   C. Trost, *Elements of Risk* (New York: New York Times Books, 1982).

21   Ibid.

22   A. H. Westing, (ed)., *Herbicides in war. The long-term ecological and human conse-
     quences. Stockholm International Peace Rearch Institute*, (London & Philadelphia:
     Taylor & Francis, 1984).

23   M. S. Meselson, A. H. Westing, J. D. Constable, R. R. Cook, "Preliminary Report
     of the Herbicides Assessment Commission of the American Association for the
     Advancers of Science," Washington DC, December 30, 1970.

24   Fransson P. "Control of birch in Northern Sweden with weed killers," *Statens
     skogsforskningsinstitut*, Sverige. 42(1) (1952) (In Swedish).

25 B. Kolmodin-Hedman, K. Erne, "Estimation of occupational exposure to phenoxy acids (2,4-D and 2,4,5-T). Further studies in assessment of toxic actions," *Arch. Toxicol. Suppl.* 4 (1980): 318–21.

26 W. S. Gump, "2,2′Dihydroxy-3,5,6,3′,5′,6′-hexachlorodiphenylmethane," US Patent 2,250,480, 29 July, to Burton T. Bush Inc., *Chem Abstr* 35 (1941): 7120(2).

27 Applied Research Laboratories, Inc. Dayton, NJ, "Subject Toxicity Study, Sample G-11," Pure. Index MX–155-C. September 18, 1939.

28 H. Halling, "Misstänkt samband mellan hexaklorofenexposition och missbild-ningsbörd," *Läkartidningen* 4 (1977): 542–6.

29 H Halling, "Suspected link between exposure to hexachlorophene and malformed infants," *Annals of New York Academy of Sciences* 320 (1979): 426–35.

30 G. Martin-Bouyer, R. Lebreton, M. Toga, P. D. Stolley, "Outbreak of accidental hexachlorophene poisoning in France," *Lancet* i (1982): 91–5.

31 Ibid.

32 J. Kimmig, K. H. Schultz, "Occupational chloracne caused by aromatic cyclic ethers," *Dermatologica* 115 (1957): 540–6.

33 N. E. Skelly, "Isolation and identification of possible acnegens from the caustic-insoluble portion of the products from the 2,4,5-trichlorophenol process," Dow Chemical Company, Report No. ALS 54-474, December 8, 1964.

34 Meselson, et al. Preliminary Report of the Herbicides, December 30, 1970.

35 IARC Vol 69, 1997.

36 L. Hardell, "Malignant lymphoma of histiocytic type and exposure to phenoxy-acetic acids or chlorophenols," *Lancet* i (1979): 55–6.

37 K. Hardell, M. Carlberg, L. Hardell, H. Björnfoth, I. Ericson, M. Eriksson, B. van Bavel, G. Lindström, "Concentrations of organohalogen compounds and titres of antibodies to Epstein-Barr virus antigens and the risk for non-Hodgkin lymphoma," *Oncology Reports* 21 (2009): 1567–76.

38 L. Hardell, M. Eriksson, "Is the decline of the increasing incidence of non-Hodgkin lymphoma in Sweden and other countries a result of cancer preventive measures?" *Environ Health Perspect* 111 (2003): 1704–6.

39 Socialstyrelsen. Statistikdabas för Cancer. http://www.socialstyrelsen.se/statistik/statistikdatabas/cancer (Accessed October 2, 2016).

40 Hardell, "Pesticides, soft-tissue sarcoma . . . . 2008."

41 J. Dreiher, E. Kordysh, "Non-Hodgkin lymphoma and pesticide exposure: 25 years of research," *Acta Haematol* 116 (2006): 153–64.

42 IARC Vol 69, 1997.

43 L. Hardell, M. Walker, B. Walhjalt, L. S. Friedman, E. D. Richter, "Secret ties to industry and conflicting interests in cancer research," *Am J Ind Med.* 50 (2007): 227–33.

44 Nilsson, "Chlorinated phenoxyacetic acids," 1974.

45 C. Ramel, ed. *Chlorinated phenoxyacetic acids and their dioxins. Ecological Bulletins/NFR 27*, Report from a Conference arranged by the Royal Swedish Academy of Sciences, Stockholm, Sweden, February 7–9, 1977. NFR Editorial Service, 1978.

46 Nilsson, "Chlorinated phenoxyacetic acids," 1974.

47 Westing, *Hervicides in war . . .* 1984.

48 United States of America—Before the Environmental Protection Agency. *In the matter of the hearing of 2,4,5-T and Silvex. The Dow Chemical Company, et al.* Docket No. 415, et al. 1980.

49 P. Cole, Direct testimony before the Environmental Protection Agency of the United States of America. Washington DC, 1980, Exhibit 860, pp. 2–24.

50 "Agent Orange" Product Liability Litigation. United States District Court Eastern District of New York MDL No. 381, 1984.

51 Institute of Medicine. *Veterans and Agent Orange. Health effects of herbicides used in Vietnam,* (Washington DC: National Academy Press, 1994) (updated 1996).

52 *Royal Commission on the use and effects of chemical agents on Australian personnel in Vietnam,* Final Report, Vols. 1–9. Australian Government Publishing Service, Canberra, 1985.

53 Monsanto Australia Limited. Axelson and Hardell—The odd men out. Submission to the Royal Commission on the use and effects of chemical agents on Australian personnel in Vietnam, Exhibit 1981, 1985,pp 64–9, 146–237.

54 Doll's letter to The Hon. Mr. Justice Phillip Evatt, DSC, LLB. December 4, 1985. 40-X-016. Green College, Oxford OX2 6UE, England.

55 O. Axelson, ed. *Rebuttals of the final report on cancer by the Royal Commission on the use and effects of chemical agents on Australian personnel in Vietnam.* Report No. Liu-YMED-R-6. University of Linköping, Linköping, Sweden, 1986.

56 Comments by Department of Veteran's Affairs, Attachment C, Woden, Australia, May 19, 1988.

57 Ibid.

58 M. J. Walker, 2005. *Company Men and the Public Health: Part Two, Sir Richard Doll: Death, Dioxin and PVC,* www.dipmat.unipg.it/~mamone/sci-dem/contri/walker.pdf (Accessed October 3, 2016).

59 Hardell, et al. "Secret ties to industry . . ." 2007.

60 Walker, 2016.

61 Wellcome, 1984, Doll Papers PP/DOL/B/5/3 Correspondence B. Bennett to R. Doll 16. 11. 84.

62 Wellcome, 1986, Doll Papers. PP/DOL/B/5/3. B. Gaffey to R. Doll 01/05/86. "Once again I enclose two copies of a letter extending your consulting agreement with Monsanto. We have changed the fee from $1,000 per day to $1,500 per day."

63 Wellcome, 1986b, Doll Papers PP/DOL/B/5/3. B. Doll to Gaffey, 11/07/86.

64 A. L. Young, K. H. Kang, B. M. Shepard, "Chlorinated dioxins as herbicide contaminants," *Environ Sci Technol* 17(11) (1983): 530A-40A.

65 G. Reggiani, "Localized contamination with TCDD-Seveso, Missouri and other areas. In: Halogenated Biphenyls, Terphenyls, Naphthalenes, Dibenzodioxins and related products," R. Kimborough, ed. *Elsevier/North-Holland Biomedical Press* (1980): pp 303–71.

66 A. L. Young, G. M. Reggiani, eds. *Agent Orange and its associated dioxin: Assessment of a cotroversy,* (Amsterdam:Elsevier (Biomedical Division), 1988).

67 Axelson, 1986.

68 Veteran's Affairs, 1988.

69 B. O'Keefe, F. B. Smith, eds. *Medicine at war,* (St. Leonards, Australia: Allen & Unwin, 1994).

70   L. Hardell, M. Eriksson, O. Axelson, "Agent Orange in war medicine: an aftermath myth," *Int J Health Serv.* 28 (1998): 715–24.

71   B. Walhjalt, "Greenwashing: an introduction," *Medikament* 6 (2002): 72-80, (In Swedish).

72   B. Walhjalt, *On reality-- images, experiences, and distortions: industrial ties in three acts,* https://web.archive.org/web/20070427132223/http://www.gbg.bonet.se/bwf/art/industrialTies.html (Accessed October 3, 2016).

73   L. Hardell, "From phenoxyacetic acids to cellular telephones: Is there historic evidence of the precautionary principle in cancer prevention?" *Int J Health Services* 4 (2004): 25–37.

74   Hardell, et al. "Secret ties to industry . . .," 2007.

75   See previous chapter, Egilman, The Basis of Bad Science.

76   H. O. Adami, "Can studies by a single investigator override collective evidence? The case of dioxin," *Organohalogen Compounds* 54 (2001): 403–4.

77   J. Mandel, "Epidemiology studies of Vietnam Veterans: A critical review," *Organohalogen Compounds* 54 (2001): 400–1.

78   D. Trichopoulos, "No evidence that dioxin is a human carcinogen," *Organohalogen Compounds* 54 (2001): 409–11.

79   IARC Vol 69, 1997.

80   J. Mandel, email to Trichopoulos and Adami: meeting in Korea and review of SAB report. April 26, 2001.

81   H. O. Adami, P. Cole, J. Mandel, H. Pastitides, T. B. Starr, D. Trichopolous, "Dioxin and cancer," Report, August 7, 2000, Submission to EPA.

82   S. M. Hays, L. Aylward, "Temporal trends in body-burden suggest that dioxin exposures in the general population have declined significantly," *Organohalogen Compounds* 52 (2001): 214–6.

83   S. M. Hays, L. Aylward, B. Finley, D. Paustenbach, "Implementing a cancer risk assessment for dioxin using a margin of exposure approach and an internal measure of dose," *Organohalogen Compounds.* 52 (2001) 225–8.

84   K. Connor, B. Finley, "The need for TEFs based on internal measures of dose: an assessment of body burden TEQs," *Organohalogen Compounds* 53: (2001) 53:247–50.

85   D. Paustenbach, "The United States EPA Science Advisory Board Report (2001) on the EPA dioxin reassessment," *Organohalogen Compounds* 53 (2001): 241–6.

86   K. A. Fehling, M. V. Ruby, D. J. Paustenbach, "*In vitro* bioaccessability study of low concentrations (50–350 ppt TEQ) of dioxin/furans in weatherhead soils," *Organohalogen Compounds* 52 (2001): 180–4.

87   B. Sun, A. Sarofim, E. Eddings, D. Paustenbach, "Reducing PCDD/PCDF formation and emission from a hazardous waste combustion facility: technological identification, implementation, and achievement," *Organohalogen Compounds* 54 (2001): 278–83.

88   P. Cole, D. Trichopoulos, H. Pastides, T. Starr, J. S. Mandel, J. S., "Dioxin and cancer: a critical review," *Regul Toxicol Pharmacol* 38(3) (2003): 378–88.

89   IARC Vol 69, 1997.

90   Monsanto 2002 (website). *Backgrounder: Glyphosate: Response to non-Hodgkin's Lymphoma Allegations,* www.monsanto.com—nhl_backgr.pdf (Accessed October 2, 2016).

91 L. Hardell, M. Eriksson, "A case-control study of non-Hodgin lymphoma and exposure to pesticides," *Cancer* 85 (1999): 1353–60.

92 H. O. Adami, D. Trichopolous, "Review of the study by Hardell and Eriksson on non-Hodgkin lymphoma and exposure to pesticides," published in *Cancer* 85 (1999): 1353-60. Unpublished review. Can be requested from Monsanto's Public Affairs Director for Agricultural Chemicals as 314-694-3546.

93 For more details, see E. D. Richter, Expert Opinion, February 11, 2004, for *Physicians for Human Rights v. Government of Israel.*

94 M. Dallal, Petition 2887/04 filed on 22 March 2004. On behalf of four Arab Bedouin citizens of Israel and eight human rights organizations: Physicians for Human Rights-Israel; the Association of Forty; the Forum for Co-Existence in the Negev; the Negev Company for Land & Man; Ltd.; Bustan for Peace; the Association for Support and Defense of Bedouin Rights in Israel; the Arab Association for Human Rights (HRA); The Galilee Society; and Adalah. Against: the Israel Lands Administration (ILA), the Ministry of Industry and Trade, the Ministry of Agriculture. www.court.gov.il and www.adalah.org (Accessed October 3, 2016).

95 Hardell, Eriksson, "A case-control study . . ." 1999.

96 M. Eriksson, L, Hardell, M. Carlberg, M. Akerman, "Pesticide exposure as risk factor for non-Hodgkin lymphoma including histopathological subgroup analysis," *Int J Cancer* 123 (2008): 1657–63.

97 K. Z. Guyton, D. Loomis, Y. Grosse, F. El Ghissassi, L. Benbrahim-Tallaa, N. Guha, C. Scoccianti, H. Mattock, K. Straif, "International Agency for Research on Cancer Monograph Working Group," IARC, Lyon, France. "Carcinogenicity of tetra-chlorvinphos, parathion, malathion, diazinon, and glyphosate," *Lancet Oncol* pii (March 20, 2015): S1470-2045(15)70134-8. doi: 10.1016/S1470-2045(15)70134-8.

98 B. L. Waddell, S. H. Zahm, D. Baris, D. D. Weisenburger, F. Holmes, L. F. Burmeister, K. P. Cantor, A. Blair, "Agricultural use of organophosphate pesticides and the risk of non-Hodgkin's lymphoma among male farmers (United States)" *Cancer Causes Control* 12 (2001) 509–17.

99 H. H. McDuffie, P. Pahwa, J. R. McLaughlin, J. J. Spinelli, S. Fincham, J. A. Dosman, D. Robson, L. F. Skinnider, N. W. Choi, "Non-Hodgkin's lymphoma and specific pesticide exposures in men: cross-Canada study of pesticides and health," *Cancer Epidemiol Biomarkers Prev 001* 10: 1155–63.

100 Eriksson, et al., "Pesticide exposure . . . " 2008.

101 Guyton et al., IARC, 2015.

102 J. D. Boice, Jr, J. K. McLaughlin, "Epidemiologic studies of cellular telephones and cancer risk—a review. Statens Strålskyddsinstitut rapport," *(Swedish Radiation Protection Authority Report).* 2002:16. http://www.stralsakerhetsmyndigheten.se/Publikationer/Rapport/Stralskydd/2002/200216/ (Accessed October 3, 2016).

103 L. Hardell, A. Hallquist, K. Hansson Mild, M. Carlberg, A. Påhlson, A. Lilja, "Cellular and cordless telephones and the risk for brain tumors," *Eur. J. Cancer. Prev.* 11 (2002): 377-86.

104 F. Söderqvist, M. Carlberg, L. Hardell, "Review of four publications on the Danish cohort study on mobile phone subscribers and risk of brain tumors," Rev. *Environ. Health* 27 (1) (2012): 51-8.

105 *Christopher Newman, et al. v. Motorola, Inc., et al.* In the United States District Court for the District of Maryland. Civil No. CCB-00-2609.

106 Letter from Mr. Tom Watson, defendant lawyer for Motorola, dated January 18, 2002 and referee comments from fax 301 517 4063 International Epidemiology Institute fax dated 11/19/2001.

107 Hardell, "From phenoxyacetic acids to cellular telephones . . ." 2004.

108 K. Hansson Mild, L. Hardell, M. Kundi, M-O Mattsson, "Mobile telephones and cancer: Is there really no evidence of an association?" (Review), *Int. J. Molecular Medicine* 12 (2003): 67-72.

109 O. Nyrén, L. Yin, S. Josefsson, J. K. McLaughlin, W. J. Blot, M. Engqvist, L. Hakelius, J. D. Boice, Jr, H. O. Adami, "Risk of connective tissue disease and related disorders among women with breast implants: a nation-wide retrospective cohort study in Sweden," *BMJ* 316 (1998): 417–22.

110 J. K. McLaughlin, O. Nyrén, W. J. Blot, L. Yin, S. Josefsson, J. F. Fraumeni, Jr, H. O. Adami, "Cancer risk among women with cosmetic breast implants: a population-based cohort study in Sweden," *J. Natl. Cancer Inst* 90 (1998): 156-8.

111 J. K. McLaughlin, L. Lipworth, J. P. Fryzek, W. Ye, R. E. Tarone, O. Nyren, "Long-term cancer risk among Swedish women with cosmetic breast implants: an update of a nationwide study," *J Natl Cancer Inst.* 19 (April 19, 2006): 557-60.

112 Interphone Study Group, "Brain tumor risk in relation to mobile telephone use: results of the INTERPHONE international case-control study," *Int. J. Epidemiol.* 39 (2010): 675-94.

113 R. Baan, Y. Grosse, B. Lauby-Secretan, F. El Ghissassi, V. Bouvard, L. Benbrahim-Tallaa, N. Guha, F. Islami, L. Galichet, K. Straif, "Carcinogenicity of radiofrequency electromagnetic fields," *Lancet Oncol.* 12 (2011): 624-6.

114 "IARC Monographs on the Evaluation of Carcinogenic Risks to Humans, Volume 102," *Non-Ionizing radiation, Part 2: Radiofrequency Electromagnetic Fields. International Agency for Research on Cancer,* Lyon, France, 2013, http://monographs.iarc.fr/ENG/Monographs/vol102/mono102.pdf (Accessed October 3, 2016).

115 L. Hardell, M. Carlberg, K. Hansson Mild, "Pooled analysis of two case-control studies on use of cellular and cordless telephones and the risk for malignant brain tumors diagnosed in 1997-2003," *Int. Arch. Occup. Environ. Health* 79 (2006): 630-9.

116 L. Hardell, M. Carlberg, K. Hansson Mild, "Pooled analysis of two case-control studies on the use of cellular and cordless telephones and the risk of benign brain tumors diagnosed during 1997-2003," *Int. J. Oncol.* 28 (2006): 509-18.

117 L. Hardell, M. Carlberg, K. Hansson Mild, "Pooled analysis of case-control studies on malignant brain tumors and the use of mobile and cordless phones including living and deceased subjects," *Int. J. Oncol.* 38 (2011): 1465-74.

118 Interphone Study Group, *Int. J. Epidemiol.* 39 (2010): 675–94.

119 Interphone Study Group. "Acoustic neuroma risk in relation to mobile telephone use: results of the INTERPHONE international case-control study," *Cancer Epidemiol* 35 (2011): 453-64.

120 E. Cardis, B. K. Armstrong, J. D. Bowman, G. G. Giles, M. Hours, D. Krewski, M. McBride, M. E. Parent, S. Sadetzki, A. Woodward, J. Brown, A. Chetrit, J. Figuerola, C. Hoffmann, A. Jarus-Hakak, L. Montestruq, L. Nadon, L. Richardson, R. Villegas, M. Vrijheid, "Risk of brain tumors in relation to estimated RF dose from mobile phones: results from five Interphone countries," *Occup. Environ. Med.* 68 (2011): 631-40.

121 H. O. Adami, A. Ahlbom, A. Ekbom, L. Hagmar, M. Ingelman-Sundberg, Opinion—"Experts who talk rubbish," *Bioelectromagnetics Society Newsletter* 162 (2001): 162:4-5.

122 Hardell, et al. "Secret ties to industry . . . " 2007.

123 *REFLEX. Risk Evaluation of Potential Environmental Hazards From Low Frequency Electromagnetic Field Exposure Using Sensitive in vitro Methods.* Final Report 2005, http://www.itis.ethz.ch/downloads/REFLEX_Final percent20Report_171104.pdf (Accessed October 3, 2016).

124 D. Trichopoulos, H. O. Adami, "Cellular telephones and brain tumors," *N Engl J Med* 344 (2001): 133-4.

125 P. D. Inskip, R. E. Tarone, E. E. Hatch, *et al.* "Cellular-telephone use and brain tumors," *N Engl J Med* 344 (2001): 79-86.

126 Hardell, et al. "Secret ties to industry . . . " 2007.

127 D. Michaels, *Doubt is Their Product. How Industry's Assault on Science Threatens Your Health* (New York: Oxford University Press, 2008).

128 U. Björksten, Vetenskap ur funktion. Forskningen om biologiska effekter av mobiltelefoni ("Science out of order. The research on biological effects from use of mobile phones"), Atlantis, Stockholm, Sweden 2006, page 64. (In Swedish)

129 Hardell, et al. "Secret ties to industry . . . " 2007.

130 M. Kundi, "The controversy about a possible relationship between mobile phone use and cancer," *Environ Health Perpect* 117 (2009): 316-24.

131 M. N. Mead, "Tough call: Challenges to assessing cancer effects of mobile phone use," *Environ Health Perpect* 117 (2009): A116.

132 S.K. Myung, W. Ju, D. D. McDonnell, G. Kazinets, C. T. Cheng, J. M. Moskowitz, "Mobile phone use and risk of tumors: a meta-analysis," *J. Clin. Oncol.* 27 (2009): 5565-72.

133 P. J. Mink, H. O. Adami, D. Trichopoulos, N. L. Britton, J. S. Mandel, "Pesticides and prostate cancer: a review of epidemiologic studies with specific agricultural information," *Eur J Cancer Prev* 17 (2008): 97-110.

134 D. D. Alexander, P. J. Mink, H. O. Adami, E. T. Chang, P. Cole, J. S. Mandel, D. Trichopoulos, "The non-Hodgkin lymphomas: a review of the epidemiologic literature," *Int J Cancer* 120: (2007): 1-39.

135 Guyton et al., IARC 2015.

136 P. Boffetta, H. O. Adami, S. C. Berry, J. S. Mandel, "Atrazine and cancer: a review of the epidemiologic evidence," *Eur J Cancer Prev.* 22(2) (2013): 169-80.

137 E. T. Chang, P. Boffetta, H. O. Adami, P. Cole, J. S. Mandel, "A critical review of the epidemiology of Agent Orange/TCDD and prostate cancer," *Eur J Epidemiol* 29(10) (2014): 667–723.

138 E. T. Chang, H. O. Adami, P. Boffetta, P. Cole, T. B. Starr, J. S. Mandel, "A critical review of perfluorooctanoate and perfluorooctanesulfonate exposure and cancer risk in humans," *Crit Rev Toxicol.* 44S (2014): 1:1–81.

139 E. Hardell, A. Kärrman, B. van Bavel, J. Bao, M. Carlberg, L. Hardell, "Case-control study on perfluorinated alkyl acids (PFAAs) and the risk of prostate cancer," *Environ. Int.* 63 (2014): 35–9.

140 www.socialstyrelsen.se

141 G. L. Henriksen, N. S. Ketchum, J. E. Michalek, et al. "Serum dioxin and diabetes mellitus in veterans of Operation Ranch Hand," *Epidemiology* 8 (1997): 252–8.

142 N. S. Ketchum, J. E. Michalek, *A Matched Analysis of Diabetes Mellitus and Herbicide Exposure in Veterans of Operation Ranch Hand*, (Brooks City-Base, TX: United States Air Force, 2006).

143 J. E. Michalek, N. S. Ketchum, R. C. Tripathi, "Diabetes mellitus and 2,3,7,8-etra-chlorodibenzo-p-dioxin elimination in veterans of Operation Ranch Hand. J Toxicol," *Environ Health A.* 66 (2003): 211–21.

144 J. E. Michalek, M. Pavuk, "Diabetes and cancer in veterans of Operation Ranch Hand after adjustment for calendar period, days of spraying, and time spent in Southeast Asia," *J Occup Environ Med.* 50 (2008): 330–40.

145 Institute of Medicine, *Veterans and Agent Orange: Update 2012.* (Washington, DC: National Academy Press, 2014).

146 M. Goodman, K. M. Narayan, D. Flanders, E. T. Chang, H. O. Adami, P.. Boffetta, J. S. Mandel, "Dose-response relationship between serum 2,3,7,8-Tetrachlorodibenzo-p-Dioxin and diabetes mellitus: A meta-analysis," *Am J Epidemiol.* 181 (2015): 374–84.

147 Ibid.

148 Microwave News. http://www.microwavenews.com/IARC.RF.Ahlbom.html (Accessed October 3, 2016).

149 Baan, et al., Carcinogencity of radiofrequency . . ." 2011.

150 IARC Volume 102. 2013.

151 A. Ahlbom, M. Feychting, "Mobile telephones and brain tumors," *BMJ.* Oct 19, 2011, 343:d6605. doi: 10.1136/bmj.d6605.

152 Hardell, et al. "Secret ties to industry . . ." 2007.

153 Michaels, *Doubt is Their Product,* 2008.

Chapter 4: Losing the War on Cancer, Richard Clapp

1 (http://abcnews.go.com/blogs/health/2013/12/18/outrage-at-the-increasingly-high-cost-of-cancer-drugs/).

2 "International Agency for Research on Cancer (IARC)" Press Release No. 223, 12 December 2013. *Latest world cancer statistics. Global cancer buden rises to 14.1 million new cases in 2012: Marked increase in breast cancer must be addressed. IARC.* Lyon, France.

3 F. Bray, J. S. Ren, E. Masuyer, et al. "Global estimates of cancer prevalence for 27 sites in the adult population in 2008" *Int J Cancer* 132 (2013): 1133–45.

4 Bray, et al. 2013.

5   "International Agency for Research on Cancer (IARC)," *Cancer incidence in five continents.* IARC. Lyon, France. (http://ci5.iarc.fr/ accessed on December 17, 2013).

6   A. J. Sasco, "Cancer and globalization," *Biomedicine and Pharmacotherapy* 62 (2008): 110–21.

7   P. Raskin, T. Banuri, G. Gallopin, et al., *Great transition. The promise and lure of the times ahead* (Boston:Stockholm Environment Institute, 2002).

8   V. J. Cogliano, R. Baan, K. Straif, et al., "Preventable exposures associated with human cancers," *J Natl Cancer Inst* 103 (2011): 1827–39.

9   WHO, *World Cancer Report 2008. International Agency for Research on Cancer.* Lyon, France. 2008.

10 D. Michaels, M. Jones, "Doubt is their product,"*Scientific American* 292 (2005): 96–101.

Chapter 5: Greenwashing in science–a Swedish perspective, Bo Walhjalt

1   H. Österman, *Han spionerade åt tobaksjätte (He was a spy for the giant tobacco company).* Aftonbladet 7/12 2001 and Hans Österman, *Wahren: Jag såg inga bekymmer (Wahren: I did not see any problems).* Aftonbladet 7/12 2001. Via internet: www.aftonbladet.se/vss/nyheter/story/0,2789,112166,00.html and www.aftonbladet.se/vss/nyheter/story/0,2789,112165,00.html.

2   L. Söderberg, *Nobelprofessor hyrs av kemijätte (Nobel Committee professor hired by large chemical company).* Aftonbladet, 17/12, 2001. Via internet: www.aftonbladet.se/vss/nyheter/story/0,2789,114883,00.html and www.aftonbladet.se/vss/nyheter/story/0,2789,115077,00.html.

3   B. Forsberg, *Sponsrad Forskning. Om jag kliar din rygg. (Supported Research. If I itch your back) Veckans Affärer.* 10: pp. 18-19, March 4, 2002.

4   M. Lambe, E. Hallhagen, G. Boëthius, "Cyniskt spel inom tobaksindustrin. Tvångspublicerade interna dokument avslöjar mångåriga ansträngningar att förneka eller tona ner tobakens negativa hälsoeffekter," (A cynical game within tobacco industry). *Läkartidningen.* 99 (2002): 2756–62.

5   K. E. Tallmo, *Philip Morris gav hemliga anslag till svensk professor (Philip Morris gave secret grants to a Swedish professor). Dagens Forskning.* 12: 2002. Via internet: www.dagensforskning.se/Article.asp?article_id=1190.

6   K. E. Tallmo, *Rylander: Jag har aldrig varit konsult åt Philip Morris, (Rylander: I have never been a consultant for Philip Morris) Dagens Forskning.* 12:2002. Via internet www.dagensforskning.se/Article.asp?article_id=1191.

7   R. Rylander, "*Dagens Forskning handskas vårdslöst med källmaterialet.*" (*Dagens Forskning is not careful about original data*). *Dagens Forskning.* Via internet www.dagensforskning.se/Article.asp?article_Id=1170 - Dagens Forskning has promised new articles.

8   J. Weman, *Orkar du svälja det här? (Are you enough strong to swallow this?) Aftonbladet.* 18/7, 2002. Via Internet: www.aftonbladet.se/vss/kultur/story/0,2789,185528,00.html.

9   T. Heldmark, *Universitetens dolda krafter: Allt fler "köpta" professorer. (The secret power within universities: More and more "bought" professors.* Dagens Nyheter 1/8 2002 (also another article in the same issue) and Thomas Heldmark, *"Universiteten på väg att bli bolag", (The universites are about to be companies). Dagens Nyheter 2/8, 2002.

10   B. Rothstein, *Lobbyister eller forskare?, (Lobbyists or researchers?),* Aftonbladet 1/8, 2002. Via Internet: www.aftonbladet.se/vss/kultur/story/0,2789,189450,00.html.

11   B. Sjö, *"Sponsrad forskning mindre kritisk", (Sponsored research is less critical)* Sydsvenska Dagbladet 12/8, 2002. This article is about research that gets grants from the drug industry. Similar investigations have been made about tobacco industry and the chemical industry with similar results. For tobacco industry see: Barnes D., Bero L. *Industry-funded research and conflict of interest: an analysis of research sponsored by the tobacco industry through the Center for Indoor Air Research.* J. Health Polit. Policy Law. 21: 515-542, 1996. For chemical industry: Center for Public Integrity: www.publicintegrity.org/dtaweb/index.asp?L1=20& L2=33&L3=37&L4=0&L5=0&State= This website is a complement to: Fagin D, Lavelle M, and The Center For Public Integrity: Toxic Deception: *How the Industry Manipulates Science, Bends the Law, and Endangers Your Health.* Second Edition. Common Courage Press, 1999. ISBN: 1-56751-162-7.

12   Greenwashing may be defined in different ways. For one example and a little history see for example: www.corpwatch.org/campaigns/PCD.jsp?articleid=243 and www.corpwatch.org/campaigns/PCC.jsp?topicid=102.

13   David Michaels, Eula Bingham, Les Boden, Richard Clapp, Lynn R. Goldman, Polly Hoppin, Sheldon Krimsky, Celeste Monforton, David Ozonoff, Anthony Robbins, "Advice Without Dissent," *Science* 298 (October 25, 2002): 703.

14   For much information about the Anniston case see: www.chemicalindustryar-chives.org/dirtysecrets/annistonindepth/intro.asp or the gathered information in pdf file: www.chemicalindustryarchives.org/dirtysecrets/annistonindepth/indepth.pdf.

15   Confidential Report of Aroclor, Ad Hoc Committee; October 2, 1969. The citation either in the pdf file in reference (14) or via: www.chemicalindustryarchives.org/dirtysecrets/annistonindepth/toxicity.asp.

16   (http://www.techjournal.org/2007/05/rtp percentE2 percent80 percent99s-ciit-centers-becoming-hamner-institutes/).

17   A colleague of Sir Richard Doll who was involved in organizing the CIIT then lectured there.

18   D. Fagin, M. Lavelle, and The Center For Public Integrity: *Toxic Deception: How the Industry Manipulates Science, Bends the Law, and Endangers Your Health.* Second Edition. Common Courage Press, 1999. ISBN: 1-56751-162-7, pp 31-32— here the history and strategy is related. This part may be found as an abstract form the book via Internet: www.publicintegrity.org/dtaweb/index.asp?L1=20&L2=33 &L3=20&L4=0&L5=0.

19   A more detailed commentary may be found in Peter Montague: "Let's Stop Wasting Our Time," *Rachel's Environment & Health Weekly,* #553 (July 3,

1997) Via Internet: www.rachel.org/bulletin/bulletin.cfm?Issue_ID=570 and Peter Montague: "Toxic Deception - Part 2," *Rachel's Environment & Health Weekly*, #554 (July 10, 1997) Via Internet: www.rachel.org/bulletin/bulletin. cfm?Issue_ID=569.

20 Lambe, et al. 2002.

21 *Kupé* (SJs kundtidning) (The customer newspaper from Swedish Railways) 8/2002, page 10.

22 See: http://info.ki.se/ki/organization/cmi/sbspages/ostros.htm.

23 *Science*, September 28, 2002.

24 *Dagens Nyheter*, June 7, 2002.

25 B. Walhjalt, "Greenwashing—an introduction," *Medikament*. 6 (2002a): 72–80. (In Swedish).

26 M. Starendal, *Adamis obegripliga naivitet. (It is unbelievable how naive Adami is).* Dagens Forskning 1/2003.

27 Ibid.

28 Ibid.

29 Michaels, et al., "Advice Without Dissent," 2002.

30 The setting up of Britains first medical lobby group was first discussed in the British Medical Journalists Association. This organization was the first to be sponsored by the pharmaceutical industry.

31 *Integrity in Science* keeps an updated page with links to documents related to the WHO/IARC including the letters referred to. http://cspinet.org/integrity/iarc. html.

32 Michaels, et al., "Advice Without Dissent," 2002.

33 J. Huff, "IARC Monographs, industry influence, and upgrading, downgrading, and under-grading chemicals," *Int J Occup Environ Health* 8 (2002): 249-70.

34 Ibid.

35 Starendal, 2003.

36 T. Heldmark, *Forskarprotester mot industriintressen i WHO. (Researchers protest against industrial interests in WHO).* Dagens Forskning 23/2002.

37 T. Heldmark, *Regeringens WHO-kandidat saknar stöd i forskar-Sverige. (The WHO-candidate by the government has not support among researchers in Sweden).* Dagens Forskning 5/2003.

38 E. P. Thomson book on Warwick University.

39 In Britain this question has been raised in relation to members of the now defunct Revolutionary Communist Party and their communion with pharmaceutical lobby groups and high flying liberal corporatists inside Britain's new bio-bourgeoisie.

40 Thomas Heldmark: *KI-forskare kritiserar cancerlarm på uppdrag av kemisk industri. (KI-researcher criticizes cancer alarm commissoned by the chemical industry).* Dagens Forskning 18/2002.

41 Thomas Heldmark: *Cancerfonden kollar inte forskares vandel. (The Swedish Cancer Fund does not check moral of researcher).* Dagens Forskning 19/2002.

42 Svenska Dagbladet, September 3, 2001.

43 O. Akre, H. A. Boyd, M. Ahlgren, et al., "Maternal and Gestational Risk Factors for Hypospadias," *Environ Health Perspect* 116 (2008): 1071-6.

44 *Forskning NU* s. 163, 2001, By the Swedish Cancerfonden.

45 Report of sidelines. Karolinska Institutet. Dnr 1123/01-209.

46 www.mednobel.ki.se/mednobel/assembly.html.

47 A presentation of LRI is found at Internet: www.cefic.org/lri/Templates/shwStory.asp?NID=19&HID=284.

48 In: *LRI Annual Progress Report 2001*, page 6, gives a list of the members at the scientific board. Via Internet: www.cefic.org/lri/Files/Publications/Annual Report 2001 FINAL.pdf (page. 8 in the pdf-document).

49 In one news letter from LRI with the title *Mother Nature is not what she was* . . . the start of the introduction: "Frogs growing extra limbs . . . Alligators and fish feminising. . ." and continues: "About eight years ago, American biologists noticed that male alligators near a DDT spill in Florida were feminizing. Some six years ago, British scientists found that male fish on the settlement lagoons of a sewage treatment works had become partly feminized. At the same time, five-limbed frogs started appearing and the male half of the human population was told they were only half the men their grandfathers used to be." It is an alarming description of facts and it is formulated in a way as it was taken from the environmental movement. Nobody can suspect that industry is behind this description of problems. (c.f. what Howlett says in the later part of reference no. 33 above). In the text the viewpoint of industry is given. It says: "Regarding human health, despite considerable study, there is—at this point—no evidence for a relationship between exposure to low levels of chemicals present in the environment and adverse health effects." In that way a one-sided memorial is presented when it is given as if it is a true description of how the scientific community in general considers real facts. The news letter can be found as a pdf-file: www.cefic.org/lri/Files/Publications/update2.pdf.

50 The project is presented via Internet: research.kib.ki.se/e-uven/show_project.cfm?projects_no=C81665.

51 P. Boffetta, H. O. Adami, S. C. Berry, J. S. Mandel, "Atrazine and cancer: a review of the epidemiologic evidence," *Eur J Cancer Prev.* 22 (2013): 169-80.

52 Rothstein, *Lobbyister eller forskare?*

53 E. K. Ong, S. A. Glantz, "Constructing "Sound Science" and "Good Epidemiology": Tobacco, Lawyers, and Public Relations Firms," *Am J Publ Health* 91 (2001): 1749-57. Full text via Internet: www.smokefreeforhealth.org/studies/OngGlantz.htm.

54 Soderberg, 2001.

Chapter 6: Industry influences on cancer epidemiology, Neil Pearce

1 N. Pearce, "The rise and rise of corporate epidemiology and the narrowing of epidemiology's vision," *Int J Epidemiol.* 36: (2007): 713–7.

2 N. Pearce, "Corporate influences on epidemiology, *Int J Epidemiol.* 37 (2008): 46–53.

3   N. Pearce, "The distribution and determinants of epidemiologic research," *Int J Epidemiol.* 37 (2008): 65–8.

4   This chapter is largely based on material from three papers published in the *International Journal of Epidemiology* endnotes and I thank the editors of the journal for permission to reproduce this material. The Centre for Public Health Research is supported by a program grant from the Health Research Council of New Zealand.

5   M. Porta, S. Greenland, J. Last, eds., *A dictionary of epidemiology* (Oxford: Oxford University Press, 2008).

6   G. C. Kabat, *Hyping health risks: environmental hazards in daily life and the science of epidemiology* (New York: Columbia University Press, 2008).

7   N. Pearce, "Review of: Kabat GC. Hyping health risks: environmental hazards in daily life and the science of epidemiology," *Int J Epidemiol.* 38 (2009): 1746–8.

8   P. D. Stolley, "When genius errs: Fisher, R.A. and the lung cancer controversy," *Am J Epidemiol.* 133 (1991): 416–25.

9   R. Doll, A. Bradford Hill, "Smoking and carcinoma of the lung: preliminary report," *BMJ* 2 (1950): 739–48.

10 E. L. Wynder, E. A. Graham, "Tobacco smoking as a possible etiologic factor in bronchiogenic carcinoma: a study of 684 proved cases," *JAMA* 143 (1950): 329–36.

11 S. Chapman, "The hot air on passive smoking," *BMJ* 316 (1998): 945.

12 J. A. Francis, A. K. Shea, J. M. Samet, "Challenging the epidemiologic evidence on passive smoking: tactics of tobacco industry expert witnesses," *Tobacco Control.* 15 (2006): 68–76.

13 E. K. Ong, S. A. Glantz, "Constructing 'sound science' and 'good epidemiology': tobacco, lawyers, and public relations firms," *Am J Public Health.* 91 (2001): 1749–57.

14 D. A. Savitz, S. Greenland, P. D. Stolley, J. L. Kelsey, Scientific standards of criticism: a reaction to "Scientific standards in epidemiologic studies of the menace of daily life." by A. R. Feinstein, *Epidemiology.* 1 (1990): 78–83.

15 S. Greenland, "Science versus advocacy: the challenge of Dr. Feinstein," *Epidemiology* 1 (1990): 64–72.

16 G. Davey Smith, S. Ebrahim, "Epidemiology: is it time to call it a day?" *Int J Epidemiol* 3011 (2001): 1–11.

17 A. R. Feinstein, "Scientific standards in epidemiologic studies of the menace of daily life," *Science* 242 (1988): 1257–63.

18 G. Taubes, "Epidemiology faces its limits. Science," 269 (1995): 164–9.

19 Smith, Ebrahim, 2001.

20 J. Siemiatycki, S. Wacholder, R. Dewar, L. Wald, D. Begin, L. Richardson, K. Rosenman, M. Gérin, "Smoking and degree of occupational exposure: are internal analyses in cohort studies likely to be confounded by smoking status?" *Am J Ind Med.* 13 (1988): 59–69.

21 H. Checkoway, N. Pearce, D. Kriebel, *Research methods in occupational epidemiology*, 2nd ed. (New York: Oxford University Press, 2004).

22 S. Greenland, "The need for critical appraisal of expert witnesses in epidemiology and statistics," *Wake Forest Law Rev.* 39 (2004): 291–310.

23 D. Michaels, "Scientific evidence and public policy," *Am J Public Health* 95 (2005): S5–S7.

24 D. Michaels, "Doubt is their product," *Scientific American* 292 (2005): 96–101.

25 D. Michaels, "Manufactured uncertainty: protecting public health in the age of contested science and product defense," In: Mehlman M, et al., eds. *Living in a chemical world: framing the future in light of the past*, (Oxford: Wiley-Blackwell, 2006), p. 149–62.

26 D. Michaels, E. Bingham, L. Boden, R. Clapp, L. R. Goldman, P. Hoppin, S. Krimsky, C. Monforton, D. Ozonoff, A. Robbins, "Advice without dissent," *Science.* 298 (2002): 703.

27 D. Michaels, C. Monforton, "Manufacturing uncertainty: contested science and the protection of the public's health and environment," *Am J Public Health* 95 (2005): S39–S48.

28 D. Michaels, C. Monforton, P. Lurie, "Selected science: an industry campaign to undermine an OSHA hexavalent chromium standard," *Environ Health.* 5 (2006): 5.

29 N. Pearce, *Adverse reactions: the fenoterol story* (Auckland: Auckland University Press, 2007).

30 L. Hardell, M. J. Walker, B. Walhjalt, L. S. Friedman, E. D. Richter, "Secret ties to industry and conflicting interests in cancer research," *Am J Ind Med.* 50 (2007): 227–33.

31 S. Boseley, "Renowned cancer scientist was paid by chemical firm for 20 years," *The Guardian*, December 8, 2006.

32 P. F. Infante, "The past suppression of industry knowledge of the toxicity of benzene to humans and potential bias in future benzene research," *Int J Occup Environ Health* 12 (2006): 268–72.

33 C. Monforton, "Weight of the evidence or wait for the evidence? Protecting underground miners from diesel particulate matter,"*Am J Public Health.* 96 (2006): 271–6.

34 Hardell, et al. "Secret ties to industry . . ." 2007.

35 Michael, Monforton, 2006.

36 D. Egilman, "Corporate corruption of science: the case of chromium(VI)," *Int J Occup Environ Health* 12 (2006): 169–76.

37 J. D. Zhang, S. Li, "Cancer mortality in a Chinese population exposed to hexavalent chromium in water," *J Occup Environ Med.* 39 (1997): 315–9.

38 P. Brandt-Rauf, "Editorial retraction", *J Occup Environ Med.* 48 (2006): 749.

39 Zhang, Li, 1997.

40 P. Meier, "Damned lies and expert witnesses," *J Am Stat Assoc.* 394 (1986): 269–76.

41 N. Pearce, D. Crawford-Brown, "Critical discussion in epidemiology: problems with the Popperian approach,"*J Clin Epidemiol* 42 (1989): 177–84.

42 Ibid.

43 D. E. Barnes, L. A. Bero, "Why review articles on the health effects of passive smoking reach different conclusions," *JAMA* 279 (1998): 1566–70.

44 H. T. Stelfox, G. Chua, K. O'Rourke, A. S. Detsky, "Conflict of interest in the debate over calcium-channel antagonists," *N Engl J Med.* 338 (1998): 101–6.

45 K. J. Rothman, "Conflict of interest: the new McCarthyism in science," *JAMA* 269 (1993): 2782–4.
46 K. J. Rothman, S. Evans, "Extra scrutiny for industry funded trials, JAMA's demand for an additional hurdle is unfair - and absurd," *BMJ*. 331 (2005): 1350–1.
47 Epidemiology Monitor, 1990, p.4., Epidemiology Monitor, 1990b:1–5.
48 Pearce, 2007.
49 M. Martuzzi, J. A. Tickner, eds. *The precautionary principle: protecting public health, the environment, and the future of our children* (Rome:WHO, 2004).
50 S. Greenland, "Addressing corporate influences through ethical guidelines," *Int J Epidemiol*. 37 (2008): 37:57–9.
51 Monforton, "Weight of the evidence . . . " 2006.
52 Michaels, et al, "Advice without dissent," 2002. Ibid new 26 (old 24)
53 R. Clapp, P. Hoppin, D. Kriebel, "Erosion of the integrity of public health science in the USA," *Occup Environ Med*. 63 (2006): 367–8.
54 R. Horton, "Vioxx: the implosion of Merck, and aftershocks at the FDA," *Lancet*. 364 (2004): 1995–6.
55 E. J. Topol, "Failing the public health: Rofecoxib, Merck, and the FDA," *N Engl J Med*. 351 (2004): 1707–9.
56 E. K. Ong, S. A. Glantz, "Tobacco industry efforts subverting International Agency for Research on Cancer's second-hand smoke study,"*Lancet* 355 (2000): 1253–9.
57 O. Axelson, B. Castleman, S. Epstein, F. Giannasi, P. Grandjean, M. Greenberg, et al., "WHO handling of conflicts of interest," *Int J Occup Environ Health* 9 (2003): 92.
58 L. Tomatis, "The IARC monographs program: changing attitudes towards public health," *Int J Occup Environ Health* 8 (2002): 144–52.
59 L. Tomatis, "The IARC must maintain its important role in the protection of public health," *Int J Occup Environ Health* 9 (2003): 82.
60 N. Pearce, E. Matos, H. Vainio, P. Boffetta, M. Kogevinas, "Occupational cancer in developing countries," *Lyon: IARC* (1994).
61 L. Tomatis, "Asbestos and international organizations," *Environ Health Perspect*. 112 (2004): A336–7.
62 S. Foliaki, T. Fakakovikaetau, L. Waqatakirewa, N. Pearce, "Health research in the Pacific," *Pac Health Dialog*. 11 (2004): 199–203.
63 S. Foliaki, N. Pearce, "Changing pattern of ill health for indigenous people: control of lifestyle is beyond individuals and depends on social and political factors," *BMJ*. 327 (2003): 406–7.
64 J. Last, "Epidemiology and ethics," *Lancet* 336 (1990): 497.
65 R. R. Neutra, A. Cohen, T. Fletcher, D. Michaels, E. D. Richter, C. L. Soskolne, "Toward guidelines for the ethical reanalysis and reinterpretation of another's research," *Epidemiology* 17 (2006): 335–8.
66 R. J. Prineas, K. Goodman, C. L. Soskolne, G. Buck, M. Feinleib, J. Last, et al. "Findings from the American College of Epidemiology's survey on ethics guidelines," *Ann Epidemiol*. 8 (1998): 482–9.
67 C. L. Soskolne, L. E. Sieswerda, "Implementing ethics in the professions: examples from environmental epidemiology," *Sci Eng Ethics* 9 (2003): 181-90.

68 C. L. Soskolne, "Epidemiology: questions of science, ethics, morality, and law," *Am J Epidemiol* 129 (1989): 1–18.

69 J. Olsen, "Good epidemiological practice: proper conduct in epidemiologic research,"*International Epidemiological Association*, 2007.

70 Clapp, et al. "Erosion of the integrity . . ." 2006.

71 G. Davey Smith, "Reflections on the limitations to epidemiology," *J Clin Epidemiol.* 54 (2001): 325–31.

72 P. Vallance, "Developing an open relationship with the drug industry,"*Lancet* 366 (2005): 1062–4.

Chapter 7: Serving Industry, Kathleen Ruff

1 Margaret Chan. Address to the Sixty-sixth World Health Assembly. May 20, 2013. http://www.foodnavigator.com/Legislation/WHO-director-general-slams-industry-involvement-in-health-policy.

2 Caroline Scott-Thomas. WHO director-general slams industry involvement in health policy. July 4, 2013, http://www.foodnavigator.com/Legislation/WHO-director-general-slams-industry-involvement-in-health-policy.

3 A. M. Brandt, "Inventing conflicts of interest: a history of tobacco industry tactics," *Am J Public Health* 102 (2012): 63–71.

4 http://scholar.google.ca/citations?user=BcSVQxoAAAAJ&hl=en.

5 The International Agency for Research on Cancer (IARC) is the expert committee on causes of cancer for the World Health Organization (WHO). The organization invites a "Working Group" comprised of scientists from throughout the world twice a year to evaluate data on the causes of cancer. These cancer evaluations have policy implications for countries worldwide.

6 P. Boffetta, H. O. Adami, P. Cole, D. Trichopoulos, J. S. Mandel, "Epidemiologic studies of styrene and cancer: a review of the literature," *J Occup Environ Med.* 51 (2009): 1275–87.

7 J. Huff, P. F. Infante, "Styrene exposure and risk of cancer,"*Mutagenesis.* 26 (2011): 583–4.

8 Request for NTP to Fully Consider New Styrene Epidemiology Review Prior to Finalizing Styrene Draft Substance Profile. Letter of Dec. 16, 2008 from Jack Snyder, Executive Director, SIRC, to Samuel Wilson, M D, Acting Director, National Institute of Environmental Health Sciences / National Toxicology Program.

9 See, for example: Lamb JC 4th, P. Boffetta, W. G. Foster, J. E. Goodman, K.L. Hentz, L. R. Rhomberg, et al. Critical comments on the WHO-UNEP State of the Science of Endocrine Disrupting Chemicals - 2012. Regul Toxicol Pharmacol. 2014;69:22–40.

10 D. Michaels, *Doubt is their product: how industry's assault on science threatens your health* (Oxford: Oxford University Press, 2008).

11 An example of Boyle's defensiveness of the status quo is his extraordinary review in the *Lancet* of the book by Devra Davis, *The secret history of the war on cancer.* While the journal *Nature* and health experts, such as David O Carpenter, Director of the Institute for Health and the Environment, State University of New York at

Albany, Lorenzo Tomatis, a former director of IARC, James Huff, of the National Institute of Environmental Health Sciences, praised the book and recommended that it be widely read, Boyle trashed the book as gossip and innuendo, lacking only a "steamy sex section, but perhaps this is being held back for a further volume." (Boyle, P. Conspiracy theories of cancer. Lancet. 2007;370:1751.)

12   International Prevention Research Institute. *About Us,* http://www.i-pri.org/about/.

13   P. Boyle, et al., eds. *The State of Oncology 2013.* International Prevention Research Institute. http://www.i-pri.org/oncology2013/.

14   Kate Kelland. Oncologists call for industry-led global fund to fight cancer. Reuters. September 30. 2013, http://www.reuters.com/article/2013/09/30/us-cancer-global-fund-idUSBRE98T0EO20130930.

15   International Advisory Panel, University of Strathclyde, Glasgow. http://www.strath.ac.uk/research/researchapproach/healthtechnologies/internationaladvisorypanel/.

16   World Prevention Summit, http://www.i-pri.org/world-prevention-summit-2014/.

17   World Prevention Alliance, Missions. http://www.prevention-alliance.org/Missions.html. It is incredible that if you go to the Summit website - http://prevention-summit.org/conf/index.php/wps/wps2014/schedConf/program - there is zero info about the program, the speakers, the funders.

18   Roughly 180,000 deaths worldwide linked to sugary drink consumption. Harvard School of Public Health. http://www.hsph.harvard.edu/news/hsph-in-the-news/roughly-180000-deaths-worldwide-linked-to-sugary-drink-consumption/.

19   P. Boyle, A. Koechlin, P. Autier, "Sweetened carbonated beverage consumption and cancer risk: meta-analysis and review," *Eur J Cancer Prev.* 23 (2014): 481–90.

20   Public health takes aim at sugar and salt. Harvard School of Public Health [Fall 2009]. http://www.hsph.harvard.edu/news/magazine/sugar-and-salt/.

21   P. Boffetta, K. A. Mundt, H. O. Adami, P. Cole, J. S. Mandel, "TCDD and cancer: a critical review of epidemiologic studies," *Crit Rev Toxicol.* 41 (2011): 622–36.

22   P. Boffetta, H. O. Adami, S. C. Berry, J. S. Mandel, "Atrazine and cancer: a review of the epidemiologic evidence," *Eur J Cancer Prev.* 22 (2013): 169–80.

23   J. Huff, "Industry influence on occupational and environmental health," *Int J Occup Environ Health* 13 (2007): 107–17.

24   H. Checkoway, P. Boffetta, D. J. Mundt, K. A. Mundt, "Critical review and synthesis of the epidemiologic evidence on formaldehyde exposure and risk of leukemia and other lymphohematopoietic malignancies," *Cancer Causes Control* 23 (2012): 1747–66.

25   "International Agency for Research on Cancer (IARC)," Monographs. Vol:100F; 2012.

26   P. Boffetta, J. P. Fryzek, J. S. Mandel, "Occupational exposure to beryllium and cancer risk: a review of the epidemiologic evidence," *Crit Rev Toxicol.* 42 (2012): 107–18.

27   "International Agency for Research on Cancer (IARC)," Monographs. Vol. 100C; 2012. http://monographs.iarc.fr/ENG/Monographs/vol100C/mono100C-11.pdf.

28   C. Pelucci, C. La Vecchia, C. Bosetti, P. Boyle, P. Boffetta, "Exposure to acrylamide and human cancer: a review and meta-analysis of epidemiologic studies,"*Ann Oncol.* 22 (2011): 1487-99.

29   P. Boffetta, M. Dosemeci, G. Gridley, H. Bath, T. Moradi, D. Silverman, "Occupational exposure to diesel engine emissions and risk of cancer in Swedish men and women," *Cancer Causes Control* 12 (2001): 365-74.

30   E. Garshick, F. Laden, J. E. Hart, M. E. Davis, E. A. Eisen, T. J. Smith, "Lung cancer and elemental carbon exposure in trucking industry workers," *Environ Health Perspect.* 120 (2012): 1301–6.

31   D. T. Silverman, J. H. Lubin, A. E. Blair, R. Vermeulen, P. A. Stewart, P. L. Schleiff, et al., "The Diesel Exhaust in Miners Study: a nested case–control study of lung cancer and diesel exhaust," *J Natl Cancer Inst.* 104 (2012): 1–14.

32   J. F. Gamble, M. J. Nicolich, P. Boffetta, "Lung cancer and diesel exhaust: an updated critical review of the occupational epidemiology literature," *Crit Rev Toxicol.* 42 (2012): 549–98.

33   World Health Organization. United Nations Environment Programme (WHO-UNEP). A. Bergman, J. J: Heindel, S. Jobling, K. A. Kidd, R. T. Zoeller, editors. *State of the science of endocrine disrupting chemicals – 2012,* http://www.who.int/ceh/publications/endocrine/en/index.html.

34   J. C. Lamb IV, P. Boffetta, W. G. Foster, J. E. Goodman, L. Karyn, K. L. Hentz, et al. "Critical comments on the WHO-UNEP State of the science of endocrine disrupting chemicals – 2012," *Regul Toxicol Pharmacol.* 60 (2014): 22–40.

35   C. La Vecchia, P. Boffetta,, "Role of stopping exposure and recent exposure to asbestos in the risk of mesothelioma," *Eur J Cancer Prev.* 21 (2012): 227–30.

36   C. Magnani, D. Ferrante, F. Barone-Adesi, M. Bertolotti, A. Todesco, D. Mirabelli, et al., "Cancer risk after cessation of asbestos exposure: a cohort study of Italian asbestos cement workers," *Occup Environ Med.* 65 (2008): 164–70.

37   M. I. Colnaghi, Scientific Director, Italian Association for Cancer Research (AIRC). Letter to Alessandro Pugno. Familiari e vittime dell'amianto di Casale Monf.to (Afeva). January 20, 2014.

38   Alfredo Faieta. Amianto, tra gli imputati del processo Pirelli anche l'ex presidente dell'Airc. il Fatto. 2014 June 5. http://www.ilfattoquotidiano.it/2014/06/05/amianto-tra-gli-imputati-del-processo-pirelli-anche-lex-presidente-dellairc/1015561/.

39   Joint Letter, January 28, 2014, to Professor Jaak Ph Janssens, President, European Cancer Prevention Organization and Editor-in-Chief, European Journal of Cancer Prevention. http://www.rightoncanada.ca/wp-content/uploads/2014/02/Letter-to-European-Cancer-Prevention-Organization.pdf.

40   "Role of stopping exposure and recent exposure to asbestos in the risk of mesothelioma," Erratum. Eur J Cancer Prev. 2015, 24:68. http://journals.lww.com/eurjcancerprev/Fulltext/2015/01000/Role_of_stopping_exposure_and_recent_exposure_to.10.aspx.

41   C. La Vecchia, P. Boffetta, Lo Studio SENTIERI - Elementi di critica. June 19, 2013; Boffetta P, La Vecchia C, et al. Commenti al documento "Valutazione del Danno Sanitario Stabilimento ILVA di Taranto ai sensi della LR 21/2012—Scenari emissivi pre-AIA (anno 2010) e post-AIA (anno 2016)" dell'ARPA Puglia. June 7, 2013.

42   L'Associazione Italiana di Epidemiologia, Epidemiologia e Prevenzione. Comunicato stampa dell'AIE sull'ILVA di Taranto. July 15, 2013. http://www.epiprev.it/comunicato-stampa-dellaie-sullilva-di-taranto.

43   Stéphane Fourcart. Epidémiologie: des liaisons dangereuses. Le Monde. 2013 December 18.

44   Agence française de sécurité sanitaire des produits de santé. Press Release. Use of medications containing Pioglitazone (Actos®, Competact®) suspended. June 9, 2011. http://ansm.sante.fr/S-informer/Presse-Communiques-Points-presse/Suspension-de-l-utilisation-des-medicaments-contenant-de-la-pioglitazone-Actos-R-Competact-R-Communique.

45   Jean Paul Moatti. Position de l'ISP sur la Direction du CESP. January 18, 2014.

46   T. Rabesandratanat, "Top choice for French post drops out in industry flap," *Science* 343 (February 7, 2014): 586–7.

47   P. Boffetta, J. K. McLaughlin, C. La Vecchia, R. E. Tarone, L. Loren Lipworth, W. J. Blot, "False-positive results in cancer epidemiology: a plea for epistemological modesty," *J Natl Cancer Inst.* 100 (2008): 988–95.

48   V. Cogliano, K. Straif, "Re: False-positive results in cancer epidemiology: a plea for epistemological modesty," *J Natl Cancer Inst.* 102 (2010): 134.

49   P. Vineis, "The skeptical epidemiologist," *Int J Epidemiol,* 38 (2009): 675–7.

50   P. Boffetta, J. K. McLaughlin, C. La Vecchia, R.E. Tarone, L. Lipworth, W.J. Blot, "A further plea for adherence to the principles underlying science in general and the epidemiologic enterprise in particular," *Int J Epidemiol.* 38 (2009): 628–9.

51   J. K. McLaughlin, L. Lipworth, R. E. Tarone, C. La Vecchia, W.J. Blot, P. Boffetta, Authors' response, *Int J Epidemiol.*39 (2010): 1679–80.

52   Caroline Scott-Thomas, op cit. http://www.foodnavigator.com/Legislation/WHO-director-general-slams-industry-involvement-in-health-policy.

53   Rachel Aviv. "After Tyrone Hayes said that a chemical was harmful, its maker pursued him," *New Yorker*, February 10, 2014, http://www.newyorker.com/reporting/2014/02/10/140210fa_fact_aviv?currentPage=all.

54   J. B. Sass, A. Colangelo, "European Union bans atrazine, while the United States negotiates continued use," *Int J Occup Environ Health.* 12 (2006): 2:260-7.

55   Boffetta, et al., "Atrazine and cancer . . . " 2013.

56   J. Ladou, D. T. Teitelbaum, D. S. Egilman, A. L. Frank, S. N. Kramer, J. Huff, "American College of Occupational and Environmental Medicine (ACOEM): a professional association in service to industry," *Int J Occup Environ Health.* 13 (2007): 404–26.

57   D. S. Egilman, T. Bird, C. Lee, "Dust diseases and the legacy of corporate manipulation of science and law," *Int J Occup Environ Health.* 20 (2014): 115–25.

58   R. Moodie, D. Stuckler, C. Monteiro, N. Sheron, B. Neal, T. Thamarangsi, et al., "Profits and pandemics: prevention of harmful effects of tobacco, alcohol, and ultra-processed food and drink industries,"*Lancet* 381 (2013): 670–9.

Chapter 8: Secret Ties in Asbestos, Geoffrey Tweedale

1   M. Lalonde, Scientists, MDs, "Labour groups sound the alarm," *Montreal Gazette.* January 30, 2010.

2   A. Lippmann. McGill Dept. of Epidemiology, Biostatics & Occupational Health, to Charest, February 10, 2010.

3   J. LaDou. "The asbestos cancer epidemic," *Environ Health Perspect.* 112 (2003): 285–90.

4   L. Kazan-Allen, *Killing the future: asbestos use in Asia* (London: International Ban Asbestos Secretariat, 2007) p. 38. http://www.lkaz.demon.co.uk/ktf_web_fin.pdf.

5   P. Brodeur. "Outrageous misconduct: the asbestos industry on trial," *New York: Pantheon,* 1985.

6   B. I. Castleman, *Asbestos: medical and legal aspects.* 5th ed. (New York: Aspen Publishers, 2005).

7   D. Ozonoff, *Failed warnings: asbestos-related disease and industrial medicine,* In: Bayer R., ed. *The health and safety of workers,* (New York: Oxford University Press, 1988). p. 139–218.

8   D. E. Lilienfeld, "The silence: the asbestos industry and early occupational cancer research—a case study," *Am J Public Health* 81 (1991): 791–800.

9   D. Rosner, G. Markowitz, *Deadly dust: silicosis and the on-going struggle to protect workers' health.* 2nd ed. (Ann Arbor, MI: Michigan University Press, 2006).

10   J.C. Wagner, C. A. Sleggs, P Marchand, "Diffuse pleural mesotheliomas and asbestos exposure in the North-Western Cape Province," *Br J Ind Med.* 17 (1960): 260–71.

11   J. McCulloch, G. Tweedale, "Science is not sufficient: Irving J. Selikoff and the American asbestos tragedy," *New Solutions* 17 (2007): 293–310.

12   J. McCulloch, G. Tweedale, *Defending the indefensible: the global asbestos industry and its fight for survival* (Oxford: Oxford University Press, 2008).

13   J. McCulloch, *Asbestos blues: labour, capital, physicians and the State in South Africa* (Oxford: James Currey, 2002).

14   M. Greenberg, "Re. Call for an international ban on asbestos: Trust me I'm a doctor," *Am J Ind Med.* 37 (2000): 37:232–4.

15   M. Greenberg, "A report on the health of asbestos, Quebec miners 1940," *Am J Ind Med.* 48 (2005): 230–7.

16   J.C. McDonald, McGill asbestos research priorities since 1964. In: Mitastein M, editor. Memorias/Proceedings.Meeting on Asbestos and Health in Latin América, México, 31 October–1 November 1985. México: ECO; 1987. p.137-70.

17   McDonald to Kenneth W. Smith, Johns-Manville Corporation, November 27, 1964.

18   A. Dalton, *Asbestos killer dust.* (London: BSSRS Publications, 1979).

19   J.C. McDonald, A.D. McDonald, "Chrysotile, tremolite and carcinogenicity," *Ann Occup Hyg.* 41 (1997): 699–705.

20   G. Tweedale, "Science or public relations? The inside story of the Asbestosis Research Council," *Am J Ind Med.* 38 (2000): 723–34.

21   G. Tweedale, *Magic mineral to killer dust: Turner & Newall and the asbestos hazard* (Oxford: Oxford University Press, 2001).

22   F. D. K. Liddell, "Magic, menace, myth and malice," *Ann Occup Hyg.* 4 (1997): 1-12.

23   BOHS. Brief history. c.1967.

24   Selikoff letter to Sheldon Samuels, AFL-CIO, May 29, 1973.

25   G. Tweedale, "Hero or villain? Sir Richard Doll and occupational cancer," *Int J Occup Environ Health* 13 (2007): 233–5.

26   WHO. Occupational exposure limit for asbestos. Report prepared by a WHO meeting, Oxford, 10–11 April 1989.

27 J. C. Wagner, "Mesothelioma and mineral fibers," [Charles Mott Prize paper]. *Cancer* 57 (1986): 1905–11.

28 R.P. Nolan, A.M. Langer, M. Ross, F.J. Wicks, R.F. Martin, editors, T*he health effects of chrysotile asbestos: contribution of science to risk-management decisions* (Ottawa: Mineralogical Association of Canada, 2001).

29 J. McCulloch, "Saving the industry1960-2006,"*Public Health Rep.* 121 (2006): 609–14.

30 J. C. McDonald, A.D. McDonald,, "The epidemiology of mesothelioma in historical context," *Eur Respir J.* 9 (1996): 1932–42.

31 J. C. McDonald, "Letter to Editor. Re. Call for an international ban on asbestos," *Am J Ind Med.* 37 (2000): 235.

32 B. I. Castleman, "WTO confidential: the case of asbestos," *Int J Health Serv.* 32 (2002): 489–501.

33 WTO. European Community—measures affecting asbestos and asbestos-containing products. Report of the Appellate Body, WT/DS135/AB/R, March 12, 2001; Report of the Panel, WT/DS135/R, 18 September 2000.

34 International Conference on Chrysotile, Montreal, 23-24 May 2006. Available from: http://www.chrysotile.com/en/conferences/default.aspx.

35 Paradis address to International Conference on Chrysotile. p. 1–2.

36 J. Brophy, The public health disaster Canada chooses to ignore. In: Chrysotile asbestos: hazardous to humans, deadly to the Rotterdam Convention. London: Building & Woodworkers International and International Ban Asbestos Secretariat; 2006. p. 17–20. Available from: www.lkaz.demon.co.uk/chrys_hazard_rott_conv_06.pdf.

37 "Asbestos kept off global list of toxic substances," *Reuters,* October 13, 2006.

38 Letter by Richard Wiles (Environmental Working Group) to Vivian Turner, Environmental Protection Agency, May 2007. Available from: http://www.ewg.org/node/20960.

39 D. Bernstein, *Asbestos*, In: H. Salem, S.A. Katz, editors. *Inhalation toxicology.* 2nd ed. (London: Taylor & Francis, 2006). p. 647–67.

40 Trial on the merits of Dr. David Bernstein. In: Emma Josephine Maloney Martin et al *vs.* Quigley Company et al, in District Court Ellis County, Texas, 40th Judicial District, 16 October 2000. Transcript p. 95–9.

41 "Asbestos panellists accuse Government of misusing science," *CMAJ* 179 (2008): 886–7.

42 D. Bernstein, A. Gibbs, F. Pooley, A. Langer, K. Donaldson, J. Hoskins, J. Dunnigan, "Misconceptions and misuse of International Agency for Research on Cancer 'Classification of Carcinogenic Substances': the case of asbestos," *Indoor Built Environ.* 16 (2007): 94–8.

43 D. Michaels, *Doubt is their product: how industry's assault on science threatens your health.* (New York: Oxford University Press, 2008). p. 53.

44 R. Nolan, editor, "International Symposium on the Health Hazard Evaluation of Fibrous Particles Associated with Taconite and the Adjacent Duluth Complex," *Regul Toxicol Pharmacol.* 52 (2008): S1–S248.

45 D. Michaels, *Doubt is their product: how industry's assault on science threatens your health.* (New York: Oxford University Press, 2008). p. 53.

46   S. Milloy, "Asbestos could have saved WTC lives," Fox News. September 14, 2001, Available from: http://www.foxnews.com/story/0,2933,34342,00.html.

47   A. Schlafly, "Did flawed science and litigation help bring down the World Trade Center?" *J Am Phys Surg*. 8 (2003): 89–93.

48   J. H. Lange, "Emergence of a new policy for asbestos: a result of the World Trade Center tragedy," *Indoor Built Environ*. 13 (2004): 21-33.

49   G. Tweedale, "Fire and risk: the controversy over the role of fire-retardants in the World Trade Center disaster," *J Risk Governance* 1 (2008): 219-32.

50   R. N. Proctor, *Cancer wars: how politics shapes what we know and don't know about cancer*, (New York: Basic Books, 1995).

51   D. S. Egilman, S. Bohme, editors. "Corporate corruption of science," *Int J Occup Environ Health*. 11 (2005): 331–7.

52   J. Huff, "Industry influence on occupational and environmental health," *Int J Occup Environ Health* 13 (2007): 107–17.

53   D. Davis, *The secret history of the war on cancer* (New York: Basic Books, 2007).

54   T. O. McGarity, W. E. Wagner, *Bending science: how special interests corrupt public health research* (Cambridge: Harvard University Press, 2008).

55   N. Pearce, "Corporate influences on epidemiology," *Int J Epidemiol* 37 (2008): 46–53.

56   Letter from Corbett McDonald to David Kotelchuck, March 10, 1976.

57   Selikoff letter to Dr. Morris Greenberg, June 17, 1983.

58   Selikoff to Greenberg, December 31. 1979.

Chapter 9: Kidding a Kidder, Martin Walker

1   B. Woffinden, "Cover-up," *The Guardian*, August 25, 2001, Available from: http://www.theguardian.com/education/2001/aug/25/research.highereducation.

2   As with a great many such situations, it is the most powerful group that defined the illness and gave it its name. Every time the label is used it endorses the idea that, in this case "toxic oil" was responsible. I don't want to continue this fantasy: in fact, I want from the beginning of the chapter to do the opposite and inform people that it was not toxic oil that was responsible. However, changing the name of the illness is very difficult and likely to detract from the clarity of the text. Given this problem I have chosen to deploy a line through the official title of the illness as a reminder of its status in this chapter.

3   Such cases vary in size and potency, from the underlying explanation for the cause of AIDS-related illnesses and the "discovery" of HIV, to the official explanation of the collapse of the third tower on 9/11, to much smaller matters such as, how Dr. Andrew Wakefield was turned from a highly qualified, award-winning medical research worker to an abomination, on the word of a free-lance journalist working for Rupert Murdoch's *Sunday Times*.

4   Woffinden, "Cover-up."

5   M. J. Walker, Sir Richard Doll: Death, Dioxin and PVC. Available from: http://www.whale.to/v/walker_doll.pdf.

6   The results of Doll's study were published, no questions asked—no statement of the funding from the Chemical Industries Association—by the *Scandinavian*

Journal of Work, Environment and Health, recommended to Doll by Bennett the Medical Advisor to ICI, a producer of PVC.

7   Walker. Death. Dioxin, and PVC.

8   *Daily Telegraph*, February 7,1983.

9   *Daily Mail*, June 3, 1992.

10 Ibid.

11 American Council of Science and Health (ACSH). Sir Richard Doll, ACSH Advisor, RIP. 2005 Jul 25. Available from: http://web.archive.org/web/20120204012541/https://www.acsh.org/healthissues/newsID.1150/healthissue_detail.asp.

12 M. J. Walker, *Dirty Medicine: Science, Big Business and the Assault on Natural Health Care* (London: Slingshot Publications, 1993).

13 In 2007 the CIIT became the Hamner Institutes for Health Sciences

14 Covington & Burling served as "corporate affairs consultants" to the Philip Morris group of companies. According to a 1993 internal budget review document that indicated the firm was paid $280,000 to advise the company on litigation. They were also involved in organizing Philip Morris's Whitecoat Project, designed to help obscure the health effects of exposure to secondhand tobacco smoke. (SourceWatch. Covington & Burling. Available from: http://www.sourcewatch.org/index.php?title=Covington_ percent26_Burling).

15 There were two major cases brought by workers and their families in Italy and the US against PVC-producing companies.

In Italy, Greenpeace declared today to be "a dark day for environmental justice" as twenty-eight senior managers of petrochemical companies Enichem and Montedison were acquitted of charges of mass manslaughter and environmental disaster by an Italian court. After, the companies paid off the claimants. The managers had been accused of mismanaging their VCM and PVC production plants, causing cancer among PVC workers and environmental disaster in the Venice Lagoon.

The case was instigated by the workers when, in 1994, a retired PVC worker, Gabriele Bortolozzo, approached public prosecutor Felice Casson in Venice.

In the United States, in a trial for which Doll gave evidence, for the defense, from London, in 2000, *Ross v. Conoco*, Inc. his legal fees were paid by Monsanto. Ross a worker suffering from brain cancer, won his case against Conoco.

16 Woffinden, "Cover-up."

17 Letter from William R. Gaffey, Epidemiological Director at Monsanto, St. Louis, dated May 1st 1986, to Sir Richard Doll, Clinical Trial Service Unit, University of Oxford. "Once again I enclose two copies of a letter extending your consulting agreement with Monsanto. We have changed the fee from $1,000 to $1,500 per day."

Gaffey goes on to invite Doll and Lady Doll to Monsanto later that year, where they were "particularly interested in pursuing the general topic of what we ought to be doing in the long run at Monsanto." So, far from being funded by a corporation to carry out studies, Doll was being paid to help with Monsanto's scientific and business strategy. The relevance of this is that it must have increasingly endangered his independence in any research he did on their products.

18 On behalf of Monsanto, Gaffey waged a long-term libel law suit against Peter Montague and Rachel's Environment & Health Weekly. Its founder Peter

Montague a giant of an activist, campaigner and writer, had said that Gaffey had distorted information on one of his studies of dioxin. Fortunately, after years in the pipeline, the case ended when Gaffey died in 1995. http://www.planetwaves. net/dioxin_critic.html.

Gaffey's career and work is well summed up in an obituary by Montague in his Environmental Research Foundation newsletter no. 494, 1996 May 15. http://www. rachel.org/?q=es/node/3947.

19   This prospective study began in 1951 ended with a paper entitled: *Mortality in relation to smoking: 50 years' observations on male British doctors* and was authored by Richard Doll, emeritus professor of medicine Richard Peto, professor of medical statistics and epidemiology, Jillian Boreham, senior research fellow, Isabelle Sutherland, research assistant and was Published in June 2004. (*BMJ* 2004;328:1519) (http://dx.doi.org/10.1136/bmj.38142.554479.AE) The objective of the study was to compare the hazards of cigarette smoking in men who formed their habits at different periods. It that continued from 1951 to 2001.

20   C. Beckett, "An epidemiologist at work: The personal papers of Sir Richard Doll" *Med Hist.* 46 (2002): 403–21.

21   B. L. Castleman, *Asbestos: Medical and Legal Aspects*. 4th ed., (Englewood Cliffs, NJ: Aspen Law and Business 1996).

22   Doll's official biographer, Conrad Keating, published Doll's bizarrely titled: *Smoking kills: the revolutionary life of Richard Doll*. Keating began writing under Doll's guidance before Doll died and the final book fails to mention or even refer to the most-notable, most-publicized and controversial case of European poisoning in history at which Doll gave seminal evidence.

23   This impromptu research was brushed up and published in the Lancet. Tabuenca JM. "Toxic-allergic syndrome caused by ingestion of rapeseed oil denatured with aniline," *Lancet* 2 (1981): 567–8.

24   J. G. Rigau-Pérez, L. Pérez-Alvarez, S. Dueñas-Castro, K. Choi, S.B. Thacker, J.L. Germain, et al. "Epidemiologic investigation of an oil-associated pneumonic paralytic eosinophilic syndrome in Spain," *Amer J Epidemiol.* 119 (1984): 250–60.

25   Gaston Vettorazzi, of the Joint FAO/WHO Meeting on Pesticide Residues from the beginning showed complete intellectual opposition to the simplistic idea that the oil was responsible. In February 1985 (Cambio16, no 689, 11-2-1985) interviewed by Rafael Cid, Vettorazzi said "there is absolutely no possibility that oil was responsible for this epidemic." Vettorazzi was then Executive and Technical Secretary of the Joint FAO/WHO Meeting on Pesticide Residues (JMPR) and the Joint FAO/WHO Expert Committee on Food Additives since 1972. From 1980 to 1988 Vettorazzi had also been the senior toxicologist with the WHO/UNEP/ILO International Programme on Chemical Safety. He retired from the WHO in 1988. He then set up, in San Sebastián, Spain, the International Toxicology Information Centre (ITIC). (Information obtained from the WHO website).

26   G. Greunke, J. Heimbrecht, El montaje del Síndrome Tóxico [The Toxic Syndrome cover up]. Barcelona: Ediciones Obelisco; 1988.

27   Ibid.

28 Peralta Serrano A. La neumonía atípica. Diario Ya, 1981 May 12. Available from: http://free-news.org/aperal01.htm.
29 http://www.mapperleyplains.co.uk/oprus/npu.htm See: The truth about the National Poisons Unit, that suggests staff of the Unit are sometimes trained by, and even sometimes salaried by, the chemical industry.
30 Goulding communication with Doll after visiting Madrid in August 1984. PP/DOL/C/2/1/18. PP/DOL, List of papers in the Wellcome Library for The History and Understanding of Medicine, compiled by Chris Beckett.
31 Greunke, Heimbrecht, 1988.
32 Greunke, Heimbrecht, 1988.
33 Communication from Goulding to Doll at Green College Oxford, 1984 Aug 29. PP/DOL/C/2/1/18. PP/DOL, List of papers in the Wellcome Library for The History and Understanding of Medicine, compiled by Chris Beckett.
34 PP/DOL/C/2/1/18. PP/DOL, List of papers in the Wellcome Library for The History and Understanding of Medicine, compiled by Chris Beckett.
35 Beckett, "An epidemiologist at work . . ." 2002.
36 R. Doll, The Aetiology of the Spanish Toxic Syndrome: Interpretation of the epidemiological evidence. Gac Sanit. 2000;14:72-88. Available from: http://lbe.uab.es/vm/sp/old/docs/problemas/gs-sd-toxico-epi.pdf.
37 Ibid.
38 Ibid.
39 Communication from Doll to Goulding, Dec 1985. PP/DOL/C/2/1/18. PP/DOL, List of papers in the Wellcome Library for The History and Understanding of Medicine, compiled by Chris Beckett.
40 Ibid.
41 Woffinden, "Cover-up."
42 E. M. Kilbourne, LinkedIn website. Available from: https://www.linkedin.com/in/emkmd.
43 Correspondence between Doll and Kilbourne. PP/DOL/C/2/1/18. PP/DOL, List of papers in the Wellcome Library for The History and Understanding of Medicine, compiled by Chris Beckett.
44 Ibid.
45 Kilbourne, www.linkedin.com/in/emkmd.
46 The Cancer Research Campaign and the Imperial Cancer Research Fund joined in February 2002 to make a massive part corporately funded cancer "charity," Cancer Research UK.
47 E. M. Kilbourne, "Toxic-oil syndrome. Epidemic with an elusive etiology," Chest. 88 (1985): 324–5.
48 Walker, Death, Dioxin, and PVC.
49 G. Greene, The Woman who Knew Too Much: Alice Stewart and the Secrets of Radiation (Ann Arbor, MI: The University of Michigan Press, 1999).
50 S. Garfield, "The man who saved a million lives," The Guardian, April 24, 2005, Available from: http://www.theguardian.com/society/2005/apr/24/smoking.medicineandhealth.

51 Doll's letter to Medical History in the issue following Beckett's case history.

52 Doll to Goulding. PP/DOL/C/2/1/18. PP/DOL, autumn 1987. List of papers in the Wellcome Library for The History and Understanding of Medicine, compiled by Chris Beckett.

53 Greunke, Heimbrecht, 1988.

54 Greunke, Heimbrecht, 1988.

55 Woffinden, "Cover-up."

56 R. Riding, "Trial in Spain on Toxic Cooking Oil Ends in Uproar," *The New York Times*, May 21, 1989. Available from: http://www.nytimes.com/1989/05/21/world/trial-in-spain-on-toxic-cooking-oil-ends-in-uproar.html

57 Greunke, Heimbrecht, 1988.

58 Centers for Disease Control and Prevention (CDC). 1980–1995 History by Subject. Available from: http://www.cdc.gov/nceh/history/history.htm

59 Doll's letter to Medical History.

60 Even now, thirty years later, there is a complete belief in the official corporate media presentation of the epidemic and the trial. I spoke with a Madrilenian family in 2009 about the epidemic and they immediately became angry when I talked about alternative theories.

61 Woffinden, "Cover-up."

62 N. Davis, *Flat Earth News: An Award-winning Reporter Exposes Falsehood, Distortion and Propaganda in the Global Media* (London: Vintage Books, 2009).

63 Ibid new 62 (old 41).

64 Woffinden, "Cover-up."

Chapter 10: Escaping Electrosensitivity, Christian Blom

1 Spaceweather.com, Available at: http://spaceweather.com/.

2 Auroras now.com, Available at: http://aurora.fmi.fi/public_service/.

3 Statistics showing the highly increased magnetic values in Helsinki during the period of 29–31 October, 2003 available at: http://aurora.fmi.fi/public_service/NURdercol.txt.

4 Clay Ericsson H. Big Data—Big Deal? Forum for economy and technology. 6/2014 (In Swedish). [Internet]. Available at: http://www.forummag.fi/big-data-big-deal/.

Chapter 11: Ignoring chronic illness caused by new chemicals and technology, Gunni Nordström

1 *Research Advisory Committee on Gulf War Veterans' Illnesses. Gulf War Illness and the Health of Gulf War Veterans: Scientific Findings and Recommendations.* (Washington DC: US Government Printing Office, November 2008).

2 R. Andersson, K. Göransson, G. Andersson, S. Marklund, P.A. Zingmark, "Occupational photodermatosis of the face," *Lancet* I(8322) (1983): 472.

3 P. A. Zingmark, A.K. Norlér, B. Stenberg, A. Hedén. "Fläktsjukan" 10 år senare—Medicinska och sociala konsekvenser. Arbetarskyddsstyreisens.1990:2. ("Fläktsjukan" 10 years later—Medical and social consequences. Swedish Work Environment Authority. 1990:2.)

4   H. Allen, K. Kaidbey, "Persistent photosensitivity following occupational exposure to epoxy resin," *Arch Dermatol.* 115 (1979): 1307–10.
5   A. M. Hornblum, *Acres of skin: human experiments at Holmesburg Prison. A true story of abuse and exploitation in the name of medical science* (New York: Routledge, 1999).
6   L. Hardell, M. Carlberg, F. Söderqvist, K. Hardell, H. Björnforth, B. van Bavel, G. Lindström. Increased concentration of certain persistent organic pollutants in subjects with self-reported electromagnetic hypersensitivity—a pilot study. Electromagn Biol Med. 2008;27:197–203.

Chapter 12: A Tale of Two Scientists, Gayle Greene

1   A version of this article was published as G. Greene, "Richard Doll and Alice Stewart: reputation and the creation of scientific 'truth,'" *Persp Biol Med.* 54 (2011): 504–31.
2   D. Giles, D. Hewitt, A. Stewart, J. Webb, "Malignant disease in childhood and diagnostic irradiation in utero," *Lancet.* 271 (1956): 447.
3   A. Stewart, J. Webb, D. Hewitt, D. "A survey of childhood malignancies," *Br Med J.* 1 (1958): 1495–508.
4   C. Keating, *Smoking kills: The Revolutionary Life of Richard Doll* (Oxford: Signal Books, 2009), p. 211.
5   A. D. Espinosa-Brito, "Honour to Sir Richard Doll, *BMJ* 331 (2005): 295. Available from: http://www.bmj.com/rapid-response/2011/10/31/honour-sir-richard-doll
6   A. Tucker. 2005. Obituary: Sir Richard Doll. *The Guardian*, 2005 Jul 25. Available from: http://www.theguardian.com/news/2005/jul/25/guardianobituaries.obituaries/print
7   S. Boseley, "Renowned cancer scientist was paid by chemical firm for 20 years," *The Guardian*, December 8, 2006, Available from: http://www.theguardian.com/science/2006/dec/08/smoking.frontpagenews.
8   C. Talbot, Medical research and big business: The case of Sir Richard Doll. World Socialist Website, 2007 Jan 9. Available from: http://www.wsws.org/en/articles/2007/01/doll-j09.html.
9   Keating, *Smoking Kills,* 2009, p 211.
10 Ibid., p. 205, 454.
11 G. Greene, *The woman who knew too much: Alice Stewart and the secrets of radiation,* (Ann Arbor, MI: University of Michigan Press, 1999).
12 Keating, *Smoking Kills,* 2009, p 439
13 Ibid., p. 218.
14 W. M. Court-Brown, R. Doll, Leukaemia and aplastic anaemia in patients irradiated for ankolysing spondylitis. Spec Rep Ser Med Res Counc (GB). 1957;295:1–135.
15 (Interview, Oxford, October 9, 1998).
16 R. Doll, R. Wakeford, "Risk of childhood cancer from fetal irradiation," *Br J Radiol.* 70 (1997): 130–9.
17 G. Ferry, "No smoke without fire," *Oxford Today,* 5(3) (1993): 11–2.

18   Keating, *Smoking Kills,* 2009, p. 273.

19   Ibid., p. 304.

20   U.K. Co-ordinating Committee. "Unique national survey of children's cancer to begin in April," Press release, March 12, 1992.

21   R. Doll, "A conversation with Sir Richard Doll,"*Epidemiology*.14 (2003): 375–9.

22   Green, *The woman who knew too much,"* 1999.

23   S. Wing, D. Richardson, A. Stewart, "The relevance of occupational epidemiology to radiation protection standards," *New Solut.* 9 (1999): 133–51.

24   Green, *The woman who knew too much,"* 1999, p 183–84.

25   K. Schneider, "Radiation Records of 44,000 Released," *The New York Times,* July 18, 1990, Available from: http://www.nytimes.com/1990/07/18/us/radiation-records-of-44000-released.html.

26   K. Schneider, "Scientist Who Managed to 'Shock the World' on Atomic Workers' Health," *The New York Times,* May 3, 1990. Available from: http://www.nytimes.com/1990/05/03/us/scientist-who-managed-to-shock-the-world-on-atomic-workers-health.html.

27   M. L. Wald, "U.S. Acknowledges Radiation Killed Weapons Workers," *The New York Times,* January 29, 2000. Available from: http://www.nytimes.com/2000/01/29/us/us-acknowledges-radiation-killed-weapons-workers.html

28   A. M. Stewart, "Risk of childhood cancer from fetal irradiation: 1. Correspondence," *Br J Radiol.* 70 (1997): 769–70.

29   Wing, Stewart, "The relevance of occupational epidemiology . . . " 1999, p 147.

30   B. W. Jacobs, "The politics of radiation: When public health and the nuclear industry collide," *Greenpeace.* 1986 (July–Aug.):6–9.

31   C. Caulfield, *Multiple exposures: Chronicles of the Radiation Age* (New York: Harper and Row, 1989).

32   M. S. Lindee, *Suffering Made Real: American Science and the Survivors at Hiroshima.* (Chicago, IL: University of Chicago Press, 1994).

33   Keating, *Smoking Kills,* 2009p 221.

34   Ibid. p. 275.

35   Ibid. p. 305.

36   Ibid. p. 270–6.

37   R. Doll, R. Peto, "The causes of cancer: Quantitative estimates of avoidable risks of cancer in the United States today," *J Natl Cancer Inst.* 66 (1981): 1195–308.

38   Ibid.

39   R.W. Clapp, G.K. Howe, M.M. Jacobs. Environmental and Occupational Causes of Cancer: A Review of Recent Scientific Literature. Cancer Working Group of the Collaborative on Health and the Environment, Lowell Center for Sustainable Production. University of Massachusetts, Lowell, 2005 Sept.

40   I. U. Selikoff, "Influence of age at death on accuracy of death certificate disease diagnosis: Findings in 475 consecutive deaths of mesothelioma among asbestos insulation workers and asbestos factory workers," *Am J Ind Med.* 22 (1992): 505–10.

41   D.L. Davis, A.D. Lilienfeld, A. Gittelsohn, M.E. Scheckenbach, "Increasing trends in some cancers in older Americans: Fact or artifact?" *Toxicol Ind Health.* 2 (1986): 127–44.

42 S. Epstein, *The Politics of Cancer Revisited* (Fremont City, NY: East Ridge Press, 1998).

43 Clapp, et al., Environmental and Occupational Causes of Cancer, 2005, p 4–5.

44 P. Boffey, "Cancer Experts Lean Toward Vigilance, But Less Alarm, on Environment," *The New York Times*, March 2, 1982, Available from: http://www.nytimes.com/1982/03/02/science/cancer-experts-lean-toward-vigilance-but-less-alarm-on-environment.html.

45 R. N. Proctor,. *Cancer Wars: How Politics Shapes What We Know and Don't Know about Cancer* (New York: Basic Books, 1995).

46 C. Cookson, "The weapons of a killer: The search for what causes cancer has thrown up hundreds of suspects, from smoking to driving," *Financial Times*, December 13, 1994.

47 *The Times*, June 8, 1967.

48 *The Daily Telegraph*, Feb 7, 1983.

49 *Daily Mail*, June 3, 1992.

50 M. Walker, "Sir Richard Doll: A Questionable Pillar of the Cancer Establishment," *The Ecologist*, Mar 1, 1998. Available from: http://www.theecologist.org/investigations/health/268974/sir_richard_doll_a_questionable_pillar_of_the_cancer_establishment.html.

51 R. O'Neill, editor of Injury Watch, personal communication, 2008 Aug 20.

52 M. J. Walker, "Scoop! A Strange Tale of Plagiarism, Journalists and Damage Limitation But Not Necessarily in That Order," 2011. Available from: http://www.whale.to/a/walker.pdf.

53 L. Hardell, M.J. Walker, B. Walhjalt, L.S. Friedman, E.D.Richter, "Secret ties to industry and conflicting interests in cancer research, " *Am J Ind Med.* 50 (2007): 227–33.

54 M. J. , Sir Richard Doll: Death, Dioxin, and PVC. Available from: http://www.whale.to/v/walker_doll.pdf.

55 Walker, Scoop!, 2004.

56 E. Marshall, "Experts clash over cancer data," *Science* 250 (1990): 900–2.

57 "Sex and the Scientist: Our Brilliant Careers" [TV Documentary]. Channel 4, UK, screened August 19, 1996.

58 Keating, *Smoking Kills*, 2009.

59 Ibid. p. 311.

60 Greene, 1999.

61 Ibid.

62 Keating, *Smoking Kills*, 2009, p. 310

63 Ibid. p. 309

64 Greene 1999. p. 256.

65 Keating, *Smoking Kills*, 2009, p. 143, 447.

66 Ibid. p. 284.

67 Ibid. p. 284.

68 Ibid. p. 143.

69 Ibid. 256–7.

70 "Sex and the Scientist."

71   Keating, *Smoking Kills,* 2009, p. 312.

72   M. Greenberg, The evolution of attitudes to the human hazards of ionizing radiation and its investigators. Am J Ind Med. 1991;20:717–21.

73   I. Greene, 1999, p. 230.

74   Keating, *Smoking Kills,* 2009, p. 292.

75   Ibid. p. 303.

76   Ibid. p. 108, 230.

77   R. M. Park, Doll's Contribution. Occ-Env-Med-L Internet Mail-list. December 15, 2006, Available from: http://lists.unc.edu/read/messages?id=3704073#3704073

78   G. Tweedale, "The Rochdale asbestos cancer studies and the politics of epidemiology: What you see depends on where you sit," *Int J Occup Environ Health.* 13 (2007): 70–9.

79   C. Cook, "Oral history - Sir Richard Doll," *J Public Health* (Oxf). 26 (2004): 327–36.

80   Clapp, et al., Environmental and Occupational Causes of Cancer, 2005.

81   Walker, "A Questionable Pillar of the Cancer Establishment," 1998.

82   Committee for the Compilation of Materials on Damage Caused by the Atomic Bombs in Hiroshima and Nagasaki, *Hiroshima and Nagasaki: The Physical, Medical and Social Effects of the Atomic Bombings,* (New York: Basic Books, 1981).

83   M. V. Malko, Chernobyl Accident: the Crisis of the International Radiation Community. Research Activities about the Radiobiological Consequences of the Chernobyl NPT accident and Social Activities to Assist the Sufferers by the Accident. KURR-KR-2, 1998 Mar. Available from: http://www.rri.kyoto-u.ac.jp/NSRG/reports/kr21/kr21pdf/Malko1.pdf.

84   Y. Shimizu, Kato, W. J. Schull, D. G. Hoel, "1992. Studies of the mortality of A-bomb survivors. 9. Mortality, 1950–1985: Part 3. Noncancer mortality based on the revised doses (DS86)" *Radiat Res.* 130 (1992): 249–66.

85   R. Alvarez, "Statement before the NAS Advisory Committee on the Biological Effects of Ionizing Radiations. BEIRV," *Environmental Policy Institute,* 1987 Mar 2.

86   R. Doll. "A tentative estimate of the leukaemogenic effect of test thermonuclear explosions," *J Radiol Prot.* 16 (1996): 3–5. Accepted for publication in 1955.

87   Cook, "Oral history . . ." 2004. Ibid new 79 (old 44).

88   Doll, *J. Radiol Prot),* 1955.

89   Page 335.

90   Biological Effects of Ionizing Radiation (BEIRV). *Health Effects of Exposure to Low Levels of Ionizing Radiation* (Washington, DC,: The National Academies Press, 1990). Available from: http://www.nap.edu/catalog/1224/health-effects-of-exposure-to-low-levels-of-ionizing-radiation.

91   J. Strather, C. Muirhead, R. Cox, "Radiation-induced cancer at low doses and low dose rates," *Radiol Protect Bull.* 167 (1995): 8–12.

92   M. Drabble, *The Sea Lady* (New York: Harcourt, 2007).

93   Ibid.

94   Medical Research Council (MRC). 1947. Conference on Cancer of the Lung, Feb 6, Report to MRC meeting March 21;A. Bradford Hill, Memorandum, "Proposed Statistical Investigation of Cancer of the Lung," MRC Nov 10.

95 Cook, "Oral history . . ." 2004, p. 33.

96 R. Doll, A. B. Hill, "Smoking and carcinoma of the lung: Preliminary report," *Br Med J* 2 (1950): 739–48.

97 Keating, *Smoking Kills*, 2009.

98 J. Lilburne, "Comment on: Smith R. Scientists are only human," *The Guardian*, 2006 Dec 8. Available from: http://www.theguardian.com/commentisfree/2006/dec/08/scientistsareonlyhuman#comment-1847826.

99 G. Tweedale, "Hero or villain? Sir Richard Doll and occupational cancer," *Int J Occup Environ Health* 13 (2007): 233–5.

100 Tweedale, "Hero or villain?" 2007.

101 D. Simpson, Sir Richard Doll, 1912–2005. Obituary. Tob Control. 2005;14:289–90. Available from: http://tobaccocontrol.bmj.com/content/14/5/289.full.

102 Ibid.

103 D. Davis, *The Secret History of the War on Cancer* (New York: Basic Books, 2007).

104 Ibid. p. 257, 262.

105 Tweedale, "Hero or villain?" 2007.

106 p. 234.

107 P. Levi, *The Memory of the Offense*, In: Levi P. *The Drowned and the Saved*, (New York: Summit Books, 1988). p. 23–35.

108 Epstein, 1998.

109 Keating, *Smoking Kills*, 2009.

110 R. Horton, Cancer: Malignant Maneuvers. Review of *Devra Davis The Secret History of the War on Cancer*. The New York Review of Books, 2008 Mar 6. Available from: http://www.nybooks.com/articles/archives/2008/mar/06/cancer-malignant-maneuvers/.

111 G. Greene. 2008. "Malignant Maneuvers." In response to: Cancer: Malignant Maneuvers from the March 6, 2008 issue. The New York Review of Books, 2008 Jun 26. Available from: http://www.nybooks.com/articles/archives/2008/jun/26/malignant-maneuvers/.

112 Greene, 1999.

113 Walker, "A Questionable Pillar of the Cancer Establishment," 1998.

114 A. J. McMichael, "Smoking Kills: The Revolutionary Life of Richard Doll," Book Review, *Int J Epidemiol*. 39 (2010): 1123–6.

115 J. Samet, B. Pineles, "Smoking Kills: The Revolutionary Life of Richard Doll," Book Review, *Am J Epidemiol*. 171 (2010) 848–50.

116 P. Shetti P, "Richard Doll's smoking gun," Review, *New Sci*. 2743 (January 15, 2010).

117 Medical Research Council (MRC, "Science chiefs defend cancer pioneer," *Press release. Sunday Times*, 2006 Oct 9).

118 R. Doll, "Are we winning the fight against cancer? An epidemiological assessment," *Eur J Cancer*. 26 (1990): 500–8.

119 Walker, "A Questionable Pillar of the Cancer Establishment," 1998.

120 p. 82

121 Keating, *Smoking Kills*, 2009.

122 p. xi

123 Talbot, Medical research and big business, 2007.

124 R. Stott, "Cloud over Sir Richard," *Sunday Mirror*, 2006 Dec 10. Available from: http://www.thefreelibrary.com/Cloud+over+Sir+Richard percent3B+STOTTY +ON+SUNDAY.-a0155701671.

125 A. V. Yablokov, V.B. Nesterenko, A.V. Nesterenko, *Chernobyl: Consequences of the Catastrophe for People and the Environment.* Annals of the New York Academy of Sciences, Volume 1181, (Boston, MA: Blackwell Publishing, 2009).

126 D. Grady, "Radiation Is Everywhere, but How to Rate Harm?" *The New York Times*, 2011 Apr 5. Available from: http://www.nytimes.com/2011/04/05/ health/05radiation.html?_r=0.

127 W. J. Broad, "Radiation Over U.S. Is harmless, Officials Say," *The New York Times*, 2011 Mar 21. Available from: http://www.nytimes.com/2011/03/22/world/ asia/22plume.html.

128 Democracy Now! "Prescription for Survival": A Debate on the Future of Nuclear Energy Between Anti-coal Advocate George Monbiot and Anti-Nuclear Activist Dr. Helen Caldicott. Transcript, 2011 Mar 30. Available from: http://www.democ-racynow.org/2011/3/30/prescription_for_survival_a_debate_on.

129 D. Grady, "Precautions Should Limit Health Problems From Nuclear Plant's Radiation," *The New York Times*, 2011 Mar 15. Available from: http://www. nytimes.com/2011/03/16/world/asia/16health.html.

130 E. Rosenthal, "Experts Find Reduced Effects of Chernobyl" *The New York Times*, 2005 Sep 6. Available from: http://www.nytimes.com/2005/09/06/world/europe/ experts-find-reduced-effects-of-chernobyl.html.

131 I. Fairlie, D. Sumner, The Other Report on Chernobyl (TORCH). Berlin, Brussels, Kiev: MEP Greens/EFA; 2006. Available from: http://www.chernobylreport.org/ torch.pdf.

132 Greenpeace. The Chernobyl Catastrophe: Consequences on Human Health. Amsterdam: Greenpeace; 2006. Available from: http://www.greenpeace.org/inter-national/Global/international/planet-2/report/2006/4/chernobylhealthreport. pdf.

133 Yablokov, et al., *Consequences of the Catastrophe for People and the Environment*, 2009.

134 Ibid. p. 2.

135 Ibid. p. 255.

136 Ibid.

137 Ibid. p. 3, 33.

138 E. Cardis, A. Kesminiene, V. Ivanov, I. Malakhova, Y. Shibata, V. Khrouch, et al., "Risk of thyroid cancer after exposure to 131I in childhood," *J Natl Cancer Inst*. 97 (2005): 724–32.

139 Yablokov, et al., *Consequences of the Catastrophe for People and the Environment*, 2009, p. 130, 125.

140 Ibid. p. 133.

141 Ibid. p. 211.

142 Ibid. p. 323, 237.

143 Ibid. p. 42.

144 R. H. Nussbaum, "Childhood leukemia and cancers near German nuclear reactors: significance, context, and ramifications of recent studies," *Int J Occup Environ Health.* 15 (2009): 318–23.

145 p. 321.

146 D. J. Brenner, R. K. Sachs, "Estimating radiation-induced cancer risk as at very low doses: Rationale for using a linear no-threshold approach," *Radiat Environ Biophys.* 44 (2006): 253–6.

147 Committee Examining Radiation Risks of Internal Emitters (CERRIE). 2004. Report. Oct. 20. Available from: http://webarchive.nationalarchives.gov. uk/20140108135436/http://www.cerrie.org/pdfs/cerrie_report_e-book.pdf.

148 Malko, Chernobyl Accident.

149 C-Span. Japan Nuclear Plant Crisis and Chernobyl Anniversary [video, press conference]. 2011 Mar 15. Available from: http://www.c-span.org/video/?298667-1/japan-nuclear-plant-crisis-chernobyl-anniversary.

Chapter 13: The Corporate Hijack of the UK Vaccine Programme, Martin Walker

1   N. Chomsky, M. Foucault, *The Chomsky - Foucault Debate: On Human Nature.* (New York: The New Press, 2006).

2   M. Foucault, *The Birth of the Clinic: An Archaeology of Medical Perception.* (London: Tavistock, 1973) (originally in French, 1963).

3   B. S. Hooker, "Measles-mumps-rubella vaccination timing and autism among young African American boys: a reanalysis of CDC data," *Transl Neurodegener.* 3 (2014): 16. (Retracted).

4   F. DeStefano, T. K. Bhasin, W. W. Thompson, C. Yeargin-Allsopp M. Boyle, "Age at first measles-mumps-rubella vaccination in children with autism and school-matched control subjects: a population-based study in metropolitan Atlanta," *Pediatrics.* 113 (2004): 259–66.

5   A. J. Wakefield, S. H. Murch, A. Anthony, J. Linnell, D. M. Casson, M. Malik, et al. "Ileal-lymphoid-nodular hyperplasia, non-specific colitis, and pervasive developmental disorder in children," *Lancet.* 351 (1998): 637–41.

6   M. J. Walker, *The Urabe Farrago: A Recent Historical Account of Corporations and Governments Hiding Vaccine Damage for the Greater Good.* (London: Slingshot Publications, 2009).

7   Ibid.

8   In the wake of the withdrawal, accompanied by claims that meningitis wasn't after all that serious a childhood illness, the most elaborate conspiracy was practised to protect those who had been a part of the Committee in 1987 and 1988 and ensure that no one was brought to account. Christine England, Martin Walker, Lisa Blakemore-Brown.

9   ClinicalTrials.gov. Analysis of the Immune Response to Respiratory Syncytial Virus (RSV) Exposure in a Paediatric Population [Internet]. Available from: http://clinicaltrials.gov/show/NCT01922648.

10 Joint Committee on Vaccination and Immunisation (JVCI). Minute of the meeting on Wednesday 6 February 2013, 102A-124A, Skipton House, Department of Health, 80 London Road, London SE1 6LH. Available from: https://www.gov.uk/government/uploads/system/uploads/attachment_data/file/223498/JCVI_minutes_February_2013_meeting_-_final.pdf.

11 H. Burns, M. McGuire, Announcement of Phase Two Priority Groups for the Influenza A (H1N1) Vaccination Programme. The Scottish Government; 2009. Available from: http://www.show.scot.nhs.uk/App_Shared/pdf/H1N1vaccinationprogrammeCMOCNOletteronPhaseTwo3December2009.pdf.

12 Houses of the Oireachtas. Written Answers - Vaccination Programme. Dáil Éireann Debate. Vol. 768 No. 2, 2012. Available from: http://debates.oireachtas.ie/dail/2012/06/13/00204.asp.

13 Läkemedelsverket (Medical Products Agency; MPA). Occurrence of narcolepsy with cataplexy among children and adolescents in relation to the H1N1 pandemic and Pandemrix vaccinations. Results of a case inventory study by the MPA in Sweden during 2009–2010. MPA 2011 Jun 30. Available from: https://lakemedelsverket.se/upload/nyheter/2011/Fallinventeringsrapport_pandermrix_110630.pdf.

14 R. Smith, Change in swine flu virus is my biggest fear: Liam Donaldson. The Telegraph 2009 Dec 3. Available from: http://www.telegraph.co.uk/news/health/swine-flu/6719861/Change-in-swine-flu-virus-is-my-biggest-fear-Liam-Donaldson.html.

15 ClinicalTrials.gov. Swine Flu (Influenza A H1N1) Follow on Vaccine Study [Internet]. Available from: https://clinicaltrials.gov/ct2/show/NCT01239537.

16 Daily Mail Reporter. "Glaxo profits soar as drug firm charges NHS £6 for swine flu vaccine that costs £1 to make," *Mail Online* 2009 Jul 23. Available from: http://www.dailymail.co.uk/news/article-1201450/GlaxoSmithKline-accused-profiteering-drug-giant-charges-NHS-6-flu-vaccine-costs-1-make.html.

17 House of Commons. Hansard Written Answers for 18 Jan 2010. Available from: http://www.publications.parliament.uk/pa/cm200910/cmhansrd/cm100118/text/100118w0030.htm.

18 World Health Organization. Statement on narcolepsy and Pandemrix. 2011 Jul 27. Available from: http://www.who.int/vaccine_safety/committee/topics/influenza/pandemic/h1n1_safety_assessing/narcolepsy_statement_Jul2011/en/.

19 R. Knowlson, Swine flu vaccine "caused narcolepsy" admits Government. Pulse 2013 Sep 24. Available from: http://www.pulsetoday.co.uk/clinical/therapy-areas/immunisation/swine-flu-vaccine-caused-narcolepsy-admits-government/20004418.article#.U_yQx6Npu1s.

20 D. O'Flanagan, A.S. Barret, M. Foley, S. Cotter, C. Bonner, C. Crowe, et al. Investigation of an association between onset of narcolepsy and vaccination with pandemic influenza vaccine, Ireland April 2009–December 2010. Euro Surveill. 2014;19:15-25.

21 The group action will be brought against GSK, but Todd said the drug company had an indemnity clause in its contract to provide the vaccine, which means government will ultimately foot the bill.

22   How seriously we view meningitis depends on who is claimed to have caused it; when it was created by the Urabe strain MMR, it was said by the DoH to be not dangerous at all.

23   Joint Committee on Vaccination and Immunisation (JCVI). Update on the outcome of consultation about use of Bexsero® meningococcal B vaccine in the UK. 2013 Oct 25. Available from: https://www.gov.uk/government/uploads/system/uploads/attachment_data/file/252859/JCVI_MenB_Update.pdf.

24   Novartis. Novartis meningitis B vaccine Bexsero® receives FDA Breakthrough Therapy designation in the US. Media releases 2014 Apr 7. Available from: http://www.novartis.com/newsroom/media-releases/en/2014/1774805.shtml.

25   ClinicalTrials.gov. Investigating the Immune Response to 4CMenB in Infants [Internet]. Available from: http://clinicaltrials.gov/show/NCT02080559.

26   UK Clinical Research Network. Investigating the immune response to 4CMenB in infants (EUCLIDS)2+1. Available from: http://public.ukcrn.org.uk/search/StudyDetail.aspx?StudyID=16339.

27   Ibid.

28   PMlive. Novartis gets EU approval for Bexsero meningitis B shot. 2013 Jan 23. Available from: http://www.pmlive.com/pharma_news/novartis_gets_eu_approval_for_bexsero_meningitis_b_shot_459938.

29   D. Tyer, Novartis pays $16bn for GSK's oncology portfolio. PMlive 2014 Apr 22. Available from: http://www.pmlive.com/pharma_news/novartis_pays_$16bn_for_gsks_oncology_portfolio_562086.

30   Most recently this has applied to the claims of parents in the MMR case, which took ten years to prepare before legal aid was withdrawn.

31   In the UK, Getting Ahead of the Curve: A strategy for combating infectious diseases (including other aspects of health protection), A report by the Chief Medical Officer Sir Kenneth Calman published in 1992 advocated government policy of combined vaccines.In the US, one major vaccine researcher and patent holder, Paul Offit has frequently stresses the possibility of using combined strain vaccines containing up to 10,000 viral Strains. Offit claims 10,000 viral Strains would have no adverse effect whatsoever on a young child.

      This bogus science is also propagated by the Oxford Vaccine Group, chaired by Professor Andrew Pollard, and can be found on the group's website. "The Vaccine Knowledge Project; Authoritative Information For All"; published on the Internet by Oxford University and the Oxford Vaccine Group. Overseen by Professor Andrew Pollard can be found at:

      http://www.ovg.ox.ac.uk/combination-vaccines-and-multiple-vaccinations.

32   N. Z. Miller, G. S. Goldman, "Infant mortality rates regressed against number of vaccine doses routinely given: Is there a biochemical or synergistic toxicology?" Hum Exp Toxicol. 30 (2011): 1420–8.

33   National Vaccine Information Centre (NVIC). Forty-nine doses of 14 Vaccines before age 6? Sixty-nine doses of 16 vaccines by age 18? Before you take the risk, find out what it is. Available from: http://www.nvic.org/CMSTemplates/NVIC/pdf/49-Doses-PosterB.pdf.

34   Netdoctor. Childhood vaccinations. Available from: http://www.netdoctor.co.uk/ health_advice/facts/childhoodvaccinations.htm.

35   J. Deckoff-Jones, "The Fox Guarding The Henhouse - The CDC & Vaccine Safety. GreenMedInfo," 2014 Sep 4. Available from: http://www.greenmedinfo.com/blog/ fox-guarding-henhouse-cdc-vaccine-safety.

36   That logic might make sense if the health of the species had actually improved during the period in question, but it is quite the opposite. More than half of the people in the US have a chronic disease, including our children. Our infant mortality rate is thirty-fourth in the world, despite, or perhaps because of, the fact that we give more vaccine doses before the age of 1 than the 33 countries ahead of us.

37   There are now so many books that outline vested interests in research and science that it is difficult to cite only one reference. Chapter 1 of this book cites many of these works, including the last three of these references. The first one puts the case succinctly.

      Arthur Schafer *The University as Corporate Handmaiden: Who're ya gonna trust* http:// umanitoba.ca/ University of Manitoba faculties/arts/departments/philosophy/ ethics/media/University_as_Corporate_Handmaiden.pdf.

      J. Strauber, S. Rampton, Trust *Us We're Experts! How Industry Manipulates Science and Gambles with Your future.* (New York: Tarcher, 2002).

      D. Fagin, M. Lavelle, *Toxic Deception: How the Chemical Industry Manipulates Science, Bends the Law and Endangers Your Health* (New Jersey: Carol Publishing Group, 1996).

      J. Strauber, S. Rampton, *Toxic Sludge is Good for You! Lies, Damn Lies and the Public Relations Industry.* (Monroe: ME: Common Courage Press, 1995).

38   Ibid.

39   Wakefield, et al., "Ileal-lymphoidmodular hyperplasia . . . " 1998.

Chapter 14: Exponent and Dioxin in Sweden in the Early 2000s, Martin Walker and Bo Walhjalt

1   B. Ramel. Jag går forskningens och sanningens ärende," *Läkartidningen.* 100(4) (2003): 206–7. Available from:http://www.lakartidningen.se/ OldPdfFiles/2003/26043.pdf.

2   H-O .Adami, A. Ahlbom, A. Ekbom, L. Hagmar, M. Ingelman-Sundberg. Forskare som pratar strunt. Svenska Dagbladet 2001 Sep 3. Available from: http://web. archive.org/web/20030222001824/http://www.svd.se/dynamiskt/Brannpunkt/ did_1601568.asp.

3   L. Söderberg. Nobelprofessor hyrs av kemijätte (Nobel Committee professor hired by large chemical company). Aftonbladet. 2001 Dec 17. Available from: http:// www.aftonbladet.se/nyheter/article10248592.ab and http://www.aftonbladet.se/ nyheter/article10248731.ab.

4   L. Hardell, "Pesticides, soft-tissue sarcoma and non-Hodgkin lymphoma: historical aspects on the precautionary principle in cancer prevention," Acta Oncol. 47 (2008): 347–54.

5   L. Hardell, Maligna mesenkymala mjukdelstumorer och exposition for fenoxisy-
      ror—en klinisk observation. Lakartidningen. 1977;71:2753–4.
6   L. Hardell, A. Sandstrom, "Case control study: soft tissue sarcomas and exposure
      to phenoxyacetic acids or chlorophenols," *Br J Cancer*. 39 (1979): 711–7.
7   Adami, et al., www.svd.se.
8   Söderberg, 2001.
9   H-O. Adami, P. Cole, J. Mandel, H. Pastides, T. B. Starr, D. Trichopoulos. Dioxin and
      cancer. The first Exponent review to be presented to the EPA Science Advisory Board.
      There are more versions circulating, because it has also been used in legal processes.
10   2,3,7,8-tetrachlorodibenzo-p-dioxin (TCDD) and chemically similar compounds,
      collectively known as dioxins.
11   Alongside the humans serving in Vietnam, there were 3.895 military working dogs,
      almost all of them pure bred German shepherds. (H. M. Hayes, et al. US military
      working dogs with Vietnam service: definition and characteristics of the cohort. Mil
      Med. 1994;159:669–75.) About 91 percent of these dogs were "intact" (uncastrated)
      males. When a military working dog dies, regardless of the circumstances of death
      or the duty location, an autopsy is performed by a veterinarian, and a standard-
      ized set of tissue specimens and organs are sent to the Armed Forces Institute of
      Pathology in Washington, DC. During the late 1980s, in two studies, the autopsy
      records of dogs with Vietnam service were compared with dogs which served in the
      continental US (Hayes HM, et al. Excess of seminomas observed in Vietnam service
      US military working dogs. J Natl Cancer Inst. 1990;82:1042–6.). The studies showed
      that dogs that served in Vietnam were about twice as likely (1.8 times as likely) to
      have cancer of the testicles, compared to military working dogs that served only in
      the States. Likewise, military dogs that died in Okinawa were about twice as likely
      (2.2 times as likely) to have testicular cancer as dogs that served only in the States.
      (Rachel's Environment and Health Weekly. #436, 1995 Apr 6.
12   See accounts of the Australian Royal Commission.
13   Earthjustice Legal Defense Fund. Press release dated 1999 Nov 29.
14   This paragraph and those that follow, on waste incinerators and dioxin, are
      based on paragraphs in the book *Behind closed doors,* published by the Center
      for Health, Environment and Justice's Stop Dioxin Exposure Campaign, 2000.
      Available from Center For Health, Environment and Justice, P.O. Box 6806, Falls
      Church, VA 22040, 703-237-2249, chej@chej.org. The Center is also responsible
      for publishing *America's choice: children's health or corporate profit. The American
      people's Dioxin Report,* and for distributing the brilliant *Dying from dioxin: a citi-
      zen's guide to reclaiming our health and rebuilding democracy,* by Lois Mary Gibbs
      and the Citizen's Clearinghouse for Hazardous Waste, published by South End
      Press, Boston, 1995.
15   L. Hardell, . Sandström, "Case-control study: Soft tissue sarcomas and exposure to
      phenoxyacetic acids or chlorophenols," *Br J Cancer* 39 (1979): 711–7.
16   J. Müntzing. Forskare eller olycksprofet (Researcher or Doomsday Prophet).
      Svenska Dagbladet 1979 Sep 3.

17   Polychlorinated dibenzo-*para*-dioxins and polychlorinated dibenzofurans. IARC Monographs on the evaluation of carcinogenic risks to humans. Vol 69. Lyon: International Agency for Research on Cancer; 1997.

18   J. Mandel, Epidemiological studies of Vietnam veterans: a critical review. Organohalogen Compounds 2001;54:400–1.

19   H-O, Adami, "Can studies by a single investigator override collective evidence? The case of dioxin," *Organohalogen Compounds* 54 (2001): 403–4.

20   Ibid.

21   D. Trichopoulos, "No evidence that dioxin is a human carcinogen," *Organohalogen Compounds* 54 (2001): 409–11.

22   Adami, et al. EPA Science Advisory Board.

23   H-O. Adami. Bespara människor okritiska larm. Dagens Forskning. 2002(20).

24   Ibid.

25   Ibid.

26   M. Eriksson, L. Hardell, H. O. Adami, "Exposure to dioxins as a risk factor for soft tissue sarcoma: a population-based case-control study," *J Natl Cancer Inst.* 82 (1990): 486–90.

27   Exponent. About Us [Internet]. Available from: http://www.exponent.com/about/.

28   See Tweedale.

29   Given recent problems with Gulf War Syndrome and depleted uranium ammunition, the US Government needs these companies as much as the companies need them.

30   Rachel's Environment & Health Weekly. Nationwide Dioxin Campaign. Number 479, 1996 Feb 1. Available from: http://www.ejnet.org/rachel/rehw479.htm.

31   L. M. Gibbs, *The Citizens Clearinghouse for Hazardous Waste. Dying from Dioxin: A Citizen's Guide to Reclaiming Our Health and Rebuilding Democracy* (Boston, MA: South End Press, 1995).

32   Chemicals that are suspected of interfering with the normal functioning of sex hormones in humans and wildlife.

33   Another company officer who plays a leading part in regulatory and toxicity matters is Corporate Vice President Dennis J. Paustenbach, PhD, CIH, DABT.

34   The manner in which National Semiconductor have responded to women's health issues at their plant in Greenock appears to be a classic case of censure, dirty tricks, and intrigue. Having brought in the big guns of Exponent they then turned to a similar but much smaller local company, Beattie Media, who devised a strategy to defeat the workers that included "utilizing Beattie Media female staff members to pose as clean room workers in order to dupe journalists investigating the company's health record. Beattie Media also planned intelligence gathering on Jim McCourt and PHASE II, with the intention of `undermining the credibility of individuals and groups involved." McCourt claims that his office was burgled and he was intimidated in the street [Hazards 76. 2001, PO Box 199 Sheffield S1 4YL].

35   Luanne Jenkins, spokeswoman for National Semiconductor.

36   In an unbelievable irony, the EPA website, which reported this third meeting in 2000, left out the word chemical in its introductory paragraph, defining the Report Program as the Voluntary Children's Evaluation Program! (VCCEP).

37   Ninth Report on Carcinogens, Revised January 2001, US Department of Health and Human Services, National Toxicology Program, citing IARC Vol. 63, 1995 and ATSDR, 1995-H008.

38   EPAStopStalling.org. Citations for PCRM's Comprehensive Report on the EPA's Voluntary Children's Chemical Evaluation Program [Internet]. Available from: http://web.archive.org/web/20020116010259/http://www.epastopstalling.org/cite_trichloroethylene.htm.

39   Ninth Report on Carcinogens, Revised January 2001, US Department of Health and Human Services, National Toxicology Program.

40   One of the groups opposed to the time-wasting exercise by the chemical companies is PETA, the animal rights organization. PETA estimated from the EPA's own figures that the tests will use "between six hundred thousand and 1.2 million animals."

41   US EPA, 1994.

42   EPA Science Advisory Board. A Second Look at Dioxin. Available from: http://yosemite.epa.gov/sab/sabproduct.nsf/0D86745602ADB6C68525719B006B0260/$File/ec95021.pdf.

43   US EPA, 2000.

44   In 1999, the Sierra Club filed a lawsuit aimed at reducing the amount of harmful chemicals dumped into the air by toxic waste incinerators and waste-burning cement kilns. The Sierra Club stated that, although hazardous waste incinerators are among America's most dangerous polluters, the federal government has failed to monitor and control the pollution they release into our air (including dioxins, furans, mercury, and organic hazardous air pollutants). "Toxic waste incinerators foul our air, land, and food. These incinerators make it tougher for kids with asthma to breathe, fill our lungs with toxic chemicals, and poison the food we eat," said Dr. Neil Carman, clean air program director of Sierra Club's Lone Star Chapter in Texas. "The government has been looking the other way again, letting the toxic waste industry pollute at outrageous levels and then self-monitor their incinerators for violations." (Earthjustice Legal Defense Fund; Press release dated November 29, 1999.)

45   See reports and statements of the Virginia-based Center for Health, Environment and Justice.

46   Behind closed doors, published by Center for Health, Environment and Justice's Stop Dioxin Exposure Campaign 2000. Available from Center For Health, Environment and Justice, P.O. Box 6806, Falls Church, VA 22040, 703-237-2249, chej@chej.org.

47   Ibid.

48   M. J. Walker. "Sir Richard Doll: a questionable pillar of the cancer establishment," Ecologist. 28 (1998) 82–92.

49   Institute of Medicine. Veterans and Agent Orange. Health effects of herbicides used in Vietnam (Washington, DC: National Academy Press, 1994) (updated 1996).

50   Established in 1976 as the Chemical Industry Institute of Toxicology, in 2001 the organization changed its name to CIIT, Centers for Health Research. Appearing to operate like one of the National Institutes for Health, and cited by its President,

William F. Greenlee, as "positioned to become one of the pre-eminent environmental and human health research institutes with a global role in benefiting the public," CIIT is wholly funded by the Chemical Industry for which it carries out research. Funded initially by the American Chemistry Council Long Range Research Initiative (LRRI), its backers now include government agencies, any corporate clients while its member companies include: Bayer, BASF, Chevron, Dow, Du Pont, Kodak, Exxon, Novartis and GEC.

Chapter 15: References Burying the Evidence, O'Neill, Pickvance, Andrew Watterson

1   Health and Safety Executive (HSE). Estimated attributable fractions, deaths, and registrations by cancer site (based on Table at p11 in The Burden of Occupational Cancer in Great Britain - Rushton cancer burden report). Available from: http://web.archive.org/web/20100430204851/http://www.hse.gov.uk/statistics/tables/can01.htm.

2   Health and Safety Executive (HSE). Cancer Statistics. Available from: http://web.archive.org/web/20070610175912/http://www.hse.gov.uk/statistics/causdis/cancer.htm.

3   "HSE blocks new rights, says lives are not worth saving," *Hazards magazine*, 2007 Apr–Jun. Available from: http://www.hazards.org/safetyreps/crosswords.htm.

4   R. Doll, R. Peto, "The causes of cancer: quantitative estimates of avoidable risks of cancer in the United States today," *J Natl Cancer Inst.* 66 (1981): 1191–308.

5   R. W. Clapp, G. K. Howe, M. Jacobs, "Environmental and occupational causes of cancer re-visited," *J Public Health Policy* 27 (2006): 61–76.

6   L. Fritschi, T. Driscoll, "Cancer due to occupation in Australia: *Aust N Z J Pub Health* 30 (2006): 213–9.

7   L. Hardell, M. J. Walker, B. Walhjalt, L. S. Friedman, E. D. Richter. "Secret ties to industry and conflicting interests in cancer research," *Am J Ind Med* 50 (2007): 227–33.

8   "Hazards Work Cancer Prevention Kit," *Hazards magazine*, Mar. 2007 Available from: http://www.hazards.org/cancer/preventionkit/.

9   P. Hämäläinen, J. Takala, K. L. Saarela, "Global estimates of fatal work-related diseases," *Am J Ind Med.* 50 (2007): 28–41.

10   T. Kauppinen, J. Toikkanen, D. Pedersen, R. Young, W. Ahrens, P. Boffetta, et al. "Occupational exposure to carcinogens in the European Union" *Occup Environ Med.* 57 (2000): 10–8.

11   Health and Safety Laboratory (HSL). Powertrain Occupational Respiratory Disease Outbreak: Report of Immunological Investigation. MU/06/01, 2007 Mar. Available from: http://www.hse.gov.uk/aboutus/meetings/iacs/acts/watch/190607/p5ann3.pdf.

12   F. Mirer, "Updated epidemiology of workers exposed to metalworking fluids provides sufficient evidence for carcinogenicity," *Appl Occup Environ Hyg.* 18 (2003): 902–12.

13   "Come clean," *Hazards magazine*, 2006 Jul-Sep. Available from: http://www.hazards.org/commissionimpossible/comeclean.htm.

14   HSE Chief in York. World of work has changed but ill-health still claims 24 million working days. HSE Press release 2007 Jul 5. YH /26307. GNN ref 14902M.

15   M. Greenberg, "Three tears for EMAS," *Occup.Med* (Lond), 55 (2005): 73–4.

16   Politics.co.uk. Industry Facts & Figures. Chemical Industries Association (CIA), 2006 Jan. Available from: http://web.archive.org/web/20071021223851/http://www.politics.co.uk/campaignsite/chemical-industries-association-cia-$364291$4.htm.

17   The Global Occupational Health Network (GOHNET). Prevention of occupational cancer. World Health Organization (WHO), GOHNET newsletter, 11, 2006. Available from: http://www.who.int/occupational_health/publications/newsletter/gohnet11e.pdf.

18   P. Vineis, L. Simonato, "Proportion of lung and bladder cancers in males resulting from occupation: a systematic approach," *Arch Environ Health*. 46 (1991): 6-15.

19   "Hazards Work Cancer Prevention Kit," March 2007.

20   Kauppinen, et al., "Occupational Exposure . . ." 2000.

21   International Association of Labour Inspection. Summary report of conference: "Labour Inspection and Chemicals and Carcinogens." 17th–18th May 2004, Dublin, Ireland. Available from: http://www.iali-aiit.org/resources/conferences/ReportEN(FINAL).doc.

22   Federation of Small Businesses (FSB). Health Matters: a small business perspective. London: FSB; 2006. Available from: http://www.fsb.org.uk/documentstore/filedetails.asp?ID=367.

23   Health and Safety Executive (HSE). About metalworking fluids. Available from: http://www.hse.gov.uk/metalworking/about.htm

24   E.J. Malloy, K.L. Miller, E.A. Eisen, "Rectal cancer and exposure to metalworking fluids in the automobile manufacturing industry," *Occup Environ Med*. 64 (2007): 244–9.

25   "Burying the evidence," *Hazards magazine*, 2005 Nov. Available from: http://www.hazards.org/cancer/report.htm.

26   "International Agency for Research on Cancer (IARC)," Recent Meetings. Volume 88: Formaldehyde, 2-Butoxyethanol and 1-tert-Butoxy-2-propanol. 2004 Jun 2–9. Available from: http://web.archive.org/web/20081209093129/http://monographs.iarc.fr/ENG/Meetings/vol88.php.

27   "International Agency for Research on Cancer (IARC)," IARC Monographs on the Evaluation of Carcinogenic Risks to Humans. Formaldehyde, 2-Butoxyethanol and 1-tert-Butoxy-2-propanol. Volume 88. Lyon (France): WHO Press; 2006. Available from: http://monographs.iarc.fr/ENG/Monographs/vol88/mono88.pdf.

28   Centers for Disease Control and Prevention. NIOSH Current Intelligence Bulletin No 20. Tetrachloroethylene. 1978 Jan 20. Available from: http://web.archive.org/web/20120516005531/http://www.cdc.gov/niosh/78112_20.html.

29   Health and Safety Executive (HSE). Drycleaners—Are you in control? HSE; 2000. Available from: http://www.hse.gov.uk/pubns/indg310.pdf.

30   United Nations Economic Commission for Europe (UNECE). Facts about women & men in Great Britain 2006. Equal Opportunities Commission; 2006 May.

Available from: http://www.unece.org/fileadmin/DAM/stats/gender/publications/UK/Facts_about_W&M_GB_2006.pdf.

31 Breast Cancer UK. Breast cancer—an environmental disease: the case for primary prevention. UK Working Group on the Primary Prevention of Breast Cancer; 2005. Available from: http://www.breastcanceruk.org.uk/uploads/Breast_cancer_-_an_environmental_disease.pdf.

32 "International Agency for Research on Cancer (IARC)," IARC Monographs on the Evaluation of Carcinogenic Risks to Humans. Some organic solvents, resin monomers and related compounds, pigments and occupational exposures in paint manufacture and painting. Volume 47. Lyon (France): WHO Press; 1989. Available from: http://monographs.iarc.fr/ENG/Monographs/vol47/mono47.pdf.

33 C. H. Barcenas, G. L. Delclos, R. El-Zein, G. Tortolero-Luna, L. W. Whitehead, M.R. Spitz, "Wood dust exposure and the association with lung cancer risk," *Am J Ind Med.* 47 (2005): 349–57.

34 "Hazards Work Cancer Prevention Kit," March 2007.

35 J. T. Brophy, M. M. Keith, K. M. Gorey, E. Laukkanen, I. Luginaah, H. Abu-Zahra, et al., "Cancer and construction: what occupational histories in a Canadian community reveal," *Int J Occup Environ Health* 13 (2007): 32–8.

36 K. Kjaerheim, "Occupational cancer research in the Nordic countries, *Environ Health Perspect.* 107 (1999): (Suppl 2):233–8.

37 E. Kellen, M. P. Zeegers, E. D. Hond, F. Buntinx, "Blood cadmium may be associated with bladder carcinogenesis: the Belgian case-control study on bladder cancer," *Cancer Detect Prev.*, 31 (2007): 77–82.

38 A. J. Darnton, D. M. McElvenny, J. T. Hodgson, "Estimating the number of asbestos-related lung cancer deaths in Great Britain from 1980–2000, *Ann Occup Hyg.* 50 (2006): 29–38.

39 Toxics Use Reduction Institute. Available from: http://www.turi.org/

40 Toxics Use Reduction Institute. Five Chemicals Alternatives Assessment Study. Lowell (MA): TURI; 2006 Jun 30. Available from: http://www.turi.org/TURI_Publications/TURI_Methods_Policy_Reports/Five_Chemicals_Alternatives_Assessment_Study._2006/Full_Report.

41 Canadian Strategy for Cancer Control (CSCC). Prevention of Occupational and Environmental Cancers in Canada: A best Practices Review and Recommendations. 2005 May. Available from: https://web.archive.org/web/20070206081247/http://www.cancercontrol.org/cscc/pdf/BestProactiseReview.pdf.

42 European Environment Agency (EEA). Late lessons from early warnings: The precautionary principle 1896–2000. Environmental issue report 22. Copenhagen (Denmark): EEA; 2001 Jan 9. Available from: http://reports.eea.europa.eu/environmental_issue_report_2001_22/en.

43 "Silent Spring Institute. Environment and breast cancer," *Science Review*, 2007. Available from: http://sciencereview.silentspring.org/index.cfm.

44 H. A Wakelee, E. T. Chang, S. L. Gomez, T. H. Keegan, D. Feskanich, C. A. Clarke, et al., "Lung cancer incidence in never smokers," *J Clin Oncol.* 25 (2007): 472-8.

45 "A little compensation," *Hazards magazine*, 2005 May. Available from: http://www.hazards.org/compensation/briefing.htm.

46 V. W. Popp, K. Bruening, *Straif, Berufliche Krebserkrankungen—Situation in Deutschland*, In: J. Konietzko, H. Dupuis, editors, *Handbuch der Arbeitsmedizin* (Landsberg, Germany: Ecomed, 2002) p. 1–14.

47 *Science Review*, 2007 ·

48 Research International (UK) Ltd. Industry's perception & use of occupational exposure limits. Contract Research Report 144. HSE Books; 1997. Available from: http://www.hse.gov.uk/research/crr_pdf/1997/crr97144.pdf.

49 D. Provost, A. Cantagrel, P. L.ebailly, A. Jaffré, V. Loyant, H. Loiseau, et al., "Brain tumors and exposure to pesticides: a case-control study in southwestern France," *Occup Environ Med.* 64 (2007): 509–14.

50 R. W. Clapp, "Mortality among US employees of a large computer manufacturing company: 1969–2001," *Environ Health.* 2006; 5:30.

51 A. Watterson, "Regulation of occupational health and safety in the semiconductor industry: enforcement problems and solutions,"*Int J Occup Environ Health,* 12 (2006): 72–80.

52 J. LaDou, J. C. III Bailar, "Cancer and reproductive risks in the semiconductor industry," *Int J Occup Environ Health* 13 (2007): 376–85.

53 R. O'Neill, "Not dead yet," *Hazards magazine*, Number 96, 2006 Oct/Dec. Available from: http://www.hazards.org/olderworkers/.

54 (UNECE), Facts about women & men in Great Britain 2006, May 2006.

55 "Get a life!" *Hazards magazine*, Available from: http://www.hazards.org/getalife/index.htm.

56 "Smoking and the workplace," *Hazards magazine*, Available from: http://www.hazards.org/smoking/index.htm.

57 "Drugs and alcohol," *Hazards magazine*, Available from: http://www.hazards.org/drugs/.

58 "Testing times," *Hazards magazine*, Available from: http://www.hazards.org/testingtimes/.

59 European Monitoring Centre for Drugs and Drug Addiction. Drug Demand Reduction in the Workplace. Final Report. EMCDDA; 1997 Nov. Available from: https://web.archive.org/web/20040224160651/http://www.emcdda.eu.int/multimedia/project_reports/ddr_workplace_report.pdf.

60 Barcenas, et al., "Wood dust exposure . . . " 2005.

61 T. Gouveia-Vigeant, J. Tickner, *Toxic chemicals and childhood cancer: a review of the evidence* (Lowell, MA: Lowell Center for Sustainable Production, University of Massachusetts Lowell, 2003 May), Available from: http://www.sustainableproduction.org/downloads/Child percent20Canc percent20Exec percent20Summary.pdf.

62 J. J. Heindel, "Role of exposure to environmental chemicals in the developmental basis of disease and dysfunction," *Reprod Toxicol.*, 23 (2007): 257–9.

63 "Asbestos," *Hazards magazine*, Available from: http://www.hazards.org/asbestos/.

64 J. Carlin, J. Knight, S. Pickvance, A. Watterson, "A worker-driven and community-based investigation of the health of one group of workers exposed to vinyl chloride monomer," (VCM), *J Risk Govern.*, 1 (2009): 105–24.

Chapter 16: Spin in the Antipodes, Don Maisch

1   The International Committee of Medical Journal Editors (ICMJE): Uniform Requirements for Manuscripts Submitted to Biomedical Journals: Writing and Editing for Biomedical Publication, 2007.

2   S. Krimsky, Science in *the Private Interest: Has the Lure of Profits Corrupted Biomedical Research?* (Rowman & Littlefield publishers, 2003).

3   East Sydney Private Hospital, Sydney & Epworth Richmond Hospital, Melbourne.

4   Prince of Wales Private Hospital, New South Wales, Australia.

5   Royal Melbourne Hospital and the Alfred Hospital, Victoria, Australia.

6   V. G. Khurana, C. Teo, R. G. Bittar. "Health risks of cell phone technology," *Surgical Neurology* 72 (2009): 436–7.

7   V. G. Khurana, C. Teo, M. Kundi, L. Hardell, "Cell phones and brain tumors: a review including the long-term epidemiologic data," *Surgical Neurology* 72 (2009): 205–14.

8   *60 Minutes* transcript, "Wake Up Call," Reporter L. Bartlett, April 3, 2009.

9   "Correspondence with Khurana," *VG*, July 5, 2009.

10   Brain Tumour Research (UK) Press Release, "Brain Tumours: Leading Cause of Cancer Death in Children," April 28, 2009.

11   L. Slesin, "Are Brain Cancer Rates Rising Among Young Adults? Striking Increase Cited at Congressional Hearing," *Microwave News*, Sept. 30, 2008. Available at: http://www.microwavenews.com/kucinich.html.

12   P. Allen, F. Macrae, "France cracks down on children's mobile phone use, but Britain still ignoring warnings,"*The Daily Mail*, 12 January 2009. Available at: http://www.dailymail.co.uk/health/article-1112123/France-cracks-childrens-mobile-phone-use-Britain-ignoring-warnings.html.

13   Y. Grigoryev, "Memorandum, The opinion of the Russian National Committee on Non-Ionizing Radiation Protection (RNCNIRP)," Mar. 4, 2009. Available at: http://www.radiationresearch.org/pdfs/20090320_grigoriev_memo.pdf.

14   ABC Lateline transcript, "Scientists speak out on mobile phone, cancer link," April 4, 2009. Available at: http://www.abc.net.au/lateline/content/2008/s2533725.htm.

15   G. Haddad, (testimony), The Australian Senate Environment, Communications, Information Technology and the Arts References Committee: Inquiry into Electromagnetic Radiation, June 2000.

16   D. Maisch, "Children and Mobile Phone Use . . . Is There a Health Risk?" *JACNEM*, 2003 Aug; 22(2): 3-8. Available at: http://www.emfacts.com/download/children_mobiles.pdf.

17   ABC Lateline transcript.

18   ACRBR main page. Available at: http://www.acrbr.org.au/.

19   IARC, Press release #200, Interphone study reports on mobile phone use and brain cancer risk , 17 May 2010, Available at:https://www.iarc.fr/en/media-centre/pr/2010/pdfs/pr200_E.pdf.

20   S. Curwood. "Cell Phone Use May Take Toll," (transcript), *PRI's Environmental News Magazine*, 12 May, 2010, Available at: http://newsletters.environmental-healthnews.org/t/40560/1038/49945/0/.

21 IARC, Press release #200.

22 D. Rose, "Experts deny mobile phones cause tumours," *The Sydney Morning Herald*, May 17, 2010, Available at: http://www.smh.com.au//breaking-news-national/experts-deny-mobile-phones-cause-tumours-20100517-v6ut.html.

23 IARC, Press Release # 208, IARC Classifies Rediofrequency Electromagnetic Fields as Possible Carcinogenic to Humans, 31 May, 2011, Available at: http://www.iarc.fr/en/media-centre/pr/2011/pdfs/pr208_E.pdf.

24 Denoted as radiofrequency and microwave frequencies (RF/MW) sometimes simply as RF.

25 CSIRO History, Available at: http://www.csiro.au/Portals/About-CSIRO/Who-we are/History/CSIROHistoryOverview.aspx. Accessed July 12, 2006.

26 Spectrum Management Agency (SMA) was a Commonwealth statutory agency within the portfolio of Communications and Arts. The primary function of SMA was to manage and allow access to the radiofrequency spectrum. On July 1, 1997 SMA was merged with the telecommunications regulator, AUSTEL, to later become the Australian Communications and Media Authority (ACMA).

27 Ibid.

28 This is defined as an obvious detrimental biological effect (tissue heating) from exposure to acute (high-level) RF/MW exposure levels.

29 Defined as possible biological effects from RF/MW exposures at levels (intensities) too low to cause a heating effect.

30 S. Barnett, Status of Research on Biological Effects and Safety of Electromagnetic Radiation:Telecommunications Frequencies , CSIRO Report, CSIRO Division of Radiophysics, June 1994.

31 D. Maisch, Fields of Conflict: The EMF Health Hazard Controversy, Australian Democrats, Aug. 1995, Anomous letter from a Telecom employee to Senator Robert Bell, Mar. 30, 1995, pp. 56–58.

32 S. Jasanoff, in *Organizational Encounters with Risk*, eds. Hutter and Power, (Cambridge University Press, 2005)."Restoring reason: causal narratives and political culture," pp. 209–232.

33 In 1996, the Division of Radiophysics was merged with the Division of Applied Science to become the Division of Telecommunications and Industrial Physics (TIP).

34 Maisch, 1995.

35 S. Barnett, circulated letter, September 22, 2003.

36 ABC Online, Inside Business—CSIRO heads toward commercialisation, November 11, 2003.

37 CEO Insight, Making change happen: Geoff Garnett at CSIRO , October 30, 2005.

38 J. Cribb, T. S. Hartomo, *Sharing knowledge: a guide to effective science communication,* (CSIRO Publishing, 2002).

39 *The ABC Science Show, Science Funding & CSIRO*, Saturday 24 April 2004, Available at: http://www.abc.net.au/radionational/programs/scienceshow/science-funding—csiro/3377284#transcript.

40 Correspondence with Stewart Fist, October 14, 2005.

41 *The ABC Science Show.*

42 P. Pockley, "Tobacco Statement "Disingenuous," *Australasian Science,* 2004 July: p. 44. Available at: http://connection.ebscohost.com/c/articles/13922373/tobacco-statement-disingenuous.

43 *The ABC Science Show.*

44 http://wwwdstaunton.com/experience.htm, Assessed October 29, 2005.

45 CSIRO Executive Team, Resume of Ms Donna Staunton: Executive Director of Communications, Available at: http://www.csiro.au/csiro/content/standard/psh4,,.html , Accessed February 16, 2006.

46 *The ABC Science Show.*

47 G. Nolch, "Smokescreen on CSIRO Science," *Viewpoint, Australasian Science,* Mar. 30, 2004 http://www.thefunneled-web.com/Old_Viewpoints/V-P-30_03_04.htm, Accessed Feb 6, 2006.

48 G. Nolch, "Critical Comment of CSIRO by Australasian Science Evokes Executive Outrage and a Threatened Boycott," *Australasian Science News & Views* item, June 2, 2004. Available at: http://math.haifa.ac.il/yair/The-Funneled-Web-archive-%282001-2013%29RIP/N&V_2004%28jun-Dec%29/N&V_0406/news__views_item_june_2004-040602.htm.

49 B. Carter, "All the signs of full-blown Mother Earthism," *Sydney Morning Herald,* Sept. 29, 2005. Available at: http://www.smh.com.au/news/opinion/all-the-signs-of-fullblown-mother-earthism/2005/09/28/1127804546992.html.

50 CSIRO, Available at: http://www.marine.csiro.au/iawg/impacts2001.pdf.

51 Correspondence with Stewart Fist, September 1, 2009.

52 S. Barnett, CSIRO Report, 1994, op. cit.

53 Letter from Richard Morris, Assistant Secretary, Health Research Branch, NH&MRC, to Sarah Benson, researcher for Senator Lyn Allison, 30 Dec. 1996.

54 The Australian Academy of Science, Available at: http://www.ncrs.org.au/annual/2005.pdf.

55 Standards Australia, Committee TE/7: Human Exposure to Electromagnetic Fields, meeting No. 1/98, 12 August 1998. Minutes.

56 Australian Senate Inquiry, 2002, Section 4.68, Available at: http://www.aph.gov.au/senate/committee/ecita_ctee/completed_inquiries/1999-02/emr/report/c04.htm. Oct 2, 2005.

57 K. Joyner, Australian Government Action on Electromagnetic Energy Public Health Issues. Bioelectromagnetics Society Newsletter. 1998 July/Aug; 143.

58 Mobile Phone Emissions: Research Grants, Australian Senate Hansard , page 2603, May 12,1998.

59 L. Slesin,, "The Talk of Long Beach: Motorola Takes Center Stage as Carlo Makes His Exit," *Microwave News,* 1999 July/Aug; 19(4).

60 Senate Hansard, 12 March 1998, p. 1012.

61 Ibid.

62 C. Althaus, AMTA CEO, Dr Ken Joyner to leave AMTA Committee roles, AMTA Snapshot , Edition 141, Jan. 16, 2009.

63 NH&MRC, Peer Reviewers and External Assessors (2009), Available at: https://www.nhmrc.gov.au/grants/peer-review/peer-review-honour-roll-2009.

64 Victorian Radiation Advisory Committee, Committee members. Available at: http://www.health.vic.gov.au/radiation/committee.htm.

65 RMIT research & innovation, Available at: http://www.rmit.edu.au/browse/Our%20Organisation%2FResearch%2FResearch%20Centres/#nhmrc.

66 D. Maisch, Notes from the Final Standards Australia TE/7 meeting, March 1999.

67 Burson Marsteller, Tobacco Documents, Available at: http://tobaccodocuments.org/profiles/bm.html.

68 AMTA's 2003 Annual Report, pp 28.

69 "Mobile Phone Debate," *Insight archives*, July 5, 2001, Available at: http://news.sbs.com.au/insight/trans.php?transid=225.

70 Ibid.

71 Ibid.

72 V. Anderson, "Mobile Telephony and the Precautionary Principle – A Phoney Debate?" *Radiation Protection in Australasia*, 18(2) (Dec. 2, 2001): 71–76.

73 Ibid.

74 RMIT University, Industry and Business // Get your strategic advantage, Available at: http://www.rmit.edu.au/advantage/.

75 RMIT University, Telstra Home Team, A different way of thinking, Available at: http://www2.rmit.edu.au/departments/rd/case/case8.htm.

76 RMIT Research Specialties, Available at: http://www.rmit.edu/sece/research.

77 RMIT conflict of interest policy, Available at: http://131.170.40.30/redirect?URL=http%3A%2F%2Fprodmams.rmit.edu.au%2Ffgznvzyjv4qi.doc.

78 M. Kenney, *Biotechnology: The University-Industrial Complex*, (New Haven: Yale University Press, 1986).

79 S. Krimsky.

80 Telstra Annual Report (2004). Available at: http://www.telstra.com.au/abouttelstra/investor/docs/companyoverview.pdf.

81 Telstra/Australian Government joint DVD, "Mobile Communications and Health," 2004.

82 S. Krimsky, 2003, Also see Corporate Influence in Academic Science. Available at: http://www.tufts.edu/~skrimsky/PowerPoint/COIAcademicSci4.pdf.

83 T. Bodenheimer, R. Collins, "Integrity in Science, Telling the Truth: What Drug Companies Don't Want You to Know," Available at: http://www.cspinet.org/integrity/tell_truth.html.

84 Many similar cases of the pitfalls that can occur in university-industry partnerships are detailed in: D. B. Resnik & A. E. Shamoo, Conflict of Interest and the University, Accountability in Research: Policies and Quality Assurance, 2002 Jan 9(1): 45–64.

85 Senate adjournment speech by Australian Democrat Senator Lyn Allison, in: ADJOURNMENT: Commonwealth Scientific and Industrial Research Organisation, Hansard, Sept 10, 2003.

86 S. Barnett.

87 Mobile Phone Emissions: Research Grants, Australian Senate Hansard, p. 2603, May 12, 1998.

88 Letter from Richard Morris.

89 ACRBR website: (June 2007) Available at: http://www.acrbr.org.au/index. php?inc=about/centre/researchdirectors.

90 ACRBR website, ibid.

91 ACRBR website (June 2007), Available at: http://www.acrbr.org. au/?inc=community.

92 S. Slesin, "Industry Rules RF: Controlling Research, Setting Standards and Spinning History," *Microwave News*, July 2004.Available at: http://microwavenews. com/news-center/industry-rules-rf-controlling-research-setting-standards-and-spinning-history.

93 S. Krimsky.

94 H. Barnes, *Social Institutions—In an Era of World Upheaval*, (New York, Prentice-Hall, 1942). Taken from Resnik & Shamoo, Conflict of Interest and the University p. 52.

95 Uniform Requirements for Manuscripts Submitted to Biomedical Journals: Writing and Editing for Biomedical Publication, the International Committee of Medical Journal Editors, Section II.D. Conflicts of Interest. Available at: http:// www.ncbi.nlm.nih.gov/pmc/articles/PMC3142758/.

96 J. Pegg, Health Advocacy Group Warns of Conflicted Science, Corp Watch, July 14, 2003. Available at: http://www.corpwatch.org/article.php?id=7608.

97 Meaning "contrary to what intuition or common sense would indicate," the term "counterintuitive research" would suggest that the findings of any particular study could not have been easily predicted. For example, if an industry has reached a decision about the level of safety of its product and finds that in fact these precepts are false, these results are said to be counterintuitive.

98 L. Slesin, "Wireless Notes," *Microwave News*, 2000 Nov/Dec: 21(6):8.

99 ARPANSA, The Mobile Phone System and Health Effects, Part 1 and 2, Health Hazard Assessment, Available at: http://www.arpansa.gov.au/mph2.htm.

100 L. Slesin, *Microwave News*.

101 ARPANSA, Fact Sheet, EME Series, No. 1, Electromagnetic Energy and its effects, November 2003.

102 R. Adey, C. Byus, C. Cain, et al., "Spontaneous and Nitrosourea-Induced Primary Tumors of the Central nervous System in Fischer 344 Rats Chronically Exposed to 836 MHz Modulated Microwaves," *Radiation Research*, 152 (1999 Sept): 293–302.

103 L. Slesin, "Digital Cell Phone Signals: Protection Against Brain Tumors," *Microwave News*, 16(3) (1999 Sept/Oct): 8.

104 Correspondence from Ross Adey to this author, January 7, 2004.

105 S. Jasanoff, *In Democratization of Experts? Exploring Novel Forms of Science Advice in Political Decision Making* . Ed. Maasen and Weingart, Springer. Chapter 11, "Judgement Under Siege: The Three-Body Problem of Expert Legitimacy," pp. 209-224, 2005.

106 ACRBR, Available at: http://acrbr.org.au/.

107 Swinburne University, BPsyC Research Groups, Available at: http://www.swin-burne.edu.au/lss/bpsyc/research-groups.html#rf.

108 Radiofrequency (RF) Dosimetry At Swinburne. Available at: http://www.swin-burne.edu.au/lss/bpsyc/facilities/radiofrequencydosimetry-laboratory.html.

109 ibid.

110 Swinburne University, Bill Scales, Available at: http://www.swinburne.edu.au/chancellery/chancellor/about/about.html.

   Swinburne University, Business and Industry. Available at: http://www.industry.swinburne.edu.au/business/?utm_campaign=businessindustry&utm_medium=button-main&utm_source=swinburne-home&utm_content=business-industry.

111 Telstra Annual Report (2004).

112 About Greenwave Systems. Available at: http://www.greenwavesystems.com/#about.

113 Swinburne University, Energy Management Research Centre (EMRC). Available at: https://wiki.ict.swin.edu.au/g_emrc/index.php?title=Public_Energy_Management_Research_Centre.

114 B. Deshpande, Smart meters are at the forefront on Internet of Things. Available from: http://www.simafore.com/blog/bid/118289/Utility-smart-meter-analytics-can-energize-internet-of-things.

115 Union of Concerned Scientists, Heads They Win, Tails We Lose: How Corporations Corrupt Science at the Public's Expense, Feb. 2012. Available at: http://www.ucsusa.org/sites/default/files/legacy/assets/documents/scientific_integrity/how-corporations-corrupt-science.pdf.

116 Univ. of Wollongong media release, "UOW leads new research centre targeting mobile phone health concerns," August 6, 2012. Available at: http://media.uow.edu.au/news/UOW130536.html.

117 NHMRC Centre of Excellence: Australian Centre for Electromagnetic Bioeffects Research, Swinburne BPsyC. Available at: http://www.swinburne.edu.au/lss/bpsyc/acebr.html.

118 NH&MRC grants for EME research—grant summaries. Available at: http://www.nhmrc.gov.au/grants/outcomes-funding-rounds/nhmrc-funded-research-effects-electromagnetic-energy/nhmrc-grants-eme.

119 D. Maisch, Ten case histories of people in Melbourne who are suffering health problems after a smart meter was installed near their bedroom (or in one case their workstation). Available at: http://www.emfacts.com/download/SM_case_studies.pdf.

120 EMF Safety Network, Smart meter health complaints. Available at: http://emfsafetynetwork.org/smart-meters/smart-meter-health-complaints/.

121 D. Maisch, An incomplete Benefit-Cost analysis and the urgent need for research: Comments on the Commonwealth of Massachusetts document no. D.P.U. 12-76-A. Investigation by the Department of Public Utilities on its own Motion into Modernization of the Electric Grid, January 22, 2014. Available at: http://www.emfacts.com/download/Mass_SM2_statement.pdf.

122 M. Wood, ACEBR, Science and Wireless 2013, Powerpoint presentation, March 20, 2014. Available at: https://www.youtube.com/watch?v=yUoZdihrwpI.

123 R. Hoy, ACEBR, Science and Wireless 2013, Powerpoint presentation, March 20, 2014. Available at: https://www.youtube.com/watch?v=6AFv_ixmsLU.

124 Pacific Gas and Electricity Co. Response to Administrative Law Judge's October 18, 2011 Ruling Directing it to File Clarifying Radio Frequency Information.

Available at: http://emfsafetynetwork.org/wp-content/uploads/2011/11/PGERFDataOpt-outalternatives_11-1-11-3pm.pdf.

125 Richard Tell Associates, An Evaluation of Radio Frequency Fields Produced by Smart Meters Deployed in Vermont, January 1, 2013. Available at: http://public-service.vermont.gov/sites/psd/files/Topics/Electric/Smart_Grid/Vermont%20DPS%20Smart%20Meter%20Measurement%20Report%20-%20Final.pdf.

126 M. Markov, Y. Grigoriey, "Wi-Fi Technology—an uncontrolled global experiment on the health of mankind," *Elec Bio and Med*, 32(2) (2013 June): 200-208.

127 C. Hamilton, S. Maddison, *Silencing Dissent: How the Australian government is controlling public opinion and stifling debate*, (Allen& Unwin, 2007).

128 D. Korn, "Conflicts of interest in biomedical research," *JAMA* 284 (17) (2000 Nov1): 2234–2237.

Chapter 17: Westlake Research Institute, Janine Allis-Smith

1 M. Forwood, The Legacy of Reprocessing in the United Kingdom. International Panel on Fissile Materials; 2008 Jul. IPFM Research Report #5.

2 L. Arnold, *Windscale 1957: Anatomy of a Nuclear Accident*, 3rd ed. (Palgrave: Macmillan, 2007).

3 M. J. Crick, G. S. Linsley, "GS. An assessment of the radiological impact of the Windscale reactor fire, October 1957," *Int J Radiat Biol Relat Stud Phys Chem Med*. 46(5) (1984): 479–506.

4 S. D'Arcy, R. Edwards, *Still Fighting for Gemma. Bloomsbury* (Publishing PLC, 1995).

5 R. J. Parker, *The Windscale Inquiry: Report* (London: H.M. Stationery Office, 1978).

6 P. Taylor, The impact of nuclear waste disposals to the marine environment. Oxford: Political Ecology Research Group; 1982 Mar. PERG RR-8.

7 Yorkshire Television: *Windscale - the Nuclear Laundry* [television documentary]. 1983 Nov 1 [cited 2015 Mar 23]. Available from: https://www.youtube.com/watch?v=UQmFeAGCpC0.

8 J. May, *The Greenpeace Book of the Nuclear Age: The Hidden History, the Human Cost*. (Greenpeace Books, 1989) [cited 2015 Mar 23]. Available from: http://www.greenpeace.org/international/Global/international/planet-2/report/2006/2/the-greenpeace-book-of-the-nuc.pdf.

9 D. Black, *Investigation of the Possible Increased Incidence of Cancer in West Cumbria: Report of the Independent Advisory Group* (London: H.M. Stationery Office, 1984 Dec).

10 M. Bobrow, *The implications of the new data on the releases from Sellafield in the 1950s for the conclusions of the report on the investigation of the possible increased incidence of cancer in West Cumbria 1986: First report* (London: H.M. Stationery Office, 1986). Committee on Medical Aspects or Radiation in the Environment (COMARE).

11 M. J. Gardner, M. P. Snee, A. J. Hall, C. A. Powell, S. Downes, J. D. Terrell, "Results of a case-control study of leukaemia and lymphoma among young

people near Sellafield nuclear plant in West Cumbria," *BMJ* 300(6722) (1990 Feb 17): 423–9.

12   M. Bobrow, *Investigation of the possible increased incidence of leukaemia in young people near the Dounreay Nuclear Establishment, Caithness, Scotland. Second report.* (London: H.M. Stationery Office, 1988). Committee on Medical Aspects of Radiation in the Environment (COMARE).

13   Letter Freshfields to Legal Aid Fund, 22.12.1988.

14   L. Kinlen, "Evidence for an infective cause of childhood leukaemia: comparison of a Scottish new town with nuclear reprocessing sites in Britain," *Lancet.* 2(8624) (1988): 1323–7.

15   Letter from Richard Doll to Janine Allis-Smith 15.5.1989.

16   Letter from Richard Doll to Jean McSorley 16.5.1989.

17   United Kingdom Clinical Research Collaboration (UKCRC) Research Programme Press briefing 24th May 1995.

18   CERRIE (Committee Examining Radiation Risk of Internal Emitters) [cited 2015 Mar 23]. Available from: http://webarchive.nationalarchives.gov. uk/20140108135436/http://www.cerrie.org/.

19   K. J. Bunch, T. J. Vincent, R. J. Black, M. S. Pearce, R. J. McNally, P. A. McKinney, et al. "Updated investigations of cancer excesses in individuals born or resident in the vicinity of Sellafield and Dounreay," *Br J Cancer.* 111(9) (2014): 1814-23.

20   Arte TV: *Radioactive Waste: Dumped and Forgotten* [television documentary]. 2013 May 25 [cited 2015 Mar 23]. Available from: https://www.youtube.com/ watch?v=oX_lzoYl9AU.

21   Merlin and another v. British Nuclear Fuels plc [1990] 2 QB 557. http://www. econ.cam.ac.uk/dae/repec/cam/pdf/cwpe1207.pdf.

22   Gardner, "Results of a case-control study . . ." 1990.

23   B. Wynne, C. Waterton, R. Grove-White, *Public Perceptions and the Nuclear Industry in West Cumbria 2007* (Lancaster: Centre for the Study of Environmental Change, Lancaster University, 2007) [cited 2015 Mar 23]. Available from: http:// www.csec.lancs.ac.uk/docs/Public%20Perceptions%20Nuclear%20Industry.pdf.

24   H. Bolter, *Inside Sellafield*, 1st ed. (Quarter Books, 1996).

25   In 1994, Professor John Fyfe was appointed to the Board of Westlakes Research (Trading) Limited, and in 1995 joined the Westlakes Research Institute's Board of directors. Seen "As a champion of West Cumbria" in 2010 and serving on the board of Cumbria Vision through the Energy Coast Masterplan, Fyfe was awarded a CBE for his services to West Cumbria. In October 2014, the nuclear industry also recognised his services. Named in his honor, John Fyfe House in Whitehaven will eventually be home to 1,000 Sellafield workers.

26   By 2015, the Westlakes Science & Technology Park plays host to 66 business tenants. A large majority, around 70 percent, which includes major national engineering and construction companies that took up residence at the Park many years ago, are directly involved with work at Sellafield and other nuclear industry contracts. The minority itself includes a number of smaller organizations with interests (property, accountancy, IT, and project planning consultancies) in both

the nuclear and other sectors, and raises the percentage of tenants either directly or indirectly related to Sellafield to at least 85 percent.

27 "Editorial," *Whitehaven News,* 1992 Oct 22.

28 Westlakes Research Institute, published on behalf of the WRI by Corporate Publicity, BNFL, Risley.

29 View from the Park, project partly funded by the Rural Development Commission and the European Development Fund.

30 High Court of Justice Transcripts days 47, 48.

31 High Court of Justice Transcripts days 60, 60A, 61, 62.

32 High Court of Justice Transcripts, days 6, 7, 8, 9.

33 High Court of Justice Judgement October 8th 1993 http://www.heraldscotland. com/sport/spl/aberdeen/cancer-cluster-actions-rejected-by-high-court-1.738635; http://www.independent.co.uk/news/uk/sellafield-families-lose-cancer-dam- ages-fight-high-court-rejects-genetic-link-between-disease-and-nuclear-plant- heather-mills-and-ian-mackinnon-report-on-a-landmark-judgment-1509547. html.

34 Ibid.

35 E. I. Evans, *Environmental characterisation of particulate-associated radioactivity deposited close to the Sellafield works* [thesis], (University of London, 1998).

36 In 2013, he questioned why it had taken a Freedom of Information request to Imperial College to gain access to his research findings. The thesis is now available through the British Library.

37 R. Waterhouse. The balance of power: Disturbing questions persist about the effects of the Sellafield nuclear plant on people who work there or live in the area. Research at a new state-of-the-art centre could provide the answers. So should it matter that it is funded by British Nuclear Fuels? *The Independent.* 1994 Oct 2 [cited 2015 Mar 24]. Available from: http://www.independent.co.uk/ arts-entertainment/the-balance-of-power-disturbing-questions-persist-about- the-effects-of-the-sellafield-nuclear-plant-on-people-who-work-there-or-live-in- the-area-research-at-a-new-stateoftheart-centre-could-provide-the-answers-so- should-it-matter-that-it-is-funded-by-british-nuclear-fuels-1440351.html.

38 L. Parker, M. S. Pearce, H. O. Dickinson, M. Aitkin, A. W. Craft, "Stillbirths among offspring of male radiation workers at Sellafield nuclear reprocessing plant," *Lancet* 354 (9188) (1999): 1407-14.

39 Newcastle University Press Release 20.5.1994.

40 Minutes West Cumbria Health Authority meeting 1984.

41 Letter from Louise Parker to Janine Allis-Smith 31/5/1994.

42 Sellafield Newsletter No.356; http://www.heraldscotland.com/sport/spl/aberdeen/ british-nuclear-fuels-backs-genetic-experiments-as-mps-demand-curbs-on- drugs-and-laboratories-outcry-over-baby-research-plan-1.670665).

43 Responses to CORE from Prof June Lloyd and Prof Angus Clarke.

44 *Whitehaven News,* 1994 Jun 23.

45 *Whitehaven News,* 1994 Dec 15.

46 Public Meeting on the NCCGP Notes for participants John Burns 7.11.1994.

47 The Proposed DNA Bank in West Cumbria Statement by Dr. David King 13.12.1994.

48 *Whitehaven News* 1994 Dec 15.

49 D. King, Glycophorin: a somatic mutation assay. 1995 Apr 24.

50 Minutes North Cumbria Health Authority 21.12.1994 http://www.ncbi.nlm.nih.gov/pmc/articles/PMC1051317/pdf/jmedgene00234-0061.pdf; See also: Chase DS, Tawn EJ, Parker L, Jonas P, Parker CO, Burn J. The North Cumbria Community Genetics Project. J Med Genet. 1998;35(5):413–6.

51 C. P. Daniel, A. Fisher, L. Parker, J. Burn, E. J. Tawn, "Individual variation in somatic mutations of the glycophorin-A gene in neonates in relation to pre-natal factors," *Mutat Res.* 467 (2) (2000): 153–9.

52 North Cumbria Community Genetics Project. Report 1996–2000. Cumbria: Westlakes Research Institute; 2000 Sep.

53 E. Haimes, M. Barr, *Levels and styles of participation in genetic databases: A case study of the North Cumbria Community Genetics Project,* In: Tutton R, Corrigan O, editors. *Genetic Databases: Socio-ethical issues in the collection and use of DNA.* (London: Routledge, 2004). p. 57–77.

54 *The Redfern Inquiry into human tissue analysis in UK nuclear facilities.* (London: The Stationery Office, 2010) Nov [cited 2015 Mar 24]. Report HC 571. Available from: https://www.gov.uk/government/uploads/system/uploads/attachment_data/file/229155/0571_i.pdf.

55 *Whitehaven News.* 2010 Jul 16.

56 John Burn response to EHSC. North Cumbria Genetics Project 1994: Fate/Future of Samples—May 2011.

57 Email from John Haywood to JAS.

58 Cumbrians Opposed to a Radioactive Environment (CORE). Radioactive Particles on West Cumbrian Beaches—the case for the provision of signs to advise the public. Cumbria; 2013 Aug [cited 2015 Mar 24]. Available from: http://wcssg.co.uk/wp-content/uploads/2014/10/CORE-beach-report-2013.pdf.

Further Reading

"Childhood Cancer and Nuclear Installations" ed. Valerie Beral, Eve Roman, and Martin Bobrow, *BMJ* (1993).

The Greenpeace Book of the Nuclear Age, John May. (Victor Gollanez: 1989).

Britain's Nuclear Nightmare, James Cutler & Rob Edwards, *Sphere Books,* (1988).

Living in the Shadow of Sellafield, the story of the people of Sellafield. Jean McSorley, (Pan Book: 1990).

Still Fighting for Gemma, Susan D'Arcy & Rob Edwards. (Bloomsbury Publishing PLC: 31 Aug.1995).

Films & Documentaries available on Youtube

Windscale the Nuclear Laundry, First Tuesday, 1 November 1983
https://www.youtube.com/watch?v=UQmFeAGCpC0
Windscale, Britain's worst nuclear accident

https://www.youtube.com/watch?v=vZ4vtUzG6sQ

Fighting for Gemma - Granada TV film

http://youtu.be/pIYdjKEK44M

Nuclear Waste, dumped and forgotten- ARTE TV documentary:
https://www.youtube.com/watch?v=oX_lzoYl9AU

Chapter 18: Wilhelm Hueper and Robert Kehoe–Epidemiological War Crimes, Devra Davis

1   Adapted from *The Secret History of the War on Cancer*, (New York, 2007), Chapter 4 pg 73–105.

2   R. Proctor, *The Nazi war on cancer. Princeton*, (NJ: Princeton University Press, 1999).

3   David Michaels, "When science isn't enough: Wilhelm Hueper, Robert A. M. Case, and the limits of scientific evidence in preventing occupational bladder cancer," *Int J Occup Environ Health* 1 (1995): 278–88.

4   Archival documents from University of Cincinnati, Kehoe papers, provided to author.

5   Office of Military Government for Germany, Field Information Agency Technical FIAT Review of German Science, 1939–1946

6   Ibid.

7   W. C. Hueper, Autobiography. Unpublished, on file in National Library of Medicine Also cited in Michaels, p. 282–3.

8   Ibid.

9   Ibid.

10   W. C. Hueper, *Occupational tumors and allied diseases* (Springfield, IL: Charles C. Thomas, 1942).

11   W. C. Hueper, *Environmental cancer* (Washington, DC: US Government Printing Office, 1950).

12   Ibid.

13   Ibid.

14   The Halifax Project. Available from: http://gettingtoknowcancer.org/.

Chapter 19: The Precautionary Principle, Pierre Mallia

1   World Commission on the Ethics of Scientific Knowledge and Technology (COMEST). The Precautionary Principle. Paris: UNESCO; 2005. Available from: http://unesdoc.unesco.org/images/0013/001395/139578e.pdf.

2   Commission of the European Communities. Communication from the Commission on the Precautionary Principle. Brussels: EU; 2000. Available from: http://ec.europa.eu/dgs/health_consumer/library/pub/pub07_en.pdf.

3   International Commission for Electromagnetic Safety (ICEMS). Workshop on possible biological and health effects of RF electromagnetic fields. Vienna EMF-Resolution. Vienna, 1998 Oct 25-28. Available from: http://www.icems.eu/docs/resolutions/Vienna_Resolution_1998.pdf.

4   Salzburg Resolution on Mobile Telecommunication Base Stations. International Conference on Cell Tower Siting Linking Science & Public Health Salzburg, 2000 Jun 7-8. Available from: http://www.salzburg.gv.at/salzburg_resolution_e.pdf.

5   REFLEX. Risk Evaluation of Potential Environmental Hazards From Low Frequency Electromagnetic Field Exposure Using Sensitive in vitro Methods. Final report, 2004. Available from: http://www.iaff.org/hs/PDF/REFLEX percent20Final percent20Report.pdf.

6   Independent Expert Group on Mobile Phones (IEGMP). Mobile Phones and Health. Chairman Sir William Stewart. 2000. Available from: http://webarchive.nationalarchives.gov.uk/20101011032547/http:/www.iegmp.org.uk/report/text.htm.

7   "Joint Committee on Bioethical Issues of the Bishops" Conferences of Scotland, Ireland, England and Wales. Use of the "Morning-After pill" in Cases of Rape. Origins. 1986;15:635–7.

8   Paragraph entitled "Judicial review of the morning after pill." In Howard PK, Bogle J. Lecture Notes: Medical Law and Ethics. London: Blackwell Publishing; 2005. p. 96.

9   "Joint Committee on Bioethical Issues of the Bishops," 196.

10 "Mallia P. The use of emergency hormonal contraception in cases of rape-revisiting the Catholic position," Hum Reprod Genet Ethics. 2005;11:35–42.

11 http://www.parliament.gov.mt/sacmeetings11?l=1 (meeting 74).

12 P. Le Ruz. Third communications seminar on health, Environment and Society; Risk assessment, risk evaluation, deployment risks, November 2006, in where more than 400 international studies as showing health risks to those living close to relay masts are pointed out.

13 L-Isqof Grech dwar ic-censura—discors lill-gurnalisti. (Bishop Grech on Censor—a talk to journalists). Il-Paci Maghkom, 2010 Mar, p.1.

14 UNESCO; 2005.

15 Ibid.

16 Ibid.

17 Ibid.

18 Ibid.

19 Ibid.

20 Ibid.

21 Ibid.

22 Ibid.

Chapter 20:The Precautionary Principle in the Protection of Wildlife – the Tasmanian Devils and the Beluga Whales, Jody Warren

1   World Wildlife Fund (WWF). Living Planet Report 2006. Available from: http://d2ouvy59p0dg6k.cloudfront.net/downloads/living_planet_report.pdf.

2   The Greenwashing of atrazine is referred to in Chapter Greenwashing in Sweden.

3   E. Young, "Pollution blamed for cancer ravaging Quebec's whales," New Scientist, (2002 Feb 27).

4   S. Steingraber, "Living with cancer," Earth Island Journal, (1998 Mar.).

5   "Cancer: Tasmania's highest rate," Tasmanian Times 2008 Dec 22. Available from: http://tasmaniantimes.com/index.php?/weblog/article/cancer-tasmanias-highest-rate/.

6   World Commission on the Ethics of Scientific Knowledge and Technology (COMEST). The Precautionary Principle. Paris: UNESCO; 2005. Available from: http://unesdoc.unesco.org/images/0013/001395/139578e.pdf.

7   Ibid.

8   Ibid.

9   Ibid.

10   S. Beder, *Environmental Principles and Policies. An Interdisciplinary Approach,* (Sydney: UNSW Press, 2006).

11   P. Harremoes, D. Gee, M. MacGarvin, A. Stirling, J. Keys, B. Wynne, S. G. Vaz, editors. *The Precautionary Principle in the Twentieth Century. Late Lessons from Early Warnings.* (London: Earthscan Publications Ltd, 2002).

12   D. Kriebel, J. Tickner, P. Epstein, J. Lemons, R. Levins, E. L. Loechler, et al. "The precautionary principle in environmental science. Environ Health Perspect," 109 (2001): 871-6.

13   Ibid.

14   Ibid.

15   Ibid.

16   Ibid.

17   M. Breitholtz, C. Rudén, S. O. Hansson, B. E. Bengtsson, "Ten challenges for improved exotoxicological testing in environmental risk assessment," *Ecotoxicol Environ Saf.* 63 (2006): 324–35.

18   R. Dworkin quoted in S. Marr, *The Precautionary Principle in the Law of the Sea, Modern Decision Making in International Law* (The Hague: Martinus Nijhoff Publishers, 2003), p. 12.

19   M. Karlsson, "The Precautionary Principle, Swedish Chemicals Policy and Sustainable Development," *Journal of Risk Research* 9 (2006): 337–60.

20   Ibid.

21   Stockholm Convention on Persistent Organic Pollutants (POPs). Available from: http://web.archive.org/web/20070411012604/http://www.pops.int/.

22   Wingspread Statement on the Precautionary Principle. Available from: http://www.gdrc.org/u-gov/precaution-3.html.

23   S. Loewenberg. "Precaution is for Europeans," *The New York Times*, 2003 May 18. Available from: http://www.nytimes.com/2003/05/18/weekinreview/precaution-is-for-europeans.html.

24   J. DiGangi, REACH and the Long Arm of the Chemical Industry. Multinational Monitor, Vol 25, No 9, 2004 Sep. Available from: http://www.multinationalmonitor.org/mm2004/092004/digangi.html.

25   C. Raffensperger, An Interview: Precautionary Precepts, The Power and Potential of the Precautionary Principle, Multinational Monitor, 2004, Vol 25, No 9 pp 1–9. Available from: http://multinationalmonitor.org/mm2004/09012004/september-04interviewraffen.html.

26   Loewenberg, "Precaution is for Europeans."

27   Karlsson, p. 337–60.

28 N. Myers, C. Raffensperger, "A Precaution Primer. An ounce of prevention is worth a pound of cure," *YES! Magazine*, 2001 Sep 30. Available from: http://www.yesmagazine.org/issues/technology-who-chooses/461.

29 DiGangi, 2004.

30 World Wildlife Fund (WWF). A Precautionary Approach to Toxic Chemicals. 2001 Mar. Available from: http://assets.panda.org/downloads/prectox.doc.

31 J. G. Morone, E. J. Woodhouse. Averting Catastrophe: Strategies for Regulating Risky Technologies. Berkeley (CA): University of California Press; 1986.

32 S. Milmo, Precautionary Principles. European Chemical Producers Question Precautionary Rules. Ecoglobe, 2000. Available from: http://www.ecoglobe.org/nz/precprin/prec0410.htm.

33 Loewenberg, "Precaution is for Europeans."

34 D. Knight, Environment: WTO Attacked for Ignoring "Precautionary Principle," IPS Correspondents, 1999 Dec 3. Available from: http://www.ipsnews.net/1999/12/environment-wto-attacked-for-ignoring-precautionary-principle/

35 Milmo, Ecoglobe, 2000.

36 Loewenberg, "Precaution is for Europeans."

37 DiGangi, 2004.

38 Ibid.

39 Ibid.

40 P. Montague, "Critiques of the Precautionary Principle," *Rachels Environment Health News*, No 781, 2003 (December 4).

41 J. Thornton, *Chemicals Policy and the Precautionary Principle: The Case of Endocrine Disruption*. In: Tickner JA, editor. *Precaution, Environmental Science, and Preventive Public Policy*. (Washington, DC: Island Press, 2003). p. 103–26.

42 Beder, 2006.

43 R. Carson, *Silent Spring - with an Introduction by Vice President Al Gore* (New York: Houghton Mifflin, 1994).

44 Takasugi & Bern quoted in T. Colborn, D. Dumanoski, J. P. Myers, *Our Stolen Future: Are We Threatening Our Fertility, Intelligence, and Survival?—A Scientific Detective Story*. (Boston, MA: Little, Brown and Company, 1996). p. 57–58.

45 D. Fagin, M. Lavelle, *Toxic Deception: How the Chemical Industry Manipulates Science, Bends the Law, and Endangers Your Health*. (Secaucus, NJ: Carol Publishing Group, 1996).

46 Corporate Watch. Syngenta: Overview. 2005 Jun 2. Available from: http://www.corporatewatch.org/company-profiles/syngenta-overview.

47 Lexdon: The Business Library. Syngenta Full Year Results 2005. Available from: http://www.lexdon.com/article/Syngenta_Full_Year_Results_2005/32618.html.

48 Sygenta. Products & Services: Product Line Performance. 2007. Available from: http://web.archive.org/web/20071215143026/http://www.syngenta.com/en/products_services/index.aspx.

49 S. Krimsky, *Hormonal Chaos. The Scientific and Social Origins of the Environmental Endocrine Hypothesis*. (Baltimore, MD: John Hopkins University Press, 2000).

50 J. M. Kiesecker, "Synergism between trematode infection and pesticide exposure: A link to amphibian limb deformities in nature?" *Proc Natl Acad Sci USA.* 99 (2002): 9900–4.

51 C. Cox, "Atrazine: Environmental Contamination and Ecological Effects," *Journal of Pesticide Reform.* 21 (2001): 12–20.

52 Guillette LJ Jr, Crain DA, editors. Environmental Endocrine Disrupters: An Evolutionary Perspective. New York (NY): Taylor & Francis; 2000.

53 Ibid new 52 (old 34).

54 Ibid new 52 (old 34).

55 W. Fan, T. Yanase, H. Morinaga, S. Gondo, T. Okabe, M. Nomura, et al. "Atrazine-Induced Aromatase Expression Is SF-1 Dependent: Implications for Endocrine Disruption in Wildlife and Reproductive Cancers in Humans," *Environ Health Perspect.* 115 (2007): 720–7.

56 J. B. Sass, A. Colangelo, "European Union Bans Atrazine, While the United States Negotiates Continued Use," *Int J Occup Environ Health.* 12. (2006): 260–7.

57 Ibid.

58 Australian Government. National Health and Medical Research Council. Australian Drinking Water Guidelines. 2004. Available from: http://www.nhmrc.gov.au/_files_nhmrc/publications/attachments/eh34_adwg_11_06.pdf.

59 Ibid.

60 Canadian Council of Ministers of the Environment. Canadian Water Quality Guidelines for the Protection of Aquatic Life. Atrazine. 1999. Available from: http://ceqg-rcqe.ccme.ca/download/en/144.

61 T. Hayes, K. Haston, M. Tsui, A. Hoang, C. Haeffele, A .Vonk, "Atrazine-induced hermaphroditism at 0.1 ppb in American leopard frogs (Rana pipiens): Laboratory and field evidence," *Environ Health Perspect.* 111 (2003): 568–75.

62 G. Blumenstyk, The Story of Syngenta & Tyrone Hayes at UC Berkeley. The Price of Research. The Chronical of Higher Education. 2003;50. Available from: http://www.mindfully.org/Pesticide/2003/Syngenta-Tyrone-Hayes31oct03.htm.

63 Ibid.

64 S. Stachura, "Mayo docs hear from researcher on suspected atrazine, cancer links," *MPR News,* 2007 Jan 4. Available from: http://www.mprnews.org/story/2007/01/02/hayesmayo.

65 Blumenstyk, 2003.

66 A. Avery, Rachel Carson Syndrome Case 4: Leopard Frogs and Atrazine Accusations. Hudson Institute, Centre for Global Food Issues. Available from: http://web.archive.org/web/20071022120313/http://cgfi.org/materials/key_pubs/rachel-carson-syndrome-leapard-frogs-atrazine-accusations.htm.

67 SourceWatch. Center for Regulatory Effectiveness. Available from: http://www.sourcewatch.org/index.php?title=Center_for_Regulatory_Effectiveness.

68 SourceWatch, Hudson Institute. Available from: http://www.sourcewatch.org/index.php?title=Hudson_Institute.

69 R. Weiss, "Data Quality" Law is Nemesis of Regulation. *The Washington Post,* 2004 Aug 16. Available from: http://www.washingtonpost.com/wp-dyn/articles/A3733-2004Aug15.html.

70   C. K. Yoon, "Studies Conflict on Common Herbicide's Effects on Frogs," *The New York Times*, 2002 Nov 19. Available from: http://www.nytimes.com/2002/11/19/science/studies-conflict-on-common-herbicide-s-effects-on-frogs.html.

71   Ibid.

72   Weiss, "Data Quality."

73   Ibid.

74   Sass, Colangelo, "European Union Bans Atrazine . . ." 2006.

75   T. S. McMullin, M. E. Andersen, A Nagahara, T. D. Lund, T Pak, R. J. Handa, et al. "Evidence That Atrazine and Diaminochlorotriazine Inhibit the Estrogen/Progesterone Induced Surge of Luteinizing Hormone in Female Sprague-Dawley Rats Without Changing Estrogen Receptor Action," *Toxicol Sci*. 79 (2004): 278–86.

76   L. T. Wetzel, L. G. Luempert, C. B. Breckenridge, M. O. Tisdel, J. T. Stevens, A. K. Thakur, et al. "Chronic effects of atrazine on estrus and mammary tumor formation in female Sprague-Dawley and Fisher 344 rats," *J Toxicol Environ Health*. 43 (1994): 169–82.

77   J. T. Stevens, C. B. Breckenridge, L. Wetzel, "A risk characterization for atrazine: oncogenicity profile," *J Toxicol Environ Health A*. 56 (1999): 69-109.

78   Environment News Service. Enviros Seek Stricter Atrazine Regulation. 2003 Oct 14. Available from: http://www.ens-newswire.com/ens/oct2003/2003-10-14-09.html#anchor3.

79   Natural Resources Defense Council (NRDC). EPA Won't Restrict Toxic Herbicide Atrazine, Despite Health Threat. 2004 Jan 23. Available from: https://web.archive.org/web/20100410015505/http://www.nrdc.org/health/pesticides/natrazine.asp.

80   Fan, et al., Atrazine-Induced Aromatase Expression . . . , 2007.

81   Australian Pesticides & Veterinary Medicines Authority (APVMA). The reconsideration of approvals of the active constituent atrazine, registration of products containing atrazine, and their associated labels. Second Draft Final Review Report. 2004 Oct. Available from: http://apvma.gov.au/sites/default/files/publication/14336-atrazine-second-draft-final-review-report.pdf.

82   Krimsky, 2000.

83   N. Lubick, "EPA Releases List of Endocrine-disrupter Candidates," *Environmental Science & Technology*, 2007 Jul 5.

84   Sass, "European Union Bans Atrazine . . ." 2006.

85   Ibid.

86   Natural Resources Defense Council (NRDC). EPA Failing to Protect Public from Weed Killer's Cancer Threat, says NRDC. 2003 Oct 14. Available from: http://www.nrdc.org/media/pressreleases/031014.asp.

87   Sass, "European Union Bans Atrazine . . ." 2006.

88   Ibid.

89   Ibid.

90   United States Environment Protection Agency. Atrazine Update. Available from: https://web.archive.org/web/20080908115012/http://www.epa.gov/oppsrrd1/reregistration/atrazine/atrazine_update.htm.

91   Ibid.

92   APVMA, October 2004.

93 Ibid.

94 Ibid.

95 Health Canada. Pest Management Regulatory Agency. Proposed acceptability for continuing registration PACR2003-13. Re-evaluation of Atrazine. Ottawa (ON): Pest Management Regulatory Agency; 2003.

96 Environment Canada. CEPA Environmental Registry. ARCHIVED - Draft Entry Characterization of trifluralin; atrazine; chlorothalonil; chlorophacinone; methoxychlor; and pentachlorophenol. Available from: https://ec.gc.ca/lcpe-cepa/default.asp?lang=En&n=EE479482-1&wsdoc=8AC3F404-B736-6B14-609E-69031E430883.

97 CEPA, Characterization of trifluralin . . .

98 Health Canada, Endocrine Disrupting Chemicals—Canada's Perspective. Science for Sustainable Development 13, Government of Canada, Ottawa, Ontario. Available from: http://badc.nerc.ac.uk/community/poster_heaven_old/Poster13E.pdf.

99 Environment Canada. Endocrine Disrupting Substances in the Environment. Available from: https://web.archive.org/web/20070715130410/http://www.ec.gc.ca/eds/fact/broch_e.htm.

100 Ibid.

101 Health Canada, Endrocrine Disrupting Chemicals.

102 Canada's Chemical Producers. What is the endocrine issue? Available from: http://web.archive.org/web/20060923193838/http://www.ccpa.ca/Issues/Enviro/Endocrine.asp.

103 Ibid.

104 CNTC. Research Priorities. Reproductive and Endocrine Ecotoxicology Project Goals 2002 -2003. Available from: http://web.archive.org/web/20050421235824/http://www.uoguelph.ca/cntc/archive/research2002_2003/endocrine/summaries.shtml.

105 Yoon, *New York Times*, 2002.

106 J. A. Carr, L. H. De Preez, J. P. Giesy, T. S. Gross, R. J. Kendall, E. E. Smith, K. R. Solomon, G. J. Van Der Kraak, Critique of: Hayes, et al., "Hermaphroditic, demasculinized frogs after exposure to the herbicide arazine at low ecologically relevant doses," *Proc. Nat. Acad. Sci.* 99 (2002): 5476-5480. The Atrazine Endocrine Ecological Risk Assessment Panel, EcoRisk, Inc, 2002 Aug 16. Available from: http://www.thecre.com/pdf/exhibit-j-20020808_syngenta.pdf.

107 K. Solomon, Pesticides are safe: Proving the improvable. Parry Sound Beacon Star, 2001 Apr 28. Available from: http://www.24d.org/newsarticles/Solomon-Parry-Sound-2001.pdf.

108 Natural Sciences and Engineering Research Council of Canada (NSERC). NSERC: A strategic partner in managing risk. Innovating through Partnerships, Vol 2. Available from: http://web.archive.org/web/20070822001452/http://www.nserc-crsng.gc.ca/about/cme_pub_06_e.pdf.

109 University of Guelph. Total Research Funds Received by Department in the College of Biological Science May 1, 2005—April 30, 2006. Available from: http://www.uoguelph.ca/research/summaries/2006/Table percent208.pdf 05.02.09.

110 C. J. Swanton, R. H. Gulden, K. Chandler, 2007, "A Rationale for Atrazine Stewardship in Corn," *Weed Science*. 55 (2007): 75-81.

111 Australian Government. Department of the Environment, Water, Heritage and the Arts. Intergovernmental Agreement on the Environment. 1992 May 1. Available from: http://web.archive.org/web/20090927094310/http://environment.gov.au/esd/national/igae/index.html.

112 Australian Government. Environment Protection and Biodiversity Conservation Act 1999. Available from: http://www.austlii.edu.au/cgi-bin/download.cgi/cgi-bin/download.cgi/download/au/legis/cth/consol_act/epabca1999588.txt.

113 Ibid.

114 M. Scammell, *Environmental Problems* (Georges Bay, Tasmania: Tasmanian Seafood Industry Council, 2004).

115 S. Percival, 2004, "Oyster Health in Georges Bay, Collation and Analysis of Data," Tasmanian Department of Primary Industries, Water and Environment, Hobart.

116 Three previous expert studies by Professor B. Noller, Dr. M. Scammell, and Dr. M. Mortimer were collated and reviewed in Percival S. Oyster Health in Georges Bay: Collation and analysis of data. Tasmania: Department of Primary Industries and Water; 2004.

117 Brief Communications has been withdrawn due to submissions being in part too preliminary. See: Editorial. "The brief goodbye," *Nature*. 2006;443:246.

118 A. M. Pearse, K. Swift, "Allograft theory: Transmission of devil facial-tumor disease," *Nature*. 2006;439:549.

119 H. V. Siddle, A. Kreiss, M. D. Eldridge, E. Noonan, C. J. Clarke, S. Pyecroft, et al. "Transmission of a fatal clonal tumor by biting occurs due to depleted MHC diversity in a threatened carnivorous marsupial," *Proc Natl Acad Sci USA* 104 (2007): 16221-6.

120 Scientific Blogging. Atrazine Herbicide Disrupts Human Hormone Activity— Study. 2008 May 6. Available from: http://www.science20.com/news_releases/atrazine_herbicide_disrupts_human_hormone_activity_study.

121 S. Krimsky, *Science in the Private Interest: Has the Lure of Profits Corrupted Biomedical Research?* (Lanham, MD: Rowman & Littlefield Publishing, Inc, 2003).

122 Australian Grain Industry. Directory of Linkages in the Australian Grains Industry. 2004 Feb. Available from: http://web.archive.org/web/20110218100801/http://www.grainexchange.com.au/documents/media_directory_0204.pdf.

123 AWB Limited. New Commercial Focus for Grain Research. Media Release, 2003 Mar 5. Available from: http://www.awb.com.au/investors/companyannouncements/mediareleases/2003mediareleases/05.03.03NewCommercialFocusForGrainResearch.htm.

124 The University of Sydney. William James Peacock. Science Hall of Fame. Available from: http://sydney.edu.au/science/about_us/fame_peacock.shtml.

125 Tasmania's Pulp Mill. The Approval. Media Release, 2007 Oct 4. Available from: http://web.archive.org/web/20090327101649/http://tasmaniapulpmill.info/the_approval.

126 Government of Canada. Endangered Species Act 1998, Chapter 11. 1999 May 1. Available from: http://web.archive.org/web/20081230141346/http://www.gov.ns.ca/legislature/legc/statutes/endspec.htm.

127 Government of Canada. Canadian Environmental Protection Act, 1999. Available from: http://www.ec.gc.ca/lcpe-cepa/default.asp?lang=En&n=CC0DE5E2-1&toc=hide.

128 Ibid.

129 Government of Canada. Chemical Substances—an ecoACTION initiative. Available from: http://web.archive.org/web/20090124012120/http://chemicalsubstanceschimiques.gc.ca/manage-gestion/what-quoi/index_e.html.

130 L. Armstrong, G. Dauncey, A. Wordsworth, *Cancer: 101 Solutions to a Preventable Epidemic.* (Gabriola Island, BC: New Society Publications, 2007).

131 Envirodesic. Diseases of Beluga Whales in the Saint Lawrence Estuary. Available from: http://www.ecogent.ca/enviro/env_stle.htm.

132 D. Martineau, K. Lemberger, A. Dalaire, P. Labelle, T. P. Lipscombe, M. Pascal, et al., "Cancer in wildlife, a case study: Beluga from the St. Lawrence Estuary, Québec, Canada," *Environ Health Perspect* 110 (2002): 285–92.

133 Ibid.

134 Ibid.

135 SeaWorld of California. Beluga Whales. 2009. Available from: http://web.archive.org/web/20101223124414/http://seaworld.org/animal-info/info-books/beluga/pdf/ib-beluga.pdf.

136 Martineau, et al, "Cancer in wildlife, a case study," 2002.

137 Whales online. Research projects. St. Lawrence beluga. Available from: http://baleinesendirect.org/en/scientific-exploration/research-projects/st-lawrence-beluga/.

138 C. Lemieux, K. R. Lum, "Sources, distribution and transport of atrazine in the St Lawrence River (Canada)," *Water, Air, & Soil Pollution.* 90 (1996): 355–74.

139 Ibid.

140 Environment Canada. St Lawrence Centre. Monitoring Water Quality at Quebec. Available from: http://web.archive.org/web/20090507141209/http://www.qc.ec.gc.ca/csl/inf/inf006_e.html.

141 Environment Canada. Great Lakes-St Lawrence Ecosystem. Water Quality in the Great Lakes - St. Lawrence Basin: Contamination by Toxic Substances. Available from: http://www.on.ec.gc.ca/csl/fich/fich005_002_e.html.

142 St. Lawrence National Institute of Ecotoxicology (SLNIE). The institute. Available from: http://web.archive.org/web/20050924084602/http://www.inesl.org/eng/6/6-1.html.

143 I. Mikaelian, P. Labelle, M. Kopal, S. De Guise, D. Martineau, "Adenomatous hyperplasia of the thyroid gland in beluga whales (Delhinapterus leucas) from the St. Lawrence Estuary and Hudson Bay, Quebec, Canada," *Vet Pathol.* 40 (2003): 698–703.

144 SourceWatch. Donner Canadian Foundation. Available from: http://www.sourcewatch.org/index.php?title=Donner_Canadian_Foundation

145 Natural Sciences and Engineering Research Council of Canada. Chairholder Profile. Available from: http://www.nserc-crsng.gc.ca/Partners-Partenaires/Chairholders-TitulairesDeChaire/Chairholder-Titulaire_eng.asp?pid=528.

146 M. A. McKinney, A. Arukwe, S. De Guise, D. Martineau, P. Béland, A. Dallaire, et al., "Characterization and profiling of hepatic cytochromes P450 and phase II

xenobiotic-metabolizing enzymes in beluga whales (Delphinapterus leucas) from the St. Lawrence River Estuary and the Canadian Artic," *Aquat Toxicol.* 69 (2004): 35–49.

147 M. A. McKinney, S. De Guise, D. Martineau, P. Béland, A. Arukwe, R. J. Letcher, "Biotransformation of polybrominated diphenyl ethers and polychlorinated biphenyls in beluga whale (Delphinapterus leucas) and rat mammalian model using an in vitro hepatic microsomal assay," *Aquat Toxicol.* 77 (2006): 87–97.

Chapter 21: Dust, Labor and Capital, Jock McCulloch

1   E. Katz, *The white death: silicosis on the Witwatersrand gold mines 1886-1910.* (Johannesburg: Witwatersrand University Press, 1994).

2   D. Rosner, G. Markowitz, *Deadly dust: Silicosis and the On-going Struggle to Protect Workers' Health.* 2nd ed. (Ann Arbor, MI: University of Michigan Press, 2006).

3   Mankayi Mbini and Anglo American Corporation of South Africa Ltd. High Court of South Africa (Witwatersrand Local Division) Case No: 04/18272 2004 Aug 2.

4   "Anglo being sued for R20m," *The Sunday Independent,* 2007 Sep 30.

5   N. Segal, S. Malherbe, A perspective on the South African Mining Industry in the Twenty-First Century: An independent report prepared for the Chamber of Mines of South Africa by the Graduate School of Business of the University of Cape Town in association with Genesis Analytics. 2000. Available from: http://pmg-assets.s3-website-eu-west-1.amazonaws.com/docs/segal.pdf.

6   The Mining Sector, Tuberculosis and Migrant Labour in Southern Africa. Johannesburg: Aids and Rights Alliance for Southern Africa; 2008. Available from: http://www.tac.org.za/community/files/Mines,_TB_and_Southern_Africa.pdf.

7   Katz, 1994.

8   I. Donsky, *A History of Silicosis on the Witwaterstrand Gold Mines, 1910–1946* [PhD thesis]. (Johannesburg: Rand Afrikaans University, 1993).

9   G. E. Barry, In: Silicosis: records of the International Conference held at Johannesburg 13–27th August 1930. London: International Labour Organization; 1930. p. 4.

10 Sampson HW. In: Silicosis: records of the International Conference held at Johannesburg 13–27th August 1930. London: International Labour Organization; 1930. p. 14.

11 Miners' Phthisis Prevention Committee. The Prevention of Silicosis on the Mines of the Witwatersrand. Pretoria: Government Printer; 1937. For a parallel narrative presented at the 1930 Silicosis Conference, see: I. G. Irvine, A. Mavrogardato, H. Pirow. A review of the history of silicosis on the Witwatersrand goldfields. Silicosis: records of the International Conference held at Johannesburg 13–27th, August 1930. London: ILO; 1930. p. 178–208.

12 Ibid.
13 Ibid.
14 Ibid.
15 Ibid.
16 Ibid.

17 M. Malan, *The Quest of Health: The South African Institute for Medical Research, 1912-1973.* (Johannesburg: Lowry Publishers, 1988).

18 A. Mavrogordato, Contributions to the study of miners' phthisis. Typescript. Johannesburg: Adler Medical Library, University of the Witwatersrand; 1926. An abridged version of this paper was published under the same title as a monograph by the South African Institute of Medical Research, 19; December 1926.

19 Ibid.

20 Ibid.

21 G. A. Turner, *Report on the Prevalence of Pulmonary Tuberculosis and Allied Diseases in the Kraals of the Natives of Portuguese East African Territory, South of Latitude 22°.* (Johannesburg: Hayne & Gibson, 1906).

22 Tuberculosis Research Committee. *Tuberculosis in South African Natives with Special Reference to the Disease Among the Mine Labourers of the Witwatersrand.* (Johannesburg: South African Institute for Medical Research, 1932).

23 Mavrogordato, Contributions to the study of miners' phthisis.

24 Ibid.

25 T. W. Steen, K. M. Gyi, N. W. White, T. Gabosianelwe, S. Ludick, G. N. Mazonde, et al., "Prevalence of occupational lung diseases among Botswana men formerly employed in the South African mining industry," *Occup Environ Med.* 54 (1997): 19–26.

26 B. V. Girdler-Brown, N. W. White, R. I. Ehrlich, G. J. Churchyard, "The burden of silicosis, pulmonary tuberculosis and COPD among former Basotho goldminers," *Am J Ind Med.* 51 (2008): 640–7.

27 A. Trapido, *An Analysis of the Burden of Occupational Lung Disease in a Random Sample of Former Gold Mineworkers in the Libode District of the Eastern Cape* [PhD thesis]. (Johannesburg: University of the Witwatersrand, 2000).

28 G. J. Churchyard, R. Ehrlich, J. M. teWaterNaude, L. Pemba, K. Dekker, M. Vermeijs, et al. "Silicosis prevalence and exposure-response relations in South African goldminers," *Occup Environ Med.* 61 (2004): 811–6.

29 N. White, *Is the ODMW Act fair? A Comparison of the Occupational Diseases in Mines and Works Amendment Act, 1993 and the Compensation of Occupational Injuries and Diseases Act, 1993 with Respect to Compensation of Pneumoconiosis.* (Cape Town: University of Cape Town, 2004). Available from: http://www.publichealth.uct.ac.za/sites/default/files/image_tool/images/8/A percent20Comparison percent20of percent20the percent20Occupational percent20Diseases percent20in percent20Mines percent20and percent20Works percent20Amendment percent-t20Act, percent201993.pdf.

30 Report of the Commission of Enquiry into the Functioning of the Silicosis Medical Bureau and the Silicosis Medical Board of Appeal. Pretoria: Government Printer; 1952.

31 Malan, 1988.

32 M. A. Felix, *Environmental asbestos and respiratory disease in South Africa* [PhD thesis]. (Johannesburg: University of the Witwatersrand, 1997).

33 A. J. Orenstein, In: *Silicosis: records of the International Conference* held at Johannesburg 13–27th August 1930. London: International Labour Organization, 1930. p. 32.

34 Donsky, 1993.

35 M. J. Smith, "'Working in the Grave': the development of a health and safety system on the Witwatersrand gold mines, 1900-1939" [MA thesis]. (Grahamstown: Rhodes University, 1993).

36 Donsky, 1993.

37 R. H. Davies, *Capital, State and White Labour in South Africa 1900-1960* (New Jersey: Humanities Press, 1979).

38 Rosner, Markowitz, 2006.

39 Ibid.

40 F. Wilson, *Labour in the South African Gold Mines 1911-1969*. (Cambridge: Cambridge University Press, 1972).

41 Report of the Witwatersrand Mine Native Wages Commission on the Remuneration and Conditions of Employment of Natives on the Witwatersrand Gold Mines. (Pretoria: Government Printer, 1943).

42 Annual Medical and Sanitary Reports. Zomba, Nyasaland, 1928 to 1940. Malawi National Archive.

43 The Mining Sector; www.tac.org.za.

44 *The Sunday Independent*, September 2007.

45 J. McCulloch, "Beating the odds: the quest for justice by South African asbestos mining communities," *Review of African Political Economy*. 32 (2005): 63–77.

46 Rosner, Markowitz, 2006.

47 A. Derickson, *Black lung: Anatomy of a Public Health Disaster*. (Ithaca, NY: Cornell University Press, 1998).

48 A. McIvor, *Johnston R. Miners' Lung: a History of Dust Diseases in British Coal Mining*. (London: Ashgate, 2007).

Chapter 22: Community Epidemiology, Andrew Watterson

1 This article first appeared in more summary form in *Pesticides News* No. 30, December 1995, pages 8–9.

2 Anne Isabella Thackeray Ritchie in Mrs. Dymond, 1885.

3 A. E. Watterson, "Chemical Hazards and Public Confidence," *Lancet* 342 (1993): 131–2.

4 P. Brown, ed., *Perspectives in Medical Sociology* (Belmont, California: Wadsworth, 1989).

5 Phil Brown, Edwin J. Mikkelsen, Chapter 4 *Taking Control: Popular Epidemiology. No Safe Place. Toxic Waste, Leukemia, and Community Action*, (University of California Press, October 1997).

6 Workers Health International Newsletter (1994/5), When it comes to their health, workers always know best, 42:10–11.

7 Jonathan Harr, *Civil Action* (Vintage Books, USA, 1996).

8   P. Brown, "Popular Epidemiology and Toxic Waste contamination: lay and professional ways of knowing," *Journal of Health and Social Behavior* 33 (1992): 267–81.

9   S. Hernberg, *Introduction to Occupational Epidemiology*. (Michigan: Lewis Publishers, 1992).

10   J. Olsen, F. Merletti, D. Snashall, K. Vuylsteek, *Searching for the Causes of Work-related Diseases*, (Oxford University Press, Oxford, 1991).

11   H. Burrage, "Epidemiology and Community Health: a strained connection," *Soc Sci Med* 25 (1987): 895–903.

12   A. Scott-Samuel, *Building the new public health: a public health alliance and a new epidemiology* In C. Martin, and D. McQueen, *Readings for a New Public Health*, (Edinburgh University Press, 1989), p. 29–44.

13   Ibid.

14   R. Loewenson, C. Laurell, C. Hogstedt, Participatory approaches in occupational health research, 1994. National Institute of Occupational Health. Sweden World Health Organization, European Charter on Environment and Health. Copenhagen, WHO, 1989.

15   World Health Organization, Environment and Health: The European Charter and Commentary, Copenhagen, WHO, 1994, 1990:68 WHIN.

16   T. Beritic, "Workers at Risk: the right to know," *Lancet* 341 (1993): 933-4.

17   G. Rose, "Environmental health: problems and prospects," *Journal Roy Coll Physicians* 25 (1991): 48–52.

18   Op. cit. 8.P. Brown, "Popular Epidemiology and Toxic Waste contamination: lay and professional ways of knowing," *Journal of Health and Social Behavior* 33 (1992): 267–28

19   A. and J. Watterson, Public *Health Research Tools in Public Health in Practice*. (Pagrave Macmillan: Basingstoke, 2003), pp24–49.

Chapter 23: Downplaying Radiation Risk, Nicola Wright

1   Press Release N° 208, 31 May 2011 IARC Classifies Radiofrequency Electromagnetic Fields as Possibly Carcinogenic to Humans. Available from: http://www.iarc.fr/en/media-centre/pr/2011/pdfs/pr208_E.pdf.

2   "Teens in mobile phone danger," Daily Mail Dec 2000 Available from: http://www.dailymail.co.uk/health/article-7049/Teens-mobile-phone-danger.html.

3   Statement made by Barry Trower, physicist and ex-government advisor on microwaves, who trained at the Government's Microwave Warfare establishment in the 60's. Available from: http://www.tetrawatch.net/main/choice.php.

4   ICNIRP Guidelines. Basis for Limiting Exposure "these guidelines are based on short-term, immediate health effects," Available from: http://www.icnirp.de/documents/emfgdl.pdf.

5   Powerwatch. International Guidance Levels. Available from: http://www.powerwatch.org.uk/science/intguidance.asp.

6   Electromagnetic fields and public health: mobile phones WHO Fact sheet N°193, June 2011. Available from: http://www.who.int/mediacentre/factsheets/fs193/en/.

7   WHO Electromagnetic fields (EMF) Standards and Guidelines. Available from: http://www.who.int/peh-emf/standards/en/index.html.

8   *Federal Gazette* Nr. 43, 3 March 1992,—Publications of the Federal Radiation Protection Commission, Volume 24, Page 6. Available from: http://www.hese-project.org/hese-uk/en/niemr/health.php?content_type=R&list=frequency.

9   Lymphomas in E mu-Pim1 transgenic mice exposed to pulsed 900 MHZ electromagnetic fields. Repacholi 1997. Available from: http://www.ncbi.nlm.nih.gov/pubmed/9146709.

       Comments on above. Available from: http://electricwords.emfacts.com/re22596.html

10   A Report on Non-Ionizing Radiation, *Microwave News* November 17, 2006. Vol. XXVI No. 9. Available from:http://www.microwavenews.com/docs/MWN.11(9)-06.pdf.

11   WHO Electromagnetic fields. Available from: http://www.who.int/peh-emf/en/.

12   The international EMF project Progress Report June 2006-2007 p. 8. Available from: www.who.int/peh-emf/project/IAC percent20progress percent20report_final.pdf.

13   July 2007 RF gateway interview with Michael Repacholi p. 6. Available from: http://www.next-up.org/pdf/GatewayInterviewMichaelRepacholi20070726.pdf.

14   12 July 2005, *Microwave News* Available from: http://www.microwavenews.com/nc_jul2005.html.

15   University of California: Legacy Tobacco Documents Library. Tobacco documents no 2023329725/9728. Available from: http://www.legacy.library.ucsf.edu/action/document/page?tid=uca90b00.

16   Public Hearings on the WHO Framework Convention on Tobacco Control, Geneva, Switzerland 12–13 October 2000. Available from: www.who.int/geneva-hearings/inquiry.html.

17   Vodafone Group Plc. Corporate Social Responsibility Report 2001–02 p13. Available from: http://www.vodafone.com/content/dam/vodafone/about/sustainability/reports/2001-02_vodafonecr.pdf.

       Vodafone Research Programs. Available from: http://www.vodafone.com/content/index/about/sustainability/mpmh/scientific_research/research_programmes.html.

18   Overloading of Towns and Cities with Radio Transmitters (Cellular Transmitter): a hazard for the human health and a disturbance of eco-ethics. Karl Hecht, Elena N. Savoley. Available from: http://www.natur-med.com.tr/index.php?page=haber Detay&id=9&lang=en.

19   Evidence that Electromagnetic Radiation is Genotoxic: The implications for the epidemiology of cancer and cardiac, neurological and reproductive effects by Dr. Neil Cherry June 2000. Available from: http://www.whale.to/b/cherry_h.html.

20   Criticism of the Proposal to Adopt The ICNIRP Guidelines for cellsites in New Zealand, p5. Dr. Neil Cherry, Lincoln University. Available from: www.salzburg.gv.at/ICNIRP-Kritik1.pdf.

21   WHO Standards and Guidelines. Available from: http://www.who.int/peh-emf/standards/en/index.html.

22 The International Commission on Non-Ionising Radiation Protection. Available from: http://www.hese-project.org/hese-uk/en/niemr/icnirp.php.

23 Biologische Wirkungen Elektromagnetischer Felder im Frequenzbereich 0—3 GHz auf den Menschen. Studie russischer Literatur von 1960—1996. Bearbeiter Prof. em. Prof. Dr. med. Karl Hecht Dr. rer. nat. Hans-Ulrich Balzer. Available from: http://www.iddd.de/umtsno/profhecht.pdf.

24 Freiburg Appeal 2002. Available from: http://www.feb.se/NEWS/Appell-021019-englisch.pdf

 Dr. Cornelia Waldmann Selsam. Available from: http://www.tetrawatch.net/links/links.php?id=stoiberlet

 International doctors appeals. Available from: http://www.elektrosmognews.de/Appelle/inhalt.html

 The London Resolution. Available from: http://www.mastsanity.org/the-london-resolution.html

 Irish Doctors Environmental Association Position on Electro-Magnetic Radiation. Available from: http://www.ideaireland.org/emr.htm

 The Venice Resolution. The International Commission for Electromagnetic Safety, 2008. Available from: http://www.icems.eu/resolution.htm.

25 2006 WHO Research Agenda for Radio Frequency Fields p. 25. Available from http://www.who.int/peh-emf/research/rf_research_agenda_2006.pdf.

26 Mobile Phones and Health. Independent Expert Group on Mobile Phones, IEGMP. Report of the Group (The Stewart Report). Available from: http://www.iegmp.org.uk/report/text.htm.

27 Ref: *Documents of the NRPB: Volume 14, No. 2 2003. Health Effects from Radiofrequency Electromagnetic Fields: Report of an Advisory Group on Non-Ionising Radiation*

 Some other members of Advisory Group on Non-Ionising Radiation (AGNIR) were Chairman until March 2003, Sir Richard Doll, Imperial Cancer Research Fund Cancer Studies Unit, Oxford until 31/3/03 / Professor A J Swerdlow, Chairman, Institute of Cancer Research, London, ICNIRP / Professor C Blakemore, University of Oxford / Professor L J Challis, University of Nottingham, MTHR/

 Professor D. N. M. Coggan, University of Southampton

 Professor E. H. Grant, Microwave Consultants Limited, London /

 Secretariat: Dr. R. D. Saunders, NRPB, ICNIRP/ Dr. Simon Mann, NRPB post 2005, ICNIRP/

 Observer: Dr. H. Walker, Department of Health, London / Assessors: Dr. A. F. McKinlay, NRPB, ICNIRP / Dr. C. R. Muirhead, NRPB / Dr. J. W. Stather, NRPB /

 Consultant: Dr. Zenon Sienkiewicz NRPB/ Mr S G Allen, NRPB/. Available from: http://www.hpa.org.uk/webc/HPAwebFile/HPAweb_C/1194947334474.

28 "Risk from mobile masts was hidden from the Stewart Committee," *The Observer* 14 May 2000. Available from: http://www.tetrawatch.net/science/hidden.php.

29 A. A. Kolodynski, V. V. Kolodynska, "Motor and psychological functions of school children living in the area of the Skrunda Radio Location Station in Latvia," *Sci Total Environ.* 180(1) (Feb. 2, 1996): 87–93. Available from: http://www.ncbi.nlm.nih.gov/pubmed/8717320.

30 Criticism of the NRP Report by Roger Coghill. Available from: http://www.cogre-slab.co.uk/nrpb_rvw.asp.

31 Power Frequency Electromagnetic Fields, Melatonin and the Risk of Breast Cancer. June 2006 Critique by Prof Henshaw. P. 1. Available from: www.electric-fields.bris.ac.uk/CritiqueAGNIRMelatonin.pdf.

32 Report on TETRA for the Police Federation 2001. P. 14. Available from: http://www.tetrawatch.net/papers/trower_report.pdf.

33 The members of the Biological Effects Policy Advisory Group, BEPAG, IET were the following:

Professor Anthony Barker (Chair), Department of Medical Physics and Clinical Engineering, Royal Hallamshire Hospital;

Dr. Leslie Coulton, Bone Biology Group, University of Sheffield Medical School;

Dr. Camelia Gabriel, Microwave Consultants Limited;

Dr. Patricia McKinney, Paediatric Epidemiology Group, University of Leeds;

Dr. Zenon Sienkiewicz, NRPB, MTHR, ICNIRP

Dr. John Swanson, National Grid Transco.

Available from: www.theiet.org/factfiles/bioeffects/emf-position-page.cfm?type=pdf.

34 Mobile Telecommunications and Health, Review of the current scientific research in view of precautionary health protection, April 2000. ECOLOG-Institute. Available from: http://www.hese-project.org/hese-uk/en/papers/ecolog2000.pdf.

35 Statement by Dr. Hans-Peter Neitzke, ECOLOG-Institute. Available from: http://www.hese-project.org/hese-uk/en/niemr/ecologsum.php.

36 Daniel Foggo, Phone Cancer report "Buried." *The Sunday Times*. April 15th 2007, Available online by subscription.

37 "Do Cellphones Cause Brain Cancer?" *New York Times* 11/4/2011. Available from: http://www.nytimes.com/2011/04/17/magazine/mag-17cellphones-t.html?pagewanted=all.

38 Dr. George Carlo interview 12.01.2006 on Mast-vicitms.org. Available from: http://www.mast-victims.org/index.php?content=resources.

39 Cell Phones: Invisible Hazards in the Wireless Age. Dr. Carlo. Available from: http://www.amazon.com/gp/product/0786708182/103-6240875-9082223?v=glance&n=283155.

40 BioInitiative Report: A Rationale for a Biologically based Public Exposure Standard for Electromagnetic Fields (ELF and RF). Available from: www.bioinititive.org.

41 EU watchdog calls for urgent action on Wi-Fi radiation. By Geoffrey Lean. Sunday Independent. 16/9/2007. Available from: http://www.independent.co.uk/environment/green-living/eu-watchdog-calls-for-urgent-action-on-wifi-radiation-402539.html.

42 "Electromagnetic Fields (EMF)" Special Issue: *Journal of Pathophysiology* Volume 16, Issues 2–3, Pages 67–250 (August 2009). Available from: http://www.sciencedirect.com/science/journal/09284680/16/2-3.

43 MTHR Report 2007. Available from: www.mthr.org.uk/documents/MTHR_report_2007.pdf.

44   Science Media Centre Press Release on MTHR Report. Available from: 2007http://www.sciencemediacentre.org/pages/press_briefings/index. php?showArticle=26&year=2007

Powerwatch: How was the MTHR report so misreported? Available from: http://www.powerwatch.org.uk/news/20070926_mthr_update.asp

Mast Sanity: MTHR Publication vs. BioInitiative Report. Available from: http://www.mastsanity.org/index.php?option=com_content&task=view&id=166&Itemid=1.

45   Science Media Centre. "About us" Available from: http://www.sciencemediacentre.org/pages/about/.

46   Science Media Centre. "Funding" Available from: http://www.sciencemediacentre.org/pages/about/funding.htm.

47   "Mobile phone studies find no short-term health problems," *The Guardian* 12/9/07. Available from: http://www.guardian.co.uk/uk/2007/sep/12/mobile-phones.health.

48   Mobile phones "safe in the short-term" There is evidence suggesting the long-term use of mobile phones could be linked to an increased risk in cancer, scientists revealed. The Telegraph 12/9/07. Available from: http://www.telegraph.co.uk/news/uknews/1562894/Mobile-phones-safe-in-the-short-term.html.

49   Mobile phone use and risk of glioma in adults: case-control study. BMJ 2006.   Available   from: http://www.bmj.com/content/332/7546/883.full?view=long&pmid=16428250.

50   REFLEX: Risk Evaluation of Potential Environmental Hazards from Low Energy Electromagnetic Field Exposure Using Sensitive in vitro Methods. Available from:http://www.verum-foundation.de/eu-projekte/reflex.html.

51   "EU watchdog calls for urgent action on Wi-Fi radiation" *The Independent* 16/9/07. Available from: http://www.independent.co.uk/environment/green-living/eu-watchdog-calls-for-urgent-action-on-wifi-radiation-402539.html.

52   Scientists claim radiation from handsets are to blame for mysterious "colony collapse" of bees. *The Independent* 15/4/07. Available from: http://www.independent.co.uk/environment/nature/are-mobile-phones-wiping-out-our-bees-444768.html.

53   Bees, Birds and Mankind Destroying Nature by `Electrosmog´ Dr. Ulrich Warnke. Available from: http://www.kompetenzinitiative.net/broschuerenreihe/brochure-series/english/bees-birds-and-mankind.html.

54   The New Thought Police—Suppressing Dissent in Science. Institute of Science in Society ISIS. Available from: http://www.psrast.org/thoughtpolice.htm.

55   MTHR New Mobile Phone Research announced 6/8/08. Available from: http://www.mthr.org.uk/documents/MTHRP9.pdf.

56   "The Cellphone Industry shamelessly tries its hardest to keep health effects from cellphone radiation quiet," *Toronto Star* 11/7/05. Available from: http://www.powerwatch.org.uk/news/20050711_industry.asp.

57   Benevento Resolution 19/9/06. Available from: http://www.icems.eu/benevento_resolution.htm.

58   Which Science or Scientists Can You Trust? ISIS 25/2/05. Available from: http://www.i-sis.org.uk/WSoSCYT.php.

59   Hutchison/MRC Research Centre open 2002. Available from: http://www.lksf.org/en/media/press/20020520.
      http://www.lksf.org/en/media/press/20070205.

60   Li Ka Shing Foundation and Hutchison Whampoa. Available from: http://www.lksf.org/en/media/press.

61   When corporations rule the world ISIS. Available from: http://www.i-sis.org.uk/isisnews/sis26.php.

62   Dr. Alastair McKinlay MTHR. Available from: http://www.mthr.org.uk/members/mckinlay.htm.

63   Barrie Trower Evidence. Available from: http://www.whale.to/a/trower_q.html.

64   Available from: www.theiet.org/factfiles/bioeffects/emf-position-page.cfm?type=pdf.

65   Available from: http://www.hpa.org.uk/Publications/Radiation/NPRBArchive/DocumentsOfTheNRPB/Absd1504/.

66   Available from: http://www.hpa.org.uk/webc/HPAwebFile/HPAweb_C/1194947334474.

67   Some members of the UK's Mobile Telecommunication and Health Research Programme, MTHR, at the time of writing (2011) are as follows: Prof. Challis, Physics; also on the AGNIR and Stewart Committee, Niels Kuster, an electrical engineer. In 1992, he was Invited Professor at the Electromagnetics Laboratory of Motorola Inc. in Florida, USA. His research interest is currently focused on the area of reliable and safe on/in-body wireless communications and related topics. Zenon Sienkiewicz, neurobiology. ICNIRP works for the HPA-NRB. Professor D. N. M. Coggon, Prof Medicine, Southampton, Chairman of the Depleted Uranium Oversight Board. From 2000 to 2005, he was Chairman of the Advisory Committee on Pesticides, on AGNIR, and was on IEGMP, IARC monograph committee. Professor J. Metcalfe, cell Biochemistry Cambridge. He was seconded part-time to the Cancer Research Campaign as Chairman of the Scientific Committee from 1995 to 2000. Chairman of the scientific advisory committee for the EMF Biological Research Trust (funded by National Grid) Professor P. Haggard, Psychology, Institute of Cognitive Neuroscience, University College, London, ICNIRP, AGNIR Dr. T. E. van Deventer, electrical engineer. Chairman IEEE Toronto section. Chairman WHO EMF Project,

      Former members:

      Professor Grant. He retired from King's College London in 1996 and joined Microwave Consultants Ltd, MCL as Principal Scientific Consultant and Non-Executive Director. He used to be on the NRPB and the AGNIR.

      * Professor C. Blakemore

      * Professor P. Elliott, Professor of Epidemiology and Public Health Medicine at Imperial College of Science, Technology, and Medicine, London. He was a member of the Health Advisory Group on Chemical Contamination Incidents (Dept Health, 1990-2001), and is a member of the UK Medical Research Council Advisory Board (1997-)

      * Dr. A. McKinlay, former Chairman of ICNIRP

      * Dr. M. Repacholi Ex Chairman of the WHO EMF Project, ex-Chairman of ICNIRP

Available from: http://www.mthr.org.uk/members/members.htm.

68 Available from: www.sirc.org/publik/revised_guidelines.shtml

69 Available from: http://www.icr.ac.uk/press/press_archive/press_releases_2011/21212.shtml

70 Available from: http://www.iop.kcl.ac.uk/staff/profile/default.aspx?go=10206

71 Available from: http://www.sciencemediacentre.org/pages/about/sap.htm

72 Available from: http://www.mast-victims.org/index.php?content=news&action=view&type=newsitem&id=4651

73 Available from: http://www.who.int/peh-emf/publications/riskenglish/en/index.html

74 Available from: http://www.who.int/peh-emf/meetings/base_stations_june05/en/index2.html
http://www.who.int/entity/peh-emf/meetings/archive/salomon_borraz_bsw.pdf

75 Available from: http://www.thelancet.com/journals/lancet/article/PIIS0140-6736(00)02098-5/abstract

76 Available from: http://www.guardian.co.uk/environment/2006/sep/19/ethicalliving.g2

77 Available from: http://www.amazon.com/Doubt-Their-Product-Industrys-Threatens/dp/019530067X

78 Available from: http://ajph.aphapublications.org/doi/full/10.2105/AJPH.91.11.1749

79 Available from:
http://broschuerenreihe.net/britannien-uk/assets/ki_heft-5_eng_screen.pdf
http://www.pandora-foundation.eu/
http://www.profil.at/articles/0847/560/226363/rufunterdrueckung-das-sittenbild-handystudien

80 Available from: http://www.powerwatch.org.uk/news/20041222_reflex.asp

81 Available from: http://www.mthr.org.uk/press/p7/p7_2007.htm

82 Available from: http://www.nature.com/bjc/journal/v103/n11/full/6605948a.html

83 Available from: http://www.bmj.com/content/340/bmj.c3077.abstract
http://www.powerwatch.org.uk/news/20100623_cancer_phone_mast_bmj.asp

84 A study published in the BMJ on June 23 found no link between childhood cancer and mobile phone masts. *The Guardian* 23 June 2010.
Available from: http://www.guardian.co.uk/science/2010/jun/22/mobile-phone-masts-cancer

85 Available from: http://www.mthr.org.uk/research_projects/mthr_funded_projects/documents/RUM1FinalReport.pdf

86 Available from: www.mthr.org.uk/research_projects/documents/Rum4FinalReport.pdf

87 Available from: http://www.mthr.org.uk/research_projects/funded_projects.htm

88 Available from: http://www.iarc.fr/en/research-groups/RAD/RCAd.html

89 Available from: http://www.dailymail.co.uk/health/article-374620/Mobile-phones-dont-raise-brain-cancer-risk.html

90 Available from: http://www.ncbi.nlm.nih.gov/pubmed/16428250

http://www.powerwatch.org.uk/columns/morgan/20060125_glioma.asp

91 Available from: http://www.economist.com/node/12295222

92 Available from: http://www.ncbi.nlm.nih.gov/pubmed/18493271

93 2064229233/9247

A proposal to explore the role of memory in epidemiologic studies, develop practical standards of significance, and improve scientific communication.

Available from: http://legacy.library.ucsf.edu/tid/ayv93c00

Tobacco and health research procedural memo.

Timn0071488/1491.

Available from: http://legacy.library.ucsf.edu/tid/upv92f00

94 Available from: http://www.ncbi.nlm.nih.gov/pubmed/19513546

95 Available from: http://www.ncbi.nlm.nih.gov/pubmed/19328536

96 *Sixty Minutes*. Wake Up Call Friday, April 3, 2009. Available from: http://sixtyminutes.ninemsn.com.au/stories/liambartlett/797215/wake-up-call

97 Available from: http://www.iarc.fr/en/media-centre/pr/2011/pdfs/pr208_E.pdf

98 Available from: http://www.bbc.co.uk/news/health-15387297

99 Available from: http://news.bbc.co.uk/1/hi/health/3742120.stm

100 Available from: http://www.microwavenews.com/Ahlbom.html; http://www.nfp57.ch/e_index.cfm

101 Available from:

http://www.guardian.co.uk/science/2011/may/31/mobile-phone-radiation-cancer-risk

http://www.independent.co.uk/life-style/health-and-families/health-news/mobile-phone-users-warned-over-cancer-link-2291515.html

http://www.bbc.co.uk/news/health-13608444

102 Available from: http://www.telegraph.co.uk/health/healthnews/8548725/Mobile-phones-possibly-carcinogenic-say-World-Health-Organization-experts.html

103 Available from: http://www.powerwatch.org.uk/news/20111021-danish-mobile-phone-study.asp

104 Available from: http://www.telegraph.co.uk/technology/news/8436831/Student-addiction-to-technology-similar-to-drug-cravings-study-finds.html

105 Brain Tumor UK Information Pack, "The numbers of those dying from brain tumors is increasing by 2 percent p.a. and more children and young people die from a brain tumor than from any other cancer."

106 Wi-Fi: A warning signal, Available from:, http://news.bbc.co.uk/1/hi/programmes/panorama/6674675.stm

107 The Naila Study, Germany: 10-year Study of Residents near Mobile Telephone Mast. One thousand case notes were studied of patients living within 400m of the mast for 10 years. The doctors found a trebling of cancer risk after 5 years exposure.

Available from: http://www.tetrawatch.net/papers/naila.pdf

"Cancer near a cell phone transmitter station," Tel Aviv University. Wolf MD and Wolf MD. They found a 4-fold increase in cancer within 350m of a normal mast.

Available from: http://www.powerwatch.org.uk/news/20050207_israel.pdf

108 Available from: http://www.guardian.co.uk/science/2007/may/21/bbc. broadcasting

109 Available from:http://www.powerwatch.org.uk/news/20090915_hpa_wifi.asp

110 Available from:
http://www.buergerwelle.de/pdf/wlan_dect_in_schools_and_kindergardens.pdf
http://omega.twoday.net/stories/3974159/
http://www.icems.eu/benevento_resolution.htm
http://www.wifiinschools.org.uk/4.html
http://www.next-up.org/pdf/FranceNationalLibraryGivesUpWiFi07042008.pdf

111 The potential dangers of electromagnetic fields and their effect on the environment. Resolution 1815 (2011) Final version. http://assembly.coe.int/nw/xml/XRef/Xref-XML2HTML-en.asp?fileid=17994&

112 Available from: http://www.tuc.org.uk/extras/occupationalcancer.pdf

113 Available from: www.bemri.org

Chapter 24: You Have Cancer: It's Your Fault, Janette Sherman

1 V. Packard, *The Hidden Persuaders* (New York: McKay, 1957).

2 Federal Radiological Preparedness Coordinating Committee. Subcommittee on Potassium Iodide. Interagency Technical Evaluation Paper for Section 127(f) of the Bioterrorism Act of 2002. Available from: https://www.whitehouse.gov/sites/default/files/microsites/ostp/ki-evaluation-2007.pdf.

3 Ibid. p. 46.

4 Ibid. p. 54.

5 P. Montague, T. Montague, Editorial: A new and slightly different view from Rachel's. Rachel's Democracy & Health News #829, 2005 Oct 27. Available from: http://www.rachel.org/files/document/Rachels_829_Why_We_Cant_Prevent_Cancer.htm.

BIOGRAPHIES

Andrew Watterson is a Professor of Health at Stirling University in Scotland where he is Director of the Centre for Public Health and Population Health and head of the Occupational and Environmental Health Research Group in the Faculty of Health Sciences at Stirling University, Scotland. He has published widely in the field of global occupational health, safety, and the environment. He has particular interests in occupational cancer prevention, health impact assessments, and participatory action research and lay epidemiology with workers and communities.

Bo Walhjalt: The late Bo Walhjalt BA, was a freelance writer with a background in social work, medicine, and theory of science. For more than thirteen years, his interest was focused on controversial issues concerning health and environment. More recently, his investigative work was centered on conflicts of interest issues. Around 2000, a friend introduced Bo to the Philip Morris Documents. Bo also became aware of the conflict of interests of a Swedish epidemiologist involved in studying Dioxin. After some research, Bo found that the epidemiologist worked closely with the Chemical industry although very firmly denied any health effects from dioxins. Later, Bo described a network of risk-denying consultants providing the chemical industry with the results they needed for the legal defense of their business interests. These consultants within scientific organizations appeared with their friends on editorial boards of journals and as peer reviewers. They grant access to scientific media within their own control and according to accepted scientific standards. Bo passed away in January 2016 while finishing his contributions to this book. Bo was a driven, independent, and truthful investigator. He will be sorely missed.

Christian Blom was born in 1948 and is electrohypersensitive since 2003. He graduated from high school in 1968 and studied after that at Svenska

Handelshögskolan (Swedish School of Economics) at Helsinki University, Sibelius Academy, and The Theatre Institute of Advanced Studies (University of the Arts Helsinki). He has worked as a politician, Head of printing works, Head of theatre, and Lecturer at Institute of Advanced Studies (Arts Management). Christian Blom was on sick leave from 2003 to 2008 and is retired since 2008. He has worked since the 1960s and still does as a freelance journalist. He still does research within cultural politics and history.

Dr. David O. Carpenter: David O. Carpenter is a public health physician, the director of the Institute for Health and the Environment, a Collaborating Centre of the World Health Organization, as well as a professor of environmental health sciences at Albany University School of Public Health. He previously served as Director of the Wadsworth Center of the New York State Department of Health, and as Dean of the University at Albany School of Public Health. Carpenter, who received his medical degree from Harvard Medical School, has more than 370 peer-reviewed publications, six books, and fifty reviews and book chapters to his credit.

David Egilman: Dr. David Egilman, MD MPH, is Clinical Professor of Family Medicine at the Alpert School of Medicine at Brown University. He received his Bachelors of Science in Molecular Biology and his MD from Brown University. He is board certified in internal medicine and preventive-occupational medicine and graduated from the NIH Epidemiology Training program. He received his Masters in Public Health from Harvard. Dr. Egilman does research on corporate corruption of science and the impact of the manufacture and sale of products on the health of workers and customers. He serves as an expert witness in court cases at the request of injured parties and companies on these issues. He has also published on the duty to test and warn about product hazards. He is the founder and President of the Board of Directors of Global Health through Education, Training and Service (GHETS), a nonprofit organization dedicated to improving health in developing countries through innovations in education and service (www.ghets.org). He has published on warnings, asbestos, US human radiation experiments, benzene, beryllium, Vioxx, and other toxic exposures and medical products.

Devra Davis, PhD, MPH, is President of Environmental Health Trust, a nonprofit scientific and policy think tank. Currently Visiting Professor of Medicine at The Hebrew University, Hadassah Medical Center, and Ondokuz Mayis University Medical School, she was Founding Director of the Board on

Environmental Studies and Toxicology of the US National Research Council and Founding Director, Center for Environmental Oncology, University of Pittsburgh Cancer Institute. Dr. Davis served under President Clinton as an appointee to the Chemical Safety and Hazard Investigation Board and also was a member of the Board of Scientific Counselors of the National Toxicology Program. See her other relevant publications.

Don Maisch: Dr. Maisch received his PhD from the University of Wollongong, New South Wales, Australia. He has been involved in the issue of health impacts of electromagnetic fields (EMF) since the early 1990s when he was a science writer for Australian Senator Robert Bell. He has served on government and industry EMF standard-setting committees on behalf of the Consumers Federation of Australia. He is a member of the Australasian College of Nutritional and Environmental Medicine, a training College offering postgraduate education for health professionals. His thesis examined the historical development of Western radiofrequency and microwave exposure standards and how vested interests have influenced those standards. He has published a number of papers on the health effects of electromagnetic radiation as well as numerous submissions. These are available online at www.emfacts.com/papers/.

Gayle Greene, Professor of English at Scripps College, has published widely about Shakespeare and women writers. She's published a biography of pioneering radiation epidemiologist Dr. Alice Stewart, *The Woman Who Knew Too Much,* reissued in a second edition (spring 2017).*Insomniac,* a first-person account of living with insomnia and an exploration of the science of sleep was Amazon's #1 pick of March 2008 and was shortlisted for the Gregory Bateson Prize in Cultural Anthropology. A memoir, *Missing Persons,*will be published by the University of Nevada Press, fall 2017.

Geoffrey Tweedale: Formerly Professor of Business History at Manchester Metropolitan University Business School, he has been studying the history of asbestos since 1996 and has published several articles on the subject and a book: *Magic Mineral to Killer Dust: Turner & Newall and the Asbestos Hazard* (Oxford, 2nd edition, 2001). A global study of the asbestos industry (with Jock McCulloch), *Defending the Indefensible: The Global Asbestos Industry and Its Fight for Survival*, was published in 2008 by Oxford University Press.

Gunni Nordström is a journalist, presently living in Finland where she was born. She has spent most of her life in Sweden. For a large part of her professional life she has been employed by the Swedish journal of the Confederation of Professional Employees, TCO. As a union, TCO was involved during the 1980s in the debate on electromagnetic fields from computer screens. This resulted in the TCO labeling of computer screens, well known in the world as the TCO Label. For many years she has written about the health issues of new technology. Together with her colleague Carl von Schéele, she has written two books on the subject, *Sjuk av bildskärm* 1989 (*Made Sick by computer screen*) and *Fältslaget om de elöverkänsliga* 1995 (*The Battle against Electrohypersensitivity*). In 2000, she wrote the book *Mörkläggning*. The English version of this book, *Invisible Disease*, was published in 2004 and the French version, *Ménaces Invisibles*, in 2005. She has also written books about the Roma people in Finland.

Janette D. Sherman, MD, is Research Colleague and Lecturer for the Radiation and Public Health Project. Dr. Sherman's experience includes research at Michigan State University, the Atomic Energy Commission at the University of California Berkeley, consultant to the US Environmental Protection Agency for the Toxic Substances Control Act from 1976 to 1982, and Clinical Assistant Professor at Wayne State University Medical School. She publishes and lectures in the field of toxicology and currently is an Adjunct Professor of Environmental Studies at Western Michigan University in Kalamazoo where she consults with graduate students and faculty on workers' illnesses. She is the author of *Life's Delicate Balance: Causes and Prevention of Breast Cancer* as well as *Chemical Exposure and Disease*. Visit her website at www.janettesherman.com.

Janine Allis-Smith: Janine was born in the Netherlands, she visited the United Kingdom in the early 1960s to improve her English. Captivated by the United Kingdom's Lake District, its mountains, and the outdoor life, she stayed, married, and had two sons. On a small hill farm, she tended her Herdwick sheep and spent many sunny days on the nearby West Cumbrian beaches. She began to question the safety of these beaches following Yorkshire TV's 1983 documentary "Windscale, the Nuclear Laundry," which not only exposed the extent of coastal contamination by the radioactive discharges from Sellafield's reprocessing operations but also linked the radiation to the area's exceptionally high incidence of childhood cancers.

In 1984, her twelve-year-old son was diagnosed with leukemia. After three long years of hospital stays, painful chemotherapy, and life-threatening infections, he won his battle against leukemia. Her struggle against Sellafield's radioactive discharges—prompted by her son's diagnosis—led her to become a volunteer with local group Cumbrians Opposed to a Radioactive Environment

(CORE) and one of the first local parents willing to talk to the media about the link between Sellafield's discharges and childhood leukemia. She has continued to work with CORE since 1990.

Jock McCulloch has worked as a Legislative Research Specialist for the Australian parliament and has taught at various universities. His principal research interest is in the politics of health in Southern Africa. He is the author of a history of asbestos mining in South Africa *Asbestos Blues* (2002), a study of occupational disease *South Africa's Gold Mines and the Politics of Silicosis* (2012), and with Geoff Tweedale *The Global Asbestos Industry and its Fight for Survival* (2010).

Jody Warren: is an Honorary Postdoctoral Research Associate at the University of Wollongong, Australia. Her PhD thesis at the University examined the political sociology of the scientific research into the Tasmanian devil cancer. Her research interests include why particular groups have different perspectives on research findings and how the concept of "undone" science fits into the current literature on ignorance. She runs a website, jodeswarren.wix.com/devils advocate, advocating for the protection of wildlife from environmental toxins.

John Zorabedian: John Zorabedian, BA, is a writer and blogger with a background in journalism, publishing, and marketing. He covers topics from health and the environment to politics and technology, and his writing has been published by many newspapers, magazines, and websites, including the *Jewish Journal*, the *Providence Phoenix*, *Northshore Magazine*, *American Executive*, *Naked Security*, AOL's Patch.com, and the International Journal of Occupational and Environmental Health. A native of Massachusetts, he graduated from Wesleyan University in 1999 with a Bachelor of Arts in Government.

Kathleen Ruff: Kathleen Ruff, BA, MA, has worked extensively in the area of human rights, both inside and outside government. She was director of the British Columbia Human Rights Commission and founding publisher of the *Canadian Human Rights Reporter.* She is co-coordinator of the Rotterdam Convention Alliance, director of the human rights website RightOnCanada.ca and Senior Advisor on Human Rights to the Rideau Institute. Her report, Exporting Harm: How Canada markets asbestos to the developing world (www.rideauinstitute.ca/wp-content/uploads/2011/01/exportingharmweb.pdf) brought to public attention Canada's shameful conduct as propagandist for the global asbestos industry. She organized an international campaign, involving scientists, civil society activists, and asbestos victims, which succeeded in ending Canada's mining and export of asbestos. In 2011, she received the Canadian Public Health Association's National Public Health Hero Award and the Appreciation Award from the Asian Citizens Center for Environmental Health. She received the 2012 Cancer Prevention Award from the organization Prevent Cancer Now. In 2013, she received a Special Award from the Collegium Ramazzini (www.collegiumramazzini.org/news1.asp?id=109) for her work for a global ban on asbestos. In 2016, she was awarded the medal of the Quebec National Assembly for her work to ban asbestos and protect workers' health. She has published numerous articles in scientific journals, civil society publications, and the media on public health policy and human rights.

Lelia M. Menendez: Lelia M. Menendez, JD, received her degree from the University of Iowa College of Law in 2013 and her MA from Brown University in 2003.

Lennart Hardell: Lennart Hardell, MD, PhD, has a long career as a clinical and medical research doctor, currently at the Department of Oncology, University Hospital, Örebro, Sweden. He has also served as a professor at the Örebro University. He is specialized in oncology with a focused interest in environmental risk factors for cancer that he has studied in epidemiological investigations. He was a Research fellow at School of Public Health, University of California, Berkeley, United States, in 1985. Over the years, he has been awarded several scientific prizes for his research. He was the first to show an increased risk for cancer in persons exposed to phenoxy herbicides and contaminating dioxins. His research group has also made studies on persistent organic pollutants and cancer risks, such as TCDD and PCB, and the risk for malignant lymphoma. In recent years, much research has focused on use of mobile phones and cordless phones and the risk of brain tumors. His research has contributed to the cancer classification of different agents such as TCDD, PCB, the herbicide glyphosate, and radiofrequency fields. He has published more than three hundred peer-reviewed scientific articles.

Martin Walker MA: Since 1990, Martin Walker has concentrated on campaigning and writing books and essays about lobby groups and the influence of multinational corporations in medicine, public health, and medical research. He has authored ten books on critical social issues, especially in relation to medicine and pharmaceutical lobby groups. His last four books looked at the denial of undiagnosed illnesses such as ME, Multiple Chemical Sensitivity, Gulf War Syndrome, and serious adverse reactions to pharmaceutical drugs and vaccines.

He is particularly interested in those groups that promote this denial on behalf of the State, pharmaceutical corporations, and others. He spent four years working on behalf of the parents of MMR vaccine–damaged children and attended every day but two of the intermittent three year General Medical Council (GMC) trial of Dr. Andrew Wakefield and two other consultants in London.

Professor Neil Pearce: Since the completion of his PhD in epidemiology in 1985, he has been engaged in a wide range of epidemiological research with a particular emphasis on epidemiological methods. He is the co-author of a textbook of occupational epidemiology, published by Oxford University Press in 1989, and author of a textbook of asthma epidemiology, which was published by Oxford University Press in 1998. He was director of the Asthma Research Group of the Wellington School of Medicine from 1996 to 2000, and of the Massey University Centre for Public Health Research from 2000 to 2010. Since 2011, he has been Professor of Epidemiology and Biostatistics at the London School of Hygiene and Tropical Medicine. He was President of the International Epidemiological Association from 2008 to 2011.

Nicola Wright: She has a degree in Natural Science (Physics and Theoretical Physics Pt2) from Cambridge. She became aware of the harm of human exposure to man-made microwave radiation in 2005 when her mother became ill with Hashimoto's disease and chronic fatigue syndrome from living in the main beam of a mobile phone mast. Her son also suffered severe migraines and severely disturbed sleep from exposure to microwave radiation in his school after it installed a Wi-Fi system. Since then, she has worked with various organizations to bring the dangers of constant exposure to wireless signals to public attention.

Pierre Mallia: Professor Pierre Mallia teaches Bioethics and Clinical Ethics in various faculties of the University of Malta, including Medicine & Surgery, Dentistry, Laws, Theology, Philosophy, Science, and the Faculty of Health Science. His publications include peer-reviewed journals and books. His latest is on the Phenomenon of the Doctor-Patient Relationship, published by Elsevier. He has put forward various concepts, including distinguishing between "Public Health" and "Health of the Public" as this can have and justify different ethical approaches to decisions. He has also suggested the PUME matrix in ethical teaching and debate, as it helps to clarify arguments by separating the pragmatic and consequential. He lectures also at Leannec University of Lyon and has been invited by several universities, including Maastricht and Linkoping in Sweden. He is keen on global ethics and dialogue in bioethics.

Pierre Mallia is chairman of the National Health Ethics Committee, Coordinator of the Bioethics Research Programme of the Faculty of Medicine and Surgery, and Chairs the Medicine and Law Programme of the Faculty of Laws. He is now coordinating the Mater Dei Hospital Ethics Committee in Malta. He is keen on developing the role of Clinical Ethicist and has implemented the first Masters in Clinical Ethics and Law, which besides philosophy is a comprehensive course that trains candidates in communication skills, medical leadership, anthropology of ethics, conflict resolution, etc.

He is President of the Malta College of Family Doctors and has introduced the MRCGP(INT) qualification in Malta, putting family medicine on the Specialist Register. He is working with patient groups to see how Family Medicine can help to be a voice for patients to have a say in political and research matters.

Professor Mallia is also an Expert Evaluator for projects sponsored by the European Union. At the moment he is running an Erasmus+ project to improve and harmonize End of Life care in European countries.

Professor Richard Clapp has recently retired from the position of Professor of Environmental Health, Boston University School of Public Health and Adjunct Professor at UMass Lowell Prof. Clapp is an epidemiologist with over thirty years of experience in public health practice, research, teaching, and consulting. He has an MPH from Harvard School of Public Health and a DSc in Epidemiology from Boston University School of Public Health. He served as the founding Director of the Massachusetts Cancer Registry from 1980–1989, and worked in two environmental health consulting groups. He has been on the Faculty at BU since 1993, where he currently teaches graduate courses in environmental health. He is also an Adjunct Professor at the University of Massachusetts, Lowell and a staff member in the Environmental Health Initiative at the Lowell Center for Sustainable Production. His research has included studies of cancer around nuclear facilities, in workers and military veterans, and in communities with toxic hazards. He recently conducted an analysis of causes of death among IBM workers that the company called "junk science," but which was published in a peer-reviewed journal and has been widely cited.

Professor Rory O'Neill edits *Hazards Magazine*, an award-winning magazine geared to the needs of workers, and is Visiting Professor at the Occupational and Environmental Health Research group at Stirling University, Scotland. He has produced numerous guides and reports on occupational health and safety for trade unions and other bodies across Europe and internationally.

Simon Pickvance was Senior Occupational Health Adviser and Development Consultant at SOHAS. He worked as an adviser at SOHAS beginning in 1979. He published a number of books on OH topics and was an Honorary Research Fellow in the School of Health and Related Research at the University of Sheffield. He died from mesothelioma while the book was in preparation.

Susanna Rankin Bohme: The work of Susanna Rankin Bohme, PhD, bridges the academic and the activist in the fields of public health and environmental history and policy. Currently Associate Director of Research at Corporate Accountability International, she has taught at Harvard, Brown, and the Rhode Island School of Design, and served as Deputy Editor of the *International Journal of Occupational and Environmental Health*. Her book on the history of the pesticide DBCP in the US and Central America, *Toxic Injustice: A Transnational History of Exposure and Struggle*, was published by the University of California Press in 2014. She has published in the academic and lay press on topics including national and transnational pesticide policy, corporate corruption of science, and public health and consumer warnings. She received her doctorate in American Studies from Brown University in 2008.

ACKNOWLEDGMENTS

Firstly, we would like to thank all the contributors to this book for having the patience and tenacity to stick with the project, which has taken several years to complete.

The individuals who have helped both the principles Martin Walker and Lennart Hardell to finish the project are many; they include those who have voluntarily donated money, especially to Martin Walker's work.

The project began after Lennart Hardell, Martin Walker, and Bo Walhjalt were co-authors of a paper in the *American Journal of Industrial Medicine* in 2007 and then met in Sweden. (1) (Am J Ind Med. 2007 Mar;50(3):227-33. Secret ties to industry and conflicting interests in cancer research. Hardell L, Walker MJ, Walhjalt B, Friedman LS, Richter ED.) We would especially like to thank the late Bo Walhjalt who was involved from the beginning. Bo was utterly committed to the publication of vested interests and often worked night and day to the detriment of his health. He died in January 2016 before seeing his chapters in print—you are in our memory Bo.

Those who have contributed practically to the book include Andy Dark, who worked with great technical skill on the images, Michael Carlberg, who worked with incredible absorption on the references, Dr. Samuel Epstein, who contributed ideas to the work before it got out of hand, and Louis Conte, who shared his opinion and authority over the project with SkyHorse.

Finally, the families and friends of Martin and Lennart, who put up with a roller coaster ride of diminishing and expanding concerns over various aspects of the book during the project.